LIVER PHYSIOLOGY AND TREATMENT OF LIVER DISEASES

Dr. Shipra Chandra

ALLIED HEALTH PRESS

Liver Physiology and Treatment of Liver Diseases

Author: **Dr. Shipra Chandra**

Allied Health Press
4164 Lakeshore Road
Burlington ON L7L 1A4
Canada
www.alliedhealthpress.com
Email: orders@arclereducation.com

ISBN: 978-1-77956-267-8

ABOUT THE AUTHOR

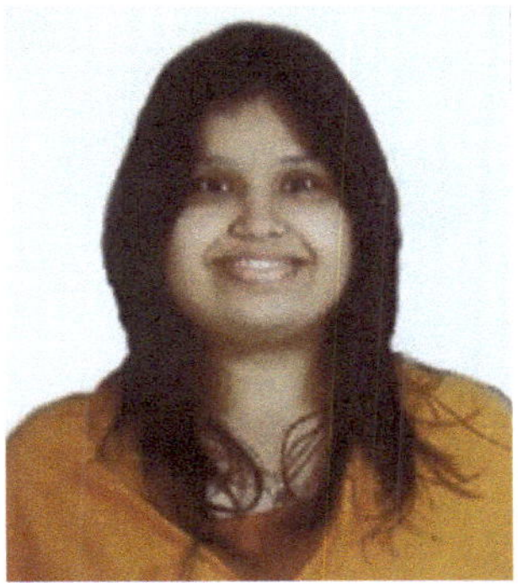

Dr. Shipra Chandra born in Delhi in 1983, completed school from a government school in Delhi in 2001 with First division. Being a science student , took admission in Chemistry Honors at Kirori Mal College, Delhi University. But the wonders of Human Body always fascinated me and I continued preparing for Pre Medical Test (PMT) despite being in a reputed college and course.

By the Grace of God and blessings of my family I secured 5th rank in CPMT 2002 along-with being waitlisted at DPMT and securing rank in AIEEE exam. Joined MBBS on 14/11/2002 at the most prestigious King George Medical College, Lucknow, U.P. Completed MBBS in First division in 2008 and joined AIIMS, New Delhi Department of Emergency Medicine for work experience in 2009 but continued the preparation for Post Graduation Entrance Test and cracked the UP-PGME in 2010 and was allotted MD Physiology from King George Medical University.

After completing the MD in 2013, I again cleared AIIMS, New Delhi entrance test for Senior Residency. Learned a lot during my 3 year tenure from 2013 to 2016 at AIIMS. Following which I joined Fortis Hospital Shalimar Bagh and continued search for a Government Job. Gave the interview at U.P. Public Service Commission in 2017, cracked it and joined as Assistant Professor at Sarojini Naidu Medical College, Agra in 2017. I have 7 research publications , one book chapter and guided 3 MD students during my tenure . Promoted to the post of Associate Professor in 2022 and currently working in the same capacity.

Word Roots, Prefixes, and Suffixes by Chapter

Chapter 1 The Liver: General Aspects and Epidemiology

Gastr/o Gastroenterologist

abdom- abdomen

hepato- hepatotoxin

-oma which means mass, tumor, cyst

Chapter 2 Structure and Ultrastructure of the Normal and Diseased Liver

Hist/o- Histology

Hepat- Hepatomegaly (enlargement of the liver)

Intra- Within

-itis Inflammation

Chapter 3 Autoimmune Hepatitis

Peri- Periportal

Chol- Cholestasis

Auto- Autoimmune

Hepat- Hepatitis

-osis Abnormal condition or process

Chapter 4 Amebic Liver Abscess

Colo- relating to the colon, where Entamoeba histolytica originates

-lysis meaning breaking down or destruction

Py- relating to pus (e.g., pyogenic)

Necro- referring to death, especially of tissue (necrosis)

-genic meaning causing or producing (e.g., pathogenic)

Chapter 5 Pathogenesis of Idiosyncratic Drug-Induced Liver Injury and Liver Regeneration

Patho-disease (e.g., pathogenesis)

-genesis origin, formation

Idio- personal, distinct (e.g., idiosyncratic)

Toxi- poison (e.g., toxic)

-opathy disease or disorder (e.g., hepatopathy)

Chapter 6 The Pathophysiology of Alcoholic Liver Disease

Steato- Steatosis (fatty liver, common in alcoholic liver disease)

Necro- Necrosis

Fibro- Fibrosis (formation of excess fibrous connective tissue, common in cirrhosis)

-megaly Hepatomegaly (enlargement of the liver)

-emia Hyperbilirubinemia (excess bilirubin in the blood)

Chapter 7 Complications of Cirrhosis and Ascites

Edema swelling

Portal- referring to the portal vein

Bili- bile

-pathy disease or disorder

Asc- bag, bladder, or sac

-centesis surgical puncture to remove fluid

Chapter 8 Hepatorenal Syndrome, Hepatopulmonary Syndrome, and Portopulmonary Hypertension

Renal kidney

-logy study of

-uria urine condition

-trophy growth

-stenosis narrowing

Chapter 9 Monitoring of Liver Fibrogenesis and Biochemical Diagnosis of Fibrosis

Angi/o - blood vessel (e.g., angiogenesis)

-cyte cell (e.g., hepatocyte)

-stasis stopping (e.g., cholestasis)

-phage eating (e.g., macrophage)

Chapter 10 N-Acetylcysteine and Resveratrol as Effective Treatments for Liver Disease

Lapar/o Refers to the abdomen (e.g., laparotomy)

Splanchn/o Refers to the viscera or internal organs (e.g., splanchnic)

Anti- against

Table of Contents

LIST OF FIGURES

stained with toluidine blue. Hepatocytes (H) show some of the intracellular organelles. (C) Electron microscopy of hepatocyte shows abundant round mitochondria (M). Part of a nucleus (N) is seen at the right. (D) A round nucleus (N) of hepatocyte is observed with a conspicuous nucleolus (Nu) is shown

Figure 2.4. Ultrastructure of hepatocyte showing some of the organelles. (A) Tangential section of the nucleus shows the presence of the nuclear membrane pores (arrows). Mitochondria (M). (B) Hepatic cytoplasm presents several membranous organelles, such as mitochondria (M), lysosomes (L), smooth endoplasmic reticulum (SER), Golgi complex (G). (C) Round mitochondria (M) and peroxisomes (P) are shown. (D) Elongated mitochondria (M) and a lysosome (L) and glycogen (Gl) associated with a tubular structure (arrow) are observed

Figure 2.5. Ultrastructure of hepatocyte organelles. (A) Transmission electron microscopy of a Golgi complex showing a pile of flat membranes and micro- and macrovesicles. (B) Scanning electron microscopy of a hepatocyte Golgi complex shows a 3D profile of this organelle. (C) Bile canalicular channel (longitudinal section) localized between hepatocytes presents small microvilli in the lumen. (D) A bile canaliculi (arrow) sectioned transversally and observed with scanning electron microscopy

Figure 2.6. Panoramic electron microscopic view of hepatic parenchyma with an associated sinusoid. Hepatocytes (H) are lining a sinusoid (Si) with some cells such as endothelial (E), Kupffer cell (K), Stellate cell (S). Table on the right shows some data of the liver volume occupied by different parenchymal (PC) and nonparenchymal (NPC) cells. E, endothelial cells; IHL, intrahepatic lymphocytes; K, Kupffer cells; S, stellate cells

Figure 2.7. (A) Diagram of a sinusoid with associated cells. Endothelial (E), Kupffer (K), stellate (S) cells. Lumen is occupied by red blood cells (RBC), neutrophils (Nø), Macrophage (Mø), hepatocytes (H). (B) Transmission electron microscopy of a sinusoid sectioned transversally. A red blood cell (RBC) occupies the sinusoid lumen totally. Endothelial cells (E) with fenestrae are enfolded by the cytoplasmic processes of hepatic stellate cells (S). A naked nerve ending (N) closely faces also the process of hepatic stellate cells. Hepatocyte (H)

Figure 2.8. Ultrastructure of nonparenchymal sinusoidal cells. (A) An endothelial cell with an elongated nucleus and thin cytoplasmic processes is seen surrounding the sinusoid and above the hepatocytes (H) separated by the Disse space. (B) Kupffer cell (K) shows a kidney-shaped nucleus, and a cytoplasm with abundant dense phagocytic granules. Hepatocyte (H). (C) Typical stellate cell (S) with many clear vacuoles is seen closely associated to Kupffer cell (K). (D) Ductular cells (D) associated to hepatocytes (H) constitute the wall of a Hering channel, which connects the canaliculi with the bile duct

Figure 2.9. Histopathology of acute viral hepatitis. (A) Portal tracts and parenchyma show a strong lymphocyte infiltration with damaged hepatocytes. (B) Acidophilic bodies with loss of nuclei are seen (arrow). Hyperplasia of Kupffer cell (arrow heads). (C) Ballooning degeneration of hepatocyte with pale cytoplasm and small nucleus is seen

Figure 2.10. (A) Alcoholic liver cirrhosis. Steatosis with intrahepatic inflammation and fibrosis are seen. (B) Nonalcoholic steatohepatitis (NASH). Ballooning of hepatocytes are present with perivenular and pericellular fibrosis. Histological features are similar to those of alcoholic hepatitis

Figure 2.11. (A) Low magnification of a biopsy of a nonalcoholic steatohepatitis (NASH). (B) Nonalcoholic steatohepatitis with ballooning degeneration, macro- and microvescicular steatosis, Mallory-Denk body (arrows) and megamitochondria are shown

Figure 2.12. (A) Electron microscopy of nonalcoholic steatohepatitis (NASH). Macro- and microvesicles

LIST OF TABLES

PREFACE

In recent times, significant strides have been made in the diagnosis and treatment of liver diseases, including viral hepatitis, liver cirrhosis, and liver cancer. Despite these advancements, current diagnostic and treatment modalities remain insufficient, with liver diseases continuing to be a leading cause of death worldwide. There is an urgent need for further advancements in liver disease management to reduce mortality rates associated with these conditions. Continued research in this field is expected to yield new insights and enhance our understanding of liver diseases.

Recent reports have highlighted the role of sarcopenia, the gut-liver axis, and blood coagulation in the pathophysiology of liver diseases. These findings hold promise for improving the diagnosis and treatment of liver diseases, offering potential avenues for further exploration and development of novel therapeutic strategies.

The management of gastrointestinal and hepatic diseases is in a state of constant evolution, driven by an increasing understanding of pathogenic mechanisms that improve daily management. This progress exemplifies translational medicine in action.

For instance, the deepened comprehension of the mechanisms behind HCV virus infection has led to the development of Direct-Acting Antivirals (DAAs), boasting a remarkable 98% cure rate among patients. Despite this success, individuals with advanced liver disease, while cured of HCV infection, remain susceptible to developing hepatocellular carcinoma (HCC), presenting a lasting medical challenge.

Ongoing efforts are focused on developing new antiviral agents for the treatment of chronic delta hepatitis (CHD). The aim is to, hopefully, control the progression of liver disease in patients with CHD, which represents the most severe form of chronic viral hepatitis.

Looking ahead, nonalcoholic fatty liver disease/nonalcoholic steatohepatitis (NAFLD/NASH) is expected to surpass viral hepatitis as the primary cause of chronic liver damage in the coming decades. Extensive work is underway to identify novel biomarkers and tools for detecting liver fibrosis and stratifying the risk of liver disease progression. Additionally, researchers are investigating novel molecules that target various pathways involved in the onset and progression of NAFLD.

The prevalence of *Helicobacter pylori* (*H. pylori*) infection has declined significantly, thanks to factors such as the widespread use of proton pump inhibitors and improved access to gastroscopies. Consequently, the incidence of peptic disease and stomach cancer, once dominant gastrointestinal pathologies, has decreased. However, *H. pylori* infection remains prevalent in many regions, highlighting the need for continued efforts to enhance eradication strategies.

In inflammatory bowel disease, understanding of inflammatory pathways has led to the development of targeted therapies, such as anti-TNF, anti-IL12/23, anti-JAK, and S1P1 modulators. Furthermore, as our understanding of the microbiome deepens, its applications are expected to extend beyond the gut. However, the ongoing COVID-19 pandemic continues to impact the management of all diseases, emphasizing the need for adaptability and innovation in healthcare practices.

This book aims to demystify the complexities of liver physiology and diseases, offering a clear and accessible overview of the liver's vital functions, common liver diseases, and the latest advancements in treatment options. By providing in-depth explanations supported by current research, the book seeks to empower patients, caregivers, and healthcare professionals with the knowledge needed to understand, manage, and treat liver diseases effectively. It also aims to inspire curiosity and interest in liver health, encouraging readers to take proactive steps towards liver disease prevention and early intervention.

This book is tailored for a wide range of readers, including patients diagnosed with liver diseases seeking to understand their condition better and make informed decisions about their health. Caregivers looking after individuals with liver diseases will also find valuable insights and practical advice. Healthcare professionals, including clinicians, nurses, and students, will benefit from its comprehensive coverage of liver physiology, pathology, and treatment modalities. Additionally, researchers in hepatology and related fields will find this book a valuable resource for understanding the latest developments in liver disease research and treatment.

Chapter 1

THE LIVER: GENERAL ASPECTS AND EPIDEMIOLOGY

Contents

Introduction

The liver, an important organ in the abdomen's right upper quadrant, is required for many physiological functions, such as metabolism, detoxification, and the production of the proteins and biochemicals needed for digestion. It is the biggest gland and internal organ in the human body, weighing between 1.4 and 1.6 kilograms in adults. The falciform ligament divides the liver structurally into the right and left lobes, and its vascular and biliary anatomy divides it functionally into eight segments.

Nutrient processing from the digestive tract is one of the liver's main jobs. It transforms fats, proteins, and carbs into energy and necessary compounds. In addition, the liver is essential for drug metabolism, detoxification of dangerous substances, and blood filtering from the digestive tract before it reaches the bloodstream. It also synthesizes vital proteins like albumin and clotting factors and produces bile, which is essential for the digestion and absorption of fat. Significant global health challenges are revealed by the epidemiology of liver diseases. Hundreds of millions of people worldwide suffer from chronic liver disease caused by the hepatitis B and C viruses, which can result in complications like cirrhosis and hepatocellular carcinoma (HCC). Both non-alcoholic fatty liver disease (NAFLD) and alcoholic liver disease (ALD) are common, especially in Western nations where obesity and alcohol consumption are common lifestyle factors. As obesity and diabetes become more common, non-alcoholic steatohepatitis (NAFLD), which can range from simple steatosis to non-alcoholic steatohepatitis (NASH), is increasingly becoming a major reason for liver transplantation.

Liver diseases contribute significantly to morbidity and mortality. The World Health Organization (WHO) estimates that liver cirrhosis and liver cancer are among the top causes of death globally. Advances in medical research and public health interventions aim to reduce the burden of liver diseases through vaccination programs for hepatitis B, antiviral treatments for hepatitis B and C, and lifestyle interventions to manage and prevent NAFLD and alcoholic liver disease.

The liver's multifaceted roles are vital to human health, and understanding the epidemiology of liver diseases is crucial for developing effective prevention and treatment strategies. Continued research and public health efforts are essential to combat the global impact of liver-related conditions.

Orientation and Directional Terms

Term	Definition	Illustration
Liver	Liver is an organ that sits just under the rib cage on the right side of the abdomen. It can weigh up to 4 pounds (1.8 kilograms). The liver is needed to help digest food, rid the body of waste products and make substances, called clotting factors, that keep the blood flowing well, among other tasks.	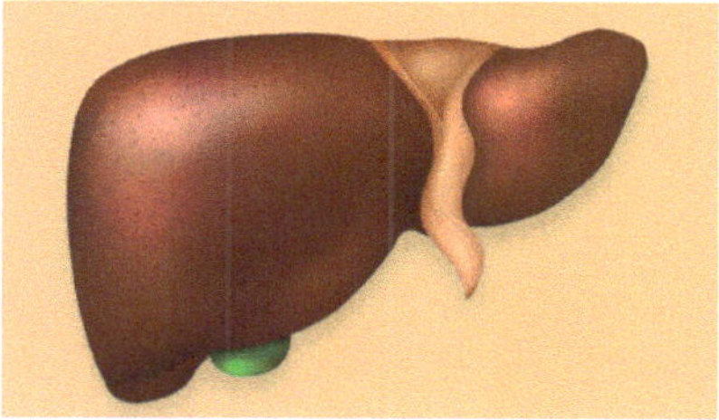
Hepatocellular carcinoma (HCC)	Hepatocellular carcinoma most commonly occurs in people with liver disease, particularly in people with chronic hepatitis B and C & Cirrhosis. Symptoms often don't appear in the early stages of the cancer. Later, symptoms include weight loss, upper abdominal pain or yellowing of the skin (jaundice). Treatments may include surgery, transplant, freezing or heating the cancer cells and chemotherapy.	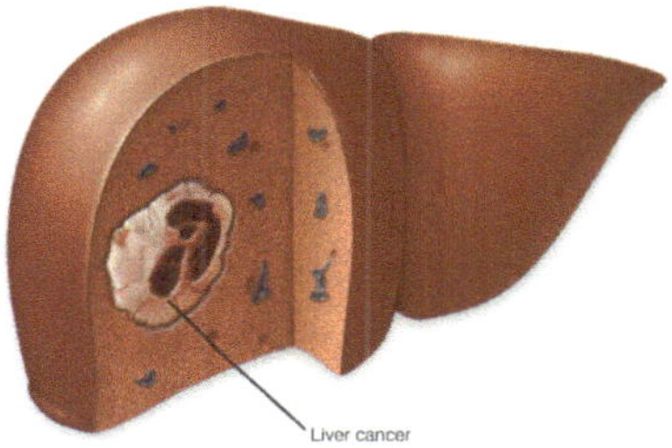
Kupffer cells (KCs)	Kupffer cells, also known as stellate macrophages and Kupffer–Browicz cells, are specialized cells localized in the liver within the lumen of the liver sinusoids and are adhesive to their endothelial cells which make up the blood vessel walls.	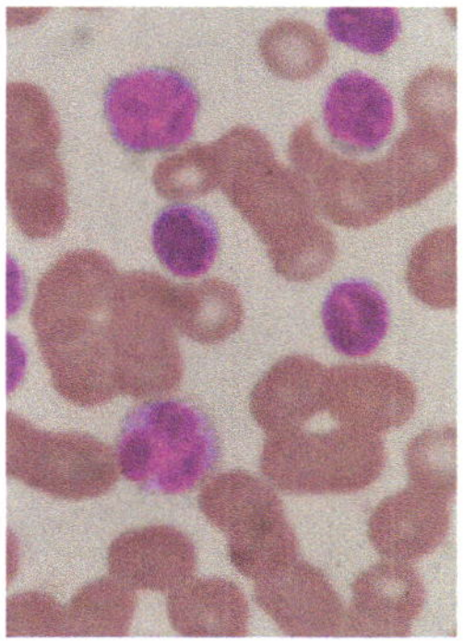
Nonalcoholic fatty liver disease (NAFLD)	Nonalcoholic fatty liver disease (NAFLD) is a condition in which fat builds up in your liver. Nonalcoholic fatty liver (NAFL) and nonalcoholic steatohepatitis (NASH) are types of NAFLD. If you have NASH, you have inflammation and liver damage, along with fat in your liver.	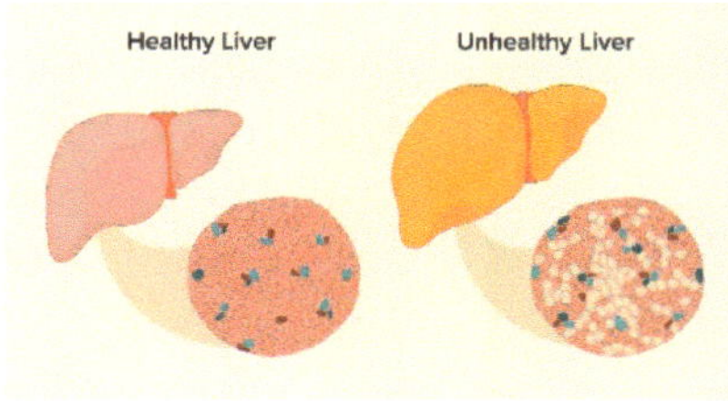

1.1. Abbreviated History of Hepatology

The liver was recognized as the body's most potent and blood-rich organ even in prehistoric times. This remarkable portion of the intestines was linked to multiple processes. It was considered the "seat of life" as well. "Lîp," an Indo-Germanic word, denoted both life and liver. Additionally, there are parallels between the German phrase "Leber-Leben" and the English terms "liver," "live," and "life" (Old English: "lifer-lıf"). The word "leb (a) ra" in Old High German refers to the liver. The Greek word "hepar" is most likely derived from the Hebrew "kábe (r), kábe (d)" (or "cheber") (Kuntz & Kuntz, 2006).

The liver's anatomy was described by Mondino de Luzzi (Bologna) in his "Anatomia Mundini," which was published in 1316. This was during the Middle Ages. Based on autopsies performed for the first time in public in 1306 and 1315, this work was created. For nearly two centuries, this unique anatomy textbook was considered canonical. Figure 1.1, which is derived from "Anatomia Mundini," depicts the liver as having multiple lobules (Kuntz & Kuntz, 2006).

The first thorough monograph on the liver was published by Glisson in 1654, and for the following two centuries, his work was regarded as an authoritative source of information. The liver's inner structure, which includes its intrahepatic vascular vessels, the portal vein's role in the differentiation of liver segments, the terminal regions of the blood and bile capillaries as functional pathways, and the dynamics of bile flow, was thoroughly explained in "Anatomia hepatis.." The intrahepatic connective tissue known as "Glisson's capsule" was identified as branching and tree-like. By Figure 1.2. The bile and blood vessels from a liver are shown in Glisson. Referred to as "Glisson's triangle," or portal trias, the vessels are encircled by connective tissue (1659). Glisson discovered nerves exclusively within the liver capsule, not within the parenchyma. The liver parenchyma was thought to play the role of using "affinity" mechanisms to separate the blood and bile. Kiernan (1833) produced one of the first illustrations of the liver lobule, demonstrating the fine anastomoses between the bile capillaries and the parenchyma's hexagonal architecture.

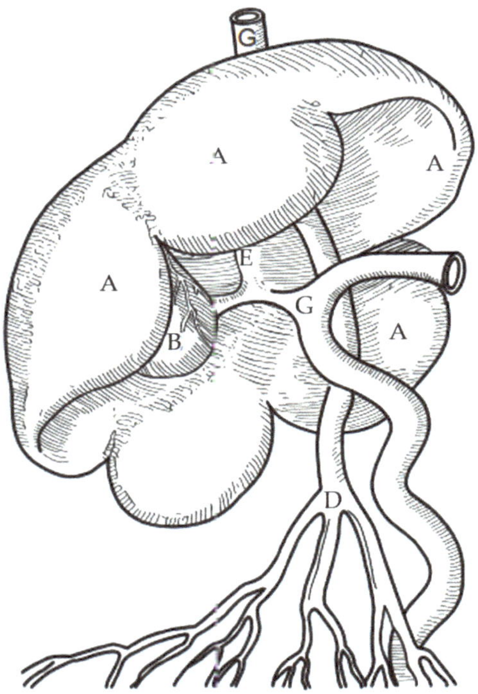

Figure 1.1. *The visceral surface of the multiple-lobed liver (A), with the gall bladder (B), portal vein (D), and bile duct, bile system (C, E) ("Anatomia Mundini," 1316) (Mondino de Luzzi, Bologna).*

Source: Reproduced from Kuntz, E., Kuntz, H.D., 2006. History of Hepatology. Hepatology, Principles and Practice. History, Morphology, Biochemistry, Diagnostics, Clinic, Therapy, second ed. Verlag Berlin Heidelberg, Springer, pp. 1–13.

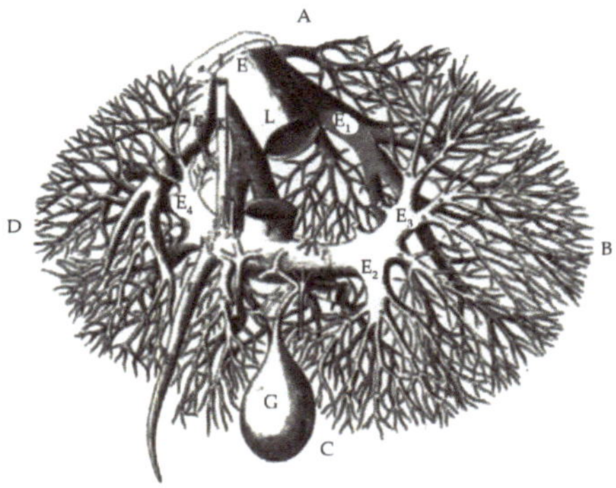

Figure 1.2. *Illustration of the blood and bile vessels of the liver by F. Glisson (1654). (A) dorsal region, (B) right aspect, (C) ventral region, (D) left aspect, (E) hepatic veins, (H) umbilical vein, (K) duct of Arantius, (G) gall bladder, (I) bile duct, (F) portal vein. (Univ. Library, Freiburg).*

Source: Reproduced from Kuntz, E., Kuntz, H.D., 2006. History of Hepatology. Hepatology, Principles and Practice. History, Morphology, Biochemistry, Diagnostics, Clinic, Therapy, second ed. Verlag Berlin Heidelberg, Springer, pp. 1–13.

1.2. Liver Anatomy and Physiology

Before examining the pathophysiology of the liver and potential treatments for the various hepatic illnesses, it is necessary to describe the liver's components (anatomy) and their interactions and functions (physiology) because the liver is an ecosystem (Rojkind & Greenwel, 1988). These two topics make up this book's main topics. To emphasize the applicability of this book, it is also necessary to discuss how liver diseases affect morbidity and mortality globally. It is imperative to acknowledge that free radicals, oxidative stress, and nitrosative stress are now acknowledged as playing a crucial role in the emergence, progression, and ultimately, the management and prevention of these illnesses. Furthermore, the development of future tactics to combat acute or chronic liver disease, which affects dozens of millions of people worldwide and is a major cause of death, depends on several models and evaluation techniques for the various hepatic pathologies.

1.2.1. Liver Anatomy

Under the diaphragm, the liver is a triangular organ that spans the abdominal cavity. The largest gland in the body, it makes up about 2.5% of the total weight of an adult human, which is approximately 1500 g. It is composed of extremely soft, pinkish-brown tissues that are encased in a connective tissue capsule. There are four lobules in the liver, with the falciform ligament dividing the lobules on the right and left. This organ receives blood-containing materials from the portal vein and oxygen-rich blood from the hepatic artery. It is anatomically positioned to fulfill its dual roles as a metabolic and biochemical transformation factory. Then, the liver utilizes the substances from both blood sources to synthesize new chemicals. These are, in turn, returned to the blood stream through the hepatic vein or to bile for excretion by the biliary system (Figure 1.3).

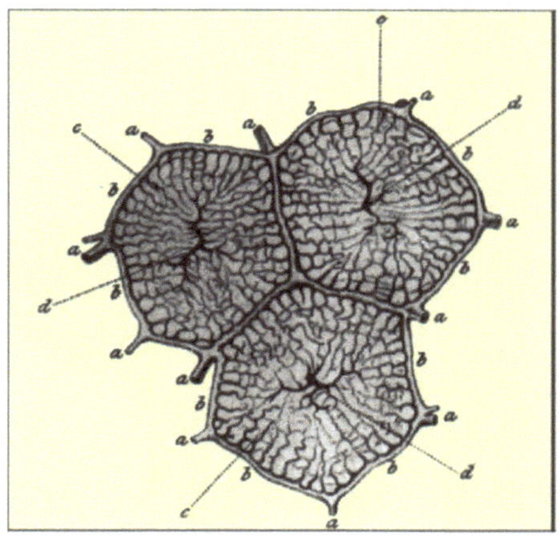

Figure 1.3. *Illustration of liver lobules and vessels by F. Kiernan (1833). (A, B) Interlobular veins, (C) intralobular vein plexus, (D) intralobular branch of the central hepatic vein.*

Source: Reproduced from Kuntz, E., Kuntz, H.D., 2006. History of Hepatology. Hepatology, Principles and Practice. History, Morphology, Biochemistry, Diagnostics, Clinic, Therapy, second ed. Verlag Berlin Heidelberg, Springer, pp. 1–13.

1.2.2. Bile Ducts

The biliary tree is an arrangement of branches made up of bile ducts, which are tubes that transport bile through the liver and gallbladder. Bile canaliculi are microscopic canals into which the bile produced by liver cells drains. The larger left and right hepatic ducts, which transport bile from both liver lobes, are formed when bile canaliculi connect to numerous bile ducts scattered throughout the liver. The common hepatic duct, which drains all bile from the liver, is formed when the hepatic ducts unite. The common bile duct, which transports bile to the duodenum, is ultimately formed when the common hepatic duct and the cystic duct from the gallbladder unite. Peristalsis propels the majority of the bile produced by the liver up the cystic duct, where it is stored until it is required for digestion in the gallbladder.

1.2.3. Blood Vessels

Blood is collected into the hepatic portal vein after passing through capillaries in the intestines, pancreas, spleen, gallbladder, and stomach. This nutrient-rich blood is then transported by the hepatic portal vein to the liver acinus, where its contents are separated into smaller vessels and processed before being distributed throughout the body. Blood that has left the liver's tissues gathers in the hepatic veins before returning to the heart through the vena cava. The hepatic artery supplies oxygenated blood to the liver as well.

1.3. Liver Cells

Numerous vital tasks carried out by the liver ensure that the organism's homeostasis is maintained. Serum protein and hormone synthesis, nutrition extraction and metabolism, xenobiotic and systemic waste product metabolism, lipid, bile acid, and lipoprotein metabolism, glucose storage and utilization, bile formation, and the elimination of foreign antigens and bacteria from the gut are some of these activities. Hepatocytes, cholangiocytes, liver sinusoidal endothelial cells (LSECs), Kupffer cells (KCs), natural killer (NK) cells, and hepatic stellate cells (HSC) are among the various cell types that carry out these functions.

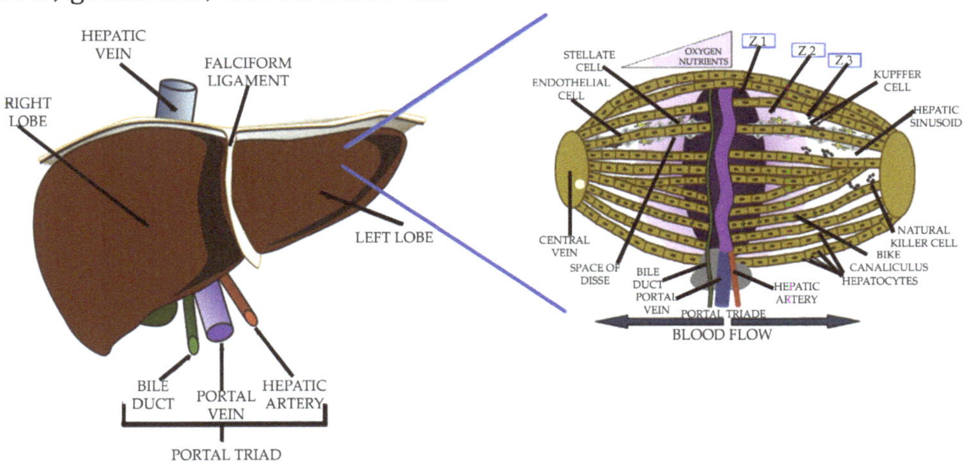

Figure 1.4. *(Left) View of the liver showing the portal triad (portal vein, hepatic artery, and the bile duct). (Right) Schematic diagram of the liver lobule and zonated liver functions (metabolic areas); representation of the bile canaliculus and hepatic sinusoid, indicating the different cell types, blood vessels, and bile duct. Arrows indicate the blood flow.*

Source: P. Muriel, The Liver: General Aspects and Epidemiology, http://dx.doi.org/10.1016/B978-0-12-804274-8.00001-1.

Two blood sources perfuse the liver parenchyma: oxygenated blood from the hepatic artery and portal venous blood, which is low in oxygen but rich in hormones, nutrients, and toxins from the spleen, pancreas, and gut (Figure 1.4). Figure 1.5 shows different types of liver cells.

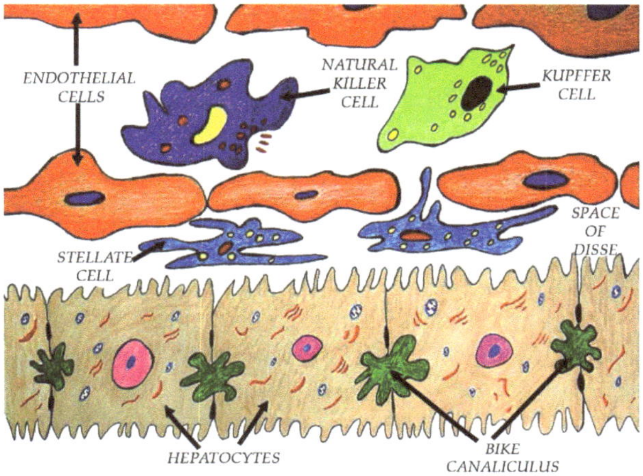

Figure 1.5. *Different types of liver cells.*

Source: P. Muriel, The Liver: General Aspects and Epidemiology, http://dx.doi.org/10.1016/B978-0-12-804274-8.00001-1.

The sinusoids, the tiniest capillary-sized blood vessels, are formed by the serial branching of these afferent blood vessels. The efferent hepatic veins, also known as central veins, are connected to sinusoids and gather sinusoidal blood that carries metabolized products and leads to the hepatic vein. The portal triad, which is made up of the hepatic artery, portal vein, and bile ducts that carry bile to the intestine and gall bladder, is another network of conduits found in the liver. According to Treyer and Müsch (2013), the hepatic lobule is the fundamental structural unit of the liver. It is composed of hepatocytes, which are abundant polarized cells arranged in single-cell thick cords lined by sinusoidal capillaries that stretch from the portal triad to the central vein. Liver zonation refers to the uneven distribution of vital metabolic and secretory functions along the portoecentral axis in the liver cell plate caused by the flow of blood from the portal vein and hepatic artery to the centrilobular vein while bile moves in the opposite direction (Torre et al., 2010).

1.3.1. The Hepatocyte and the Regenerative Capacity of the Liver

One essential feature of the liver is its capacity for metabolism and secretion. Due to the liver's pivotal role in systemic metabolism, it is frequently exposed to both endogenous and exogenous harmful agents, such as alcohol, viruses, and food ingredients, all of which can lead to hepatocellular death and are the main causes of liver disease (Blachier et al., 2013). The liver has developed an exceptional ability to regenerate itself in response to these challenges, primarily through the proliferation of hepatocytes in response to the detection of a loss of functional parenchyma. It is crucial to preserve liver function in this regard.

Hepatic parenchymal cells have a remarkable capacity for proliferation, but they can also lose their phenotype (Michalopoulos, 2013). Regrettably, a growing body of evidence indicates that the loss of hepatocellular differentiation and quiescence is the cause of liver malfunction in chronic liver disease and paves the way for the development of hepatocellular carcinoma. Therefore, in order to prevent chronic liver disease, it is imperative to identify the critical molecular factors involved in the maintenance of hepatocellular homeostasis and develop potential strategies to preserve the identity and functions of the liver. Research on this topic is presently being done, and the findings are encouraging (Avila & Moschetta, 2015; Berasain & Avila, 2015, 2016).

1.3.2. Pit Cells Exert Antitumor Functions

Pit cells are hepatic sinusoidal cells that are classified as liver-associated natural killer

(NK) cells functionally and as large granular lymphocytes morphologically. They stick to the liver sinusoidal endothelial cells (LSECs) and Kupffer cells (KCs) and are located inside the sinusoidal lumen. They have rod-cored vesicles and multivesicular dense granules. Target cells are identified by NK cells through their surface receptors, which include activating and inhibitory receptors. The primary characteristic of these cells is their ability to perform antitumor functions through the exocytosis of granules containing perforin or granzyme, induction of target cell apoptosis mediated by death receptors, and production of multiple cytokines that stimulate other immune cells (Nakatani et al., 2004). Numerous immunotherapies have been developed to combat malignant tumors, such as adoptive transfer of activated dendritic cells and lymphokine-activated killer cells, cytokines, and biological response modifiers. According to Jinushi et al. (2003), NK cells suppress the initiation of tumors in hepatoma cells in addition to preventing metastasis). Large granular lymphocytes from the liver were isolated and described: morphologically recognized as Pit cells, should consequently provide crucial hints for the treatment of liver cancers and metastases (Paschos et al., 2014).

1.3.3. LSECs Play a Prominent Role in Homeostasis

The LSECs comprise about 3% of the total liver volume, which makes 20% of the total number of liver cells. LSECs possess fenestrations, with diameters of about approximately 50–150 nm that are grouped together (Svistounov et al., 2012; Wisse, 1972). The sinusoidal endothelium lacks the basement membrane, which additionally constitutes its unique feature (Le Couteur et al., 2002). LSEC fenestrations allow for efficient transfer of lipoproteins, small chylomicron remnants, and other macromolecules between blood and the space of Disse, where they are taken up by hepatocytes (Fraser et al., 1978). LSECs have been shown to represent one of the most actively endocytosing cell types in the body mediating clearance of soluble waste macromolecules and colloid material, including bloodborne adenovirus (Ganesan et al., 2011; SimonSantamaria et al., 2014). Also, LSECs express various scavenger receptors (SR) on their surface including SR-A (also known as macrophage SR), SR-B (SR-B1 and CD36), and the most important SR-H receptor [stabilin-1/FEEL-1 (fasciclin, EGF-like, laminin-type EGF-like, and link domain-containing scavenger receptor-1) and stabilin2/FEEL-2 (fasciclin, EGF-like, laminin-type EGF-like, and link domain-containing scavenger receptor-2)/HARE (hyaluronic acid receptor for endocytosis)] (Sørensen et al., 2012). LSECs are professional pinocytic cells, clearing the blood of soluble macromolecules and small particles (<200 nm), whereas macrophages (KC) eliminate larger, insoluble particles by phagocytosis (Seternes et al., 2002). LSECs represent a structurally and functionally unique type of endothelium, which plays a fundamental role in maintaining liver homeostasis. LSEC dysfunction seems to have diagnostic, prognostic, and therapeutic significance in nonalcoholic fatty liver disease (NAFLD) and other liver diseases (Maslak et al., 2015). In addition, because LSECs are the main nitric oxide producing cells in the liver, their role in liver pathology and homeostasis is essential to this organ (Iwakiri & Kim, 2015; Iwakiri, 2015).

1.3.4. KCs are the First Line of Defense of the Organism

KCs are macrophages that reside in the liver and make up 80–90% of all tissue macrophages in the body (Gregory & Wing, 2002). They are essential for the liver's immunological and metabolic processes (Jager et al., 2016). The origin of KCs in the liver and how these cells are maintained over time are controversial. The traditional view that KCs originate from circulating monocytes that migrate into the liver where they differentiate into tissue macrophages

(Diesselhoff et al., 1979) has indeed been challenged. It is now understood that KCs originate from local intrahepatic progenitors without the assistance of hematopoietic stem cells, or from the yolk sac during embryogenesis and self-renew at the adult stage (Dey et al., 2014; Yona et al., 2013; Zigmond et al., 2014). As antigen-presenting cells, the primary job of KCs in a healthy liver is to phagocytose bacteria, microbes, and toxic substances transported by the hepatic circulation (Baffy, 2009). They are regarded as the organism's first line of defense (Baffy, 2009). KCs can move between the interstitial space (such as the space of Disse) and the vessels (such as the sinusoids) and mediate crosstalk between the recruited and resident cells of the liver. Larger KCs are found in the periportal zone, where they are immediately exposed to incoming molecular signals, while smaller KCs are found in the centrilobular regions (Baffy, 2009). In comparison to small KCs, large KCs have higher phagocytosis and lysosomal protease activity (Baffy, 2009). KCs are activated and release a variety of inflammatory mediators, including cytokines (e.g., tumor necrosis factor [TNF-a], interleukin [IL]-1b, and IL-6) and chemokines, as well as macrophage inflammatory proteins upon the recognition of a foreign substance (Kolios et al., 2006). These factors regulate the phenotype of KCs as well as that of neighboring cells, such as hepatocytes, HSCs, LSECs, and other immune cells that traffic through the liver (Bilzer et al., 2006). In turn, cytokines and chemokines secreted by KCs contribute to the recruitment of the liver cells, such as neutrophils, NKT cells, lymphocytes, NK cells, and blood monocyte-derived macrophages (Odegaard & Chawla, 2011; Swirski et al., 2007).

1.3.5. HSCs are the Main Executors in Fibrogenesis

The first HSCs were identified in 1876 by Kupffer using a gold chloride histochemical technique. Ito proposed in 1951 that KCs and HSCs were distinct cell populations. The greatest distinguishing characteristic of nonactivated HSCs is the abundance of retinoids in their cytoplasm. When the liver is damaged, the extracellular matrix (ECM) is produced, which triggers the fibrogenic process that ultimately results in cirrhosis. HSCs also become activated, lose their ability to store vitamin A, and express a number of smooth muscle markers (Yoneda et al., 2016).

Approximately 90% of ECM-producing myofibroblasts are produced by stellate cells or HSCs, which are the primary effectors in the multicellular response known as fibrogenesis (Mederacke et al., 2013) controlling many vital cell-to-cell interactions and the influx of bone marrow-derived cells via various signaling pathways. During this multicellular wound-healing response, HSCs interact closely with liver-resident cells, such as hepatocytes, KCs, cholangiocytes, LSECs, and infiltrating immune cells (Canbay et al., 2003; Duffield et al., 2005; Radaeva et al., 2006; Deleve et al., 2008; Syal et al., 2012; Pradere et al., 2013; Ding et al., 2014). These dynamic interactions are characteristic of both the development and the regression of liver fibrosis and control the activation status of HSCs and hepatic ECM content.

As the primary fibrogenesis executors, HSCs are exposed to a variety of signals from the damaged hepatic microenvironment and injured hepatocytes, the majority of which are mediated by cytokines (Schwabe & Seki, 2015; Jin et al., 2016). High sensitivity to lipopolysaccharide and cytokines causes HSCs to produce more chemokines and cytokines as well as activate proinflammatory signaling pathways like activator protein 1 and nuclear factor kappa B (NF-kB) (Seki et al., 2007). HSCs likely play a secondary role as recipients of inflammatory signals, and inflammatory pathways control their activation and maintain the viability of activated HSCs, for example through NF-kB.

However, in comparison to the pivotal role of KCs, HSCs likely contribute very little to overall hepatic inflammation in vivo (Hellerbrand et al., 1998). Additionally, during fibrogenesis (by encouraging the recruitment of cells that promote HSC activation) and during fibrosis regression (by encouraging the recruitment of cells that break down the extracellular matrix and kill HSCs), HSCs may offer particular chemotactic signals that control their interaction with different types of inflammatory cells. Additionally, because HSCs express a lot of Toll-like receptors, which promote HSC activation and fibrosis, they serve as a bridge between the gut and the liver (Seki et al., 2007).

HSCs are viewed as a potential target for creating antifibrogenic strategies by disrupting the connection between inflammation and liver fibrosis development. This involves studying the impact of inflammatory mediators on fibrogenesis and fibrosis regression (Zhang et al., 2016).

1.4. Liver Zonation Allows Functional Plasticity

The liver is a homogeneous anatomical structure made up of regular hexagon-shaped lobule arrangements resembling a honeycomb. The liver's smallest capillaries, the sinusoids, receive blood from the portal triad, which then empties into the central vein. Because blood from the portal triad is rich in these elements, Figure 1.4 demonstrates how a gradient in oxygen and nutrients is formed in the sinusoid. As blood flows to the central vein, nutrients and oxygen are consumed, resulting in the formation of three zones (Z). As a result, the biochemical and physiological roles that hepatocytes arranged along the portoecentral axis (ZI to ZIII) carry out exhibit remarkable heterogeneity. The multitude of processes required to preserve the body's metabolic homeostasis are made possible by this dynamic structural and functional heterogeneity, or metabolic zonation (Lamers et al., 1989; Gebhardt and Matz-Soja, 2014).

1.4.1. Regulation of Zonation of the Liver

Signaling molecules known as morphogens are essential to the processes of organogenesis, morphogenesis, and embryogenesis (Tabata and Takei, 2004). Numerous investigators have observed that the regulation of hepatic metabolism is associated with morphogen signaling pathways. The majority of the evidence for Wnt/b-catenin, hepatocyte growth factor (HGF), and hedgehog (Hh) signaling will be covered in this chapter, even though it is highly likely that many other morphogens also influence liver zonation.

Since it has been extensively reviewed, the significance of Wnt/b-catenin signaling in controlling liver zonation in the liver has been established (Cavard et al., 2008; Gebhardt and Hovhannisyan (2010); Gebhardt et al., 2007; Monga (2015), and Torre et al., 2011). Since it is most active in the vicinity of the liver lobules' central vein, it is especially important in controlling activities related to this zone, including heme synthesis, glutamine, bile acid, and drug metabolism (Benhamouche et al., 2006; Burke et al., 2009; Sekine et al., 2006). However, the expression of certain periportal functions (eg., Additionally, the Wnt/b-catenin signaling pathway affects ureogenesis and gluconeogenesis (Benhamouche et al., 2006). In most cases, when b-catenin signaling is activated, these portal functions are downregulated (Torre et al., 2011; Vasilj et al., 2012). It seems reasonable to think of Wnt/b-catenin as a master regulator of zonation given the pathway's wide-ranging effects on liver zonation.

It was discovered in 1991 that HGF functions as a morphogen capable of causing three-dimensional morphogenesis (Montesano et al.,

1991). Based on cell culture experiments where HGF was used as an inducer of rat sarcoma (RAS) signaling, the contribution of HGF to the regulation of zonation was proposed (Braeuning et al., 2007). Schwarz and others. developed the theory that the zonation of gene expression in the liver is determined by opposing signaling pathways that are triggered by factors that are dependent on both b-catenin and Ha-ras (Braeuning et al., 2007; Hailfinger et al., 2006). Relationships between Wnt/b-catenin and Hh signaling and RAS signaling are particularly interesting and have been reviewed in great detail, primarily in relation to tumorigenesis, proliferation, and differentiation (Guardavaccaro and Clevers, 2012; Lauth, 2011; Zeller et al., 2013). Given how context-dependent these interactions are, it is yet to be shown whether they are relevant, at least in part, for controlling zonation in adult liver.

Matz-Soja et al. (2013) have hypothesized that hepatocellular Hh signaling may contribute to liver zonation despite its low activity. Indeed, by employing transgenic mice with conditional smoothened deletion, they were able to show that even extremely low activity of this pathway has a significant impact on the function of mature liver, and as a result, on serum levels of insulin-like growth factor I (IGF-I) protein (Matz-Soja et al., 2014). Furthermore, immunohistochemistry demonstrated that Indian Hh (Ihh) is only expressed in the farthest pericentral region (Matz-Soja et al., 2014). This aligns with the established understanding that Wnt/b-catenin signaling targets Ihh (Reed et al., 2008). The pericentral distribution of Ihh in transgenic mice with increased b-catenin signaling is further evidence of the dependence of Ihh production on b-catenin signaling activity. It is still unknown how specifically Hh signaling affects the regulation of zonation, but this evidence suggests that both Wnt and Hh signaling regulate the expression of Ihh by pericentral hepatocytes.

1.4.2. Metabolic Zonal Functions

Not every hepatic function is exclusively zonal. It appears that all hepatocytes synthesize significant amounts of serum proteins, including the transporters of transthyretin and transferrin. Additionally, albumin is synthesized in every zone, but it is concentrated more in the periportal region. These days, the metabolic processes of drugs and xenobiotics, glucose metabolism, and ammonia detoxification are the most researched zonated functions. Lipid metabolism is one of the other zonated processes (Behari et al., 2014), with periportal fatty acid degradation and perivenously occurring lipogenesis (Schleicher et al., 2015). Clear perivenular (PV) zonation is seen in the synthesis of bile acids from cholesterol (Sasamoto et al., 2006; Shiue et al., 2014), such as the catabolism of serine and histidine, which primarily exhibits periportal zonation; zone III is home to glutamine synthesis, which is connected to ammonia detoxification (Bartl et al., 2015; Qvartskhava et al., 2015). One historical example of compartmentalized metabolism is glucose metabolism. The periportal zone is where most gluconeogenesis occurs (Hijmans et al., 2014), although glycolysis primarily involves PV (Dasgupta et al., 2014). One historical example of compartmentalized metabolism is glucose metabolism. The periportal zone is where most gluconeogenesis occurs (Hijmans et al., 2014), although glycolysis primarily involves PV (Dasgupta et al., 2014). The zonation of these glucose metabolism-related components appears to be influenced by hormones and nutrients, as evidenced by the different concentration gradients of these enzymes based on nutritional status. Eliminating toxic ammonia that enters the liver through the portal vein from the intestine is one of the liver's primary functions. Glutaminase, glutamine synthetase, and the urea cycle enzymes, which are represented by carbamoyl phosphate synthetase, are the three enzymes (or enzyme systems) that play a role in this process in mammals.

Using an in silico approach, numerical optimization was used to determine the distribution of these enzymes for optimal ammonia detoxification. This approach predicted that the enzymes needed to be zonated to achieve maximum removal of toxic ammonia and minimal changes in glutamine concentration. Glutaminase and carbamoyl phosphate synthetase are distributed nonhomogeneously in the periportal zone, while glutamine synthetase is only active within a limited pericentral zone (Bartl et al., 2015). Drug and xenobiotic metabolism also exhibits distinct zonation, primarily in the PV region (Monga, 2015). Excretable products are produced by the cytochrome P450 system upon the conversion of xenobiotics. This entails monooxygenation, which is followed by conjugation with sulfuric or glucuronic acid. Monooxygenation mostly takes place in the PV zone, where the predominant conjugation reaction is sulfation in periportal cells, while glucuronidation is the major conjugation reaction in these cells (Maronpot et al., 2010).

1.5. Global Liver Epidemiology

Although there has been significant advancement in the understanding and treatment of liver disease over the last 30 years, dozens of millions of people worldwide continue to experience acute or chronic liver disease. Understanding the burden of liver disease requires an understanding of the incidence and prevalence of two conditions: liver cancer and cirrhosis. They are a sign of the associated mortality because they show the final stage of liver pathology. The WHO (2015) projects that the prevalence of cirrhosis and liver cancer will rise to 2030, indicating a clear increase in these hepatic pathologies as global causes of death (Figure 1.6).

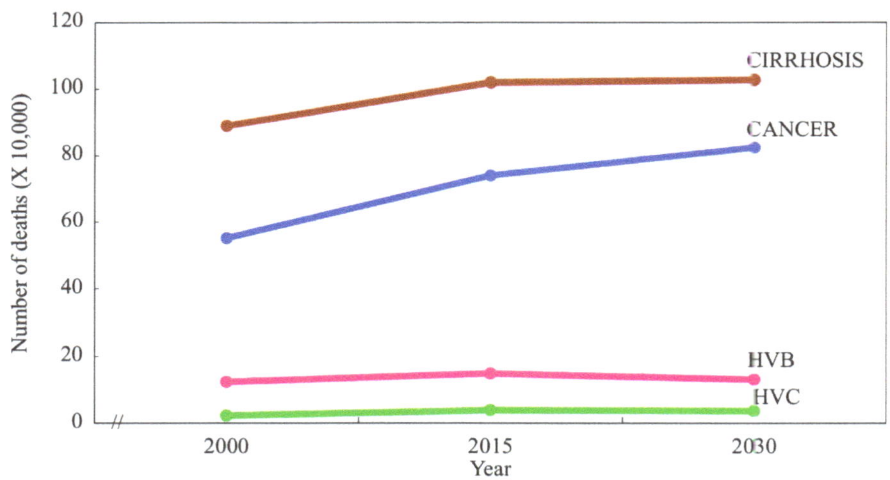

Figure 1.6. *Projection of worldwide mortality from liver cirrhosis, liver cancer, hepatitis B virus, and hepatitis C virus.*

Source: Data were obtained from WHO, 2015. http://www.who.org.

Figure 1.7 depicts the four leading causes of liver disease globally, which are NAFLD (40%), hepatitis B virus (HBV) (30%), hepatitis C virus (HCV) (15%), and harmful alcohol consumption (11%).

Global mortality from viral hepatitis, liver cancer, and cirrhosis is shown in Figure. 1.8(A). The main causes of viral hepatitis are HBV (43%), hepatitis A virus (HAV) (33%), hepatitis E virus (HEV) (18%), and HCV (5%) (Figure 1.8(B)), whereas the etiology of liver cirrhosis is HBV (30%), HCV (28%), alcohol (27%), or other (14%) (Figure 1.8(C)). The etiology of liver cancer is HBV (45%), HCV (26%), alcohol (20%), and other (39%) (Figure. 1.8(D)) (Lozano et al., 2012).

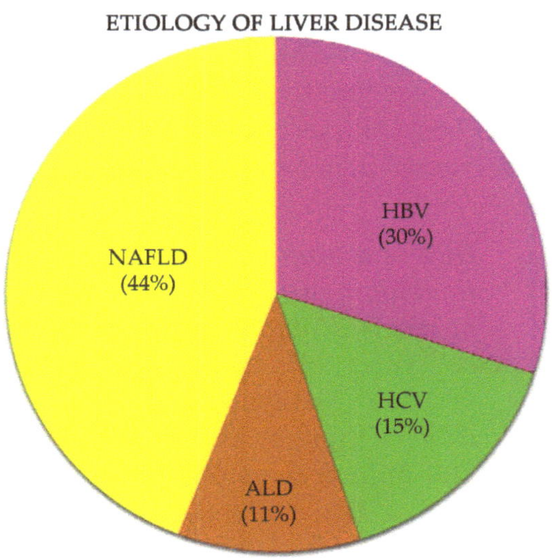

Figure 1.7. *Causes of global liver disease in 2010. NAFLD, nonalcoholic fatty liver disease, ALD, alcoholic liver disease; HBV, hepatitis B virus; HCV, hepatitis C virus.*

Source: Data were obtained from Lozano, R., Naghavi, M., Foreman, K., Lim, S., Shibuya, K., Aboyans, V., et al., 2012. Global and regional mortality from 235 causes of death for 20 age groups in 1990 and 2010: a systematic analysis for the Global Burden of Disease Study 2010. Lancet 380, 2095–2128.

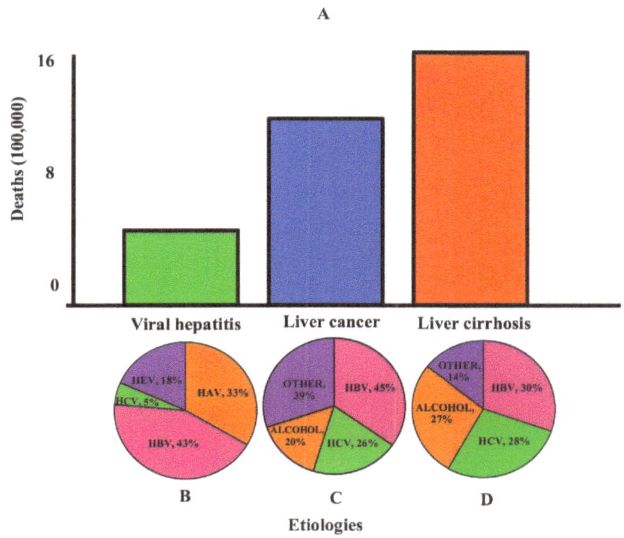

Figure 1.8. *(Panel A) Worldwide mortality from viral hepatitis, liver cancer, and liver cirrhosis in 2010. (Panel B) Etiology of viral hepatitis (HAV, hepatitis A virus; HBV, hepatitis B virus; HCV, hepatitis C virus; HEV, hepatitis E virus). (Panel C) Liver cirrhosis, and (panel D) liver cancer in 2010.*

Source: Data were obtained from Lozano, R., Naghavi, M., Foreman, K., Lim, S., Shibuya, K., Aboyans, V., et al., 2012. Global and regional mortality from 235 causes of death for 20 age groups in 1990 and 2010: a systematic analysis for the Global Burden of Disease Study 2010. Lancet 380, 2095–2128.

1.5.1. Hepatocellular Carcinoma Epidemiology

Primary liver cancer ranks second in terms of cancer mortality and is the fifth most common type of cancer globally. Between 85 and 90% of primary liver cancers are hepatocellular carcinomas (HCCs), the most prevalent histologic type of liver cancer. Patients with liver cancer have a poor overall prognosis (ratio of mortality to incidence of 0.95). Therefore, a thorough understanding of this disease and its risk factors is essential for the early detection, timely diagnosis, and screening of at-risk individuals in order to treat these patients with more effective and timely medical intervention (Ferlay et al., 2010). The majority of HCCs have a history of chronic liver disease as their underlying cause. These underlying causes are distinguished by notable differences in gender, geography, and other well-established risk factors, some of which may now be prevented (Lafaro et al., 2015).

1.5.2. Risk Factors That May Lead to HCC

A genetically diverse tumor is HCC. Because hepatocarcinogenesis is so complicated, many genetic and epigenetic changes are necessary. The involvement of known predisposing factors for HCC, such as aflatoxins, high alcohol consumption, obesity, HBV, and HCV, varies by region in terms of prevalence and contribution (Lafaro et al., 2015).

- ***Hepatitis B Virus:*** According to Tabor (2001), 70% of HCC patients in China, 41% of HCC patients in the US, and 24–27% of HCC patients in Japan had serum HBsAg (Hepatitis B surface antigen), the marker of HBV infection, without the presence of any additional risk factors. HBV raises the risk of HCC in patients with and without cirrhosis, in contrast to other risk factors. Similar to other risk factors, HBV infection causes chronic necroinflammation in the context of cirrhosis, which results in hepatocyte proliferation and fibrosis. HBV can cause hepatocarcinogenesis secondary to virus-specific factors, even in the absence of cirrhosis. The DNA virus known as HBV encodes both replicative and structural proteins through its circular genome. DNA regulatory elements are also present in it. When the virus infiltrates hepatocytes, its messenger RNAs are translated into viral proteins, viral DNA is produced, and eventually, the viral DNA can merge with the host hepatocytes' genome. In multiple ways, including the quick hepatocyte cell cycle (Chisari, 2000) and the integration of viral DNA into the genome, which results in instability (Dandri et al., 2002), this process may promote carcinogenesis; it can also introduce encoding proteins into genes that are necessary for the development of cancer (Ferber et al., 2003).

Furthermore, it has been demonstrated that HBV overexpression on its own causes malignant transformation in mice (Wu et al., 2006). A higher HBV viral load than 13 pg/mL is associated with a higher risk of developing HCC (Yang et al., 2002 ; Chen et al., 2006; Yuen et al., 2009); consequently, immunization appears to be the best course of action for combating HBV infection and, in turn, the risk of acquiring cancer.

- ***HCV is a Major Risk Factor for HCC Development:*** The Flaviviridae family of viruses includes the RNA virus known as HCV, which was discovered in 1989 (McGlynn & London, 2011). HCV is thought to infect more than 200 million people globally (Umer & Iqbal, 2016), and it is a significant risk factor for the development of HCC. According to Yoshizawa (2002), HCV infection rates in patients with HCC vary, ranging from 44–66% in Italy to 80–90% in Japan. Donato et al., (2002) conducted a meta-analysis of 21 studies showing that patients with HCV infection had a 17-fold higher risk of HCC than did controls without the virus. With sustained virologic response (SVR) and the absence of detectable HCV RNA following successful treatment, antiviral therapy of HCV fortunately eradicates the virus.

According to Singhal et al., SVR has been linked to a 54% decrease in all-cause mortality, which includes a 44% decrease in deaths from liver and HCC (2010). According to a meta-analysis, people who reached SVR had a lower incidence of HCC development (0.33% per person/year) than nonresponders (1.67% per person/year) (Morgan et al., 2013).

- ***Ethanol Abuse is Associated with HCC:*** Approximately 8–20% of chronic alcoholics develop liver cirrhosis (Zhu et al., 2012). The International Agency for Research on Cancer Working Group suggested a causal relationship between alcohol consumption and liver cancer in 1988 (IARC, 1988) and has since deemed beverages containing alcohol as carcinogenic to humans. The initial causal relationship between alcohol and HCC was subsequently confirmed by multiple studies (Donato et al., 2002; Yuan et al., 2004). Chronic excessive alcohol use (>80 g/d) for greater than 10 years has been shown to increase HCC risk fivefold (Donato et al., 2002; Grewal and Viswanathen, 2012). Naturally, cessation of alcohol consumption has been shown to decrease the risk of liver cancer. A meta-analysis showed that the risk of HCC decreases after abstinence by 6–7% per year compared with ongoing drinkers. The same study estimated that a period of 23 years of abstinence is required for the risk of HCC development to return to that of nondrinkers (Heckley et al., 2011).
- ***Aflatoxin is a Potent Carcinogen:*** The fungi *Aspergillus flavus* and *Aspergillus parasiticus* produce aflatoxin, a mycotoxin that can contaminate grains, legumes, tree nuts, maize, and groundnuts. Furthermore, the consumption of aflatoxin-contaminated feed by dairy-producing animals results in the excretion of aflatoxin M1, a metabolite, in the milk. Mozambique, Vietnam, China, and India are among the nations with a high risk of dietary aflatoxin intake due to their warm, humid climates, which encourage the growth of molds that produce aflatoxin. A risk assessment from 2010 found that aflatoxin is associated with 4.6–28.2% of HCC worldwide (Liu and Wu, 2010). There are four aflatoxins: B1, B2, G1, and G2. Aflatoxin B1 (AFB1) is the most potent carcinogen. According to an estimate from 2006, more than 55 million people worldwide suffer from uncontrolled exposure to aflatoxin (Liu and Wu, 2010). AFB1 is metabolized to the active intermediate AFB1 exo8, 9-epoxide, which in turn binds to DNA (Bressac et al., 1991; Hsu et al., 1991; Ozturk, 1991).
- ***Nonalcoholic Steatohepatitis Can Progress to Cirrhosis and HCC:*** Alcohol misuse and hepatitis viral infection are linked to the majority of HCC cases. Nonetheless, 5–20% of patients with HCC test negative for both HBV and HCV. The most frequent cause of cryptogenic chronic liver disease in the United States and other Western nations is nonalcoholic steatohepatitis (NASH), a more severe form of NAFLD that is characterized by liver disease without a history of heavy alcohol use. NASH has been reported in 1–3% of the adult Japanese population and approximately 6% in Western countries (Nishikawa & Osaki, 2013; Tokushige et al., 2011; Torres & Harrison, 2012). There is increasing evidence to support the fact that NASH and NAFLD can progress to cirrhosis and HCC, and,

a Surveillance Epidemiology and End Results Medicareebased database study showed a strong correlation between the metabolic syndrome and HCC (Lafaro et al., 2015). Also, cohort studies from Denmark and Sweden have identified an increase in HCC risk in obese males compared with those with a normal body mass index (BMI) (Wolk et al., 2001; Attner et al., 2012). Additionally, there is evidence linking obesity to a higher death rate in HCC patients. Men with a BMI of 35–40 had a five-fold higher risk of HCC mortality than men with a normal BMI, according to a large 16-year prospective cohort study conducted in the United States (Calle et al., 2003). The obesity epidemic is growing, and this could result in a marked rise in the incidence of HCC, which makes these studies crucial.

- ***Diabetes Mellitus Type 2 is an Independent Risk Factor for HCC:*** HCC has been associated with insulin resistance, a component of metabolic syndrome, most likely due to angiogenic and inflammatory alterations. Consequently, research has been done on the risk of HCC linked to diabetes mellitus (DM). As with obesity, a significant portion of DM patients (70%) have some form of fatty liver disease (Neuschwander-Tetri and Caldwell, 2003). El-Serag et al., performed a longitudinal study, including 173,643 patients with DM and 650,620 without it, to elucidate an association between DM and HCC; researchers found that DM was associated with chronic NAFLD and HCC development (El-Serag, 2007; Shimizu et al., 2013). Thus, DM was concluded to be an independent risk factor for the progression of chronic liver disease and HCC development.
- ***Tobacco Smoking Increases the Risk of Mortality in Patients With HCC:*** The association between tobacco use and HCC has been the subject of numerous research publications; sadly, the findings are mixed. According to a prospective cohort study conducted in Japan over a mean of 9 years, smokers currently smoking had a threefold higher risk of primary liver cancer than nonsmokers (Mizoue et al., 2000). A 4-year follow-up study conducted in Korea on 733,134 men revealed a significant association between current and past smokers and the development of HCC (Yun et al., 2005). In 210 patients with HCC, a prospective case-control study revealed that tobacco smokers had a higher risk of developing HCC than both nonsmoking patients and cirrhotic patients without HCC (Marrero et al., 2005).

However, a US study that used case-control data from the Selected Cancers Study discovered that current smokers did not have a higher risk of developing primary liver cancer (Zhu et al., 2007). The researchers did discover that ex-smokers had a statistically significant higher risk of developing primary liver cancer. The findings of this research could imply that smoking carries a time-dependent risk. It has been reported that alcohol intake, obesity, and tobacco use all work together to increase the risk of HCC (Marrero et al., 2005). Several studies have shown an increased risk of mortality in patients with HCC who use tobacco, even though the exact relationship between tobacco use and the development of HCC is still unknown (Jee et al., 2004; Sun et al., 2003). In conclusion, alcohol misuse, HBV, and HCV are the primary risk factors for carcinogenesis in HCC, even though NASH-associated HCC appears to be more common in Western nations. Improved cancer prevention, early detection, and treatment of HCC depend on a deeper comprehension of these risk factors and how they contribute to the development of cancer.

1.5.3. Epidemiology of Alcoholic Liver Disease

The primary cause of liver disease, viral hepatitis, can occur either in conjunction with or independently of other comorbidities like obesity or alcohol liver disease (ALD). Additionally, the liver is the organ most frequently targeted by long-term alcohol abuse. In Germany and the United States, chronic alcohol consumption is responsible for over 50% of chronic liver diseases (McCullough & O'Connor, 1998). In South Korea, 7–31% of cirrhosis cases have been attributed to alcohol abuse (Kim, 2009). The treatment of ALD causes huge costs for the health care system with nearly $3 billion per year (Maher, 2002). When the total number of deaths and disability-adjusted life years (DALYs) is taken into account, liver diseases account for 31.5% of all DALYs in Portugal. Following closely behind are traffic accidents and various cancers (Cortez-Pinto et al., 2010). China has seen the largest increase in ALD, with a 40% increase in annual per capita alcohol consumption depending on the region (Cochrane et al., 2003). Due to imprecise or lacking data regarding actual drinking patterns, it is challenging to calculate alcohol-related deaths. The risk of developing ALD is linked to alcohol consumption of 20 and 30 g per day for men and women, respectively. Even in cases with high alcohol consumption, liver cirrhosis only develops in a small percentage of cases (Maher, 2002), highlighting the significance of additional genetic factors for the progression of the disease. Approximately 5% of the whole population shows high-risk drinking behavior in the United States and Germany and 7% showed heavy alcohol consumption according to the Korean National Health and Nutrition Examination Survey (NHANES) 2009 (Park et al., 2011; Lozano et al., 2012). In the global death statistics published in 2010, liver cirrhosis and HCC are ranked at positions 12 and 16, respectively (Lozano et al., 2012) with one-third directly attributable to alcohol. Cirrhosis of the liver produces over 170,000 deaths per year in Europe and is in the fourth place in the so-called years of life lost statistics, and in ALD patients with cirrhosis, HCC is the most common fatal complication (Mueller et al., 2014; Stickel, 2015).

1.5.4. Risk Factors for ALD

The amount of alcohol consumed and the onset of liver disease do not clearly correlate with one another. Research has indicated that women are twice as vulnerable as men to alcohol-mediated hepatotoxicity and that they may experience more severe ALD with shorter half-lives and lower alcohol intake (Borro et al., 2016, Testino et al., 2014). Research has shown that individuals who drink alcohol between mealtimes have a 2.7 times higher chance of developing alcohol-related liver disease (ALD) compared to those who only drink with their meals. Men and women who consume 12 to 24 g of alcohol daily have been found to have an increased chance of dying from cirrhosis (Testino, 2013).

In alcohol-related hepatic disease, blood fasting glucose and BMI are independent risk factors for the development of fibrosis (Raynard et al., 2002). Being overweight or obese increases the risk of endotoxin-induced hepatic injury, and there is evidence linking endotoxemia to the degree of alcohol-induced liver damage.

Of all chronic liver diseases in Western countries, 70–90% are caused by alcohol consumption and chronic hepatitis C infection. Additionally, alcohol and HCV have a synergistic effect that increases the production of free radicals in the liver and weakens its antioxidant defenses. Moreover, it has been assessed that both moderate (50 g/d) increase the odds of developing oxidative stress by three times and 13–24 times, respectively (Safdar & Schiff, 2004). Additionally, chronic alcohol consumption combined with HCV infection increases hepatic lipid peroxidation and raises the expression of transforming growth factor beta (TGF-b) and TNF-a in the liver (Perlemuter et al., 2003). Fibrosis results from the overproduction of extracellular matrix (ECM) due to the activation of HSCs by TGF-b.

1.5.5. Epidemiology of NAFLD and NASH

NAFLD is a spectrum of liver disease that includes fibrosis, cirrhosis, necroinflammation, simple fat accumulation in the liver, and hepatic cancer (HCC) (Rinella & Sanyal, 2016; Zoller & Tilg, 2016). A rise in sedentary lifestyles and dietary changes could be the cause of this entity's rising prevalence. The prevalence of NAFLD in both economically developed and developing countries highlights the epidemic's global scope. While the progression of NASH to cirrhosis and HCC is well established, the progression from NAFLD to NASH is presently under investigation (Matteoni et al., 1999; Adams et al., 2005). Determining the actual incidence and prevalence of NAFLD and NASH is particularly challenging due to the asymptomatic nature of the conditions and the lack of a sensitive diagnostic method other than a liver biopsy, which is the gold standard.

However, research to date provides some understanding of the global pattern of the NAFLD/NASH pandemic. In a Japanese study that lasted 414 days and included 3147 people without NAFLD but with metabolic syndrome symptoms, 10% of the participants had new NAFLD onset (Hamaguchi et al., 2005). Another study from Japan based on large population screening reported an incidence of 31 cases per 1000 person (Suzuki et al., 2005). In an English outpatient hepatology practice setting the incidence of 29 cases per 100,000 person-years was observed (Whalley et al., 2007), whereas in an 8-year follow-up study from Italy, an incidence rate of 18.5 per 1000 person-years has been reported (Bedogni et al., 2007). The worldwide prevalence of NAFLD in the general population is estimated to be 20–30% in Western countries and 5–18% in Asia and it is increasing over time (Masarone et al., 2014). The worldwide prevalence of NASH was conservatively estimated to be between 2% and 3% (Satapathy & Sanyal, 2015). A recent meta-analysis has found that the pooled global prevalence of NAFLD was 24.24% and that it is positively correlated with economic status as represented by gross national income per capita (Zhu et al., 2015). Prevalence of NAFLD differs widely across the globe with ethnicity, population studied, and the diagnostic modalities used for the surveillance (Browning et al., 2004; Fischer et al., 2009; Mohanty et al., 2009; Saab et al., 2016; Williams et al., 2011; Younossi et al., 2011; Masarone et al., 2014; Zhu et al., 2015).

Significant differences were observed in the frequency of NAFLD according to sex (24% in white women, 42% in white men), ethnicity (45% in Hispanics, 33% in whites, and 24% in blacks), and sex (Browning et al., 2004). NHANES data from the United States between 1988 and 2008 revealed that the prevalence of nonalcoholic fatty liver disease (NAFLD) had doubled, but the prevalence of other chronic liver disease causes remained stable (Younossi et al., 2011).

1.5.6. Risk Factors for NAFLD and NASH

NAFLD has become the most common hepatic disorder in Europe and the United States (Weib et al., 2014). According to data from the US

NHANES, the proportion of NAFLD among chronic liver diseases rose from 47% to 75% between 1988 and 2008. The reason for this increase is most probably an increase in risk factors. In this sense, obesity increased from 21% to 33%; visceral obesity from 35% to 51%; type 2 diabetes from 5.6% to 9.1%; insulin resistance from 23% to 35% and arterial hypertension from 22% to 34% (Younossi et al., 2011).

Both a high body mass index (BMI) and visceral obesity increase the risk for NAFLD (Angulo, 2002). In patients with morbid obesity (BMI > 40 kg/m^2) who undergo bariatric surgery, the prevalence of NAFLD may even be over 90% (Chalasani et al., 2012). However, physical constitution and fat distribution have been found to be better indicators of mortality than BMI alone (Ahima & Lazar, 2013).

Age, sex, and ethnicity factors have also been found to play a role: male sex, older age, and Hispanic origin are associated with a significantly higher risk of developing NAFLD (Vernon et al., 2011).

1.5.7. Chronic HCV Epidemiology

In the US, hepatocellular carcinoma, cirrhosis, and chronic liver disease are all primarily brought on by HCV infection, which is also the main reason for liver transplantation (Davis et al., 2003; Lee et al., 2015; Su et al., 2016). Between 130 and 150 million people worldwide are thought to be infected with HCV (WHO, 2015). The definition of chronic HCV infection is HCV viremia that lasts longer than six months. Even though the estimated prevalence in developed nations is low (1–2%), it may be as high as 5–10% of the adult population in less developed nations. Research on the natural progression of hepatitis C, conducted through global surveillance and control, indicates that approximately 55–85% of infected individuals will develop chronic liver disease, 15–30% will progress to cirrhosis, and 1–5% will die from decompensated cirrhosis and HCC (WHO, 2015). An estimated 350,000–500,000 people die globally each year from liver disease linked to HCV (WHO, 2015). Between 45 and 85% of people with chronic HCV infection are thought to be asymptomatic and unaware of their infection (Smith et al., 2012). Several additional US studies have also predicted a twofold increase in HCV-related deaths, with direct medical expenditure exceeding $6.7 billion USD between 2010 and 2019 (Wong et al., 2000); morbidity and mortality from HCV will peak between 2030 and 2035 without intervention, forecasting for 38,600 incident cases of end-stage liver disease, 3200 referrals per year for liver transplant, and 36,100 deaths (Rein et al., 2011).

1.5.8. Risk Factors for Chronic HCV

Blood transfusions given before 1992, high-risk sexual behavior with a high number of lifetime sexual partners, and illegal drug use are the main risk factors for HCV infection. Having less than 12 years of education, being poor, and being divorced or separated were other risk factors linked to a positive HCV infection (Alter et al., 1999). Furthermore, across all risk groups and geographical areas, but particularly among injecting drug users, there is a consistently higher prevalence of HCV in HIV-positive individuals than in HIV-negative individuals (Platt et al., 2016).

1.5.9. Epidemiology of Primary Biliary Cirrhosis

An epidemiological study conducted in Europe, North America, Asia, and Australia on primary biliary cirrhosis (PBC) found that the disease affects 0.9–5.8 persons per 100,000, with women making up 92% of patients (Boonstra et al., 2012; Carey et al., 2015). Although some groups have reported increased incidence over the past 40 years (Hamlyn et al., 1983; Metcalf et al., 1997; Boonstra et al., 2014) others have not substantiated this finding (Baldursdottir et al.,

2012; McNally et al., 2014). It is unclear if these trends in incidence represent a real rise or are just a result of improvements in diagnosis and treatment. The increased survival rate following the introduction of ursodeoxycholic acid as a successful treatment, improved data collection by electronic medical records, and an increase in disease recognition are likely the causes of the increased prevalence.

1.5.10. Risk Factors for PBC

The geographic distribution suggests that environmental toxins may have a role. This is especially true in areas where toxic waste is disposed of in the United States and in low-income areas where pollution, cigarette smoking, and toxin exposure are linked in the United Kingdom (Ala et al., 2006; Boonstra et al., 2012; McNally et al., 2014). Also, PBC has been associated with infectious agents such as Escherichia coli, *Mycobacterium gordonae*, *Novosphingobium aromaticivorans*, and with hair dyes, nail polish, and cigarette smoking, although a causative role has not been demonstrated (Talwalkar & Lindor, 2003).

1.5.11. Epidemiology of Drug-Induced Liver Injury

In the majority of human and animal contexts, drugs can induce acute liver failure (ALF) in a predictable dose-dependent manner (intrinsic drug-induced liver injury [DILI]) or in an erratic, nonedose-dependent manner (idiosyncratic DILI) (Licata, 2016).

- ***Intrinsic DILI:*** About half of all cases of ALF in the US are caused by acetaminophen toxicity, which is also the most common cause of severe intrinsic DILI. Because accidental overdoses resulting from a range of patient misconceptions account for about half of acetaminophen toxicity deaths, the majority of these cases are preventable (Ostapowicz et al., 2002; Bower et al., 2007). Furthermore, the highly potent antidote N-acetyl cysteine can be used to lessen the harmful effects of an acute overdose.
- ***Idiosyncratic DILI:*** Registries of idiosyncratic DILI cases have been established in different Western (Sgro et al., 2002; Hoofnagle, 2004; Andrade et al., 2005; Björnsson et al., 2013) and Asian (Takikawa et al., 2009) countries. Patients enrolled in DILI registries are usually middle-aged women (mean age: 50 years) who require hospitalization. Hepatocellular liver damage, followed by a cholestatic or mixed presentation is the more common cause. In population-based studies, the crude annual incidence of DILI has been reported as 19.1 cases per 100,000 inhabitants in Iceland (Björnsson et al., 2013) and 13.9 cases per 100,000 inhabitants in France (Sgro et al., 2002). Risk factors include the patient's age, sex, genetics, previous episodes of DILI, and underlying chronic liver disease, patient's metabolic features (e.g., obesity), diet type, alcohol, coffee, and tobacco consumption, multidrug therapy, immune state (e.g., immunocompromised), and nutritional status (Ghabril et al., 2010; Fontana, 2014; Chen et al., 2015).

1.5.12. Epidemiology of Liver Abscess

The most relevant pathogens responsible for liver abscess (LA) are *E. coli*, *Klebsiella* spp., and *Enterococcus* spp. Among anaerobic bacteria, *Bacteroides* spp. and *Fusobacterium* spp. predominate (Rahimian et al., 2004; Romano et al., 2013). Aerobic, anaerobic, or microaerophilic streptococci are isolated in 25–

30% of cultures from LA; in a high proportion of cases polymicrobial bacterial infection is found, with a strong etiological shift toward *Klebsiella pneumoniae* (Wong et al., 2002; Siu et al., 2012). The incidence of LA is 8–15/100,000 inhabitants/year in the United States, accounting for over 80% of all LA cases; abscesses due to *Entamoeba histolytica* account for up to 10% of the cases and are more common in tropical areas and in tourists and in immigrants from developing countries, whereas abscesses due to fungi and other infectious agents are responsible for less than 10% of all LA cases (Rahimian et al., 2004).

Before the 1980s, E. coli was the most common bacterial pathogen that caused LA. During the past three decades; however, highly virulent strains of *K. pneumoniae* have emerged as a predominant cause of LA in Asian countries, especially Taiwan (Wong et al., 2002; Siu et al., 2012; Romano et al., 2013).

1.5.13. Risk Factors for LA

The peak incidence of LA is found in 50- to 65-year-old patients (Rahimian et al., 2004; Romano et al., 2013), whereas in children this is uncommon, the male-to-female ratio being approximately 1.5–2.5 (Liu et al., 2013). According to the literature, mortality ranges from 5% to 26% (Chung et al., 2007; Fung et al., 2012; Siu et al., 2012; Hennequin & Robin, 2016); however, owing to the improvement in diagnosis and treatment strategies, it has decreased in recent years and is now less than 10% (Lübbert et al., 2014; Romano et al., 2013).

The liver is an intricate organ made up of multiple cells that carry out a wide range of biochemical and molecular processes; because it is a portal for blood that comes from the intestines, it may increase the toxicity of substances that are consumed. Because of this, the liver can still regenerate after being injured, and this can result in both acute and chronic pathologies such as cirrhosis, cancer, fatty infiltration, necrosis, and cholestasis. Among the major risk factors for the development of liver damage are obesity, alcohol abuse, and hepatic viral infections. Major global causes of morbidity and mortality include diseases like liver cancer and hepatic cirrhosis. It is important to support efforts to develop novel therapeutic approaches to combat these significant causes of death, as projections show an increase in the prevalence of these liver diseases.

A Closer Look

Liver Function Tests

Liver function tests (LFTs) are a group of blood tests that provide crucial information about the state of a person's liver. They help diagnose and monitor liver disease or damage by measuring levels of proteins, liver enzymes, and bilirubin in the blood. The primary enzymes measured in LFTs include alanine aminotransferase (ALT) and aspartate aminotransferase (AST), which are released into the bloodstream when liver cells are damaged. Elevated levels of these enzymes typically indicate liver inflammation or injury, often seen in conditions such as hepatitis, cirrhosis, and liver toxicity from drugs or alcohol. Another key enzyme is alkaline phosphatase (ALP), which, when elevated, may suggest bile duct obstruction, liver cancer, or bone disease. Gamma-glutamyl transferase (GGT) is another enzyme measured, and high levels can indicate bile duct issues or alcohol-related liver disease. Bilirubin, a byproduct of red blood cell breakdown, is also measured in LFTs. High levels of bilirubin can lead to jaundice, a yellowing of the skin and eyes, and indicate possible liver dysfunction or bile duct problems. Additionally, LFTs measure albumin and total protein levels. Albumin is the main protein made by the liver, and low levels can suggest chronic liver disease or other conditions affecting protein synthesis. Total protein includes albumin and other proteins in the blood, and abnormal levels can signal liver or kidney disease.

By providing a comprehensive overview of liver health, LFTs help in diagnosing conditions like hepatitis, fatty liver disease, and alcoholic liver disease. They also monitor the progression of liver disease and the effectiveness of treatments. For example, in patients with chronic hepatitis B or C, regular LFTs can track liver inflammation and response to antiviral therapy. In patients taking medications that can affect the liver, such as statins or chemotherapy, LFTs are essential for the early detection of liver damage. Interpretation of LFT results requires understanding that levels can be influenced by factors such as age, sex, and other medical conditions. Therefore, abnormal results often lead to further testing, such as imaging studies or liver biopsy, to pinpoint the exact cause of liver dysfunction.

LFTs are a critical component of medical diagnostics, providing a non-invasive means to assess liver function and detect potential issues early. They are widely used not only in diagnosing liver diseases but also in pre-operative assessments and routine health check-ups to ensure overall well-being. Given the liver's vital roles in metabolism, detoxification, and synthesis of essential proteins, maintaining its health is crucial. Regular monitoring through LFTs, especially for individuals at higher risk of liver disease due to factors like alcohol use, obesity, or viral hepatitis, can lead to timely interventions and better health outcomes. Understanding LFT results and their implications allows healthcare providers to make informed decisions about further diagnostic procedures, treatments, and lifestyle modifications to protect and improve liver health.

Summary

- The liver is located in the upper right-hand portion of the abdominal cavity, beneath the diaphragm, and on top of the stomach, right kidney, and intestines.
- The liver regulates most chemical levels in the blood and excretes a product called bile. This helps carry away waste products from the liver. All the blood leaving the stomach and intestines passes through the liver.
- The liver is reddish-brown and shaped approximately like a cone or a wedge, with the small end above the spleen and stomach and the large end above the small intestine. The entire organ is located below the lungs in the right upper abdomen. It weighs between 3 and 3.5 pounds.
- Overall, NAFLD and ALD are emerging as important causes of CLD in the country paralleling the changes in lifestyle and social customs.
- Alcohol liver disease (ALD) is either alone or in association with other comorbidities such as obesity or viral hepatitis, the leading cause of liver disease. The liver is also the most common target organ of chronic alcohol abuse.
- Primary liver cancer is the fifth most common cancer worldwide and the second leading cause of cancer mortality. Hepatocellular carcinoma (HCC) is the most common histologic type of primary liver cancer and it accounts for between 85% and 90% of these malignancies.
- Hepatitis B still remains the major cause of CLD and liver cancer.
- The liver depicts a uniform anatomical structure composed of the regular arrangement of mainly hexagonal lobules in a honeycomb-like pattern. Blood from the portal triad enters the sinusoids, the smallest capillaries of the liver, where the blood drains into the central vein.
- The liver performs a wide variety of functions that are essential for the preservation of homeostasis in the organism.

References

1. Adams, L. A., Lymp, J. F., St Sauver, J., Sanderson, S. O., Lindor, K. D., Feldstein, A., et al. (2005). The natural history of nonalcoholic fatty liver disease: A population-based cohort study. *Gastroenterology, 129*(1), 113–121.
2. Ahima, R. S., & Lazar, M. A. (2013). Physiology. The health risk of obesity-better metrics imperative. *Science, 341*(6148), 856–858.
3. Ala, A., Stanca, C. M., Bu-Ghanim, M., Ahmado, I., Branch, A. D., Schiano, T. D., et al. (2006). Increased prevalence of primary biliary cirrhosis near Superfund toxic waste sites. *Hepatology, 43*(3), 525–531.
4. Alter, M. J., Kruszon-Moran, D., Nainan, O. V., McQuillan, G. M., Gao, F., Moyer, L. A., et al. (1999). The prevalence of hepatitis C virus infection in the United States, 1988 through 1994. *The New England Journal of Medicine, 341*(8), 556–562.
5. Andrade, R. J., Lucena, M. I., Fernández, M. C., Pelaez, G., Pachkoria, K., García-Ruiz, E., et al. (2005). Drug-induced liver injury: An analysis of 461 incidences submitted to the Spanish registry over a 10-year period. *Gastroenterology, 129*(2), 512–521.

6. Angulo, P. (2002). Nonalcoholic fatty liver disease. *The New England Journal of Medicine, 346*(16), 1221–1231.
7. Attner, B., Landin-Olsson, M., Lithman, T., Noreen, D., & Olsson, H. (2012). Cancer among patients with diabetes, obesity and abnormal blood lipids: A population-based register study in Sweden. *Cancer Causes & Control, 23*(5), 769–777.
8. Avila, M. A., & Moschetta, A. (2015). The FXR-FGF19 gut-liver axis as a novel "Hepatostat". *Gastroenterology, 149*(3), 537–540.
9. Baffy, G. (2009). Kupffer cells in non-alcoholic fatty liver disease: The emerging view. *Journal of Hepatology, 51*(1), 212–223.
10. Baldursdottir, T. R., Bergmann, O. M., Jonasson, J. G., Ludviksson, B. R., Axelsson, T. A., & Björnsson, E. S. (2012). The epidemiology and natural history of primary biliary cirrhosis: A nationwide population-based study. *European Journal of Gastroenterology & Hepatology, 24*(7), 824–830.
11. Bartl, M., Pfaff, M., Ghallab, A., Driesch, D., Henkel, S. G., & Hengstler, J. G., et al. (2015). Optimality in the zonation of ammonia detoxification in rodent liver. *Archives of Toxicology, 89*(11), 2069–2078.
12. Bedogni, G., Miglioli, L., Masutti, F., Castiglione, A., Crocè, L. S., Tiribelli, C., et al. (2007). Incidence and natural course of fatty liver in the general population: The Dionysos study. *Hepatology, 46*(5), 1387–1391.
13. Behari, J., Li, H., Liu, S., Stefanovic-Racic, M., Alonso, L., & O'Donnell, C. P., et al. (2014). β-catenin links hepatic metabolic zonation with lipid metabolism and diet-induced obesity in mice. *The American Journal of Pathology, 184*(11), 3284–3298.
14. Benhamouche, S., Decaens, T., Godard, C., Chambrey, R., Rickman, D. S., Moinard, C., et al. (2006). Apc tumor suppressor gene is the "zonation-keeper" of mouse liver. *Developmental Cell, 10*(6), 759–770.
15. Berasain, C., & Avila, M. A. (2015). Regulation of hepatocyte identity and quiescence. *Cellular and Molecular Life Sciences, 72*(20), 3831–3851.
16. Berasain, C., & Avila, M. A. (2016). Further evidence on the Janus-faced nature of the epidermal growth factor receptor: From liver regeneration to hepatocarcinogenesis. *Hepatology, 63*(1), 371–374.
17. Bilzer, M., Roggel, F., & Gerbes, A. L. (2006). Role of Kupffer cells in host defense and liver disease. *Liver International, 26*(10), 1175–1186.
18. Björnsson, E. S., Bergmann, O. M., Björnsson, H. K., Kvaran, R. B., & Olafsson, S. (2013). Incidence, presentation, and outcomes in patients with drug-induced liver injury in the general population of Iceland. *Gastroenterology, 144*(7), 1419–1425
19. Blachier, M., Leleu, H., Peck-Radosavljevic, M., Valla, D. C., & Roudot-Thoraval, F. (2013). The burden of liver disease in Europe: A review of available epidemiological data. *Journal of Hepatology, 58*(3), 593–608.
20. Boonstra, K., Beuers, U., & Ponsioen, C. Y. (2012). Epidemiology of primary sclerosing cholangitis and primary biliary cirrhosis: A systematic review. *Journal of Hepatology, 56*(5), 1181–1188.

21. Boonstra, K., Kunst, A. E., Stadhouders, P. H., Tuynman, H. A., Poen, A. C., van Nieuwkerk, K. M. J., et al. (2014). Rising incidence and prevalence of primary biliary cirrhosis: A large population-based study. *Liver International, 34*(1), 31–38.

22. Borro, P., Leone, S., & Testino, G. (2016). Liver disease and hepatocellular carcinoma in alcoholics: The role of anticraving therapy. *Current Drug Targets, 17*(2), 239–251.

23. Bower, W. A., Johns, M., Margolis, H. S., Williams, I. T., & Bell, B. P. (2007). Population-based surveillance for acute liver failure. *The American Journal of Gastroenterology, 102*(11), 2459–2463.

24. Braeuning, A., Ittrich, C., Köhle, C., Buchmann, A., & Schwarz, M. (2007). Zonal gene expression in mouse liver resembles expression patterns of Ha-ras and beta-catenin mutated hepatomas. *Drug Metabolism and Disposition, 35*(4), 503–507.

25. Bressac, B., Kew, M., Wands, J., & Ozturk, M. (1991). Selective G to T mutations of p53 gene in hepatocellular carcinoma from southern Africa. *Nature, 350*(6317), 429–431.

26. Browning, J. D., Szczepaniak, L. S., Dobbins, R., Nuremberg, P., Horton, J. D., Cohen, J. C., et al. (2004). Prevalence of hepatic steatosis in an urban population in the United States: Impact of ethnicity. *Hepatology, 40*(6), 1387–1395.

27. Burke, Z. D., Reed, K. R., Phesse, T. J., Sansom, O. J., Clarke, A. R., & Tosh, D. (2009). Liver zonation occurs through a beta-catenin-dependent, c-Myc-independent mechanism. *Gastroenterology, 136*(7), 2316–2324.

28. Calle, E. E., Rodriguez, C., Walker-Thurmond, K., & Thun, M. J. (2003). Overweight, obesity, and mortality from cancer in a prospectively studied cohort of U.S. adults. *The New England Journal of Medicine, 348*(17), 1625–1638.

29. Canbay, A., Taimr, P., Torok, N., Higuchi, H., Friedman, S., & Gores, G. J. (2003). Apoptotic body engulfment by a human stellate cell line is profibrogenic. *Laboratory Investigation, 83*(5), 655–663.

30. Carey, E. J., Ali, A. H., & Lindor, K. D. (2015). Primary biliary cirrhosis. *Lancet, 386*(10003), 1565–1575.

31. Cavard, C., Colnot, S., Audard, V., Benhamouche, S., Finzi, L., & Torre, C., et al. (2008). Wnt/beta-catenin pathway in hepatocellular carcinoma pathogenesis and liver physiology. *Future Oncology, 4*(5), 647–660.

32. Chalasani, N., Younossi, Z., Lavine, J. E., Diehl, A. M., Brunt, E. M., & Cusi, K., et al. (2012). The diagnosis and management of non-alcoholic fatty liver disease: Practice guideline by the American association for the study of liver diseases, American college of gastroenterology, and the American gastroenterological association. *Hepatology, 55*(6), 2005–2023.

33. Chen, C. J., Yang, H. I., Su, J., Jen, C. L., You, S. L., Lu, S. N., et al. (2006). Risk of hepatocellular carcinoma across a biological gradient of serum hepatitis B virus DNA level. *JAMA, 295*(1), 65–73.

34. Chen, M., Suzuki, A., Borlak, J., Andrade, R. J., & Lucena, M. I. (2015). Drug-induced liver injury: Interactions between drug properties and host factors. *Journal of Hepatology, 63*(2), 503–514.

35. Chisari, F. V. (2000). Rous-Whipple award lecture. Viruses, immunity, and cancer: Lessons from hepatitis B. *The American Journal of Pathology, 156*(4), 1117–1132.

36. Chung, D. R., Lee, S. S., Lee, H. R., Kim, H. B., Choi, H. J., Eom, J. S., et al. (2007). Emerging invasive liver abscess caused by K1 serotype Klebsiella pneumoniae in Korea. *Journal of Infection, 54*(6), 578–583.

37. Cochrane, J., Chen, H., Conigrave, K. M., & Hao, W. (2003). Alcohol use in China. *Alcohol and Alcoholism, 38*(6), 537–542.

38. Cortez-Pinto, H., Gouveia, M., dos Santos Pinheiro, L., Costa, J., Borges, M., & Vaz Carneiro, A. (2010). The burden of disease and the cost of illness attributable to alcohol drinking: Results of a national study. *Alcoholism: Clinical and Experimental Research, 34*(8), 1442–1449.

39. Dandri, M., Burda, M. R., Bürkle, A., Zuckerman, D. M., Will, H., Rogler, C. E., et al. (2002). Increase in de novo HBV DNA integrations in response to oxidative DNA damage or inhibition of poly (ADP-ribosyl) ation. *Hepatology, 35*(1), 217–223.

40. Dasgupta, T., Croll, D. H., Owen, J. A., Vander Heiden, M. G., Locasale, J. W., & Alon, U. (2014). A fundamental trade-off in covalent switching and its circumvention by enzyme bifunctionality in glucose homeostasis. *Journal of Biological Chemistry, 289*(19), 13010–13025.

41. Davis, G. L., Albright, J. E., Cook, S. F., & Rosenberg, D. M. (2003). Projecting future complications of chronic hepatitis C in the United States. *Liver Transplantation, 9*(4), 331–338.

42. Deleve, L. D., Wang, X., & Guo, Y. (2008). Sinusoidal endothelial cells prevent rat stellate cell activation and promote reversion to quiescence. *Hepatology, 48*(3), 920–930.

43. Dey, A., Allen, J., & Hankey-Giblin, P. A. (2014). Ontogeny and polarization of macrophages in inflammation: Blood monocytes versus tissue macrophages. *Frontiers in Immunology, 5*, 683.

44. Diesselhoff-Den Dulk, M. M., Crofton, R. W., & van Furth, R. (1979). Origin and kinetics of Kupffer cells during an acute inflammatory response. *Immunology, 37*(1), 7–14.

45. Ding, B. S., Cao, Z., Lis, R., Nolan, D. J., Guo, P., Simons, M., et al. (2014). Divergent angiocrine signals from vascular niche balance liver regeneration and fibrosis. *Nature, 505*(7481), 97–102.

46. Donato, F., Tagger, A., Gelatti, U., Parrinello, G., Boffetta, P., Albertini, A., et al. (2002). Alcohol and hepatocellular carcinoma: The effect of lifetime intake and hepatitis virus infections in men and women. *American Journal of Epidemiology, 155*(4), 323–331.

47. Duffield, J. S., Forbes, S. J., Constandinou, C. M., Clay, S., Partolina, M., Vuthoori, S., et al. (2005). Selective depletion of macrophages reveals distinct, opposing roles during liver injury and repair. *Journal of Clinical Investigation, 115*(1), 56–65.

48. El-Serag, H. B. (2007). Epidemiology of hepatocellular carcinoma in USA. *Hepatology Research, 37*(Suppl. 2), S88–S94.

49. Ferber, M. J., Montoya, D. P., Yu, C., Aderca, I., McGee, A., Thorland, E. C., et al. (2003). Integrations of the hepatitis B virus (HBV) and human papillomavirus (HPV) into the human telomerase reverse transcriptase (hTERT) gene in liver and cervical cancers. *Oncogene, 22*(24), 3813–3820.

50. Ferlay, J., Shin, H. R., Bray, F., Forman, D., Mathers, C., & Parkin, D. M. (2010). Estimates of worldwide burden of cancer in 2008: GLOBOCAN 2008. *International Journal of Cancer, 127*(12), 2893–2917.

51. Fischer, G. E., Bialek, S. P., Homan, C. E., Livingston, S. E., & McMahon, B. J. (2009). Chronic liver disease among Alaska-Native people, 2003–2004. *The American Journal of Gastroenterology, 104*(2), 363–370.

52. Fontana, R. J. (2014). Pathogenesis of idiosyncratic drug-induced liver injury and clinical perspectives. *Gastroenterology, 146*(4), 914–928.

53. Fraser, R., Bosanquet, A. G., & Day, W. A. (1978). Filtration of chylomicrons by the liver may influence cholesterol metabolism and atherosclerosis. *Atherosclerosis, 29*(2), 113–123.

54. Fung, C. P., Lin, Y. T., Lin, J. C., Chen, T. L., Yeh, K. M., Chang, F. Y., et al. (2012). Klebsiella pneumoniae in gastrointestinal tract and pyogenic liver abscess. *Emerging Infectious Diseases, 18*(9), 1322–1325.

55. Ganesan, L. P., Mohanty, S., Kim, J., Clark, K. R., Robinson, J. M., & Anderson, C. L. (2011). Rapid and efficient clearance of blood-borne virus by liver sinusoidal endothelium. *PLoS Pathogens, 7*(9), e1002281.

56. Gebhardt, R., & Hovhannisyan, A. (2010). Organ patterning in the adult stage: The role of Wnt/beta-catenin signaling in liver zonation and beyond. *Developmental Dynamics, 239*(1), 45–55.

57. Gebhardt, R., & Matz-Soja, M. (2014). Liver zonation: Novel aspects of its regulation and its impact on homeostasis. *World Journal of Gastroenterology, 20*(26), 8491–8504.

58. Gebhardt, R., Baldysiak-Figiel, A., Krügel, V., Ueberham, E., & Gaunitz, F. (2007). Hepatocellular expression of glutamine synthetase: An indicator of morphogen actions as master regulators of zonation in adult liver. *Progress in Histochemistry and Cytochemistry, 41*(4), 201–266.

59. Ghabril, M., Chalasani, N., & Björnsson, E. (2010). Drug-induced liver injury: A clinical update. *Current Opinion in Gastroenterology, 26*(3), 222–226.

60. Glisson, F. (1654). *Anatomia hepatis*. Typis Du-Gardianis, London.

61. Gomez Perdiguero, E., Klapproth, K., Schulz, C., Busch, K., Azzoni, E., Crozet, L., et al. (2015). Tissue-resident macrophages originate from yolk-sac-derived erythro-myeloid progenitors. *Nature, 518*(7540), 547–551.

62. Gregory, S. H., & Wing, E. J. (2002). Neutrophil-Kupffer cell interaction: A critical component of host defenses to systemic bacterial infections. *Journal of Leukocyte Biology, 72*(2), 239–248.

63. Grewal, P., & Viswanathen, V. A. (2012). Liver cancer and alcohol. *Clinics in Liver Disease, 16*(4), 839–850.

64. Guardavaccaro, D., & Clevers, H. (2012). Wnt/β-catenin and MAPK signaling: Allies and enemies in different battlefields. *Science Signaling, 5*(233), pe15.

65. Hailfinger, S., Jaworski, M., Braeuning, A., Buchmann, A., & Schwarz, M. (2006). Zonal gene expression in murine liver: Lessons from tumors. *Hepatology, 43*(2), 407–414.

66. Hamaguchi, M., Kojima, T., Takeda, N., Nakagawa, T., Taniguchi, H., Fujii, K., et al. (2005). The metabolic syndrome as a predictor of nonalcoholic fatty liver disease. *Annals of Internal Medicine, 143*(10), 722–728.

67. Hamlyn, A. N., Macklon, A. F., & James, O. (1983). Primary biliary cirrhosis: Geographical clustering and symptomatic onset seasonality. *Gut, 24*(10), 940–945.

68. Heckley, G. A., Jarl, J., Asamoah, B. O., & Gerdtham, U. G. (2011). How the risk of liver cancer changes after alcohol cessation: A review and meta-analysis of the current literature. *BMC Cancer, 11*, 446.

69. Hellerbrand, C., Jobin, C., Licato, L. L., Sartor, R. B., & Brenner, D. A. (1998). Cytokines induce NF-κB in activated but not in quiescent rat hepatic stellate cells. *American Journal of Physiology-Gastrointestinal and Liver Physiology, 275*(2), G269–G278.
70. Hennequin, C., & Robin, F. (2016). Correlation between antimicrobial resistance and virulence in Klebsiella pneumoniae. *European Journal of Clinical Microbiology & Infectious Diseases, 35*(3), 333–341.
71. Hijmans, B. S., Grefhorst, A., Oosterveer, M. H., & Groen, A. K. (2014). Zonation of glucose and fatty acid metabolism in the liver: Mechanism and metabolic consequences. *Biochimie, 96*, 121–129.
72. Hoofnagle, J. H. (2004). Drug-induced liver injury network (DILIN). *Hepatology, 40*(4), 773.
73. Hsu, I. C., Metcalf, R. A., Sun, T., Welsh, J. A., Wang, N. J., & Harris, C. C. (1991). Mutational hotspot in the p53 gene in human hepatocellular carcinomas. *Nature, 350*(6317), 427–428.
74. Huch, M., & Dollé, L. (2016). The plastic cellular states of liver cells: Are EpCAM and Lgr5 fit for purpose? *Hepatology*. https://doi.org/10.1002/hep.28469.
75. International Agency for Research on Cancer Working Group (IARC). (1988). Alcohol drinking, Lyon.
76. Iwakiri, Y. (2015). Nitric oxide in liver fibrosis: The role of inducible nitric oxide synthase. *Clinical and Molecular Hepatology, 21*(4), 319–325.
77. Iwakiri, Y., & Kim, M. Y. (2015). Nitric oxide in liver diseases. *Trends in Pharmacological Sciences, 36*(8), 524–536.
78. Jager, J., Aparicio-Vergara, M., & Aouadi, M. (2016). Liver innate immune cells and insulin resistance: The multiple facets of Kupffer cells. *Journal of Internal Medicine*. https://doi.org/10.1111/joim.12483.
79. Jee, S. H., Ohrr, H., Sull, J. W., & Samet, J. M. (2004). Cigarette smoking, alcohol drinking, hepatitis B, and risk for hepatocellular carcinoma in Korea. *Journal of the National Cancer Institute, 96*(24), 1851–1856.
80. Jin, Y., Bai, Y., Ni, H., Qiang, L., Ye, L., Shan, Y., et al. (2016). Activation of autophagy through calcium-dependent AMPK/mTOR and PKCθ pathway causes activation of rat hepatic stellate cells under hypoxic stress. *FEBS Letters, 590*(4), 672–682.
81. Jinushi, M., Takehara, T., Tatsumi, T., Kanto, T., Groh, V., Spies, T., et al. (2003). Expression and role of MICA and MICB in human hepatocellular carcinomas and their regulation by retinoic acid. *International Journal of Cancer, 104*(3), 354–361.
82. Kiernan, F. (1833). The anatomy and physiology of the liver. *Philosophical Transactions of the Royal Society of London, 123*, 711–770.
83. Kim, K. A. (2009). Current status of liver diseases in Korea: Toxic and alcoholic liver diseases. *Korean Journal of Hepatology, 15*(Suppl 6), S29–S33.
84. Kolios, G., Valatas, V., & Kouroumalis, E. (2006). Role of Kupffer cells in the pathogenesis of liver disease. *World Journal of Gastroenterology, 12*(46), 7413–7420
85. Kuntz, E., & Kuntz, H. D. (2006). History of Hepatology. In *Hepatology, Principles and Practice. History, Morphology, Biochemistry, Diagnostics, Clinic, Therapy* (2nd ed., pp. 1–13). Springer Verlag Berlin Heidelberg.

86. Lafaro, K. J., Demirjian, A. N., & Pawlik, T. M. (2015). Epidemiology of hepatocellular carcinoma. *Surgical Oncology Clinics of North America, 24*(1), 1–17.

87. Lamers, W. H., Hilberts, A., Furt, E., Smith, J., Jonges, G. N., & van Noorden, C. J. (1989). Hepatic enzymic zonation: A reevaluation of the concept of the liver acinus. *Hepatology, 10*(1), 72–76.

88. Lauth, M. (2011). RAS and Hedgehog: Partners in crime. *Frontiers in Bioscience, 16*, 2259–2270.

89. Le Couteur, D. G., Fraser, R., Cogger, V. C., & McLean, A. J. (2002). Hepatic pseudocapillarisation and atherosclerosis in ageing. *Lancet, 359*(9312), 1612–1615.

90. Lee, J., Conniff, J., Kraus, C., & Schrager, S. (2015). A brief clinical update on hepatitis C: The essentials. *WMJ, 114*(6), 263–269.

91. Licata, A. (2016). Adverse drug reactions and organ damage: The liver. *European Journal of Internal Medicine, 28*, 9–16.

92. Liu, Y., & Wu, F. (2010). Global burden of aflatoxin-induced hepatocellular carcinoma: A risk assessment. *Environmental Health Perspectives, 118*(6), 818–824.

93. Liu, Y., Wang, J. Y., & Jiang, W. (2013). An increasing prominent disease of Klebsiella pneumoniae liver abscess: Etiology, diagnosis, and treatment. *Gastroenterology Research and Practice, 2013*, 258514.

94. Lozano, R., Naghavi, M., Foreman, K., Lim, S., Shibuya, K., Aboyans, V., et al. (2012). Global and regional mortality from 235 causes of death for 20 age groups in 1990 and 2010: A systematic analysis for the Global Burden of Disease Study 2010. *Lancet, 380*(9859), 2095–2128.

95. Lübbert, C., Wiegand, J., & Karlas, T. (2014). Therapy of liver abscesses. *Viszeralmedizin, 30*(5), 334–341.

96. Maher, J. J. (2002). Alcoholic liver disease. In M. Feldman, L. S. Friedman, & M. H. Sleisenger (Eds.), *Gastrointestinal and Liver Disease* (Vol. II, pp. 1375–1391). Saunders.

97. Maronpot, R. R., Yoshizawa, K., Nyska, A., Harada, T., Flake, G., Mueller, G., et al. (2010). Hepatic enzyme induction: Histopathology. *Toxicologic Pathology, 38*(5), 776–795.

98. Marrero, J. A., Fontana, R. J., Fu, S., Conjeevaram, H. S., Su, G. L., & Lok, A. S. (2005). Alcohol, tobacco and obesity are synergistic risk factors for hepatocellular carcinoma. *Journal of Hepatology, 42*(2), 218–224.

99. Masarone, M., Federico, A., Abenavoli, L., Loguercio, C., & Persico, M. (2014). Non-alcoholic fatty liver: Epidemiology and natural history. *Reviews on Recent Clinical Trials, 9*(3), 126–133.

100. Maslak, E., Gregorius, A., & Chlopicki, S. (2015). Liver sinusoidal endothelial cells (LSECs) function and NAFLD; NO-based therapy targeted to the liver. *Pharmacological Reports, 67*(4), 689–694.

101. Matteoni, C. A., Younossi, Z. M., Gramlich, T., Boparai, N., Liu, Y. C., & McCullough, A. J. (1999). Nonalcoholic fatty liver disease: A spectrum of clinical and pathological severity. *Gastroenterology, 116*(6), 1413–1419.

102. Matz-Soja, M., Aleithe, S., Marbach, E., Böttger, J., Arnold, K., Schmidt-Heck, W., et al. (2014). Hepatic Hedgehog signaling contributes to the regulation of IGF1 and IGFBP1 serum levels. *Cell Communication and Signaling, 12*, 11.

103. Matz-Soja, M., Hovhannisyan, A., & Gebhardt, R. (2013). Hedgehog signaling pathway in adult liver: A major new player in hepatocyte metabolism and zonation? *Medical Hypotheses, 80*(4), 589–594.

104. McCullough, A. J., & O'Connor, J. F. (1998). Alcoholic liver disease: Proposed recommendations for the American College of Gastroenterology. *American Journal of Gastroenterology, 93*(12), 2022–2036.

105. McGlynn, K. A., & London, W. T. (2011). The global epidemiology of hepatocellular carcinoma: Present and future. *Clinical Liver Disease, 15*(2), 223–243.

106. McNally, R. J. Q., James, P. W., Ducker, S., Norman, P. D., & James, O. F. W. (2014). No rise in incidence but geographical heterogeneity in the occurrence of primary biliary cirrhosis in North East England. *American Journal of Epidemiology, 179*(4), 492–498.

107. Mederacke, I., Hsu, C. C., Troeger, J. S., Huebener, P., Mu, X., Dapito, D. H., et al. (2013). Fate tracing reveals hepatic stellate cells as dominant contributors to liver fibrosis independent of its aetiology. *Nature Communications, 4*, 2823.

108. Metcalf, J. V., Bhopal, R. S., Gray, J., Howel, D., & James, O. F. (1997). Incidence and prevalence of primary biliary cirrhosis in the city of Newcastle upon Tyne, England. *International Journal of Epidemiology, 26*(4), 830–836.

109. Michalopoulos, G. K. (2013). Principles of liver regeneration and growth homeostasis. *Comprehensive Physiology, 3*(1), 485–513.

110. Mizoue, T., Tokui, N., Nishisaka, K., Nishisaka, S., Ogimoto, I., Ikeda, M., et al. (2000). Prospective study on the relation of cigarette smoking with cancer of the liver and stomach in an endemic region. *International Journal of Epidemiology, 29*(2), 232–237.

111. Mohanty, S. R., Troy, T. N., Huo, D., O'Brien, B. L., Jensen, D. M., & Hart, J. (2009). Influence of ethnicity on histological differences in nonalcoholic fatty liver disease. *Journal of Hepatology, 50*(4), 797–804.

112. Monga, S. P. (2015). β-Catenin signaling and roles in liver homeostasis, injury, and tumorigenesis. *Gastroenterology, 148*(5), 1294–1310.

113. Montesano, R., Matsumoto, K., Nakamura, T., & Orci, L. (1991). Identification of a fibroblast-derived epithelial morphogen as hepatocyte growth factor. *Cell, 67*(5), 901–908.

114. Morgan, R. L., Baack, B., Smith, B. D., Yartel, A., Pitasi, M., & Falck-Ytter, Y. (2013). Eradication of hepatitis C virus infection and the development of hepatocellular carcinoma: A meta-analysis of observational studies. *Annals of Internal Medicine, 153*(5), 329–337.

115. Mueller, S., Seitz, H. K., & Rausch, V. (2014). Non-invasive diagnosis of alcoholic liver disease. *World Journal of Gastroenterology, 20*(39), 14626–14641.

116. Nakagawa, R., Nagafune, I., Tazunoki, Y., Ehara, H., Tomura, H., Iijima, R., et al. (2001). Mechanisms of the antimetastatic effect in the liver and of the hepatocyte injury induced by α-galactosylceramide in mice. *Journal of Immunology, 166*(11), 6578–6584.

117. Nakatani, K., Kaneda, K., Seki, S., & Nakajima, Y. (2004). Pit cells as liver-associated natural killer cells: Morphology and function. *Medical Electron Microscopy, 37*(1), 29–36.

118. Neuschwander-Tetri, B. A., & Caldwell, S. H. (2003). Nonalcoholic steatohepatitis: Summary of an AASLD single topic conference. *Hepatology, 37*(6), 1202–1219.

119. Nishikawa, H., & Osaki, Y. (2013). Non-B, non-C hepatocellular carcinoma (Review). *International Journal of Oncology, 43*(5), 1333–1342.

120. Odegaard, J. I., & Chawla, A. (2011). Alternative macrophage activation and metabolism. *Annual Review of Pathology, 6*, 275–297.

121. Ostapowicz, G., Fontana, R. J., Schiødt, F. V., Larson, A., Davern, T. J., Han, S. H. B., et al. (2002). Results of a prospective study of acute liver failure at 17 tertiary care centers in the United States. *Annals of Internal Medicine, 137*(12), 947–954.

122. Ozturk, M. (1991). p53 mutation in hepatocellular carcinoma after aflatoxin exposure. *Lancet, 338*(8775), 1356–1359.

123. Park, S. H., Kim, C. H., Kim, D. J., Park, J. H., Kim, T. O., Yang, S. Y., et al. (2011). Prevalence of alcoholic liver disease among Korean adults: Results from the fourth Korea national health and nutrition examination survey, 2009. *Substance Use & Misuse, 46*(14), 1755–1762.

124. Paschos, K. A., Majeed, A. W., & Bird, N. C. (2014). Natural history of hepatic metastases from colorectal cancer: Epathobiological pathways with clinical significance. *World Journal of Gastroenterology, 20*(13), 3719–3737.

125. Perlemuter, G., Lettéron, P., Carnot, F., Zavala, F., Pessayre, D., Nalpas, B., et al. (2003). Alcohol and hepatitis C virus core protein additively increase lipid peroxidation and synergistically trigger hepatic cytokine expression in a transgenic mouse model. *Journal of Hepatology, 39*(6), 1020–1027.

126. Platt, L., Easterbrook, P., Gower, E., McDonald, B., Sabin, K., McGowan, C., et al. (2016). Prevalence and burden of HCV co-infection in people living with HIV: A global systematic review and meta-analysis. *The Lancet Infectious Diseases*. https://doi.org/10.1016/S1473-3099(15)00485-5.

127. Pradere, J. P., Kluwe, J., De Minicis, S., Jiao, J. J., Gwak, G. Y., Dapito, D. H., et al. (2013). Hepatic macrophages but not dendritic cells contribute to liver fibrosis by promoting the survival of activated hepatic stellate cells in mice. *Hepatology, 58*(4), 1461–1473.

128. Qvartskhava, N., Lang, P. A., Görg, B., Pozdeev, V. I., Ortiz, M. P., Lang, K. S., et al. (2015). Hyperammonemia in gene-targeted mice lacking functional hepatic glutamine synthetase. *Proceedings of the National Academy of Sciences of the United States of America, 112*(18), 5521–5526.

129. Radaeva, S., Sun, R., Jaruga, B., Nguyen, V. T., Tian, Z., & Gao, B. (2006). Natural killer cells ameliorate liver fibrosis by killing activated stellate cells in NKG2D-dependent and tumor necrosis factor-related apoptosis-inducing ligand-dependent manners. *Gastroenterology, 130*(2), 435–452.

130. Rahimian, J., Wilson, T., Oram, V., & Holzman, R. S. (2004). Pyogenic liver abscess: Recent trends in etiology and mortality. *Clinical Infectious Diseases, 39*(11), 1654–1659.

131. Raynard, B., Balian, A., Fallik, D., Capron, F., Bedossa, P., Chaput, J. C., et al. (2002). Risk factors of fibrosis in alcohol-induced liver disease. *Hepatology, 35*(3), 635–638.

132. Reed, K. R., Athineos, D., Meniel, V. S., Wilkins, J. A., Ridgway, R. A., Burke, Z. D., et al. (2008). β-Catenin deficiency, but not Myc deletion, suppresses the immediate phenotypes of APC loss in the liver. *Proceedings of the National Academy of Sciences of the United States of America, 105*(48), 18919–18923.

133. Rein, D. B., Wittenborn, J. S., Weinbaum, C. M., Sabin, M., Smith, B. D., & Lesesne, S. B. (2011). Forecasting the morbidity and mortality associated with prevalent cases of pre-cirrhotic chronic hepatitis C in the United States. *Digestive and Liver Disease, 43*(1), 66–72.
134. Rinella, M. E., & Sanyal, A. J. (2016). Management of NAFLD: A stage-based approach. *Nature Reviews Gastroenterology & Hepatology, 13*(4), 196–205.
135. Rojkind, M., & Greenwel, P. (1988). The liver as a bioecological system. In I. M. Arias, W. B. Jacoby, H. Popper, D. Schachter, & D. A. Shafritz (Eds.), *The Liver Biology and Pathobiology* (2nd ed., pp. 1269–1285). Raven Press.
136. Romano, G., Agrusa, A., Frazzetta, G., De Vita, G., Chianetta, D., Di Buono, G., et al. (2013). Laparoscopic drainage of liver abscess: Case report and literature review. *Giornale di Chirurgia, 34*(4), 180–182.
137. Saab, S., Manne, V., Nieto, J., Schwimmer, J. B., & Chalasani, N. P. (2016). Nonalcoholic fatty liver disease in Latinos. *Clinical Gastroenterology and Hepatology, 14*(1), 5–12.
138. Safdar, K., & Schiff, E. R. (2004). Alcohol and hepatitis C. *Seminars in Liver Disease, 24*(3), 305–315.
139. Sasamoto, T., Sano, N., & Takikawa, H. (2006). Biliary excretion of sulfated bile acids and organic anions in zone 1- and zone 3-injured rats. *Journal of Gastroenterology and Hepatology, 21*(1), 26–31.
140. Satapathy, S. K., & Sanyal, A. J. (2015). Epidemiology and natural history of nonalcoholic fatty liver disease. *Seminars in Liver Disease, 35*(3), 221–235.
141. Schleicher, J., Tokarski, C., Marbach, E., Matz-Soja, M., Zellmer, S., Gebhardt, R., et al. (2015). Zonation of hepatic fatty acid metabolism: The diversity of its regulation and the benefit of modeling. *Biochimica et Biophysica Acta, 1851*(5), 641–656.
142. Schulz, C., Gomez Perdiguero, E., Chorro, L., Szabo-Rogers, H., Cagnard, N., Kierdorf, K., et al. (2012). A lineage of myeloid cells independent of Myb and hematopoietic stem cells. *Science, 336*(6089), 86–90.
143. Seki, E., & Schwabe, R. F. (2015). Hepatic inflammation and fibrosis: Functional links and key pathways. *Hepatology, 61*(3), 1066–1079.
144. Seki, E., De Minicis, S., Osterreicher, C. H., Kluwe, J., Osawa, Y., Brenner, D. A., et al. (2007). TLR4 enhances TGF-β signaling and hepatic fibrosis. *Nature Medicine, 13*(11), 1324–1332.
145. Sekine, S., Lan, B. Y. A., Bedolli, M., Feng, S., & Hebrok, M. (2006). Liver-specific loss of β-catenin blocks glutamine synthesis pathway activity and cytochrome P450 expression in mice. *Hepatology, 43*(4), 817–825.
146. Seternes, T., Sørensen, K., & Smedsrød, B. (2002). Scavenger endothelial cells of vertebrates: A nonperipheral leukocyte system for high-capacity elimination of waste macromolecules. *Proceedings of the National Academy of Sciences of the United States of America, 99*(12), 7594–7597.
147. Sgro, C., Clinard, F., Ouazir, K., Chanay, H., Allard, C., Guilleminet, C., et al. (2002). Incidence of drug-induced hepatic injuries: A French population-based study. *Hepatology, 36*(2), 451–455.
148. Shimizu, M., Tanaka, T., & Moriwaki, H. (2013). Obesity and hepatocellular carcinoma: Targeting obesity-related inflammation for chemoprevention of liver carcinogenesis. *Seminars in Immunopathology, 35*(2), 191–202.

149. Shiue, S. C., Huang, M. Z., & Su, T. S. (2014). A transgenic approach to study arginosuccinate synthetase gene expression. *Journal of Biomedical Science, 21*(1), 42.

150. Simon-Santamaria, J., Rinaldo, C. H., Kardas, P., Li, R., Malovic, I., Elvevold, K., et al. (2014). Efficient uptake of blood-borne BK and JC polyomavirus-like particles in endothelial cells of liver sinusoids and renal vasa recta. *PLoS One, 9*(7), e111762.

151. Singal, A. G., Volk, M. L., Jensen, D., Di Bisceglie, A. M., & Schoenfeld, P. S. (2010). A sustained viral response is associated with reduced liver-related morbidity and mortality in patients with hepatitis C virus. *Clinical Gastroenterology and Hepatology, 8*(3), 280–288.

152. Siu, L. K., Yeh, K. M., Lin, J. C., Fung, C. P., & Chang, F. Y. (2012). Klebsiella pneumoniae liver abscess: A new invasive syndrome. *The Lancet Infectious Diseases, 12*(12), 881–887.

153. Smith, B. D., Morgan, R. L., Beckett, G. A., Falck-Ytter, Y., Holtzman, D., Teo, C. G., et al. (2012). Recommendations for the identification of chronic hepatitis C virus infection among persons born during 1945–1965. *MMWR Recommendations and Reports, 61*(4), 1–32.

154. Sørensen, K. K., McCourt, P., Berg, T., Crossley, C., Le Couteur, D., Wake, K., et al. (2012). The scavenger endothelial cell: A new player in homeostasis and immunity. *American Journal of Physiology-Regulatory, Integrative and Comparative Physiology, 303*(10), R1217–R1230.

155. Stickel, F. (2015). Alcoholic cirrhosis and hepatocellular carcinoma. *Advances in Experimental Medicine and Biology, 815*, 113–130.

156. Su, Y. L., Woodman, R. J., Silva, M. F., Muller, K., Libby, J., Chen, J. W., et al. (2016). Good outcomes of liver transplantation for hepatitis C at a low volume center. *Annals of Hepatology, 15*(2), 207–214.

157. Sun, C. A., Wu, D. M., Lin, C. C., Lu, S. N., You, S. L., Wang, L. Y., et al. (2003). Incidence and cofactors of hepatitis C virus-related hepatocellular carcinoma: A prospective study of 12,008 men in Taiwan. *American Journal of Epidemiology, 157*(7), 674–682.

158. Suzuki, A., Angulo, P., Lymp, J., St Sauver, J., Muto, A., Okada, T., et al. (2005). Chronological development of elevated aminotransferases in a nonalcoholic population. *Hepatology, 41*(1), 64–71.

159. Svistounov, D., Warren, A., McNerney, G. P., Owen, D. M., Zencak, D., Zykova, S. N., et al. (2012). The relationship between fenestrations, sieve plates and rafts in liver sinusoidal endothelial cells. *PLoS One, 7*(12), e46134.

160. Swirski, F. K., Libby, P., Aikawa, E., Alcaide, P., Luscinskas, F. W., Weissleder, R., et al. (2007). Ly-6Chi monocytes dominate hypercholesterolemia-associated monocytosis and give rise to macrophages in atheromata. *Journal of Clinical Investigation, 117*(1), 195–205.

161. Syal, G., Fausther, M., & Dranoff, J. A. (2012). Advances in cholangiocyte immunobiology. *American Journal of Physiology-Gastrointestinal and Liver Physiology, 303*(9), G1077–G1086.

162. Tabata, T., & Takei, Y. (2004). Morphogens, their identification and regulation. *Development, 131*(4), 703–712.

163. Tabor, E. (2001). Hepatocellular carcinoma: Global epidemiology. *Digestive and Liver Disease, 33*(2), 115–117.

164. Takikawa, H., Murata, Y., Horiike, N., Fukui, H., & Onji, M. (2009). Drug-induced liver injury in Japan: An analysis of 1676 cases between 1997 and 2006. *Hepatology Research, 39*(5), 427–431.

165. Talwalkar, J. A., & Lindor, K. D. (2003). Primary biliary cirrhosis. *The Lancet, 362*(9382), 53–61.
166. Testino, G. (2013). Alcoholic hepatitis. *Journal of Medical Life, 6*(2), 161–167.
167. Testino, G., Leone, S., & Borro, P. (2014). Alcohol and hepatocellular carcinoma: A review and a point of view. *World Journal of Gastroenterology, 20*(43), 15943–15954.
168. Tokushige, K., Hashimoto, E., Horie, Y., Taniai, M., & Higuchi, S. (2011). Hepatocellular carcinoma in Japanese patients with nonalcoholic fatty liver disease, alcoholic liver disease, and chronic liver disease of unknown etiology: Report of the nationwide survey. *Journal of Gastroenterology, 46*(10), 1230–1237.
169. Torre, C., Perret, C., & Colnot, S. (2010). Molecular determinants of liver zonation. *Progress in Molecular Biology and Translational Science, 97*, 127–150.
170. Torre, C., Perret, C., & Colnot, S. (2011). Transcription dynamics in a physiological process: β-catenin signaling directs liver metabolic zonation. *International Journal of Biochemistry & Cell Biology, 43*(2), 271–278.
171. Torres, D. M., & Harrison, S. A. (2012). Nonalcoholic steatohepatitis and noncirrhotic hepatocellular carcinoma: Fertile soil. *Seminars in Liver Disease, 32*(1), 30–38.
172. Treyer, A., & Müsch, A. (2013). Hepatocyte polarity. *Comprehensive Physiology, 3*(1), 243–287.
173. Umer, M., & Iqbal, M. (2016). Hepatitis C virus prevalence and genotype distribution in Pakistan: Comprehensive review of recent data. *World Journal of Gastroenterology, 22*(5), 1684–1700.
174. Vasilj, A., Gentzel, M., Ueberham, E., Gebhardt, R., & Shevchenko, A. (2012). Tissue proteomics by one-dimensional gel electrophoresis combined with label-free protein quantification. *Journal of Proteome Research, 11*(7), 3680–3689.
175. Vernon, G., Baranova, A., & Younossi, Z. M. (2011). Systematic review: The epidemiology and natural history of non-alcoholic fatty liver disease and non-alcoholic steatohepatitis in adults. *Alimentary Pharmacology & Therapeutics, 34*(3), 274–285.
176. Weiß, J., Rau, M., & Geier, A. (2014). Non-alcoholic fatty liver disease: Epidemiology, clinical course, investigation, and treatment. *Deutsches Ärzteblatt International, 111*(26), 447–452.
177. Whalley, S., Puvanachandra, P., Desai, A., & Kennedy, H. (2007). Hepatology outpatient service provision in secondary care: A study of liver disease incidence and resource costs. *Clinical Medicine, 7*(2), 119–124. *WHO* (2015). Retrieved from: http://www.who.org (accessed on 5 August 2024).
178. Williams, C. D., Stengel, J., Asike, M. I., Torres, D. M., Shaw, J., Contreras, M., et al. (2011). Prevalence of nonalcoholic fatty liver disease and nonalcoholic steatohepatitis among a largely middle-aged population utilizing ultrasound and liver biopsy: A prospective study. *Gastroenterology, 140*(1), 124–131.
179. Wisse, E. (1972). An ultrastructural characterization of the endothelial cell in the rat liver sinusoid under normal and various experimental conditions, as a contribution to the distinction between endothelial and Kupffer cells. *Journal of Ultrastructure Research, 38*(4), 528–562.
180. Wolk, A., Gridley, G., Svensson, M., Nyrén, O., McLaughlin, J. K., Fraumeni, J. F., et al. (2001). A prospective study of obesity and cancer risk (Sweden). *Cancer Causes & Control, 12*(1), 13–21.

181. Wong, J. B., McQuillan, G. M., McHutchison, J. G., & Poynard, T. (2000). Estimating future hepatitis C morbidity, mortality, and costs in the United States. *American Journal of Public Health, 90*(10), 1562–1569.

182. Wong, W. M., Wong, B. C. Y., Hui, C. K., Ng, M., Lai, K. C., Tso, W. K., et al. (2002). Pyogenic liver abscess: Retrospective analysis of 80 cases over a 10-year period. *Journal of Gastroenterology and Hepatology, 17*(10), 1001–1007.

183. Wu, B. K., Li, C. C., Chen, H. J., Chang, J. L., Jeng, K. S., & Chou, C. K., et al. (2006). Blocking of G1/S transition and cell death in the regenerating liver of hepatitis B virus X protein transgenic mice. *Biochemical and Biophysical Research Communications, 340*(4), 916–928.

184. Yang, H. I., Lu, S. N., Liaw, Y. F., You, S. L., Sun, C. A., Wang, L. Y., et al. (2002). Hepatitis B e antigen and the risk of hepatocellular carcinoma. *New England Journal of Medicine, 347*(3), 168–174.

185. Yona, S., Kim, K. W., Wolf, Y., Mildner, A., Varol, D., Breker, M., et al. (2013). Fate mapping reveals origins and dynamics of monocytes and tissue macrophages under homeostasis. *Immunity, 38*(1), 79–91.

186. Yoneda, A., Sakai-Sawada, K., Niitsu, Y., & Tamura, Y. (2016). Vitamin A and insulin are required for the maintenance of hepatic stellate cell quiescence. *Experimental Cell Research, 341*(1), 8–17.

187. Yoshizawa, H. (2002). Hepatocellular carcinoma associated with hepatitis C virus infection in Japan: Projection to other countries in the foreseeable future. *Oncology, 62*(Suppl. 1), 8–17.

188. Younossi, Z. M., Stepanova, M., Afendy, M., Fang, Y., Younossi, Y., Mir, H., et al. (2011). Changes in the prevalence of the most common causes of chronic liver diseases in the United States from 1988 to 2008. *Clinical Gastroenterology and Hepatology, 9*(6), 524–530.

189. Yuan, J. M., Govindarajan, S., Arakawa, K., & Yu, M. C. (2004). Synergism of alcohol, diabetes, and viral hepatitis on the risk of hepatocellular carcinoma in blacks and whites in the US. *Cancer, 101*(5), 1009–1017.

190. Yuen, M. F., Tanaka, Y., Fong, D. Y. T., Fung, J., Wong, D. K. H., Yuen, J. C. H., et al. (2009). Independent risk factors and predictive score for the development of hepatocellular carcinoma in chronic hepatitis B. *Journal of Hepatology, 50*(1), 80–88.

191. Yun, Y. H., Jung, K. W., Bae, J. M., Lee, J. S., Shin, S. A., Min Park, S., et al. (2005). Cigarette smoking and cancer incidence risk in adult men: National Health Insurance Corporation Study. *Cancer Detection and Prevention, 29*(1), 15–24.

192. Zeller, E., Hammer, K., Kirschnick, M., & Braeuning, A. (2013). Mechanisms of RAS/β-catenin interactions. *Archives of Toxicology, 87*(4), 611–632.

193. Zhang, X., Zhang, J., Jia, L., & Xiao, S. (2016). Dicliptera chinensis polysaccharides target TGF-β/Smad pathway and inhibit stellate cells activation in rats with dimethyl nitrosamine-induced hepatic fibrosis. *Cellular and Molecular Biology, 62*(2), 99–103.

194. Zhu, H., Jia, Z., Misra, H., & Li, Y. R. (2012). Oxidative stress and redox signaling mechanisms of alcoholic liver disease: Updated experimental and clinical evidence. *Journal of Digestive Diseases, 13*(3), 133–142.

195. Zhu, J. Z., Dai, Y. N., Wang, Y. M., Zhou, Q. Y., Yu, C. H., & Li, Y. M. (2015). Prevalence of nonalcoholic fatty liver disease and economy. *Digestive Diseases and Sciences, 60*(11), 3194–3202.

196. Zhu, K., Moriarty, C., Caplan, L., & Levine, R. S. (2007). Cigarette smoking and primary liver cancer: A population-based case-control study in US men. *Cancer Causes & Control, 18*(3), 315–321.

197. Zigmond, E., Samia-Grinberg, S., Pasmanik-Chor, M., Brazowski, E., Shibolet, O., Halpern, Z., et al. (2014). Infiltrating monocyte-derived macrophages and resident Kupffer cells display different ontogeny and functions in acute liver injury. *Journal of Immunology, 193*(1), 344–353.

198. Zoller, H., & Tilg, H. (2016). Nonalcoholic fatty liver disease and hepatocellular carcinoma. *Metabolism.* Retrieved from: http://dx.doi.org/10.1016/j.metabol.2016.01.010.

Chapter

2

STRUCTURE AND ULTRASTRUCTURE OF THE NORMAL AND DISEASED LIVER

Contents

Introduction

The structural organization of the liver is comprised of parenchymal and vascular elements, tailored to its role as a protective barrier situated between the digestive system and the rest of the body (Elias, 1949). This strategic positioning enables the liver to process a large quantity of nutrients like amino acids, lipids, carbohydrates, vitamins, and harmful substances ingested through food and water. A defining characteristic of the liver structure is its functional tissue, which includes seven distinct types of cells: hepatocytes, sinusoidal endothelial cells, Kupffer cells, stellate cells, cholangiocytes, pit cells, and various lymphocytes (Fawcett, 1955). The fundamental unit of the liver is the hepatic lobule, a prism-shaped structure 2 mm in length and 0.7 mm in width, with a central efferent venule and surrounding portal tracts (Figure 2.1(A) and (B)).

According to Rappaport (1973), the other functional unit is known as the "acinus of Rappaport" (Figure 2.1(A)). It is based on the portal terminal tract, from which blood passes through progressively less oxygenated parenchymal zones until it reaches the efferent or terminal venules. From the perspective of the pathologist, both the classical lobular and acinar concepts have advantages in certain circumstances, despite the fact that other models have been put forth. Therefore, using the lobule as a basis, it is easier to understand the sinusoidal congestion of venous outflow obstruction, with maximum intensity at the center. In terms of the lobule, bridging hepatic necrosis is more challenging to comprehend. It has been described as the death of the hepatocytes in acinar zone 3, which is adjacent to efferent or terminal venules and has a relatively low oxygen saturation. Words from both models can be used to describe the general description of hepatic histopathology; thus, the term periportal refers to the parenchyma near the small portal tract or the portal space (Figure 2.2(A–C)), and perivenular refers to the parenchyma near an efferent terminal venule (Figure 2.2(D)).

In order to gain a better understanding of the alterations on the diseased liver, a brief review of the normal cell components of the organ will be given before analyzing the various structures and ultrastructures of liver pathologies.

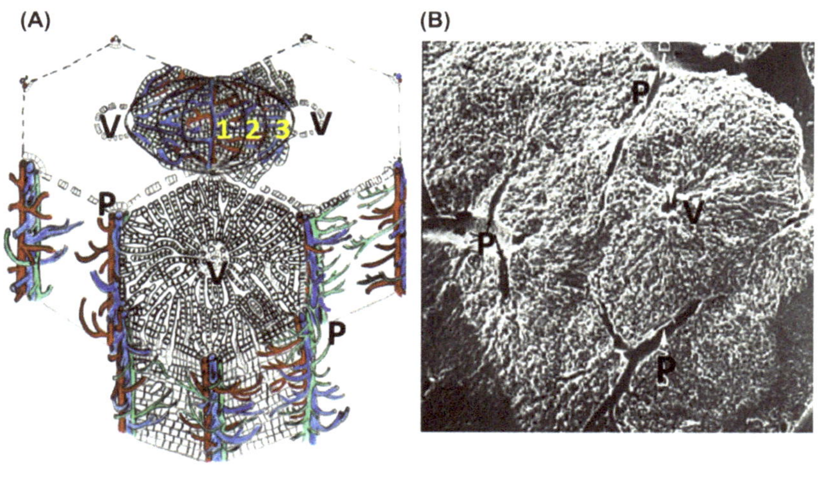

Figure 2.1. *(A) Diagram of a classic hexagonal hepatic lobule. Portal tracts (P) are formed by bile ducts, branch of hepatic arteries and portal venules. A terminal vein (V) at the center of the lobule is shown. Upper part of the same diagram shows an acinus organization lobule (Rapapport) with*

theoretical 1, 2, and 3 zones. (B) Scanning electron micrograph of a typical hepatic lobule shows a central terminal vein (V) and the vessels of the portal tracts (P) at the periphery. (A) Drawing by Francisco Sierra-López.

Source: Tsutsumi, et.al., Structure and Ultrastructure of the Normal and Diseased Liver, http://dx.doi.org/10.1016/B978-0-12-804274-8.00002-3.

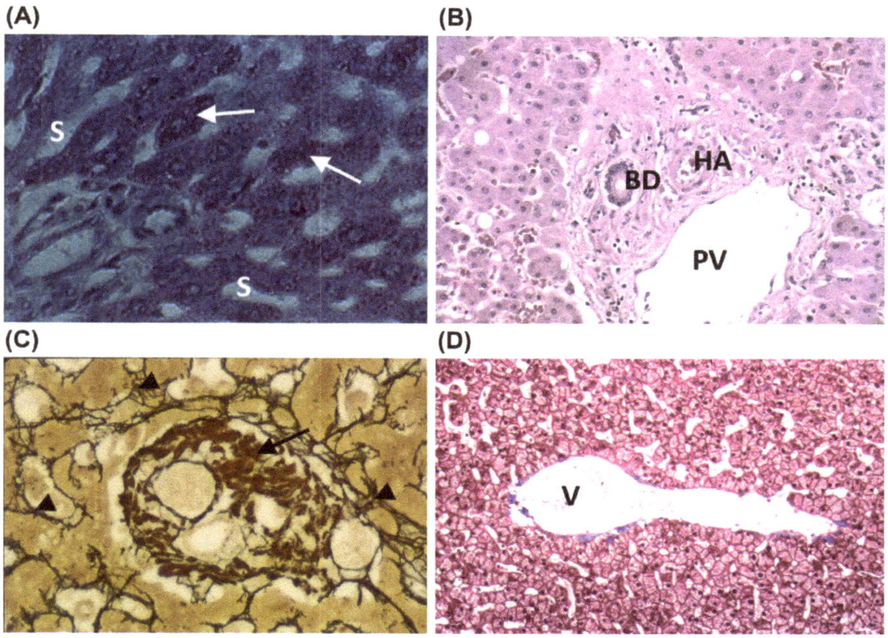

Figure 2.2. *Histology of hepatic parenchyma. (A) Cords of hepatocytes separated by sinusoids. A portal tract is seen at the lower left. Some hepatocytes show cytoplasmic glycogen (arrows) stained in red. PAS stain. (B) Part of the hepatic lobule showing a portal tract or portal space containing the triad formed by branches of portal vein (PV) containing portal vein, hepatic artery (HA), and bile duct (BD), all surrounded by connective tissue. H&E. (C) Portal tract with special stain shows its fibrillar components. Reticulin (black fibers) surrounding hepatocytes (arrow heads) and collagen (reddish) (arrow) associated to triads are observed (reticulin stain). (D) Central or terminal vein (V) at the center of the hepatic lobule. H&E.*

Source: Tsutsumi, et.al., Structure and Ultrastructure of the Normal and Diseased Liver, http://dx.doi.org/10.1016/B978-0-12-804274-8.00002-3.

Orientation and Directional Terms

Term	Definition	Illustration
Lysosomes	Lysosomes are membrane-enclosed organelles that contain an array of enzymes capable of breaking down all types of biological polymers—proteins, nucleic acids, carbohydrates, and lipids.	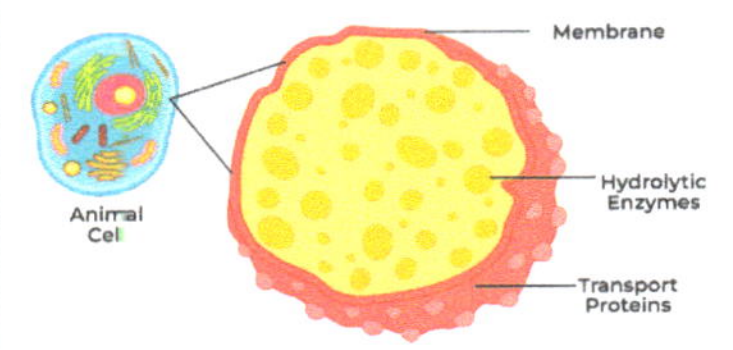
Golgi complex	A stack of small flat sacs formed by membranes inside the cell's cytoplasm (gel-like fluid). The Golgi complex prepares proteins and lipid (fat) molecules for use in other places inside and outside the cell. The Golgi complex is a cell organelle.	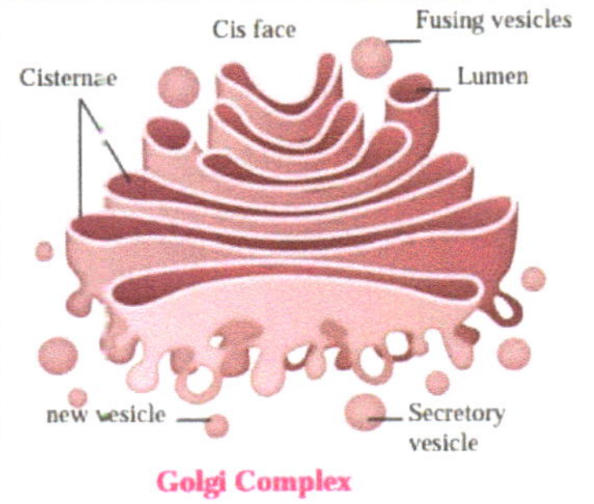
Endothelial Cells	Endothelial cells form a single cell layer that lines all blood vessels and regulates exchanges between the bloodstream and the surrounding tissues. Signals from endothelial cells organize the growth and development of connective tissue cells that form the surrounding layers of the blood-vessel wall.	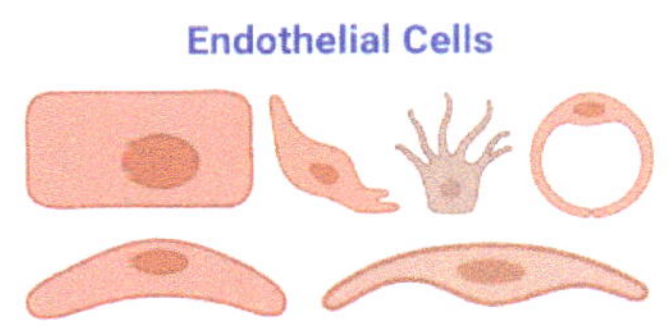
Stellate Cells	Stellate cells are star-shaped cells that were first discovered in the perisinusoidal spaces in the liver and have been found to support wound healing by the secretion of growth factors and extracellular matrix. They have since been also found to serve a similar function in the pancreas.	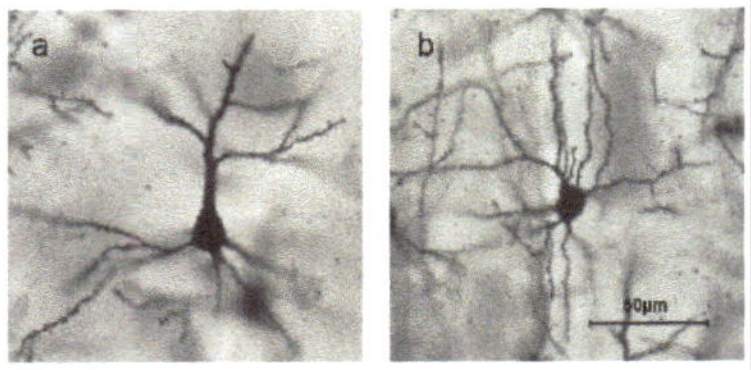
Hepatitis B virus (HBV)	Hepatitis B is an infection of the liver caused by the hepatitis B virus. The infection can be acute (short and severe) or chronic (long term). Hepatitis B can cause a chronic infection and puts people at high risk of death from cirrhosis and liver cancer.	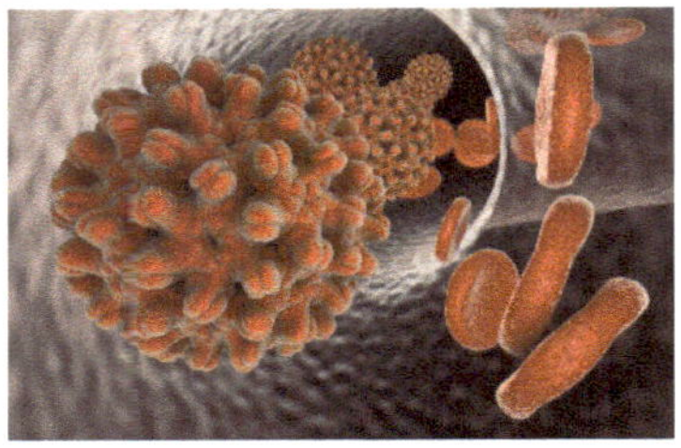

2.1. Normal Cell Types in the Liver

2.1.1. Parenchymal Cells

1. ***Hepatocytes:*** The majority of the liver's synthetic and metabolic processes are carried out by hepatocytes. These are comparatively large polygonal cells, with a cross-sectional area of 20–30 mm on average (Figure 2.3(A) and (B)). They make up the majority of the cells in the liver, accounting for roughly 80% of its mass and volume and 60–70% of all the cells in the parenchymal matrix. The area of the hepatocyte surface that faces sinusoids—roughly 35% of the total surface area—is greatly increased by the plasma membrane folding into countless microvilli that extend into the Disse space. The surface area of hepatocytes that face other hepatocytes is about 50%. Except for the location where it folds to form the bile canaliculi, the plasma membrane of these intercellular surfaces is primarily flat (Fawcett, 1955). Molecular specializations of the different surface membranes of hepatocytes, such as receptors, pumps, transport channels, and carrier proteins, polarize the cells.

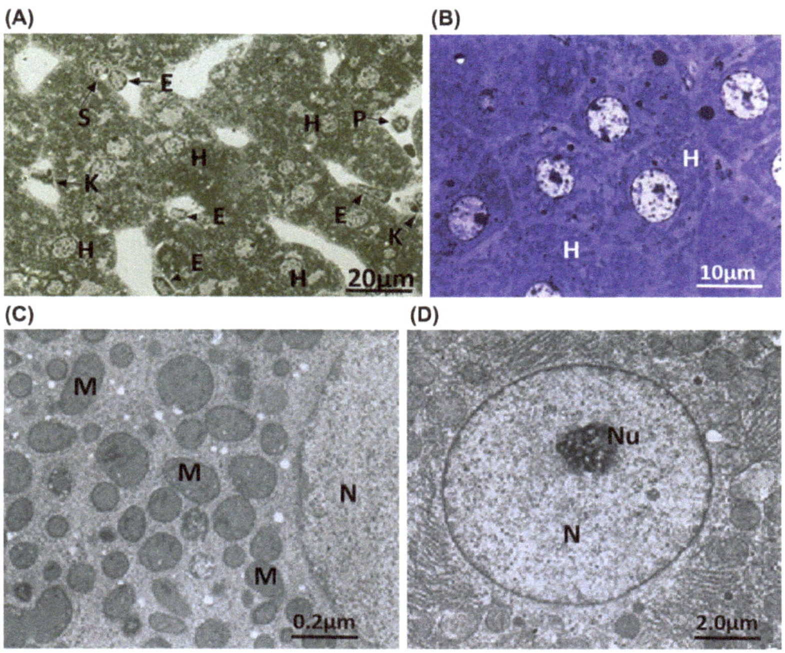

Figure 2.3. *Normal hepatocytes observed by different techniques. (A) Very low, panoramic transmission electron microscopy view of liver parenchyma shows cords of hepatocytes separated by sinusoids and some of the nonparenchymal sinusoidal cells: E, endothelial cells; H, hepatocytes; K, Kupffer cells; P, pit cell; S, stellate cells. (B) Light microscopy of liver embedded in epoxy resin. Semithin section stained with toluidine blue. Hepatocytes (H) show some of the intracellular organelles. (C) Electron microscopy of hepatocyte shows abundant round mitochondria (M). Part of a nucleus (N) is seen at the right. (D) A round nucleus (N) of hepatocyte is observed with a conspicuous nucleolus (Nu) is shown.*

Source: Tsutsumi, et.al., Structure and Ultrastructure of the Normal and Diseased Liver, http://dx.doi.org/10.1016/B978-0-12-804274-8.00002-3.

While the sinusoidal surface is capable of extracting a wide range of blood molecules and simultaneously secreting other molecules that have been altered or produced by hepatocytes into the blood, the canalicular membrane is modified for the excretion of bile. Hepatocytes have a complex array of mitochondria, peroxisomes, lysosomes, Golgi complexes, aggregates of rough and smooth endoplasmic reticulum (Figures 2.4 and 2.5), and numerous microtubules and microfilaments to carry out their numerous metabolic functions.

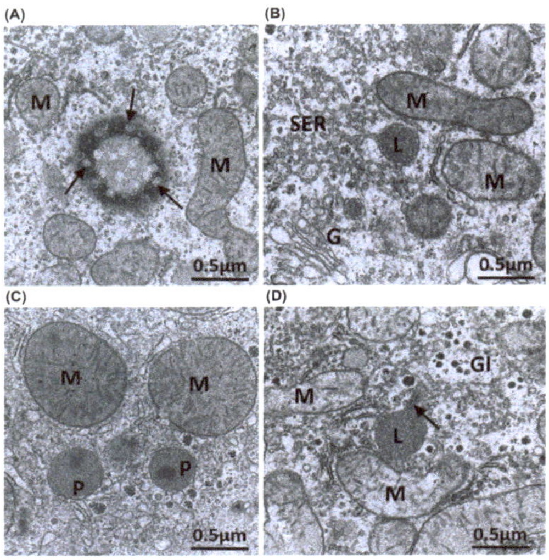

Figure 2.4. *Ultrastructure of hepatocyte showing some of the organelles. (A) Tangential section of the nucleus shows the presence of the nuclear membrane pores (arrows). Mitochondria (M). (B) Hepatic cytoplasm presents several membranous organelles, such as mitochondria (M), lysosomes (L), smooth endoplasmic reticulum (SER), Golgi complex (G). (C) Round mitochondria (M) and peroxisomes (P) are shown. (D) Elongated mitochondria (M) and a lysosome (L) and glycogen (Gl) associated with a tubular structure (arrow) are observed.*

Source: Tsutsumi, et.al., Structure and Ultrastructure of the Normal and Diseased Liver, http://dx.doi.org/10.1016/B978-0-12-804274-8.00002-3.

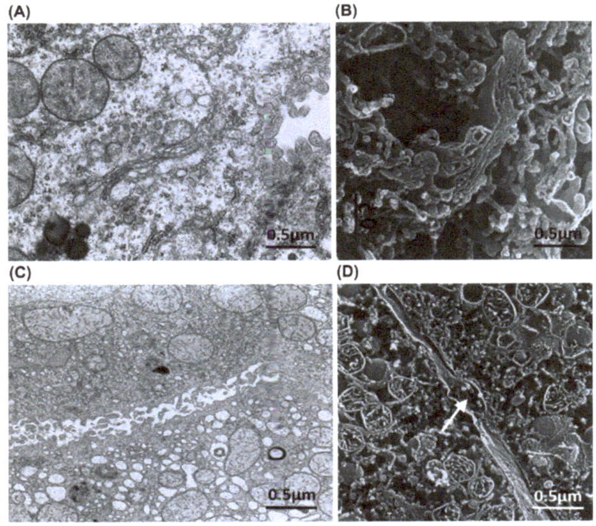

Figure 2.5. *Ultrastructure of hepatocyte organelles. (A) Transmission electron microscopy of a Golgi complex showing a pile of flat membranes and micro- and macrovesicles. (B) Scanning electron microscopy of a hepatocyte Golgi complex shows a 3D profile of this organelle. (C) Bile canalicular channel (longitudinal section) localized between hepatocytes presents small microvilli in the lumen. (D) A bile canaliculi (arrow) sectioned transversally and observed with scanning electron microscopy.*

Source: Tsutsumi, et.al., Structure and Ultrastructure of the Normal and Diseased Liver, http://dx.doi.org/10.1016/B978-0-12-804274-8.00002-3.

2.1.2. Nonparenchymal Cells

1. ***Endothelial Cells:*** The endothelial cells of the hepatic sinusoid are flat cells (Figures 2.6 and 2.8(A)), which make up the sinusoidal wall's lining. Their fenestrae, which are grouped together to form sieve plates, are scattered throughout their thin, flat cytoplasmic processes. These thin, flat sections are separated by thicker cytoplasmic arms that are filled with pinocytotic vesicles, mitochondria,

lysosomes, and other organelles. The endothelial cells form single cells in a row to form the sinusoid, the typical liver capillary, which encircles the sinusoidal lumen and forms cylindrical structures all by itself. Between sinusoidal endothelial cells, there aren't any discontinuities or open spaces under normal circumstances. Only fenestrae allow free passage of liquid, solutes, droplets, and particles from the lumen into the Disse space and vice versa. While there are traces of basal lamina components within the Disse space (Figure 2.6), a distinct basal lamina structure is absent.

A variety of vacuolar and vesicular structures, including bristle-covered pinocytotic vesicles, uncoated vesicles of similar size, bristle-covered Golgi vesicles, electron-lucent vacuoles, and vacuoles with increasing electron density up to and including numerous electron-dense lysosomes, are the prominent components of the vacuolar apparatus in addition to fenestrae. A variety of small, colloidal particles, including thorotrast, saturated iron oxide, ferric oxyhydroxide citrate, latex, colloidal gold, and horseradish peroxidase, have been shown to be absorbed by bristle-coated vesicles and macropinocytotic vesicles of endothelial cells (Wisse, 1972).

2. ***Kupffer Cells (Macrophages):*** Constitute roughly 2% of the liver's mass and volume. The majority of them are found in the portal regions of sinusoids (Figures 2.6, 2.7(A), and 2.8(B)), where they are contained by loose attachments to the sinusoidal endothelium. Via C3 and Fc receptors, Kupffer cells actively phagocyte large particles from the sinusoidal blood, such as bacteria and effete cells (dead or damaged hepatocytes, worn-out erythrocytes, etc.). They comprise the organism's main mechanism for eliminating deteriorated cells and proteins from perfusion blood, along with sinusoidal endothelial cells. Activated macrophages generate a vast array of chemokines and cytokines that are essential for the liver's acute phase response, coordinating all parenchymal cell reactions to injury (Naito et al., 1999).

Prionomic vesicles, microvilli, filopodia, pseudopodia, worm-like structures, and an abundance of lysosomes (Figure 2.8(B)) are ultrastructurally characteristic of knoppler cells. As resident macrophages, these cells exhibit an endogenous peroxidase activity localization pattern. According to van Furth (1989), Kupffer cells in adulthood are believed to be non-proliferating cells in the terminal differentiation stage, and their estimated lifespan in mice is 3.8 days. On the longevity and proliferation of Kupffer cells, however, contradictory information has been provided. Following a partial hepatectomy or the administration of multiple macrophage stimulators, these cells demonstrate a notable capacity for proliferation. The ability of Kupffer cells to proliferate increased during the monocytopenia period. These results suggest that the Kupffer cell population of resident macrophages is a long-lived and slowly proliferating population.

3. ***Stellate Cells***: These cells make up approximately 1% of the hepatic volume and are situated in the Disse (2/6, 2/7, and 2/8C) space, partially encircling the sinusoids. Stellate cells have multiple uses; they store the fat-soluble vitamin A in lipid inclusions and work with hepatocytes to participate in its metabolism.

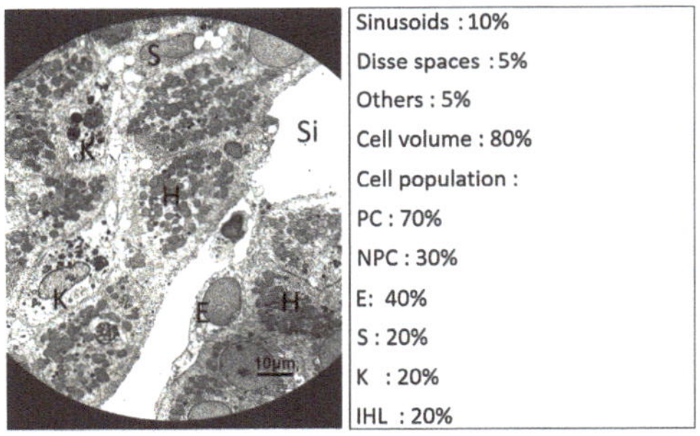

Figure 2.6. *Panoramic electron microscopic view of hepatic parenchyma with an associated sinusoid. Hepatocytes (H) are lining a sinusoid (Si) with some cells such as endothelial (E), Kupffer cell (K), Stellate cell (S). Table on the right shows some data of the liver volume occupied by different parenchymal (PC) and nonparenchymal (NPC) cells. E, endothelial cells; IHL, intrahepatic lymphocytes; K, Kupffer cells; S, stellate cells.*

Source. Tsutsumi, et.al., Structure and Ultrastructure of the Normal and Diseased Liver, http://dx.doi.org/10.1016/B978-0-12-804274-8.00002-3.

Moreover, these cells produce, secrete, and break down extracellular matrix components that are perisinusoidal. They exhibit a myofibroblastic phenotype in response to multiple cytokines, which are indicated by the expression of desmin, a-smooth muscle actin, and various neuroendocrine proteins. Stellate cells, being myofibroblasts, play a significant part in the fibrotic reactions of the liver to different types of injury (Wake, 1980; Rojkind & Reyes-Gordillo, 2009).

Stellate cells have oval or somewhat elongated nuclei that are frequently indented by vitamin A-containing lipid droplets (Figure 2.8(C)). Granular endoplasmic reticulum development is strong. Fine filamentous materials are found in the cisterns. The Golgi complex is made up of numerous vesicles connected to well-developed lamellae. Lipid droplets exist in the cytoplasm of these stellate cells, which is their most noticeable characteristic. Retinyl esters are the main form in which vitamin A is stored. In the cytoplasm of stellate cells, additional structures like microtubules, microfilaments, and intermediate filaments of desmin are noticeable.

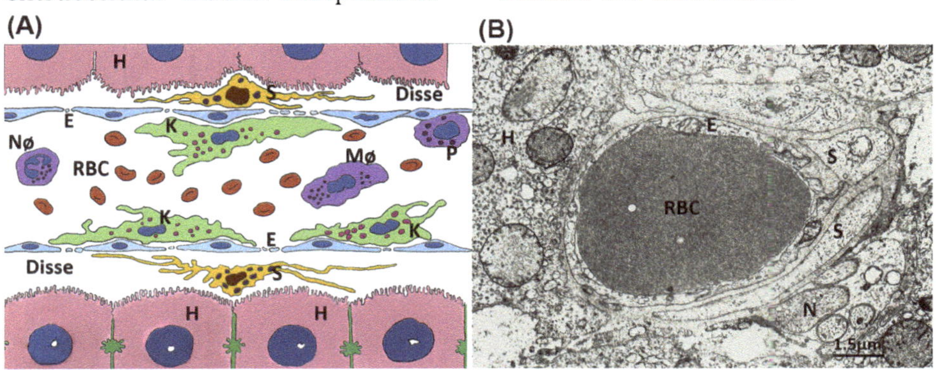

Figure 2.7. *(A) Diagram of a sinusoid with associated cells. Endothelial (E), Kupffer (K), stellate (S) cells. Lumen is occupied by red blood cells (RBC), neutrophils (Nø), Macrophage (Mø), hepatocytes (H). (B) Transmission electron microscopy of a sinusoid sectioned transversally. A red blood cell (RBC) occupies the sinusoid lumen totally. Endothelial cells (E) with fenestrae are enfolded by the cytoplasmic processes of hepatic stellate cells (S). A naked nerve ending (N) closely faces also the process of hepatic stellate cells. Hepatocyte (H).*

Source: Tsutsumi, et.al., Structure and Ultrastructure of the Normal and Diseased Liver, http://dx.doi.org/10.1016/B978-0-12-804274-8.00002-3.

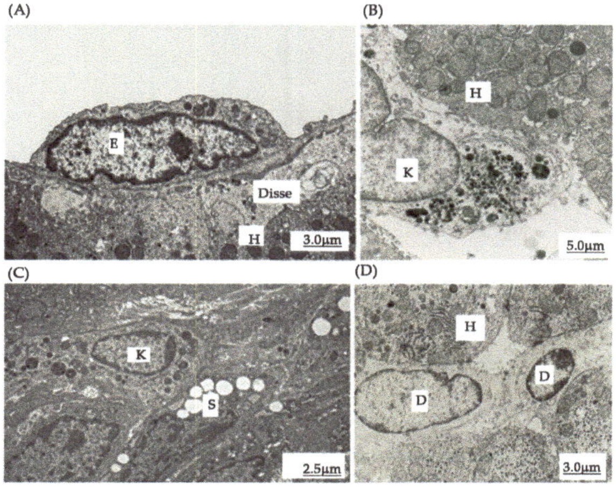

Figure 2.8. *Ultrastructure of nonparenchymal sinusoidal cells. (A) An endothelial cell with an elongated nucleus and thin cytoplasmic processes is seen surrounding the sinusoid and above the hepatocytes (H) separated by the Disse space. (B) Kupffer cell (K) shows a kidney-shaped nucleus, and a cytoplasm with abundant dense phagocytic granules. Hepatocyte (H). (C) Typical stellate cell (S) with many clear vacuoles is seen closely associated to Kupffer cell (K). (D) Ductular cells (D) associated to hepatocytes (H) constitute the wall of a Hering channel, which connects the canaliculi with the bile duct.*

Source: Tsutsumi, et.al., Structure and Ultrastructure of the Normal and Diseased Liver, http://dx.doi.org/10.1016/B978-0-12-804274-8.00002-3

4. ***Cholangiocytes:*** Similar to hepatocytes, cholangiocytes are biliary epithelial cells that develop from hepatoblasts during embryonic development (Dianat et al., 2014). The bile flows to the periphery of the classic lobule and enters small terminal bile ductules, also known as Hering channels, as part of the biliary network, which begins with the bile canaliculi, which are found between the cell membranes of neighboring hepatocytes. Two or four cells that become cuboidal line the ductules as they approach the portal channel (Figure 2.8(D)). Numerous blunt microvilli protrude from the borders of the lumen. Compared to nearby hepatocytes, the mitochondria are smaller and the nuclei are longer. These cells have vesicles thought to be pinocytotic as well as a noticeable Golgi complex. There is a basal lamina that encloses the ductules entirely. Interlobular bile ducts receive the bile that exits the terminal ductules. As they get closer to the portal tract, these ducts expand in size, creating a continuous network of passageways. Solitary cuboidal or columnar epithelial cells with microvilli on their luminal surface encircle them. Tall columnar cells enclose the extrahepatic ducts. The layers of their walls are the same as those of the intestine: adventitia, muscularis, submucosa, and mucosa.

5. ***Pit Cells:*** Liver-associated natural killer (NK) cells are the name given to these cells. They are a variant of peripheral blood NK cells with altered morphology and function. They are found inside the sinusoidal lumen, where they adhere closely to Kupffer cells and endothelial cells. They also frequently extend well-developed pseudopodia that appear to be indicative of migration along the sinusoidal wall. Pit cells often contain multivesicular body-related dense granules and rod-cored vesicles in their cytoplasm, which may play a role in their cytotoxicity towards bound tumor cells (Kaneda & Wake, 1983). Further, T, NK, NKT, and dendritic cells are examples of different phenotypes of lymphocytes. These cells are all parts of an immune system that is focused on the liver. The processes of innate (native) immunity, in particular, are involved in the antigen presentation, elimination, or neutralization of various foreign substances, including

bacteria, that enter the liver from the stomach. After cell loss and injury, the liver's natural immune system plays a crucial regulatory role in facilitating the organ's healing process. As a component of the body's acquired immune system, the tiny population of liver T lymphocytes aids in the removal of viruses, the removal of activated T cells, and the development of antigen tolerance (Ferrari and Mondelli, 2009).

2.2. Pathology of the Diseased Liver

Numerous factors contribute to the variety of diseases that affect the liver, including the organ's vast array of functions, unique structural arrangement, strategic location within the body, and unique cellular sensitivity of its various components. Liver diseases are the fourth or fifth leading cause of death globally, exhibiting a wide range of etiologies. The most prevalent liver diseases seen in pathology labs will be the primary focus of this brief review of liver histopathology. Various liver neoplasms, such as hepatocellular carcinoma (HCC), liver cirrhosis, alcoholic liver disease, nonalcoholic fatty liver disease (NAFLD), and types B and C hepatitis are among them.

2.2.1. Acute Viral Hepatitis

Hepatocellular damage and inflammatory cell infiltrations are the fundamental elements of the acute phase of hepatitis (Figure 2.9(A)). Cholestasis is one of the possible extra features. Under a light microscope, cell changes range from mild enlargement to complete cell death (Figure 2.9(B) and (C)).

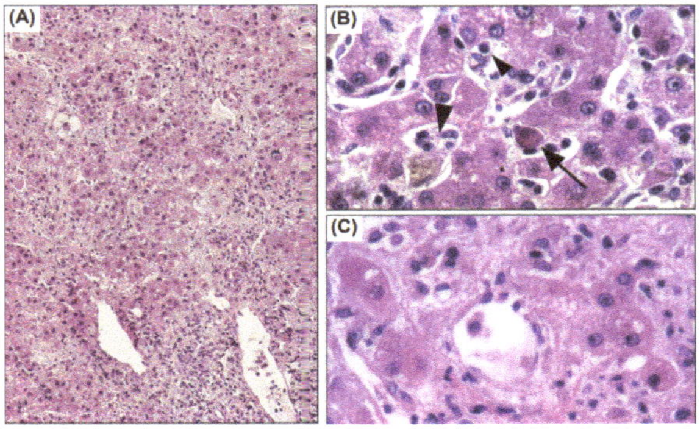

Figure 2.9. *Histopathology of acute viral hepatitis. (A) Portal tracts and parenchyma show a strong lymphocyte infiltration with damaged hepatocytes. (B) Acidophilic bodies with loss of nuclei are seen (arrow). Hyperplasia of Kupffer cell (arrow heads). (C) Ballooning degeneration of hepatocyte with pale cytoplasm and small nucleus is seen.*

Source: Tsutsumi, et.al., Structure and Ultrastructure of the Normal and Diseased Liver, http://dx.doi.org/10.1016/B978-0-12-804274-8.00002-3.

The concomitant inflammatory infiltration illustrates how crucial cellular immunity is to the pathophysiology of the majority of hepatitis types. Perivenular regions are more severely affected by inflammation and hepatocellular damage, which results in a distinctive histological pattern. It is less common to see a periportal pattern of necrosis and inflammation in cases of hepatitis A.

One of the most prevalent indicators of minor cell damage that may be remedied is swelling. Affected cells have rarified, granular, and occasionally finely vacuolated cytoplasm. Ballooning degeneration is the term for more severe cell swelling (Figure 2.9(C)). Another process of cell death in hepatitis is believed to be apoptosis, which occurs in other hepatocytes. Sometimes referred to as acidophilic change or degeneration, shrinkage and increased staining of the cytoplasm (Figure 2.9(B)) is most likely a sign of apoptosis, in which the hepatocytes become extremely dense and fragment. The largest pieces or all of the unfragmented apoptotic cells are represented by the apoptotic bodies that are visible floating freely in the sinusoids. They are frequently referred to as Councilman bodies or acidophil bodies (Klotz & Belt, 1930). Spotty necrosis is the most common type of acute hepatitis, where small clusters of macrophages and lymphocytes replace or disturb the liver plates. A "mosaic pattern" of cell organization is created on the liver cell plates as a result of focal regeneration combined with hepatocyte loss or liver cell dropout.

Hepatitis is primarily distinguished from classic acute inflammation by a lymphocytic infiltrate within the parenchyma and portal tracts (Figure 2.9(A)).

Usually, portal inflammation is the most noticeable. Portal tracts may be normal in size or enlarged, and the degree of portal inflammation varies greatly. Larger conducting tracts are frequently left undamaged. Small T lymphocytes make up the majority of the infiltrating cells in hepatitis, but plasma cells can also be noticeable, and a small number of neutrophils and eosinophils are frequently present as well. Sinusoidal endothelial cells can develop dense iron-positive granules and enlarge. Hepatic venules at the terminal stage may exhibit endothelium disruption and lymphocytic infiltration. Acute hepatitis causes a wide range of histological changes. However, some non-constant changes, such as confluent necrosis, bridging necrosis of entire lobules, and periportal necrosis, are particularly noteworthy. Significant parenchymal death is indicated by confluent necrosis. Confluent necrosis that connects terminal venules to portal tracts is referred to as bridging necrosis. This location could represent the entire zone 3 of an acinus, a theory reinforced by the curved shapes of numerous bridges. Although bridging necrosis is a sign of severe acute hepatitis, its distribution can vary, even within a single biopsy.

In multilobular necrosis, the parenchyma is replaced by collapsed stroma, inflammatory cells, and activated macrophages. Around the surviving portal tracts, there are prominent duct-like structures, some of which probably represent proliferation of pluripotential progenitor cells (Roskams et al., 1998).

There are more similarities than differences between hepatitis A, B, C, D, and E, but certain patterns are more common in one type than another, and some are described. They do not allow the pathologist to identify the cause of the hepatitis on histological appearances alone. The picture may be confused by the presence of more than one virus.

- ***Hepatitis A:*** There are two primary images described, which can appear separately or in tandem (Okuno et al., 1984). One shows minimal inflammation or damage to liver cells in the histological picture of perivenular cholestasis. Hepatitis with periportal necrosis and a dense portal infiltrate, which frequently consists of a large number of aggregated plasma cells, is the second. These two patterns—cholestasis brought on by periportal necrosis, which stops bile flow—might be connected.
- ***Hepatitis B:*** The histological features resemble other viral hepatitis types in general. It's possible that some of the variations noted in the literature are due to patient choice rather than characteristics unique to hepatitis B virus (HBV) infection. However, occasionally, hepatocytes are near lymphocytes and macrophages (peripolesis) or even deeply invaded (emperipolesis), which likely reflects

the immunological nature of the cell damage. In contrast to hepatitis C, acute hepatitis B typically causes more severe periportal inflammation (Chu et al., 2001). A moderate level of pleomorphism may be seen in the nuclei of hepatocytes. The hepatitis B surface and core antigens (HBcAg and HBsAg) are either very sparse or not detectable in the majority of acute hepatitis cases. Chronic illness is indicated by the presence of ground glass or by positive Victoria blue or orcein staining of surface material. Occult infection and mild histological abnormalities such as portal inflammation, focal necrosis, apoptosis, and fibrosis may linger for ten years or longer after acute hepatitis B has healed clinically.

- ***Hepatitis C:*** The histological characteristics of acute hepatitis are typically the same as those of any acute hepatitis; however, acute hepatitis C is distinguished by two features. First, even in the absence of significant liver cell damage, there may be a noticeable lymphocyte infiltration of the sinusoids (Bamber et al., 1981), creating an image evocative of contagious mononucleosis. Secondly, within a few weeks or months of the illness starting, lymphoid follicles and bile duct damage, which are also linked to chronic hepatitis, may be observed. Steatosis is a common finding and cholestasis may be present.

Ø *Differential Diagnosis:* The presence of characteristic hepatic alterations in the parenchyma is the primary factor used to distinguish acute hepatitis from bile duct obstruction. If the cause of the hepatitis is unclear, drug-related hepatitis should always be suspected as it may be difficult to differentiate from viral hepatitis. Characteristics that are more prevalent in drug-induced hepatitis than in viral hepatitis include granulomas, a poorly developed portal inflammatory response, a lot of neutrophils or eosinophils, and well-defined perivenular necrosis. The symptoms of hepatitis may be overshadowed by cholestasis The onset of autoimmune hepatitis (AIH) can be either clinically acute and histologically identical to viral hepatitis, or it can have the histological characteristics of chronic diseases. A noticeable fatty alteration is typically present in steatohepatitis. Hepatocytes that have ballooned may contain Mallory-Denk bodies, and neutrophils are usually included in the infiltrate. The presence of pericellular fibrosis in the afflicted areas is crucial for the diagnosis. Parenchymal alterations are more common in acute hepatitis, particularly in perivenular regions, while portal and periportal alterations are more common in chronic illness. Making the distinction can be challenging at times, particularly when significant lobular alterations are discovered during a chronic hepatitis flare-up.

2.2.2. Steatosis and Steatohepatitis

- ***Steatosis:*** When 5% or more of the hepatic cells have abnormal lipid accumulation, the condition is known as steatosis, also known as fatty change of fatty liver. The majority of steatosis is of the macrovesicular type (Figure 2.10(A) and (B)), in which the nucleus is pushed to the periphery and a single large fat vacuole or several smaller ones occupy the majority of the cell. Microvesicular steatosis is the less common but frequently more severe kind (Figure 2.11). This type of fat has a central nucleus that is finely divided. According to Brunt (2007), the two forms of steatosis can occasionally coexist (Figures 2.11(B) and 2.12(A)). Steatosis in the margins is frequent. It is often detected by noninvasive imaging and may be associated with mild abnormalities of alkaline phosphatase, gamma-glutamyl transpeptidase, and serum aminotransferases. Typically, a histological examination is insufficient to identify the cause of uncomplicated macrovesicular steatosis. However, the location of the fat could provide some information; perivenular steatosis is the most common type, but periportal steatosis can also occur in AIDS patients, people receiving parenteral nutrition, and people with kwashiorkor. Hepatocyte nuclei with glycogen vacuolation are frequently observed in patients with diabetes mellitus. Sporadic fatty change is characterized by roughly rounded foci of steatosis that are visible in an otherwise normal liver and may be misinterpreted on imaging as neoplasms. Because of either a decrease in excretion or an increase in triglyceride synthesis, hepatocytes in macrovesicular steatosis accumulate lipids. Every now and then, hepatocytes loaded with lipid burst, allowing macrophages to absorb the fat. A lipogranuloma is the lesion that results. Although lipogranulomas may fibrose and are located within lobules, frequently close to terminal venules, they do not seem to be a factor in the progression of liver disease and should be differentiated from the more significant pericellular fibrosis associated with steatohepatitis.

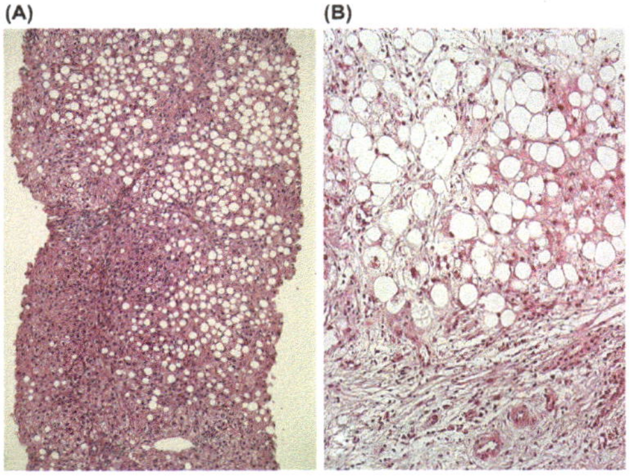

Figure 2.10. *(A) Alcoholic liver cirrhosis. Steatosis with intrahepatic inflammation and fibrosis are seen. (B) Nonalcoholic steatohepatitis (NASH). Ballooning of hepatocytes are present with perivenular and pericellular fibrosis. Histological features are similar to those of alcoholic hepatitis. H&E.*

Source: Tsutsumi, et.al., Structure and Ultrastructure of the Normal and Diseased Liver, http://dx.doi.org/10.1016/B978-0-12-804274-8.00002-3.

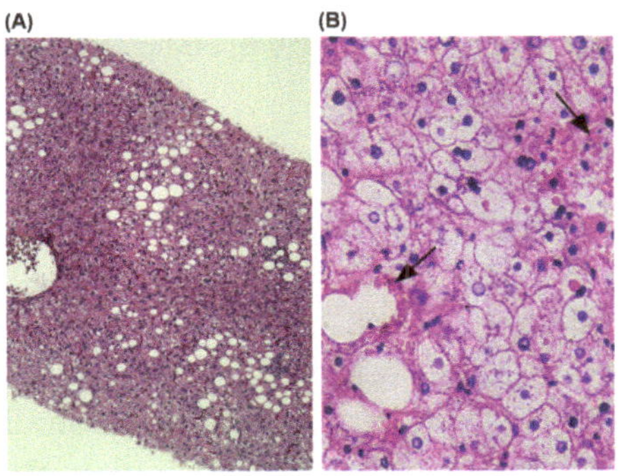

Figure 2.11. *(A) Low magnification of a biopsy of a nonalcoholic steatohepatitis (NASH). (B) Nonalcoholic steatohepatitis with ballooning degeneration, macro- and microvescicular steatosis, Mallory-Denk body (arrows) and megamitochondria are shown. H&E.*

Source. Tsutsumi, et.al., Structure and Ultrastructure of the Normal and Diseased Liver, http://dx.doi.org/10.1016/B978-0-12-804274-8.00002-3

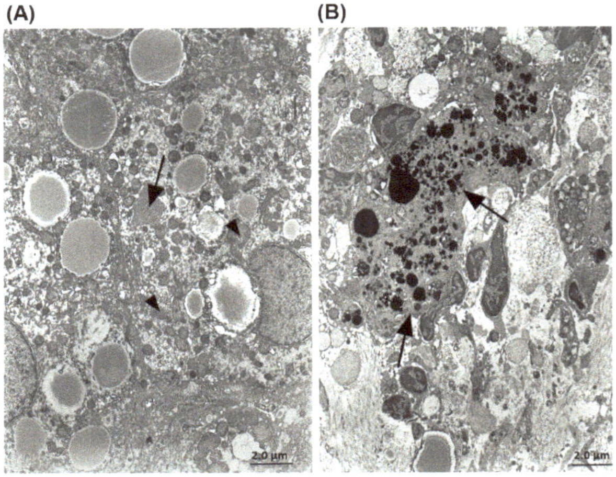

Figure 2.12. *(A) Electron microscopy of nonalcoholic steatohepatitis (NASH). Macro- and microvesicles with a small amount of Mallory-Denk body is shown (arrow) and giant mitochondria (arrow heads) are noted in the hepatocytes. (B) The portal area in NASH shows mixed inflammatory cells including polymorphonuclear cells (arrows).*

Source: Tsutsumi, et.al., Structure and Ultrastructure of the Normal and Diseased Liver, http://dx.doi.org/10.1016/B978-0-12-804274-8.00002-3.

Although macrovesicular steatosis is not a clinically significant lesion in and of itself, it does provide the framework for the development of the significant lesions associated with alcoholic and nonalcoholic steatohepatitis (NASH) (Ueno et al., 1997). A dangerous and occasionally fatal condition known as microvesicular steatosis occurs when finely divided fat builds up in the cytoplasm of hepatocytes due to mitochondrial damage that impairs b-oxidation. Acute fatty liver during pregnancy, hepatotoxic medications like valproate and nucleoside analogs, foamy degeneration in alcoholics, and complete parenteral nutrition are among the causes (Aita et al., 2001). The cytoplasmic lipid is observed to be extremely finely divided histologically, and it is not always visible in paraffin sections. In frozen sections, it can be stained with oil red O. Hepatocytes that are impacted frequently swell. They still have central nuclei.

2.2.3. Steatohepatitis, Nonalcoholic, and Alcoholic

NASH is characterized by inflammation, hepatic steatosis, and ballooning hepatocyte degeneration, either with or without fibrosis (Figure 2.11(B)). The Mayo Clinic study from 1980, which established the nonalcoholic nature of the 20 subjects with liver biopsies, is credited with coining the term NASH for fatty liver disease nomenclature (Brunt, 2007). The majority of steatohepatitis patients abuse alcohol, are overweight, have diabetes, or have all three conditions combined. The full spectrum of changes from uncomplicated steatosis to steatohepatitis and cirrhosis is referred to as alcoholic fatty liver disease (AFLD) (Figure 2.10(A)) and non-alcoholic fatty liver disease (NAFLD) (Figure 2.11(B)) (Morita et al., 2005). Alcoholic steatohepatitis (ASH) and nonalcoholic steatohepatitis (NASH) share many similarities in their alterations, making histological differences between the two conditions typically impossible (Sasaki et al., 2006).

The primary pathological characteristics include inflammation, fibrosis, and hepatocellular damage. Perivenular regions typically experience the most severe hepatocellular damage, if not exclusive to them. In addition to the appearance of Mallory-Denk bodies, it manifests as cell swelling and cytoplasmic clearing (Figures 2.11(B), 2.12(B), and 2.13(A)). These structures are made up of dense eosinophilic material skeins and clumps that can occasionally form a ring around the nucleus. Megamitochondria (Figure 2.12(A)) are elongated or rounded eosinophilic material bodies that range in size from 2 to 10 mm and are also occasionally found in hepatocytes. Megamitochondria are present in the livers of alcohol abusers without steatohepatitis (Figure

2.12(A)) and in both ASH and NASH (Le et al., 2004). Although neutrophils make up the majority of the inflammatory infiltrate, lymphocytes are also present. These are primarily CD4 and CD8 phenotype T cells, which are present in portal tracts as well as steatohepatitis-affected areas. The process involves macrophages as well as other sinusoidal cells. Vacuoles of fat may be present in Kupffer cells. One essential component of the steatohepatitis lesion is fibrosis. Pericellular fibrosis, also known as chicken-wire fibrosis, is the most prevalent type of fibrosis (Figure 2.13(B)). Collagen strands, either thinner or more delicate, encircle enlarged hepatocytes to create a network that is easily visible when using reticulin preparations or trichrome stains. The location matches that of inflammation and cell damage. Fibrosis between perivenular regions and the portal tracts itself forms fibrous bridges in cases of severe steatohepatitis. The histological characteristics of a typical, fully developed case of steatohepatitis are as follows. However, steatohepatitis is a progressive lesion that varies in severity, just like all pathological processes.

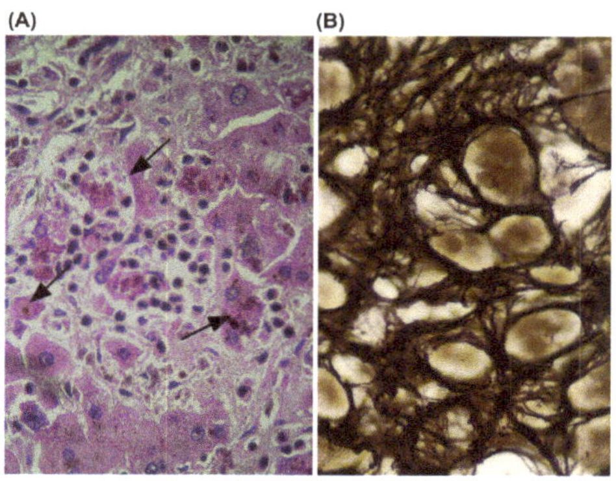

Figure 2.13. *(A) Alcoholic hepatitis with Mallory-Denk bodies (arrows) surrounded by neutrophils. (B) Chronic alcoholic hepatitis with pericelullar chicken-wire fibrosis.*

Source: Tsutsumi, et.al., Structure and Ultrastructure of the Normal and Diseased Liver, http://dx.doi.org/10.1016/B978-0-12-804274-8.00002-3.

Because of these factors, a liver biopsy may reveal less evident alterations that are difficult to identify as belonging to the entire range. Other hepatitis types are included in the histological differential diagnosis of steatohepatitis. Rather than neutrophils, lymphocytes and plasma cells infiltrate viral and AIH infections. The reticulin framework collapses in acute viral hepatitis, but pericellular fibrosis's "chicken-wire" pattern is absent. Patients with chronic hepatitis C may have steatosis, but they do not have the other characteristics of steatohepatitis. Hepatocytes close to fibrous septa in chronic cholestasis, with or without cirrhosis, are usually enlarged and may include bilirubin and Mallory-Denk bodies. Also visible are neutrophils. Paying attention to the lesion's location and the clinical circumstances helps determine the correct diagnosis.

Due to rising obesity rates in Western populations as well as increased public awareness of the illness, NASH has grown in significance in recent years. When liver function tests are abnormal but viral markers are negative, the diagnosis is now one of the most important clinical considerations. When compared to ASH, the histological lesion of NASH is rarely extremely severe. Thus, a high concentration of neutrophils and Mallory bodies ought to raise questions about alcohol misuse. In NASH, glycogen vacuolation of nuclei is frequent. The lesion may or may not progress slowly to cirrhosis. The risk of liver failure and HCC is the same as with other types of cirrhosis.

2.2.4. Chronic Hepatitis

Chronic hepatitis is a common cause of consistently abnormal liver function tests and is a precursor to the development of cirrhosis and liver cancer (HCC). It is characterized by persistent liver injury with elevated levels of aminotransferases or viral markers for more than 6 months. While this definition is somewhat arbitrary, it serves to distinguish between acute and chronic hepatitis in research studies. Chronic hepatitis is often associated with inflammatory liver diseases but is typically linked to specific causes such as hepatitis B, hepatitis C, autoimmune hepatitis (AIH), drug-induced hepatitis, and cases of unknown origin. Other conditions with pathological similarities to chronic hepatitis include Wilson disease, alpha-1 antitrypsin deficiency, primary biliary cirrhosis, and primary sclerosing cholangitis. In cases of chronic hepatitis, the inflammation in the liver is typically concentrated in portal tracts, with lymphocytes, plasma cells, and occasional segmented leukocytes infiltrating these areas. In more severe cases, the inflammation may extend into surrounding liver tissue, potentially damaging interlobular bile ducts. In milder forms, the inflammatory infiltrate remains confined to the portal tracts, while in more severe cases, there is destruction of hepatocytes in the adjacent parenchyma.

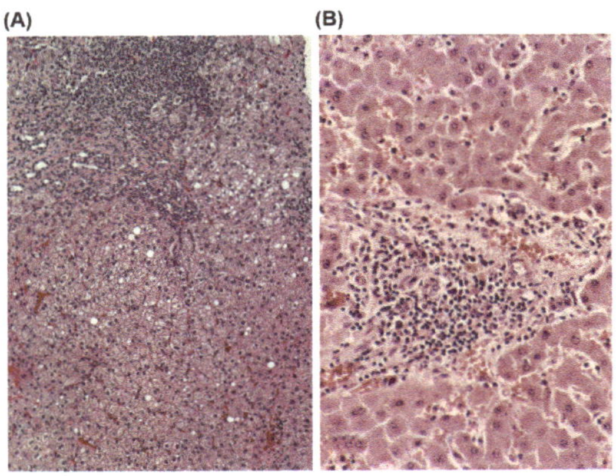

Figure 2.14. *(A) Alcoholic liver disease. Shows an intense inflammatory infiltrate with cholangiolar reaction. A mild steatosis is also observed. (B) Mild chronic hepatitis. Lymphocyte infiltration is confined to the portal tract.*

Source: Tsutsumi, et.al., Structure and Ultrastructure of the Normal and Diseased Liver, http://dx.doi.org/10.1016/B978-0-12-804274-8.00002-3.

This process, known as interface hepatitis, is characterized by irregularities in the hepatocyte limiting plates around portal tracts. In cirrhotic livers, interface hepatitis is typically observed at the edges of nodules and septa rather than surrounding portal tracts.

Sometimes referred to as the lobular component or lobular hepatitis, there are varying degrees of hepatocellular damage and inflammation deeper within the parenchyma (Liaw et al., 1982). The most typical manifestation of this is focal necrosis, although confluent and bridging necrosis can also be observed. The loss of hepatocytes in areas where lymphocytes, macrophages, and other cells have infiltrated is known as focal (spotty) necrosis.

Severe lobular hepatitis often leads to the formation of small rounded or ovoid gland-like clusters of surviving hepatocytes known as hepatitis rosettes. These rosettes are found within connective tissue and are believed to develop due to an overgrowth of hepatocytes trapped in a collapsed and inflamed area of the liver. Other changes in hepatocytes seen in chronic hepatitis include steatosis, deposition of iron, and oncocytic change. Steatosis is most common in chronic hepatitis C, while iron deposits are typically focal. If there is a substantial accumulation of iron in hepatocytes, it may indicate a possible hereditary hemochromatosis (Lefkowitch et al., 1998).

2.2.5. Chronic Hepatitis B

According to various serological, histological, and immunohistochemical results, chronic hepatitis B progresses through several phases (Fattovich, 2003). Liver biopsy results may show interface hepatitis or lobular hepatitis, depending on the histological activity. Low activity levels are more typical, though. Immunohistochemistry can be used to demonstrate the surface antigen, HBsAg (Figure 2.16). It is primarily found in the distinctive ground glass hepatocytes. At this stage of infection, the ground glass cells are usually dispersed singly throughout the parenchyma (Figure 2.15(B0).

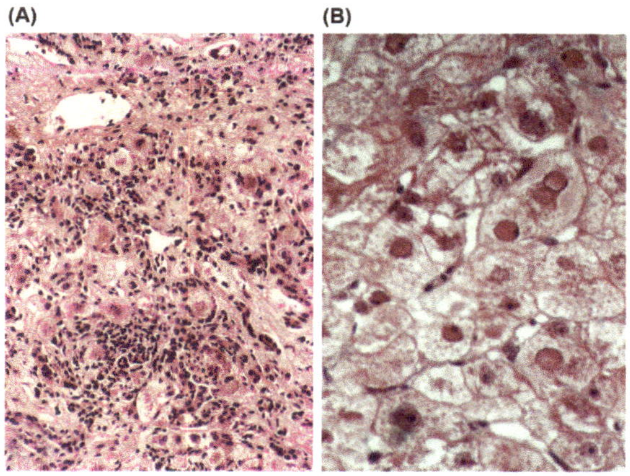

Figure 2.15. *Mild chronic hepatitis. (A) Periportal interphase hepatitis. Mononuclear infiltration is observed in the portal tract and hepatocytes in the vicinity are surrounded by lymphocytes. H&E. (B) Hepatitis by HBV. Smooth hepatic nuclei with ground glass cytoplasm is shown. H&E.*

Source: Tsutsumi, et.al., Structure and Ultrastructure of the Normal and Diseased Liver, http://dx.doi.org/10.1016/B978-0-12-804274-8.00002-3.

Immunostaining can detect the core antigen HBcAg, which is primarily found in hepatocyte nuclei (Figure 2.16). Positive nuclear staining is associated with a high viral load. Hepatocyte nuclei containing large amounts of core protein may look pale and uniform on H&E-stained sections, referred to as "sanded" (Figure 2.15(B)). The progression of hepatitis B is intricate and not always straightforward. It is characterized by varying degrees of fibrosis, depending on the severity and timing of the infection. Cirrhosis can develop at any stage, especially in patients with co-infections like hepatitis C virus (HCV) and hepatitis D virus (Mathurin et al., 2000). In chronic hepatitis B, there are additional features such as ground glass hepatocytes, HBV antigens, and variations in hepatocyte nuclei size and appearance. Close interactions between hepatocytes and lymphocytes also occur, reflecting the immunological nature of the disease (Bianchi, 1994).

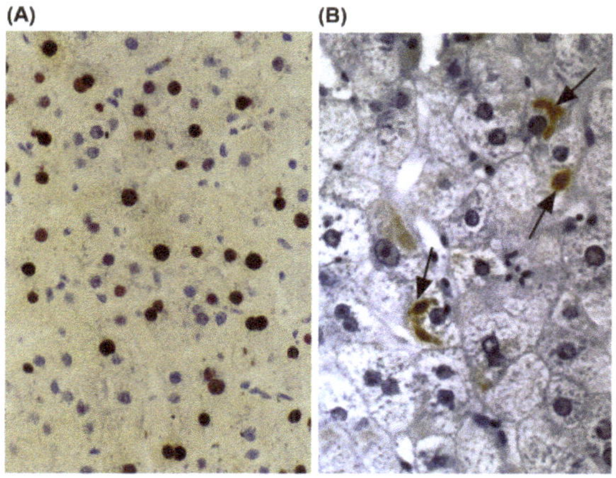

Figure 2.16. *Chronic viral hepatitis. (A) AgcHBV labels are seen in the hepatocyte nuclei. (B) Chronic viral hepatitis. AgsHBV are present in the hepatic cytoplasm (arrows). Immunoperoxidase.*

Source: Tsutsumi, et.al., Structure and Ultrastructure of the Normal and Diseased Liver, http://dx.doi.org/10.1016/B978-0-12-804274-8.00002-3.

2.2.6. Chronic Hepatitis C

Until cirrhosis manifests, which usually happens decades after hepatitis first appears, this infection is usually not fatal. The histological characteristics of chronic hepatitis C are highly characteristic, despite not being entirely diagnostic in and of themselves (Scheuer et al., 1992). Numerous lymphocytes, some of which have noticeable germinal centers, frequently assemble into aggregates or follicles within the portal infiltrate. Important characteristics also include steatosis and chronic nondestructive cholangitis. Though they are not unique to hepatitis C, the follicles are also present in hepatitis B, AIH, and primary biliary cirrhosis. In hepatitis C, however, they are more prevalent and noticeable. Acidophilic hepatocyte degeneration and the creation of acidophil bodies are common interlobular alterations.

Confluent necrosis is uncommon. Sinusoids are focally or diffusely infiltrated by lymphocytes. Iron deposition is seen not only in hepatocytes, but also in macrophages, endothelial cells, and portal tracts. Steatosis is more common in hepatitis C than in other forms of chronic hepatitis and may be quite severe (Fartoux et al., 2005). It is a risk factor for progression and can interfere with therapy. The steatosis is often associated with obesity, diabetes, and alcohol consumption. The mechanism for steatosis may be interference by the viral core protein with lipoprotein assembly and secretion. Additionally, features of steatohepatitis such as pericellular fibrosis have been reported. In biopsies taken early in the course of the disease, the hepatitis is often mild, with little interface hepatitis or fibrosis. With time, fibrous septa extend from expanded portal tracts and link vascular structures. A pericellular pattern of fibrosis in perivenular areas has been reported in children (Badizadegan et al., 1998). Spontaneous clearance of viruses or specific treatment of the infection may bring about dramatic improvement of the fibrosis and structural changes.

2.2.7. Autoimmune Hepatitis

When there are no other known causes of chronic hepatitis, serum autoantibodies, polyclonal hypergammaglobulinemia, and histological changes are the main factors used to diagnose AIH. Histological evidence is crucial for both diagnosis confirmation and the identification of other disorders that can be mistaken for AIH, such as drug-induced liver injury.

Even though AIH does not have pathognomonic histological features, many patients do have a characteristic picture before treatment. The biopsy reveals extensive hepatocellular damage and a significant lymphocyte and plasma cell infiltrate in the portal tracts, at the interface, and deep within the parenchyma, indicating active disease (Figure 2.17(A)). The amount of lymphoid follicles is lower than in hepatitis C. In cases of bridging necrosis, hepatocytes that survive frequently form hepatic rosettes. AIH may become more likely if adult hepatitis is accompanied by prominent syncytial giant hepatocytes. Although the clinical onset of AIH can occasionally be acute, all patients are thought to have a chronic illness. Corticosteroid therapy usually has a quick effect on AIH patients. After treatment, a biopsy reveals variable degrees of resolution of the necroinflammatory process as well as occasionally a marked improvement in structural changes and fibrosis. Relapse is predicted by the level of plasma cell infiltration, and fibrosis progression appears to be correlated with worsening histological activity. As a result, biopsy is still crucial to the treatment of patients.

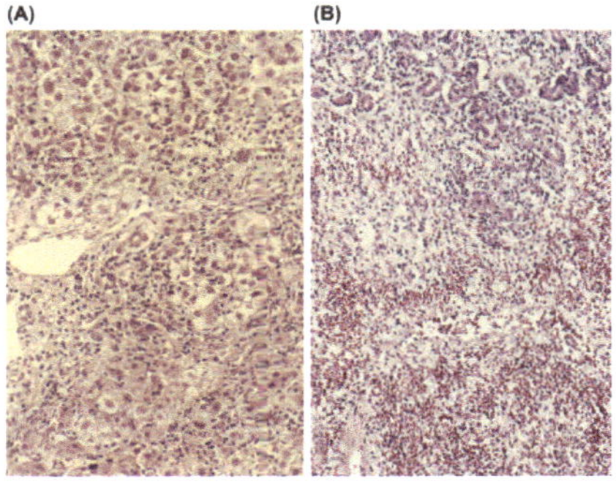

Figure 2.17. *(A) Autoimmune hepatitis. Damaged hepatocytes are forming irregular acinar groups. Inflammatory reactions are mainly by lymphocytes and monocytes. (B) Idiopathic fulminant hepatitis characterized by a panlobular hepatocellular necrosis. A cholangiolar reaction is observed at the upper part of the picture.*

Source: Tsutsumi, et.al., Structure and Ultrastructure of the Normal and Diseased Liver, http://dx.doi.org/10.1016/B978-0-12-804274-8.00002-3.

2.2.8. Cirrhosis

The diffuse process of cirrhosis results in the replacement of normal lobules with anatomically abnormal nodules divided by fibrous tissue (Anthony, 1994). The nodules, which are primarily caused by regenerative hyperplasia after hepatocellular injury, have a significant disruption of vascular relationships and are functionally less efficient than normal hepatic parenchyma.

Nodules and fibrosis are the two main histological criteria used to diagnose cirrhosis. The diagnosis is made with ease when there are distinct round nodules encircled by fibrous septa (Figure 2.20). The only possible misunderstanding relates to recent bridging necrosis, which can be handled by looking for elastic fibers in the stains and paying attention to clinical information. As a result, a pathologist and clinician must communicate in order to diagnose cirrhosis, which cannot be precisely compared to a histological stage. Simple tissue fragmentation during biopsy or laboratory processing ought to raise the suspicion of cirrhosis on its own. The assessment of structural alterations ought to be conducted through reticulin preparation, ideally without counterstaining. This might reveal characteristics that are hidden by other stains. Even in nodules that closely resemble normal liver, there are noticeable structural changes. These changes include an approximation of portal tracts and terminal venules, as well as the aberrant orientation of reticulin fibers brought on by varying patterns and rates of growth in various areas. In comparison to the number of portal tracts, which can occasionally be abnormally small and poorly formed, the number of venules may be abnormally large. Sepsis is a more noticeable anatomical abnormality in cirrhosis because it connects the portal tracts and central veins.

The livers of patients with cirrhosis may exhibit hepatocytes that appear normal in appearance and arrangement, while in other cases, there are noticeable abnormalities in growth. Regeneration is indicated by the thickening of liver cell plates. Hepatocytes in hyperplastic regions typically contain minimal to no lipofuscin pigment, even near terminal venules. Regeneration may not always be apparent in cases of cirrhosis as it is not a constant process. Therefore, the lack of evidence of regeneration does not rule out the diagnosis of cirrhosis.

The existence of neighboring populations of hepatocytes that are growing at different rates and have distinct cell and nuclear characteristics is a very distinctive feature of cirrhosis. The anomalies in reticulin pattern, most notably the propensity for reticulin fibers to lie in different directions in distinct growth areas, are caused by pleomorphism.

Nodular regenerative hyperplasia should be taken into consideration in the differential diagnosis when there is nodularity and regeneration evidence combined with minimal or absent fibrosis. Congenital hepatic fibrosis is characterized by ductal plate malformation and intact acinar architecture. The differential diagnosis between active cirrhosis and chronic hepatitis that has not progressed to the stage of cirrhosis is made in cases of chronic hepatitis with fibrosis and structural abnormalities. Well-differentiated HCC can typically be identified from cirrhotic nodules. In the latter, there are more abnormalities in the architecture of the cell plate, there may be little to no reticulin, and the cells exhibit malignant cytological traits. Furthermore, hepatocellular siderosis is usually absent in HCC tumor cells but frequently appears incidentally in cirrhosis of various etiologies.

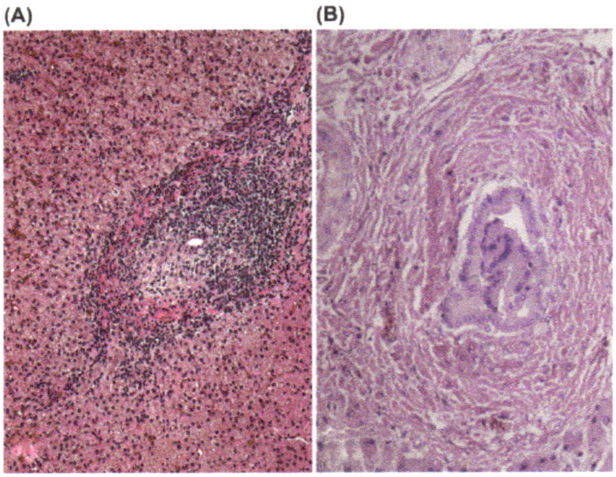

Figure 2.18. *(A) Primary biliary cirrhosis. A lymphoid aggregate and a follicle with a germinal center mark the former sites of the bile duct. The margins of the tract are blurred by fibrous and interface hepatitis. (B) Primary sclerosing cholangitis. Concentric collagen fibers surrounding biliary duct. H&E.*

Source: Tsutsumi, et.al., Structure and Ultrastructure of the Normal and Diseased Liver, http://dx.doi.org/10.1016/B978-0-12-804274-8.00002-3.

Viral hepatitis (B, C, D), alcoholism, obesity, insulin resistance/metabolic syndrome, biliary diseases, metabolic disorders (hemochromatosis, Wilson's disease, a1-antitrypsin deficiency, etc.), blockage of the venous outflow, medications and poisons, and autoimmune diseases are the primary causes of cirrhosis. Diverse patterns in nodules and fibrosis could indicate various underlying reasons. If there is perinodular edema, ductular reaction, and chronic cholestasis, irregularly shaped nodules may indicate a biliary cause (Figure 2.18). Multiple adjacent lobules are replaced by confluent fibrosis, a common feature of several types of cirrhosis, especially after steatohepatitis and chronic hepatitis with an autoimmune or viral etiology. When it comes to the bile ducts, a clear loss of them nearly invariably signifies either primary sclerosing cholangitis or primary biliary cirrhosis. In cases of primary sclerosing cholangitis, periductal fibrosis may be highly visible. Although ductular reaction is a nonspecific finding, it frequently indicates biliary disease when it is severe and focal (Figures 2.18 and 2.19).

Occluded, narrowed, or recanalized veins suggest that the cirrhosis may be the result of venous outflow block, but are also found in cirrhosis from other causes. Portal and hepatic venous thrombosis have indeed been implicated in the progression of cirrhosis in general. Neovascularization of fibrotic portal tracts, areas of confluent fibrosis, and bridging fibrosis septa in cirrhosis produces numerous lymphatic and capillary channels, particularly in chronic hepatitis B and C (Yamauchi et al., 1998).

Alcohol abusers and those at risk for NAFLD, as well as those with drug toxicity or no apparent underlying cause, can develop steatohepatitis. It is important to differentiate steatohepatitis from chronic cholestasis, which also manifests as enlarged hepatocytes containing Mallory-Denk bodies.

The presence of one of the hepatitis viruses is not always the cause of the features of chronic hepatitis, especially lymphocytic infiltration and interface hepatitis. Viral causes are also preferred for liver cell dysplasia. The diagnosis of HBV infection is aided by ground glass hepatocytes, orcein stains, and immunostains for viral antigens; however, tissue evidence of HBV antigen is not always present or detectable. The presence of lymphoid follicles or aggregates should raise the risk of hepatitis C. Excessive plasma cells can be associated with viral hepatitis, but they also increase the risk of AIH. Certain patients exhibit evident and mature cirrhosis, with clearly defined nodules and dense fibrosis suggesting a protracted illness.

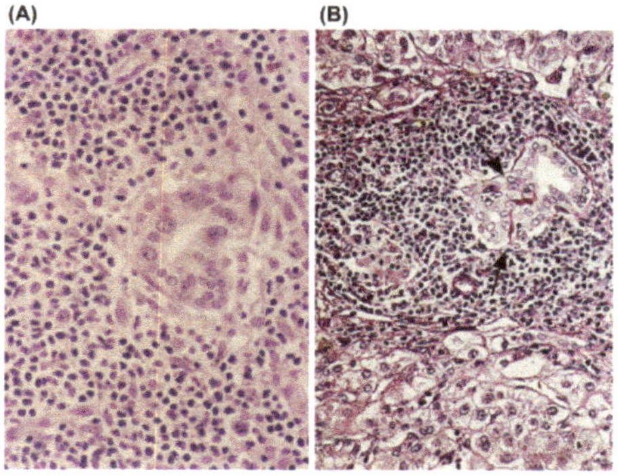

Figure 2.19. *(A) Chronic nondestructive colangitis by HCV. The bile duct shows several layers of different sizes of colangiocytes surounded by abundant mononuclear cells. H&E. (B) Chronic destructive stage I cholangitis in primary biliary cirrhosis. Partial fragmentation of basal membrane (arrows) and lymphocytes and histiocytes infiltration around the biliary duct is shown. PAS-diastase.*

Source: Tsutsumi, et.al., Structure and Ultrastructure of the Normal and Diseased Liver, http://dx.doi.org/10.1016/B978-0-12-804274-8.00002-3.

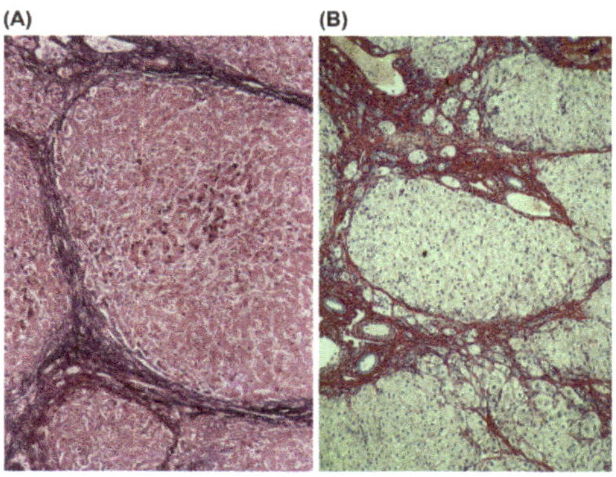

Figure 2.20. *(A) Hepatic cirrhosis by HBV. Regeneration nodules are surrounded by collagen fibers. Orcein stain. (B) Hepatic cirrhosis by nitrofurantoine, Sirian red.*

Source: Tsutsumi, et.al., Structure and Ultrastructure of the Normal and Diseased Liver, http://dx.doi.org/10.1016/B978-0-12-804274-8.00002-3.

In certain cases, it's unclear if a patient has fibrosis or cirrhosis(Figure 2.20). Cirrhosis may appear to be in its early stages of development or to be incipient (Ishak et al., 1995). Reversion to a normal lobular pattern is unlikely once cirrhosis has fully developed. Indeed, there is debate over whether cirrhosis is reversible (Friedman, 2003). Normal liver cell plate structure and vascular relationships are not always restored by therapy-induced diminished fibrosis.

2.2.9. Liver Neoplasms

Most tumor-like nodular lesions or neoplasms can be categorized based on the putative cells of origin (hepatocytes, bile duct epithelium, and endothelium) from which they originate. Histogenesis can frequently be distinguished by immunohistochemistry.

2.2.10. Liver Cell Adenoma

These benign tumors are made of hepatocytes and can be single or multiple in nature. They are typically not encapsulated, but they are clearly defined macroscopically. Tumor cells bear a striking resemblance to normal hepatocytes. Mitoses are hardly ever observed, and nuclei are tiny and regular. The cells are grouped in thickened or normal trabeculae, with prominent arteries and blood vessels with thin walls strewn throughout. As in cholestatic liver, small liver cell rosettes (acini) with an empty or bile-filled central lumen may be observed. Reticulin levels in adenomas are normal or slightly lower, but significant loss is typically limited to regions of necrosis or hemorrhage. These conditions are common in adenomas in oral contraceptive users and are the cause of pain and the potentially fatal hemoperitoneum complications (Tao, 1991).

2.2.11. Focal Nodular Hyperplasia

This type of lesion is rather common, occurring in both sexes and at any age. It is a putative preexisting artery malformation-induced reactive, hyperplastic response of polyclonal hepatocytes, fibrous stroma, and bile ductules. The nodules can clearly be distinguished macroscopically from the typical hepatic parenchyma. They have a similar appearance to cirrhosis because they are typically pale and are divided into nodules by fibrous septa. Histologically, the appearance resembles that of inactive cirrhosis quite a bit. Large, thick-walled arteries that can occasionally narrow are found within the dense fibrous septa, along with bile duct-like structures that are most likely derived from progenitor cells or metaplastic liver cell plates.

2.2.12. Nodular Regenerative Hyperplasia

Multiple hyperplastic parenchymal nodules with thickened liver cell plates are observed in this condition; however, fibrosis is either nonexistent or very minimal. This sets the lesion apart from cirrhosis. Numerous diseases, including rheumatoid arthritis, myeloproliferative disorders, and chronic venous congestion, are linked to this pathology. Therapeutic medications such as corticosteroids, anabolic steroids, oral contraceptives, antineoplastics, anticonvulsants, and immunosuppressive agents may have been administered to patients with this issue. Portal hypertension is present in certain nodular regenerative hyperplasia patients. There could be an increase in gamma glutamyl transpeptidase and serum alkaline phosphatase (Wanless, 1990). Further, Wanless (1994) categorized nodular regenerative hyperplasia, focal nodular hyperplasia, and partial nodular transformation together under the heading of "nodular transformation" because they all exhibit liver cell hyperplastic growth in the form of nodules.

2.2.13. Hemangioma

The most frequent benign tumor of the liver, a cavernous hemangioma is occasionally discovered in biopsy material and discovered by accident during an autopsy or surgery. A small number grow to a size that is clinically significant. Similar to other locations, the lesions consist of channels lined with endothelium that are held up by a fibrous stroma. This endothelial-lined channels are either empty or occasionally contain lymph and leukocytes. Peliosis is not the same as cavernous hemangiomas; it is distinguished by the absence of fibrous trabeculae and the entire endothelium layer. Although it is extremely uncommon, liver lymphphangioma has been described as a single hepatic lesion or as a component of multiorgan lymphangiomatosis.

2.2.14. Malignant Lesions

- ***Precursors of Hepatocellular Carcinoma:*** Premalignant or precursors of HCC have been identified in many hepatocellular alterations and nodular lesions. It is unclear exactly which histologic and molecular alterations occur in what is thought to be a multistep pathogenesis of human HCC. Liver cell dysplasia of the small or large cell type can be seen in varying degrees in nonneoplastic liver tissue. Enlarged, hyperchromatic nuclei found in small hepatocytes grouped in dense clusters are the hallmarks of small cell dysplasia. High rates of cellular proliferation and general cytologic similarities to HCC are present in the foci, which could be the product of progenitor cells (Nakanuma et al., 1993). Even though it is the most common, large cell dysplasia is not thought to be a strong precursor to HCC. Its distribution is haphazard within lobules or cirrhotic nodules, and it should be differentiated from the nuclear morphological variation observed in perivenular hepatocytes with aging, cholestasis, or methotrexate therapy.

Additional cellular alterations that have been linked to premalignancy include bulging nodules, irregular regeneration areas exhibiting hepatocyte glycogenosis, intracytoplasmic Mallory-Denk bodies, and oncocytic change. The macroregenerative nodule, which appears in cirrhosis or other chronic liver diseases, is an exceptionally large regenerative nodule with a diameter of 0–8 cm or more (Terada et al., 1993). The dysplastic nodule, also known as the borderline nodule, exhibits abnormal architectural and/or cytological characteristics that are incongruous with a benign macroregenerative nodule but do not meet the diagnostic criteria for a true HCC. Large and small cell dysplasia in varying degrees, increased cellularity, foci where the liver cords are less cohesive, focal loss of reticulin fibers, and pseudoacini are all possible features of dysplastic nodules (Gastaldi et al., 1995).

- ***Hepatocellular Carcinoma:*** Geographic variations in the incidence and prevalence of HCC, along with a multifactorial etiology, have been identified by epidemiological and other studies (Di Bisceglie et al., 1998). When combined with other risk factors like iron overload, exposure to aflatoxin, hepatitis B and C viral infections, and the existence of fatty liver disease, chronic liver necrosis and inflammation play a significant role in the multistep process of hepatocarcinogenesis.

The majority of HCCs develop in cirrhotic liver (Anthony, 1994). The cause of cirrhosis is usually known, even in many cases labeled as "cryptogenic," where risk factors for NAFLD become apparent. The noncirrhotic setting accounts for a substantial number of cases from North America and elsewhere (Kondo et al., 2014) and can be seen in HBV carriers or suspected occult hepatitis B and in individuals infected with HCV (el-Refaie et al., 1996). The cirrhosis associated with carcinoma is often macronodular in pattern (Figure 2.21), except for the micronodular cirrhosis seen in genetic hemochromatosis and chronic hepatitis C. The cirrhosis is usually inactive, although inflammation and necrosis may be seen near the tumor itself.

The tumor cells' similarity to normal hepatocytes and their arrangement to the trabeculae of normal liver are the most notable histological characteristics of HCC. However, reticulin is frequently sparse or nonexistent, and trabeculae are generally thicker (Figure 2.22). A network of vascular channels lined by endothelium that is positive for immunostain for CD34, factor VIII related antigen, and other molecules exists between the tumor trabeculae in HCC (Dhillon et al., 1992). In the fine needle aspirates, the endothelial lining of these channels is a very useful diagnostic feature. Although focal areas of fibrosis may occur after tumor necrosis, connective tissue stroma is rare, except fibrolamellar carcinoma. As sclerosing carcinoma, this type of HCC (Omata et al., 1981) is frequently linked to hyperkalemia; certain tumors seem to have bile duct rather than hepatocellular origins.

At a cellular level, variants include giant-cell forms with multinucleated tumor cells, spindle-cell or sarcomatoid tumors, and clear-cell carcinomas. The latter must be distinguished from metastatic renal adenocarcinoma.

When there is doubt about the hepatocellular origin of a carcinoma, further evidence can sometimes be gained from the characteristics of the tumor cells. In HCC, these often contain fat and glycogen and may also contain $\alpha 1$ -antitrypsin globules even in patients without genetic $\alpha 1$-antitrypsin deficiency.

Mallory-Denk bodies are commonly found in the cytoplasm of the tumor cells. Evidence of hepatocellular origin is also provided when immunohistochemical stains of paraffin sections are positive for albumin, fibrinogen, liver cell cytokeratins, α1-antitrypsin, or α1-antichymotrypsin.

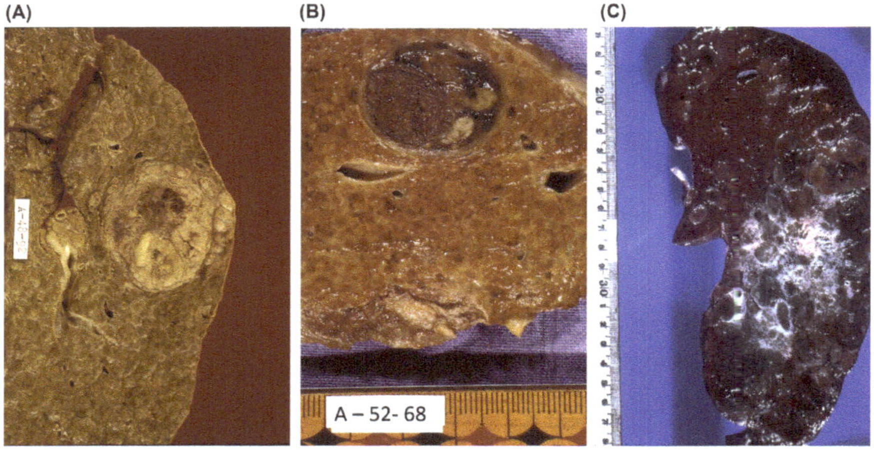

Figure 2.21. *Macroscopy. (A) Primary hepatic cell carcinoma with macronodular cirrhosis. (B) Hepatic cell carcinoma in micronodular cirrhosis. Abundant extravasated bilis is shown. (C) Fibrolaminar hepatocarcinoma. Several neoplasic nodules are seen.*

Source: Tsutsumi, et.al., Structure and Ultrastructure of the Normal and Diseased Liver, http://dx.doi.org/10.1016/B978-0-12-804274-8.00002-3.

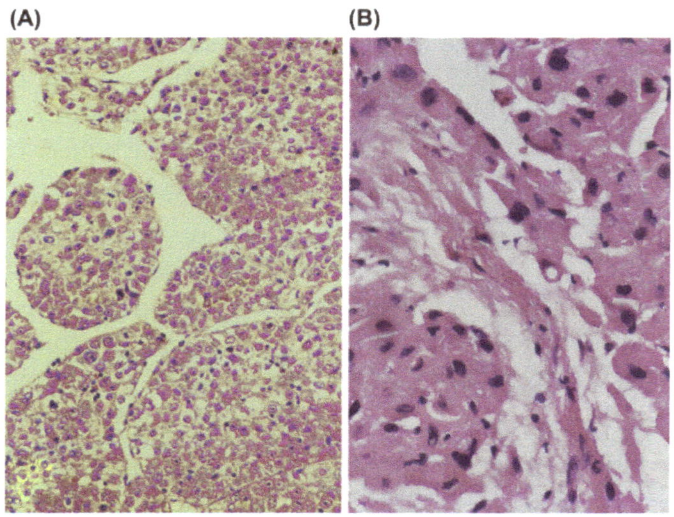

Figure 2.22. *(A) Hepatocellular carcinoma with trabecular pattern. Nodules of neoplasic cells separated by connective tissue are observed. (B) Fibrolaminar hepatocarcinoma. H&E.*

Source: Tsutsumi, et.al., Structure and Ultrastructure of the Normal and Diseased Liver, http://dx.doi.org/10.1016/B978-0-12-804274-8.00002-3.

2.2.15. Fibrolamellar Carcinoma

Because it is more resectable than a typical HCC, this tumor has a better prognosis and typically develops in noncirrhotic liver in adolescents and young adults (Craig et al., in 1980). Lesions can be solitary or multiple, with a central fibrous scar that sometimes mimics macroscopically focal nodular hyperplasia. Large, densely eosinophilic tumor cells are separated into groups by fibrous lamellae arranged in parallel; these tumor cells produce transforming growth factor-beta. The eosinophilia is caused by an abundance of mitochondria. In certain instances, the tumor exhibits characteristics of both typical HCC and fibrolamellar carcinoma, and some fibrolamellar carcinomas have neuroendocrine characteristics.

2.2.16. Bile Duct Carcinoma (Cholangiocarcinoma)

Anywhere in the liver, between the papilla of Vater and the smaller branches of the biliary tree, bile duct cancer can develop. According to Gorses (2003), there are three main anatomic types: the first is located intrahepatically, the second is at the junction of the left and right hepatic ducts (Klatskin tumor), and the third is derived from the extrahepatic bile ducts.

Bile duct carcinomas are, under a microscope, reactive, desmoplastic fibrous stroma-containing adenocarcinomas that secrete mucin. Within these tumors, a medium to small uniform gland size is frequently maintained. Tumor cells can take on a papillary pattern and are cuboidal or columnar in shape. To differentiate cholangiocarcinoma from a metastatic tumor, it is helpful to look for features such as free stromal mucin, small groups and isolated tumor cells in the fibrous stroma, the coexistence of abnormal tumor cells and seemingly normal epithelium, dysplasia, or carcinoma in situ within a duct-like structure (Weinbren & Mutum, 1983).

The histopathological information gathered from studies on liver diseases in humans serves as a crucial foundation for various experimental research projects on liver diseases at numerous reputable institutions (Figure 2.23). To refresh our understanding of the organ's histology, we first provide a brief overview of the normal structure of the liver, highlighting some of its ultrastructural features. Additionally, we succinctly discuss the most commonly observed liver pathologies in clinical settings. Given the liver's numerous vital functions, there is a significant risk of a high mortality rate associated with diseases affecting this organ.

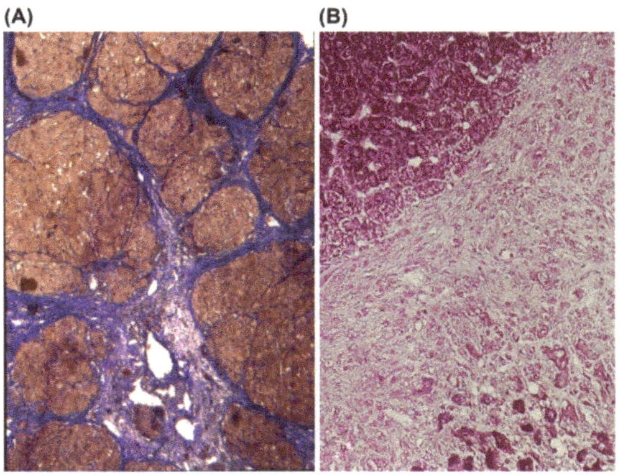

Figure 2.23. *(A) Experimental cirrhosis in rat treated with carbon tetroxide. Collagen fibers are surrounding parenchymal nodules of different sizes (Masson stain). (B) Experimental hepatocellular carcinoma produced in rat treated with diethyl nitrosamine (DEN) for 18 weeks. Neoplasic hepatocytes are seen at the lower right and surrounded by dense fibrous tissue (H&E).*

Source: Tsutsumi, et.al., Structure and Ultrastructure of the Normal and Diseased Liver, http://dx.doi.org/10.1016/B978-0-12-804274-8.00002-3.

An essential diagnostic tool for the assessment and treatment of patients with liver diseases is the histopathological examination of liver tissue taken from biopsies. Because the concepts and classification of liver diseases are based on morphology, structural studies continue to be important even in the face of an increasing number of new and sophisticated radiological methodologies, gene tests, and molecular studies. Furthermore, one of the most direct ways to see the morphologic alterations that affect the liver in disease is to look at a liver biopsy specimen under a microscope. Applying modern molecular and genomic medicine techniques to liver biopsy material can also answer questions of a more fundamental pathobiological nature.

A Closer Look

Liver Biopsy

A liver biopsy is a medical procedure in which a small sample of liver tissue is removed for examination under a microscope. This diagnostic tool is crucial for evaluating various liver conditions, including hepatitis, cirrhosis, fatty liver disease, and liver cancer. It provides detailed information that cannot be obtained through blood tests or imaging studies alone, making it invaluable for accurate diagnosis, prognosis, and treatment planning.

The procedure can be performed in several ways, with percutaneous liver biopsy being the most common. In this method, a needle is inserted through the skin into the liver to obtain the tissue sample. Ultrasound or CT guidance is often used to ensure precise placement of the needle and to minimize the risk of complications. Other techniques include transjugular liver biopsy, where the sample is taken via a catheter inserted into a neck vein, and laparoscopic liver biopsy, which involves small abdominal incisions and the use of a camera to guide the biopsy.

Before the procedure, patients typically undergo a series of pre-biopsy evaluations, including blood tests to assess clotting ability and imaging studies to identify the optimal biopsy site. Patients are usually advised to avoid certain medications, such as blood thinners, that could increase bleeding risk. On the day of the biopsy, local anesthesia is administered to numb the area, and in some cases, sedatives are given to help the patient relax. The actual biopsy takes only a few minutes, but patients are usually observed for several hours afterward to monitor for any immediate complications.

Liver biopsies, while generally safe, do carry some risks. The most common complication is pain at the biopsy site, which can usually be managed with pain relief medications. Bleeding is another concern, occurring in a small percentage of patients, and in rare cases, severe bleeding may require hospitalization or surgical intervention. Infection is a less common but potential risk, necessitating sterile techniques during the procedure. Additionally, patients may experience transient anxiety or discomfort due to the invasive nature of the biopsy.

The tissue sample obtained from a liver biopsy undergoes histopathological analysis, which can reveal the presence and extent of liver disease, including fibrosis, inflammation, and abnormal cells indicative of malignancy. This detailed examination allows healthcare providers to stage liver diseases accurately, assess the effectiveness of treatments, and make informed decisions about future therapeutic strategies. In cases of unexplained liver dysfunction, a biopsy can provide clarity and guide appropriate management.

Despite the invaluable insights provided by liver biopsies, the procedure has limitations. Sampling error is a notable issue, as the tiny tissue fragment may not represent the entire liver's condition. Moreover, the interpretation of biopsy results requires significant expertise, and there can be variability among pathologists. Advances in non-invasive diagnostic tools, such as elastography and biomarkers, are emerging as complementary methods, though they have not yet fully replaced the need for liver biopsies.

In summary, liver biopsy remains a cornerstone in hepatology, offering critical diagnostic and prognostic information for a wide range of liver disorders. Its ability to provide direct insight into liver pathology ensures it continues to be a relevant and essential procedure despite the advent of new diagnostic technologies. While it carries certain risks, careful patient selection, meticulous technique, and thorough post-procedure monitoring help mitigate these concerns, ensuring that the benefits of liver biopsy significantly outweigh the potential drawbacks.

Summary

- The structural organization of the liver, composed of parenchymal and vascular elements, is adapted to the special functions as a guardian present between the intestinal tract and the rest of the organism
- Hepatocytes are responsible for most of the synthetic and many of the metabolic functions of the liver. They are relatively large polygonal cells averaging about 20–30 mm in cross-section
- The canalicular membrane is modified for bile excretion, whereas the sinusoidal surface is equipped for the extraction of a great variety of molecules from the blood and for the simultaneous secretion into the blood of other molecules that have been modified or synthesized by hepatocytes.
- The Golgi complex consists of well-developed lamellae associated with many vesicles. The most conspicuous feature of these stellate cells is the occurrence of lipid droplets in the cytoplasm.
- These cells are named liver-associated natural killer (NK) cells. They represent a morphologically and functionally modified form of peripheral blood NK cells. They are localized inside the lumen of the sinusoid, closely adhering to the endothelial cells and Kupffer cells, and often extending well-developed pseudopodia suggestive of migration along the sinusoidal wall.
- The great number of functions that are performed by the liver, its special structural organization, its strategic localization in the human body, and the characteristic and special sensibilities of its different cellular components constitute important factors that lead to variable diseases of the organ.
- Steatosis or fatty change of fatty liver is the accumulation of abnormal amounts of lipids in 5% or more hepatic cells.
- Chronic hepatitis is a common reason for persistently abnormal liver function tests and forms the background for the development of cirrhosis and HCC. It is defined as the persistence of liver injury with raised aminotransferase levels or viral markers for more than 6 months.
- Carcinoma of the bile ducts can arise anywhere between the papilla of Vater and the smaller branches of the biliary tree within the liver.

References

1. Aita, K., Jin, Y., Irie, H., Takahashi, I., Kobori, K., Nakasato, Y., Kodama, H., et al. (2001). Are there histopathologic characteristics particular to fulminant hepatic failure caused by human herpesvirus-6 infection? A case report and discussion. *Human Pathology, 32*(8), 887–889.
2. Anthony, P. P. (1994). In *Pathology of the Liver*. Churchill Livingstone.
3. Badizadegan, K., Jonas, M. M., Ott, M. J., Nelson, S. P., & Perez-Atayde, A. R. (1998). Histopathology of the liver in children with chronic hepatitis C viral infection. *Hepatology, 28*(5), 1416–1423.

4. Bamber, M., Murray, A., Arborgh, B. A., Scheuer, P. J., Kernoff, P. B., & Thomas, H. C. (1981). Short incubation non-A, non-B hepatitis transmitted by factor VIII concentrates in patients with congenital coagulation disorders. *Gut, 22*(10), 854–859.

5. Bianchi, L., & Gudat, F. (1994). In *Chronic Hepatitis*. Churchill Livingstone.

6. Brunt, E. M. (2007). Pathology of fatty liver disease. *Modern Pathology, 20*(S1), S40–S48.

7. Chu, C. W., Hwang, S. J., Luo, J. C., Wang, Y. J., Lu, R. H., Lai, C. R., et al. (2001). Comparison of clinical, virologic and pathologic features in patients with acute hepatitis B and C. *Journal of Gastroenterology and Hepatology, 16*(2), 209–214.

8. Craig, J. R., Peters, R. L., Edmondson, H. A., & Omata, M. (1980). Fibrolamellar carcinoma of the liver: A tumor of adolescents and young adults with distinctive clinico-pathologic features. *Cancer, 45*(2), 372–379.

9. Dhillon, A. P., Colombari, R., Savage, K., & Scheuer, P. J. (1992). An immunohistochemical study of the blood vessels within primary hepatocellular tumours. *Liver, 12*(5), 311–318.

10. Di Bisceglie, A. M., Carithers Jr., R. L., & Gores, G. J. (1998). Hepatocellular carcinoma. *Hepatology, 28*(5), 1161–1165.

11. Dianat, N., Dubois-Pot-Schnider, H., Steichen, C., Desterke, C., Leclerc, P., Raveux, A., et al. (2014). Generation of functional cholangiocytes-like cells from human pluripotent stem cells and HepaRG cells. *Hepatology, 60*(2), 700–714.

12. el-Refaie, A., Savage, K., Bhattacharya, S., Khakoo, S., Harrison, T. J., el-Batanony, M., et al. (1996). HCV-associated hepatocellular carcinoma without cirrhosis. *Journal of Hepatology, 25*(3), 277–285.

13. Elias, H. (1949). A re-examination of the structure of the mammalian liver; parenchymal architecture. *American Journal of Anatomy, 85*(3), 311–333.

14. Fartoux, L., Chazouilleres, O., Wendum, D., Poupon, R., & Serfaty, L. (2005). Impact of steatosis on progression of fibrosis in patients with mild hepatitis C. *Hepatology, 41*(1), 82–87.

15. Fattovich, G. (2003). Natural history and prognosis of hepatitis B. *Seminars in Liver Disease, 23*(1), 47–58.

16. Fawcett, D. W. (1955). Observations on the cytology and electron microscopy of hepatic cells. *Journal of the National Cancer Institute, 15*(4), 1475–1503.

17. Ferrari, C., & Mondelli, M. (2009). In *The Liver: Biology and Pathobiology* (Vol. 51). Wiley-Blackwell.

18. Friedman, S. L. (2003). Liver fibrosis—From bench to bedside. *Journal of Hepatology, 38*(1), S38–S53.

19. Gastaldi, M., Massacrier, A., Planells, R., Robaglia-Schlupp, A., Portal-Bartolomei, I., Bourliere, M., et al. (1995). Detection by in situ hybridization of hepatitis C virus positive and negative RNA strands using digoxigenin-labeled cRNA probes in human liver cells. *Journal of Hepatology, 22*(4), 509–518.

20. Gores, G. J. (2003). Cholangiocarcinoma: Current concepts and insights. *Hepatology, 37*(5), 961–969.

21. Ishak, K., Baptista, A., Bianchi, L., Callea, F., De Groote, J., Gudat, F., et al. (1995). Histological grading and staging of chronic hepatitis. *Journal of Hepatology, 22*(6), 696–699.

22. Kaneda, K. D., & Wake, K. (1983). Pit cells as natural killer cells. *Biomedical Research, 4*, 567–576.

23. Klotz, O., & Belt, T. H. (1930). The pathology of the liver in yellow fever. *American Journal of Pathology, 6*(5), 663–688.

24. Kondo, R., Nakashima, O., Sata, M., Imazeki, F., Yokosuka, O., Tanikawa, K., et al. (2014). Pathological characteristics of patients who develop hepatocellular carcinoma with negative results of both serous hepatitis B surface antigen and hepatitis C virus antibody. *Hepatology Research, 44*(11), 1039–1046.

25. Le, T. H., Caldwell, S. H., Redick, J. A., Sheppard, B. L., Davis, C. A., Arseneau, K. O., et al. (2004). The zonal distribution of megamitochondria with crystalline inclusions in non-alcoholic steatohepatitis. *Hepatology, 40*(5), 1423–1429.

26. Lefkowitch, J. H., Yee, H. T., Sweeting, J., Green, P. H., & Magun, A. M. (1998). Iron-rich foci in chronic viral hepatitis. *Human Pathology, 29*(2), 116–118.

27. Liaw, Y. F., Chu, C. M., Chen, T. J., Lin, D. Y., Chang-Chien, C. S., & Wu, C. S. (1982). Chronic lobular hepatitis: A clinicopathological and prognostic study. *Hepatology, 2*(3), 258–262.

28. Mathurin, P., Thibault, V., Kadidja, K., Ganne-Carrie, N., Moussalli, J., El Younsi, M., et al. (2000). Replication status and histological features of patients with triple (B, C, D) and dual (B, C) hepatic infections. *Journal of Viral Hepatitis, 7*(1), 15–22.

29. Morita, Y., Ueno, T., Sasaki, N., Kuhara, K., Yoshioka, S., Tateishi, Y., et al. (2005). Comparison of liver histology between patients with nonalcoholic steatohepatitis and patients with alcoholic steatohepatitis in Japan. *Alcoholism: Clinical and Experimental Research, 29*(12 Suppl.), 277S–281S.

30. Naito, M., Hasegawa, G., Ebe, Y., & Mitsuyama, M. (1999). In *Liver Diseases and Hepatic Sinusoidal Cells*. Springer.

31. Nakanuma, Y., Terada, T., Ueda, K., Terasaki, S., Nonomura, A., & Matsui, O. (1993). Adenomatous hyperplasia of the liver as a precancerous lesion. *Liver, 13*(1), 1–9.

32. Okuno, T., Sano, A., Deguchi, T., Katsuma, Y., Ogasawara, T., Okanoue, T., et al. (1984). Pathology of acute hepatitis A in humans. Comparison with acute hepatitis B. *American Journal of Clinical Pathology, 82*(2), 162–169.

33. Omata, M., Peters, R. L., & Tatter, D. (1981). Sclerosing hepatic carcinoma: Relationship to hypercalcemia. *Liver, 1*(1), 33–49.

34. Rappaport, A. M. (1973). The microcirculatory hepatic unit. *Microvascular Research, 5*(3), 212–228.

35. Rojkind, M., & Reyes-Gordillo, K. (2009). In *The Liver: Biology and Pathobiology* (Vol. 28). Wiley-Blackwell.

36. Roskams, T., De Vos, R., Van Eyken, P., Myazaki, H., Van Damme, B., & Desmet, V. (1998). Hepatic OV-6 expression in human liver disease and rat experiments: Evidence for hepatic progenitor cells in man. *Journal of Hepatology, 29*(3), 455–463.

37. Sasaki, N., Ueno, T., Morita, Y., Nagata, E., & Sata, M. (2006). Usefulness of serum hepatic fibrosis markers in the diagnosis of nonalcoholic steatohepatitis (NASH). *Hepatogastroenterology, 53*(71), 678–681.

38. Scheuer, P. J., Ashrafzadeh, P., Sherlock, S., Brown, D., & Dusheiko, G. M. (1992). The pathology of hepatitis C. *Hepatology, 16*(4), 567–571.

39. Tao, L. C. (1991). Oral contraceptive-associated liver cell adenoma and hepatocellular carcinoma. Cytomorphology and mechanism of malignant transformation. *Cancer, 68*(3), 341–347.

40. Terada, T., Ueda, K., & Nakanuma, Y. (1993). Histopathological and morphometric analysis of atypical adenomatous hyperplasia of human cirrhotic livers. *Virchows Archiv A: Pathological Anatomy and Histopathology, 423*(5), 381–388.

41. Ueno, T., Sugawara, H., Sujaku, K., Hashimoto, O., Tsuji, R., Tamaki, S , et al. (1997). Therapeutic effects of restricted diet and exercise in obese patients with fatty liver. *Journal of Hepatology, 27*(1), 103–107.

42. van Furth, R. (1989). Origin and turnover of monocytes and macrophages. *Current Topics in Pathology, 81*, 125–150.

43. Van Steenbergen, W., Joosten, E., Marchal, G., Baert, A., Vanstapel, M. J., Desmet, V., et al. (1985). Hepatic lymphangiomatosis. Report of a case and review of the literature. *Gastroenterology, 89*(6), 1968–1972.

44. Wake, K. (1980). Perisinusoidal stellate cells (fat-storing cells, interstitial cells, lipocytes), their related structure in and around the liver sinusoids, and vitamin A-storing cells in extrahepatic organs. *International Review of Cytology, 68*, 303–353.

45. Wanless, I. R. (1990). Micronodular transformation (nodular regenerative hyperplasia) of the liver: A report of 64 cases among 2,500 autopsies and a new classification of benign hepatocellular nodules. *Hepatology, 12*(4), 787–797.

46. Wanless, I. R. (1994). In *Pathology of the Liver*. Churchill Livingstone.

47. Weinbren, K., & Mutum, S. S. (1983). Pathological aspects of cholangiocarcinoma. *Journal of Pathology, 141*(2), 217–238.

48. Wisse, E. (1972). An ultrastructural characterization of the endothelial cell in the rat liver sinusoid under normal and various experimental conditions, as a contribution to the distinction between endothelial and Kupffer cells. *Journal of Ultrastructural Research, 38*(5), 528–562.

49. Wisse, E., Braet, F., Luo, D., Vermijlen, D., Eddouks, M., Konstandoulaki, M., et al. (1999). In *Liver Diseases and Hepatic Sinusoidal Cells*. Springer.

50. Yamauchi, Y., Michitaka, K., & Onji, M. (1998). Morphometric analysis of lymphatic and blood vessels in human chronic viral liver diseases. *American Journal of Pathology, 153*(4), 1131–1137.

Chapter 3

AUTOIMMUNE HEPATITIS

Contents

Introduction

Autoimmune hepatitis is an inflammatory liver disease that self-perpetuates and has no known cause. It is linked to humoral and cellular immune responses that are promiscuous against homologous self-antigens (Czaja, 2001, 2007, 2015b). Through the production of neoantigens and the targeting of epitopes with increasing heterogeneity through "epitope spread," disruptions in signaling, apoptotic, and regulatory pathways can prolong and sustain innate and adaptive immune responses (Hintermann et al., 2011); Czaja & Montano-Loza, 2014; Czaja, 2015b). Major Histocompatibility Complex (MHC) genes may influence the presentation and choice of foreign antigens that mimic self-antigens (Donaldson et al., 1991; Doherty et al.,1994; Strettell et al., 1997; Czaja, 2008), and polymorphisms not located on the MHC can influence the disease's severity and clinical manifestation (Cookson et al., 1999; Agarwal et al., 2000, 2007; Hiraide et al., 2005). Age, location, and ethnicity can all affect the type, amount, and frequency of antigen exposure (Fainboim et al., 1994; Pando et al., 1999; Zolfino et al., 2002; Czaja & Carpenter, 2006; Czaja, 2009, 2013), and the protracted period of time that passes between the development of the disease and the loss of tolerance to self-antigens may restrict the ability to pinpoint the etiological trigger (Czaja, 2015b).

Homeostatic mechanisms that regulate the trafficking of inflammatory and immune cells to sites of liver injury (chemokines) (Czaja, 2014b; Marra & Tacke, 2014) or that modulate the differentiation and proliferation of activated lymphocytes (cytokines) (Montano-Loza & Czaja, 2014) may become imbalanced and strengthen cell-mediated and antibody-dependent mechanisms of liver cell injury. The receptor-mediated or extrinsic pathway of apoptosis may become overactive and promote excessive hepatocyte loss, especially in periportal areas (interface hepatitis) (Kerr et al., 1979; Fox et al., 2001; Bai & Odin, 2003; Czaja, 2014d), and the generation of apoptotic bodies may exceed the capacity for their removal and strengthen the adaptive immune response in a selfamplification loop (Savill et al., 2002; Guicciardi & Gores, 2010).

In a different self-amplification loop, reactive oxygen species (ROS) can prolong and sustain the loss of hepatocytes and encourage fibrosis. (Czaja, 2002; 2014a,c, 2015b). Kupffer cells can be activated by apoptotic bodies, and when Kupffer cells are activated, they can release reactive oxygen species (ROS), which may prompt the conversion of hepatic stellate cells into myofibroblasts (Canbay et al., 2003a,b; Zhan et al.,2006). More ROS can then be released by myofibroblasts as they expand the extracellular matrix. Additionally, oxidative stress can trigger an intrinsic apoptotic pathway and increase the permeability of the mitochondrial outer membrane (MOM) (Czaja, 2014d). Additional apoptotic bodies can be generated in order to maintain a self-amplification loop that intensifies hepatic fibrosis and liver cell death, release reactive oxygen species (ROS), encourage apoptosis, and sustain the activation of Kupffer cells (Czaja, 2014d, 2015b).

Reactive nitrogen species (RNS) have been linked to liver cell injury, and the agents of nitrosative stress—nitric oxide, peroxynitrite, nitrotyrosine, and nitrosothiols—can interact with the agents of oxidative stress, superoxide, peroxides, hydroxyl radicals, and singlet oxygen (Radi et al., 1991; Sanz-Cameno et al., (2002); Calcerrada et al., 2011; Grattagliano et al., 2014). Nitrosative stress is the overproduction or underelimination of unstable nitrogen-containing molecules, which can cause necrosis of the liver cells, inflammation, apoptosis, and changes in mitochondrial function. Autoimmune hepatitis's pathogenic mechanisms are still up for debate and conjecture. They are a patchwork of empirically supported findings from animal models, cell culture experiments, and sparse human experience (Figure 3.1).

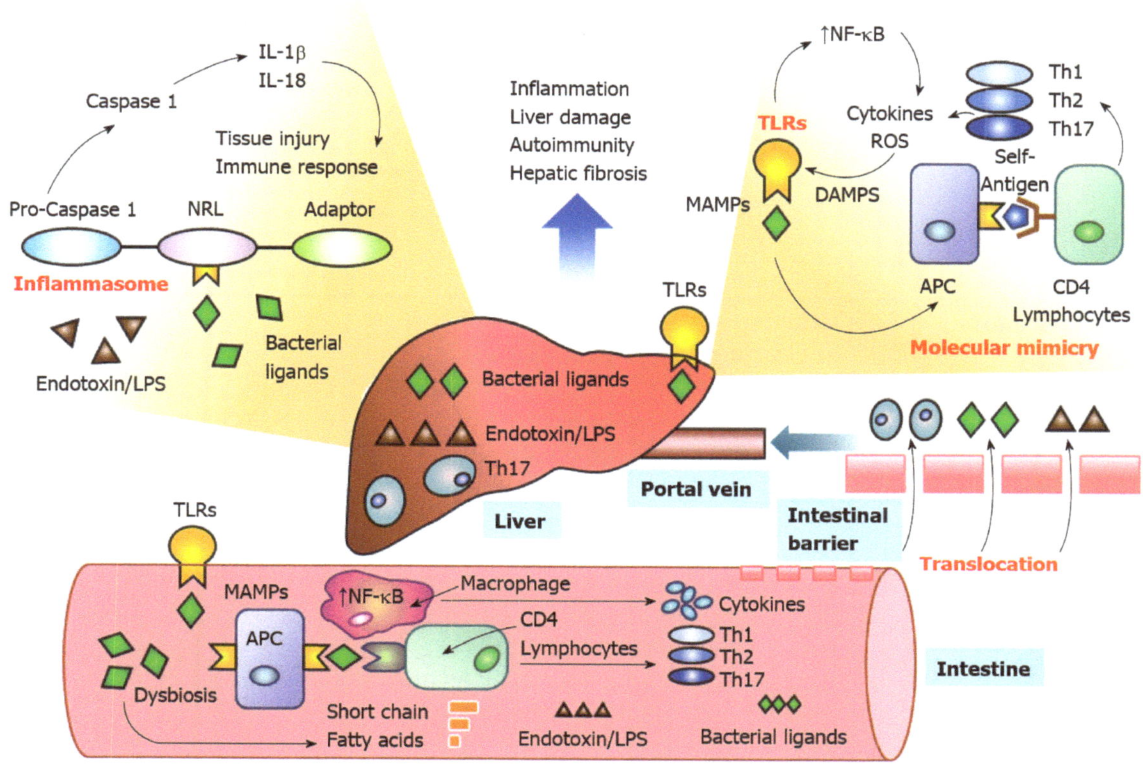

Figure 3.1. *Integrated pathogenic pathways of autoimmune hepatitis.*

Source: https://f6publishing.blob.core.windows.net/09cfc362-9344-4d6d-82c1-05387b8a3d1d/WJG-22-9257-g002.jpg

There is still speculation regarding the relationships between the mechanisms described in precise and well-defined experimental models and the real interactive network of molecular and cellular mechanisms causing the illness. The purpose of this review is to present the evidence supporting different aspects of the pathogenic process and to motivate further research aimed at combining these aspects into a comprehensive, long-lasting understanding. This allows for the design, assessment, and integration of carefully chosen therapeutic interventions into subsequent management plans.

Orientation and Directional Terms

Term	Definition	Illustration
Reactive oxygen species' (ROS)	Reactive oxygen species' (ROS) is an umbrella term for an array of derivatives of molecular oxygen that occur as a normal attribute of aerobic life. Elevated formation of the different ROS leads to molecular damage, denoted as 'oxidative distress'.	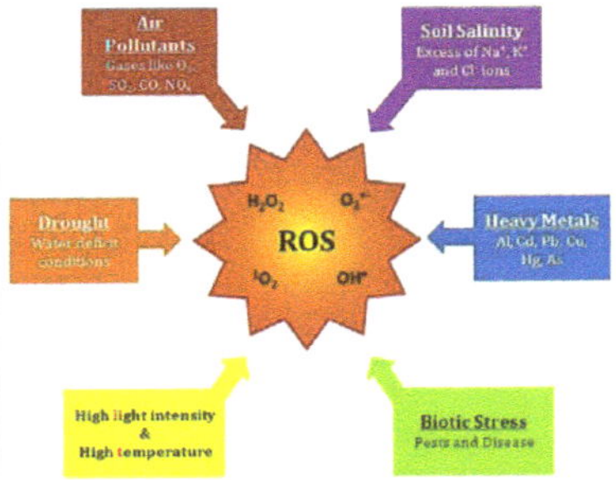
Reactive nitrogen species (RNS)	Reactive nitrogen species (RNS) are various nitric oxide-derived compounds, including nitroxyl anion, nitrosonium cation, higher oxides of nitrogen, S-nitrosothiols, and dinitrosyl iron complexes.	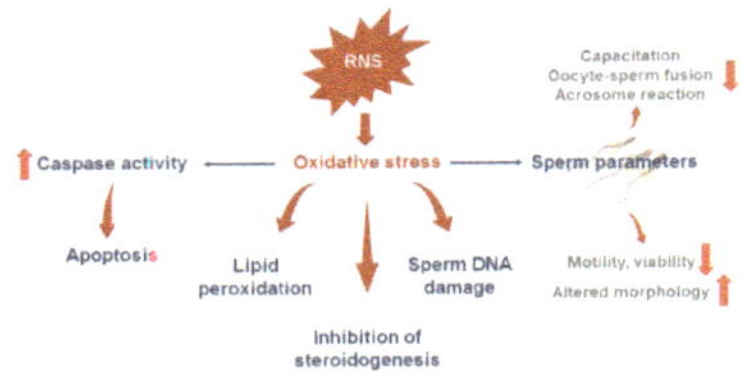
Tumor necrosis factor (TNF)	Tumor necrosis factor is a cytokine and member of the TNF superfamily, which consists of various transmembrane proteins with a homologous TNF domain. It is the first cytokine to be described as an adipokine as secreted by adipose tissue. TNF signaling occurs through two receptors: TNFR1 and TNFR2.	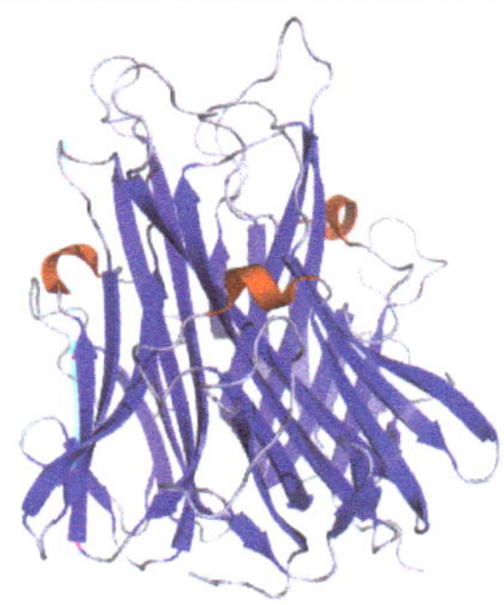
Antinuclear antibodies (ANA)	Anti-nuclear antibodies (ANA) are possible signs of autoimmune diseases, such as lupus, scleroderma, Sjögren's syndrome, juvenile arthritis, or polymyositis and dermatomyositis. White blood cells in the body's immune system make antibodies to spot and attack foreign agents that cause infections or disease.	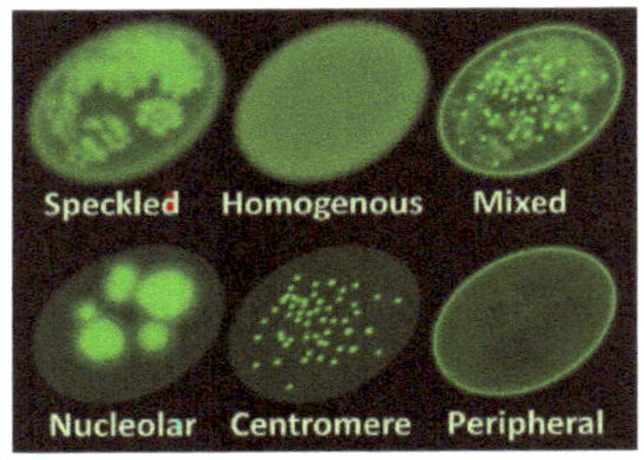
Natural killer (NK)	Natural killer (NK) cells are effector lymphocytes of the innate immune system that control several types of tumors and microbial infections by limiting their spread and subsequent tissue damage.	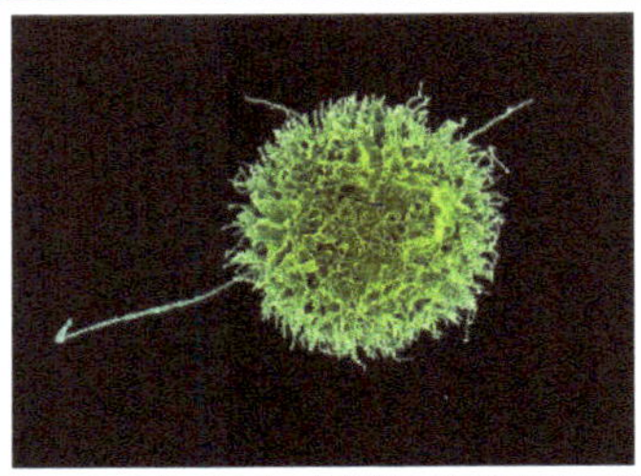

3.1. Selection and Presentation of Indigenous Foreign Antigens

Class II MHC molecules, expressed on the membrane surface of professional antigen-presenting cells (macrophages and dendritic cells), select and present foreign antigens to naïve CD4+ T helper lymphocytes (Czaja, 2008; Ganguly et al., 2013; ; Montano-Loza and Czaja, 2014; Mbongue et al., 2014). The processed antigen is positioned inside the class II MHC molecules' antigen binding groove; the composition of this groove influences the antigens that are chosen as well as the MHCeantigen complex's capacity to activate CD4+ T helper lymphocytes (Brown et al., 1988, 1993; Stern et al., 1994; Dessen et al., 1997). An invariant DRa chain and a polymorphic DRb chain constitute the class II MHC molecule, and three hypervariable regions (HVR) within the DRb chain influence the selection and presentation of antigens (Brown et al., 1988; Czaja et al., 2002a). HVR1 and HVR3 are located at the base of the antigen binding groove, and they influence the type of peptide that can be presented. HVR3 is located on the a-helical portion of the DRb chain, and it can affect peptide binding and interact with the T cell antigen receptor (TCR) of naïve lymphocytes to encourage their activation (Czaja et al., 2002a).

3.1.1. Genetic Factors

The antigen binding groove's amino acid sequences are encoded by genes found in the MHC, which also control the groove's structure and the kind of peptide that can be presented (Doherty et al., 1998; Czaja, 2008, 2002a). The class II MHC molecules' antigen selectivity is not exact or exclusive. Separate MHC molecules with similar antigen binding grooves (a "shared motif") can present the same antigen, as can MHC molecules with similar structural similarities presenting different antigens (Czaja and Donaldson, 2000; Toussirot et al., 1999). Genes that encode similar amino acid sequences within the antigen binding groove can affect susceptibility similarly, and individuals with multiple genes encoding a similar critical amino acid motif may have greater susceptibility or "gene dose" (Strettell et al., 1997; Doherty et al., 1994; Czaja & Donaldson, 2000). A hierarchy of haplotypes has been described in autoimmune hepatitis based on the number of alleles encoding similar amino acid sequences in the antigen-binding groove (Strettell et al., 1997; Doherty et al., 1994). The principal susceptibility alleles for autoimmune hepatitis in white North American and northern European patients reside on the DRB1 gene and they are DRB1*0301 and DRB1*0401 (Opelz et al., 1977; Donaldson et al., 1991; Strettell et al., 1997; Czaja et al., 1997b; Van Gerven et al., 2015). The principal susceptibility alleles in Japan (Seki et al., 1990, 1992; Yoshizawa et al., 2005, 2007), mainland China (Qiu & Ma, 2003), and Mexico (Vazquez-Garcia et al., 1998) are DRB1*0404 and DRB1*0405, and the susceptibility alleles in South Korea are DRB1*0405 and DQB1*0401 (Lim et al., 2008). At positions, DRb67–72 of the antigen binding groove, DRB1*0301 and DRB1*0401 encode a six amino acid sequence (L [leucine], L [leucine], E [glutamic acid], Q [glutamine], K [lysine], and R [arginine]). This amino acid motif has been linked to susceptibility in white North American and northern European patients (Strettell et al., 1997).

A positively charged lysine (K) at position DRb71 may be the main factor influencing susceptibility (Strettell et al., 1997). With the exception of an arginine (R) for lysine (K) at the DRb71 position, the susceptibility alleles DRB1*0404 and DRB1*0405 encode a six amino acid motif at positions DRb67–72 that is similar to that encoded by DRB1*0301 and DRB1*0401 (Czaja, 2008; Czaja & Donaldson, 2000). It is possible that the same triggering indigenous antigens will affect ethnic groups that share these similar antigen binding motifs.

However, in young Argentines, DRB1*1301 is linked to autoimmune hepatitis (Fainboim et al, 1994) and individuals from Brazil (Bittencourt et al., 1999; Goldberg et al.,2001; Czaja et al., 2002b), and the DRB1*03 and DRB1*04 alleles' preferred antigens would not be accommodated by the amino acid motif encoded by this allele. Moreover, DRB1*0405 is linked to adult susceptibility within the same ethnic group and geographic area, while the DRB1*1301 allele primarily affects susceptibility in children (Pando et al., 1999). These findings imply that exposure to structurally distinct native antigens that are preferred by various susceptibility alleles may cause adults and children to develop autoimmune hepatitis. Thus, age disparities within an ethnic group can affect the type and degree of antigen exposure, and ethnic variations can affect the susceptibility to autoimmune hepatitis.

3.1.2. Epistasis

Linkage disequilibrium (epistasis) between MHC genes can also influence the selection of foreign antigens and the incidence of autoimmune hepatitis. By forming associations with other genes that encode the same, similar, or different amino acid motifs within the class II MHC molecule, the predominant gene linked to susceptibility can have its effect strengthened or diminished. Strong linkage disequilibrium exists between DRB1*0301 and DRB3*0101, which both encode a lysine at DRb71, while DRB1*0401 and DRB4*0103, which encode an arginine at DRb71, are in strong linkage disequilibrium (Schreuder et al., 2001; Czaja, 2008). Patients with DRB1*0401 may have a less severe disease because of a decreased density of antigen-presenting molecules with lysine at DRb71, which may attenuate the immune response (Czaja et al., 1993, 1997b; Van Gerven et al., 2015; Kirstein et al., 2015). DQB1*0201, which is in strong linkage disequilibrium with DRB1*07 and DRB1*03 (Czaja et al., 1997a; Bittencourt et al., 1999; Ma et al., 2006), has been proposed as the principal genetic determinant of the autoimmune hepatitis that occurs mainly in European children (Djilali-Saiah et al., 2004). The development of antibodies against liver kidney microsome type 1 (anti-LKM1) is a characteristic of this illness (Homberg et al., 1987; Manns and Czaja, 1995). A number of closely related genes may have an epistatic effect that limits the disease to children of a particular ethnicity or geographic area by influencing antigen selection, presentation, and recognition (Czaja, 2013) (Table 3.1).

Table 3.1. *Factors Influencing Antigen Selection, Recognition, and Targeting in Autoimmune Hepatitis.*

Factor	Features	Significance
Foreign antigens	Presented by class II MHC molecules on APC (Brown et al., 1988) Main APC, dendritic cells (Montano-Loza and Czaja, 2014; Ganguly et al., 2013; Mbongue et al., 2014) Recognized by TCR of $CD4^+$ helper T cells (Doherty et al., 1998) ABG of APC genetically encoded (Toussirot et al., 1999; Strettell et al., 1997) Similar antigens presented by same ABG (Toussirot et al., 1999)	Genes affect antigen selection (Strettell et al., 1997) Multiple similar antigens and genes can trigger AIH (Czaja, 2008) Susceptibility to AIH affected by "gene dose" and epistasis (Strettell et al., 1997; Schreuder et al., 2001)
Susceptibility alleles: Type 1 AIH	North America and northern Europe (Donaldson et al., 1991; Van Gerven et al., 2015; Strettell et al., 1997): • *DRB1*0301* and *DRB1*0401* Japan, China, Mexico (Seki et al., 1990, 1992; Qiu and Ma, 2003; Vazquez-Garcia et al., 1998; Yoshizawa et al., 2005; Yokosawa et al., 2007): • *DRB1*0404* and *DRB1*0405* South Korea (Lim et al., 2008): • *DRB1*0405* and *DQB1*0401* Argentina (children) and Brazil (Fainboim et al., 1994; Pando et al., 1999; Bittencourt et al., 1999; Goldberg et al., 2001; Czaja et al., 2002b): • *DRB1*1301*	Susceptibility genes with shared amino acid motif within ABG present homologous antigenic triggers (Strettell et al., 1997) Susceptibility genes without shared motif within ABG present distinctive antigenic triggers (Czaja et al., 2002b) Antigenic triggers may differ between age groups (Czaja et al., 2002b; Pando et al., 1999)
Susceptibility alleles: Type 2 AIH	North and South America, Europe (Djilali-Saiah et al., 2004; Bittencourt et al., 1999; Czaja et al., 1997a): • *DQB1*0201* • *DRB1*07* and *DRB1*03*	Susceptibility to AIH is age- and region-related (Homberg et al., 1987; Czaja and Manns, 1995; Czaja, 2013)
Molecular mimicry	Homologous epitopes between foreign and self-antigens break immune tolerance of self (Christen and Von Herrath, 2004; Ehser et al., 2013)	Protracted or repeated exposure to viruses may trigger AIH (Fainboim et al., 2001; Kerkar et al., 2003; Manns et al., 1991)
Thymic dysfunction	Induced by drugs, genes, or surgery (Hubert et al., 2011; Watanabe et al., 1987; Hess et al., 1993) May diminish self-tolerance (Hubert et al., 2011)	Mainly conjectural (Vogel et al., 2001) Supported by animal models (Watanabe et al., 1987; Bagavant et al., 2002)
Neoantigens	Apoptotic bodies generate autoantibodies, adaptive response, and hepatic fibrosis (Canbay et al., 2003b; Savill et al., 2002)	Enhances immune response by maintaining self-amplification loop (Savill et al., 2002)
Epitope spread	Broadening of immune response to include increasingly dissimilar epitopes (Hintermann et al., 2011)	Immune response extends beyond original autoantigen (Hintermann et al., 2011)
Promiscuous lymphocytes	Imprecise targeting by activated lymphocytes (Doherty et al., 1998) TCR specificity affected by genetic factors (Manabe et al., 1994)	Adds clonal diversity to otherwise limited number of TCRs (Arenz et al., 1998)
Implicated self-antigens	Cytochrome mono-oxygenase, CYP2D6 (Manns et al., 1989, 1991) Formiminotransferase cyclodeaminase (Lapierre et al., 1999; Muratori et al., 2001)	Associated with type 2 AIH (Manns et al., 1991) Induces experimental AIH (Holdener et al., 2008; Lapierre et al., 2004)

ABG, antigen-binding groove; APC, antigen-presenting cells; *MHC*, major histocompatibility complex; *TCR*, T cell antigen receptor; *AIH*, autoimmune hepatitis.

Source: L. Dara, et al., 2017, Pathogenesis of Idiosyncratic Drug-induced Liver Injury, yhttp://dx.doi.org/10.1016/B978-0-12-804274-8.00005-9.

3.2. Breaking Immune Tolerance of Self-Antigens

The self-antigens- immune tolerance may be lost by molecular mimicry between foreign and self-antigens (Christen & Von Herrath, 2004) or by interference with tolerogenic mechanisms that either favor the induction of immune tolerance or negatively select autoreactive cells (Burnet, 1960; Vogel et al., 2001; Hubert et al., 2011). It has not been determined which mechanism causes autoimmune hepatitis.

3.2.1. Molecular Mimicry

The indigenous antigens that trigger autoimmune hepatitis are unknown, but they are likely to share a common epitope that is also found in self-antigens (molecular mimicry) (Bogdanos et al., 2001; Christen & Von Herrath, 2004). Mice that are infected with an adenovirus expressing human cytochrome, CYP2D6, lose tolerance to mouse homologs of CYP2D6, and they develop experimental autoimmune hepatitis (Ehser et al., 2013). Furthermore, mouse T cells sensitized to human CYP2D6 react to mouse homologs that have intermediate homology to human CYP2D6, whereas they tolerate mouse homologs that have close homology with the human molecule (Ehser et al., 2013). Molecular mimicry rather than molecular identity may be the key mechanism by which foreign antigens break the immune tolerance of self-antigens (Christen & Von Herrath, 2004). The intensity, duration, and frequency of exposure to the foreign antigen may also help override immune tolerance of homologous self-antigen (Fainboim et al., 2001; Vergani et al., 2002).

3.2.2. Disrupted Tolerogenic Mechanisms

The thymus's medullary epithelial cells express antigens specific to particular tissues (Miller et al., 1990; Hanahan, 1998; Hubert et al., 2011), and an autoimmune regulator gene, AIRE, can control self-tolerance of these antigens (Heino et al., 1999; Mathis & Benoist, 2009). AIRE controls how tissue-specific antigens are transferred to dendritic cells, which may then encourage the thymocytes that are specific to those antigens to be deleted (Hubert et al., 2011; Mbongue et al., 2014). Autoimmune polyendocrine syndrome type 1 (APS-1), which can include autoimmune hepatitis, has been linked to homozygous mutations in AIRE (Ahonen et al., 1990; Bjorses et al., 2000; Pitkanen et al., 2000). These findings have provided credence to the theory that AIRE mutations may either be a contributing factor to the development and clinical manifestation of autoimmune hepatitis or suggest that some patients, particularly those who have several immune-mediated disorders occurring at the same time, have an incomplete form of APS-1 (Vogel et al., 2001).

Only 1% of patients with autoimmune hepatitis and 1.7% of patients with primary biliary cholangitis (PBC) have heterozygous mutations of AIRE, and homozygous mutations typical of APS-1 have not been reported (Vogel et al., 2001). These results rule out the possibility that incomplete forms of APS-1 are present in the majority of autoimmune hepatitis patients or that AIRE mutations play a significant role in the development of autoimmune hepatitis. They do not rule out the possibility that thymic dysfunction or compromised immune tolerance in other ways may act as a predisposing factor for autoimmune hepatitis.

Drugs, especially the calcineurin inhibitors, may disrupt the tolerogenic activities of the thymus and contribute to the recurrence or de novo appearance of autoimmune hepatitis after liver transplantation (Beschorner et al., 1988; Hess et al., 1993; Bucy et al., 1993; Czaja, 2012). Neonatal thymectomy has also been an important method by which to induce acute severe (fulminant) autoimmune hepatitis in mice, mainly by depleting the emergence of regulatory T cells (Tregs) and promoting the migration of follicular helper T cells from the spleen (Watanabe et al., 1987; Bagavant et al., 2002; Kido et al., 2008; Aoki et al., 2011). Molecular mimicry has not displaced thymic dysfunction as a hypothesis for breaking self-tolerance, and both concepts require further investigation in autoimmune hepatitis.

3.3. Neoantigens and Epitope Spread

Immune cells that migrate to liver injury sites can generate or reveal new antigenic targets, known as neoantigens, and to broaden the scope of the immune response to include targets with distant homology, a process known as epitope spread. Key neoantigens known as aptotic bodies stimulate hepatic stellate cells, produce autoantibodies, and aid in the adaptive immune response (Savill et al., 2002; Canbay et al., 2003b). Promiscuous targeting by antigen-sensitized lymphocytes is a mechanism by which to spread the antigenic targets and extend the tissue damage within and outside the liver (Doherty et al., 1998).

The clonal diversity of liver-infiltrating lymphocytes' TCRs is restricted (Arenz et al., This limitation implies that TCRs might be able to target antigens with highly variable homologies (promiscuous activity), as noted by, 1998. The dominant autoantigen epitope is the target of the humoral response early in the course of autoimmune hepatitis in humans and animal models. However, later in the disease, this response broadens to include epitopes that are progressively more different from the original autoantigen (Hintermann et al., 2011). The immune response can be sustained and extended through the activation of memory cells, the emergence of new effector cells, and the promiscuous targeting of liver-infiltrating lymphocytes (Christen and Von Herrath, 2004). Genetic variables may influence the antigen specificity of the TCRs and the promiscuity of the activated lymphocytes. Polymorphisms of the TCR constant b gene have been found in patients with autoimmune hepatitis more frequently than in normal subjects (Manabe et al., 1994).

3.4. Implicated Self-Antigens

The primary self-antigen linked to autoimmune hepatitis is cytochrome mono-oxygenase, or CYP2D6 (Manns et al., 1989, 1990, 1991). Antibodies to LKM1 are directed against the recombinant molecule of CYP2D6 (Gueguen et al., 1989; Manns et al., 1991; Ma et al., 2002), and they inhibit the activity of this enzyme in vitro (Manns et al., 1990). In autoimmune hepatitis, liver-infiltrating lymphocytes are particularly sensitive to CYP2D6 (Lohr et al., 1991), and plasmids containing the CYP2D6 antigenic region have been used to immunize animals to produce models of experimental autoimmune hepatitis (Lapierre et al., 2004) or through an adenovirus infection that expresses CYP2D6 (Holdener et al., 2008).

CYP2D6 shares similarities with various foreign antigens, potentially leading to a loss of immune tolerance through molecular mimicry. The recombinant molecule contains multiple epitopes targeted by anti-LKM1 antibodies, which show similarities to amino acid sequencesmm/ in cytomegalovirus, herpes simplex virus type 1, and hepatitis C virus (Manns et al., 1991; Kerkar et al., 2003). Continued or repeated exposure to different viral antigens could be a way to disrupt immune tolerance towards this molecule.

When expressed with CYP2D6 in plasmids and given by immunization, human formiminotransferase cyclodeaminase has also been a significant antigen in the induction of experimental autoimmune hepatitis (Lapierre et al., 2004). Antibodies to liver cytosol type 1 (anti-LC1) target formiminotransferase cyclodeaminase (Lapierre et al., 1999; Muratori et al., 2001), and these antibodies are present in 14–67% of patients with autoimmune hepatitis and anti-LKM1 (Martini et al., 1988; Abuaf et al., 1992; Han et al., 1995; Muratori et al., 1995; Gregorio et al., 1997, 2001). In experimental animal models, autoimmune hepatitis can occur without reactivity to formiminotransferase cyclodeaminase (Holdener et al., 2008), and in human disease, anti-LC1 and anti-LKM1 are not consistently expressed (Han et al., 1995). However, according to Bridoux-Henno et al., (2004) antiLC1 might be the only indicator of autoimmune hepatitis (Martini et al., 1988). may change in a way that could be indicative of an active pathogenic role in relation to disease activity (Muratori et al., 1995, 1998), and could respond to an antigen (formiminotransferase cyclodeaminase) crucial to the development of an animal model for the human illness (Lapierre et al., 2004).

Only a small percentage of autoimmune hepatitis patients worldwide have autoimmune hepatitis linked to anti-LKM1 and anti-LC1 antibodies (Czaja, 2013). The majority of young European children with autoimmune hepatitis have antibodies to LKM1 (Homberg et al, 1987), and only 4% of adult white North American patients with the illness have autoantibodies (Czaja et al., 1992). The age and geographic distribution of LC1 antibodies are similar (Abuaf et al, 1992), and in adults with autoimmune hepatitis in North America, they are also uncommon (Czaja et al., 2004).

The infrequent coexistence of anti-LKM1 and anti-LC1 with the other serological markers of autoimmune hepatitis has justified their distinction as a separate type of autoimmune hepatitis (Czaja & Manns, 1995). Patients with antinuclear antibodies (ANA) and/or smooth muscle antibodies (SMA) constitute most patients with autoimmune hepatitis, and they have been designated as having type 1 autoimmune hepatitis. Patients with anti-LKM1 or antiLC1 have been classified as having type 2 autoimmune hepatitis. These designations have not been endorsed by the International Autoimmune Hepatitis Group, and their justification, especially in adults, has been challenged (Muratori et al., 2015). They have been useful mainly in research studies to ensure the selection of homogeneous study populations.

It is unclear which self-antigen is targeted in the majority of autoimmune hepatitis patients (ANA and/or SMA-positive disease). The enzymes glutathione S-transferase (Aguilera et al.), uridine triphosphate glucuronosyltransferase (Manns & Obermayer-Straub, 1997)... Dec [selenocysteine] transfer ribonucleic acid synthase: Sep [O-phosphoserine] transfer ribonucleic acid (Costa et al., 2000), alpha-actinin (Oikonomou and colleagues, 2011), as well as F1 ATPase subunits, an inner mitochondrial membrane enzyme (Preuss et al., 2012) are possibilities, but none have been proven through thorough clinical or laboratory research or employed in the development of an animal model for the illness that affects humans. Type 1 autoimmune hepatitis may be caused by a variety of self-antigens, some of which may be different in people who have the same clinical phenotype. The self-antigens that cause immunological tolerance to break down and ultimately cause the disease can be influenced by differences in immune status, age, environment, ethnicity, and exposure to antigens.

3.5. Cell Mediators of Liver Injury

Interactions between innate and adaptive immune system cells can result in autoimmune hepatitis. The primary mediators of the innate immune response are dendritic cells and natural killer (NK) cells; the primary mediators of the adaptive immune response are Tregs, gamma delta lymphocytes, natural killer T (NKT) cells, and T helper (Th) lymphocytes (Th1, Th2, and Th17 cells) (Montano-Loza & Czaja, 2014). Gamma delta T lymphocytes, dendritic cells, NK cells, and NKT cells are examples of immune cells with both innate and adaptive qualities. They can develop long-term immunological memory, which is shown by the emergence of antigen-specific TCRs and the production of autoantibodies, or they can act as first responders to liver injury in a rapid migration that is not antigen-specific (adaptive response) (Holtmeier & Kabelitz, 2005; Berzins et al., 2011; Subleski et al., 2011; Mbongue et al., 2014).

3.5.1. Dendritic Cells

Because dendritic cells have receptors for pattern recognition, they can react quickly to signals of distress, such as pathogen- or damage-associated molecular patterns (DAMPs) or PAMPs (Tang et al., 2012a). As proficient antigen-presenting cells, they can also seize, digest, and deliver both self- and foreign antigens to unresponsive CD4+ T helper lymphocytes. In addition to secreting proinflammatory interferons that maintain an inflammatory response, dendritic cells can start an adaptive immune response (Liu, 2005; Shklovskaya and Fazekas De St Groth, 2007; Coquerelle and Moser, 2010; Mbongue et al., 2014). Immune inhibitory actions counterbalance dendritic cells' proinflammatory and immune-stimulatory effects. Dendritic cells have the ability to enhance immune tolerance to endogenous antigens even in the absence of inflammatory distress signals.

Dendritic cells are instrumental in the deletion of antigen-specific precursor T lymphocytes (thymocytes) in the thymus (Mbongue et al., 2014; Hubert et al., 2011), and they can support the generation and function of immunosuppressive, interleukin (IL)-10eproducing Tregs (Ito et al., 2007). The pluripotent nature of dendritic cells positions them as key moderators in the development and maintenance of autoimmune disease, and this position has been supported in experimental animal models and humans with diverse immune-mediated diseases (Ganguly et al., 2013; Lombardi and Khaiboullina, 2014; Mbongue et al., 2014). The production of the proinflammatory cytokine, IL-18 (interferon-gamma inducing factor), by dendritic cells within the spleen and liver has characterized a murine model of fatal autoimmune hepatitis (Ikeda et al., 2014).

3.5.2. Natural Killer Cells

Tissue distress signals trigger an innate immune response in NK cells (Hudspeth et al., 2013; Montano-Loza and Czaja, 2014). Two distinct sets of receptors on NK cells influence how they react to injured cells. The NK cells' killer immunoglobulin G-like receptors (KIRs) can both stimulate and inhibit the progression of disease (Moretta et al., 1995). Stimulatory KIRs lyse stressed cells that do not identify themselves as self by expressing class I MHC molecules (Boyton and Altmann, 2007), and inhibitory KIRs suppress cytolysis and moderate disease activity (Uhrberg et al., 1997). An inherited imbalance between the stimulatory and inhibitory KIRs has been implicated in the occurrence of diverse immune-mediated diseases, and combinations of KIRs have defined haplotypes that may predispose to these diseases (Uhrberg et al., 1997; Boyton and Altmann, 2007; Takeshita et al., 2013). Natural killer group 2 member D (NKG2D) receptors constitute the second set of receptors expressed on NK cells (Gonzalez et al., 2006). These receptors bind to soluble forms of MHC class I related chains A and B (MIC A and MIC B) that are presented on the surface of distressed cells, and they prompt cell lysis (Kahraman et al., 2012). Serum levels of MIC A and MIC B have been low or absent in patients with autoimmune hepatitis, PBC, and primary sclerosing cholangitis, and the role of the NKG2D receptors in immune-mediated liver disease remains unclear (Holdenrieder et al., 2007). NK cells can also interact with antigen-presenting dendritic cells and support an adaptive immune response (Vivier et al., 2011; Barreira & Munz, 2011).

NK cells can survive an experimental viral infection and, upon reactivation, display memory in both lymphoid and nonlymphoid tissues. Adoptive transfer of these NK cells can lead to a rapid expansion of the NK cell population and protective immunity when given to naïve animals that are reexposed to viral infection (Sun et al., 2009). A high NK cell to BEC ratio in liver-derived NK cell and biliary epithelial cell (BEC) preparations will lyse BECs without the need for an autoantigen (innate response). In the presence of autoantigen, it will also activate autoreactive CD4+ T helper lymphocytes (adaptive response). BECs are not lysed if there is a low NK cell-to-BEC ratio. The autoantigen-sensitized T lymphocytes' cytopathic effect is sustained by the ongoing secretion of interferon-gamma (IFN-g) (Shimoda et al., 2015). NK cells have the potential to impact the incidence and severity of immune-mediated liver disease and may serve as a crucial link between the innate and adaptive immune responses (Table 3.2).

Table 3.2. *Principal Effector Cell Populations in Autoimmune Hepatitis*

Key Cell Population	Features	Significance
Dendritic cells	Respond rapidly to cell distress signals (Tang et al., 2012a) Professional APCs (Mbongue et al., 2014; Coquerelle and Moser, 2010; Shklovskaya and Fazekas De St Groth, 2007) Produce pro- and antiinflammatory cytokines (Mbongue et al., 2014; Ito et al., 2007) Promote tolerance to self-antigens (Hubert et al., 2011)	Innate and adaptive immunity (Mbongue et al., 2014; Lombardi and Khaiboullina, 2014) Stimulatory and inhibitory actions (Mbongue et al., 2014) Modulate disease activity (Mbongue et al., 2014; Ganguly et al., 2013) Key in fatal experimental AIH (Ikeda et al., 2014)
Natural killer (NK) cells	KIRs lyse nonself cells (stimulatory) (Moretta et al., 1995; Montano-Loza and Czaja, 2014) KIRs suppress cytolysis (inhibitory) (Moretta et al., 1995; Montano-Loza and Czaja, 2014) Inherited KIR imbalance pathogenic (Boyton and Altmann, 2007; Takeshita et al., 2013) NKG2DRs lyse distressed cells (Gonzalez et al., 2006; Kahraman et al., 2012) May develop immune memory (Sun et al., 2009) Secrete proinflammatory IFN-γ (Shimoda et al., 2015)	Innate and adaptive immunity (Hudspeth et al., 2013; Vivier et al., 2011) Activated by dendritic cells (Barreira Da Silva and Munz, 2011) Implicated in PBC (Shimoda et al., 2015) Low NKG2DR binding in AIH (Holdenrieder et al., 2007)
Th1 lymphocytes	Antigen-sensitized $CD4^+$ T helper cells (Dustin and Shaw, 1999; Montano-Loza and Czaja, 2014) Activated by dendritic cells (Greenfield et al., 1998; Montano-Loza and Czaja, 2014) Differentiate on type 1 cytokine path (Lucey et al., 1996; Peters, 1996)	Mature as cytotoxic $CD8^+$ T cells (Montano-Loza and Czaja, 2014; Lohr et al., 1991) Liver-infiltrating effector cells (Lohr et al., 1991) Induce hepatocyte loss (apoptosis) (Dardalhon et al., 2008)
Th 2 lymphocytes	Antigen-sensitized $CD4^+$ T helper cells (Dustin and Shaw, 1999; Montano-Loza and Czaja, 2014) Differentiate on type 2 cytokine path (Dardalhon et al., 2008) Mediate antibody-dependent cytotoxicity (Vergani et al., 1987)	Mature as B cells and plasma cells (Montano-Loza and Czaja, 2014; Czaja, 2015b) Antiinflammatory actions (Da Rocha Junior et al., 2013; Dardalhon et al., 2008) Expand Treg population (Tran et al., 2012; Del Prete et al., 1993)
Th 17 lymphocytes	$CD4^+$ T helper cells after stimulation by IL-6, TGF-β (Korn et al., 2009; Bettelli et al., 2008) Secrete proinflammatory cytokines (Harrington et al., 2005)	Recruit Th1 cells to injury sites (Harrington et al., 2005) Associated with severity, fibrosis (Zhao et al., 2011)
Natural killer T (NKT) cells	Respond to glycolipids on CD1d (Kitamura et al., 2000; Lalazar et al., 2006) Pro- and antiinflammatory cytokines (Nakano et al., 2012; Linsen et al., 2005)	Innate and adaptive immunity (Subleski et al., 2011; Wu and Van Kaer, 2011) Promote apoptosis and Tregs (Novak and Lehuen, 2011; Nowak and Stein-Streilein, 2007)
Gamma delta lymphocytes	TCRs have gamma and delta chains (Hammerich and Tacke, 2014) Pro- and antiinflammatory actions (Rhodes et al., 2008; Hammerich and Tacke, 2014)	Innate and adaptive immunity (Holtmeier and Kabelitz, 2005; Morita et al., 2000) Increased in AIH (Wen et al. 1992; Martins et al., 1996; Kasper et al., 2009)
Regulatory T lymphocytes	Inhibit proinflammatory genes (Da Rocha Junior et al., 2013) Secrete antiinflammatory cytokines (Fletcher et al., 2009) Induce apoptosis of immune cells (Da Rocha Junior et al., 2013) Impair Th17 and hepatic stellate cells (Marra et al., 2000; Fletcher et al., 2009)	Less number and function in AIH (Longhi et al., 2004) Corrected by steroids, drugs (Longhi et al., 2005; Czaja, 2015a) Defective galactin-9 apoptotic path (Liberal et al., 2012) Discrepant findings (Peiseler et al., 2012a)

AIH, autoimmune hepatitis; *KIR*, killer immunoglobulin G-like receptors; *PBC*, primary biliary cholangitis; *IL*, interleukin; *TGF*, transforming growth factor.

Source: L. Dara, et al., 2017, Pathogenesis of Idiosyncratic Drug-induced Liver Injury, yhttp://dx.doi.org/10.1016/B978-0-12-804274-8.00005-9.

3.5.3. Th1, Th2, and Th17 Lymphocytes

The development of autoimmune hepatitis is closely linked to three T helper lymphocyte populations: Th1, Th2, and Th17. Activated by costimulatory signals produced by their interaction with professional antigen-presenting cells (dendritic cells), Th1 lymphocytes are antigen-sensitized CD4+ T helper lymphocytes (Czaja, 2001, 2015b; Greenfield et al., 1998; Dustin and Shaw, 1999). Th1 lymphocytes differentiate and proliferate along a type 1 (proinflammatory) cytokine pathway characterized by IL-1,

IL-12, tumor necrosis factor-alpha (TNF-a), and IFN-g (Lucey et al., 1996; Peters, 1996; Czaja, 2001, 2015b). They develop into antigenspecific, liver-infiltrating, cytotoxic CD8+ T lymphocytes which can induce hepatocyte loss, mainly by apoptosis (Lohr et al., 1991). Th2 lymphocytes develop from naive CD4+ T helper lymphocytes via a type 2 cytokine pathway, leading to B lymphocytes that then become plasma cells that produce antibodies (Czaja, 2001). IL-4, IL-5, IL-10, and IL-13 are important type 2 cytokines (Lucey et al., 1996; Peters, 1996; Czaja, 2001, 2015b). Th2 lymphocytes are induced mainly by IL-4, and they also secrete IL-4 so that they can expand in an autocrine fashion (Dardalhon et al., 2008). Immunoglobulin produced by the activated plasma cells can form immune complexes on the hepatocyte surface and attract NK cells that destroy the hepatocytes (antibody-dependent cell-mediated cytotoxicity) (Vergani et al., 1987). Th2 lymphocytes produce antiinflammatory cytokines (IL-4, IL-5, IL-9, IL-10, IL-13, and IL-25), and they also inhibit the expression of proinflammatory genes (Da Rocha Junior et al., 2013; Harrington et al., 2005; Dardalhon et al., 2008). These anti-inflammatory properties inhibit Th1 and Th17 lymphocytes, whereas their production of IL-5 expands the Treg population (Del Prete et al., 1993; Tran et al., 2012).

The cytokines IL-6 and transforming growth factor-beta (TGF-b) induce naïve CD4+ T helper lymphocytes to become Th17 cells (Bettelli et al., 2008; Korn et al., 2009). They may be the first group of effector cells to migrate to liver injury sites during the adaptive immune response because of their proinflammatory qualities. Th17 lymphocytes attract Th1 lymphocytes to areas of tissue damage by secreting the proinflammatory cytokines IL-1, IL-6, and TNF-a (Harrington et al., 2005). The proinflammatory cytokine IL-17, which is produced by Th17 lymphocytes, can intensify the inflammatory response by inducing the release of IL-6 (Korn et al., 2009; Zhao et al, 2011). Together with TGF-b, IL-6 can also promote the growth of Th17 cells and suppress the production of Tregs (Bettelli et al., 2006). In addition, Th17 lymphocytes generate IL-22, an anti-inflammatory cytokine that can balance the effects of IL-17 (Ki et al., 2010).

Patients with autoimmune hepatitis have higher levels of Th17 lymphocytes in their peripheral blood and liver tissue, and these cells have been linked to severe inflammatory activity and advanced fibrosis (Zhao et al., 2011). While Th1 and Th2 lymphocytes are the main populations that affect hepatocyte loss, Th17 lymphocytes appear to primarily promote and modulate the inflammatory response.

3.5.4. Natural Killer T Cells

NKT cells have surface markers of NK cells and T lymphocytes, and they have functions that reflect these associations (Wu and Van Kaer, 2011; Montano-Loza and Czaja, 2014; Swain, 2010). NKT cells with a semiinvariant TCR (iNKT cells) are designated as type 1 NKT cells, and they have a limited number of activating antigens (Kumar, 2013). Type 1 NKT cells respond mainly to the glycolipid antigen, a-galactosylceramide, presented by class I (CD1d) MHC molecules (Kitamura et al., 2000; Lalazar et al., 2006). NKT cells without a semiinvariant receptor are designated as noninvariant (non-iNKT) or type 2 NKT cells (Kumar, 2013; Kanamori et al., 2012). Type 2 NKT cells express diverse TCRs that broaden their response to tissue-specific isoforms of sulfatide (30 - sulfogalactosylceramide) presented by CD1d molecules (Blomqvist et al., 2009; Arrenberg et al., 2010; Girardi et al., 2012).

NKT cells can migrate rapidly to sites of tissue damage (innate immune response) (Berzins et al., 2011; Subleski et al., 2011; Wu and Van Kaer, 2011). Glycolipid antigens released by the damaged tissue and presented by CD1d molecules can then sensitize the NKT cells (adaptive immune response) (Van Kaer et al., 2011; Novak and Lehuen, 2011; Zeissig and Blumberg, 2012). Antigenactivated NKT cells secrete proinflammatory (IFN-g and TNF-a) and antiinflammatory (IL-4 and IL-13) cytokines depending on the nature of the antigen (Linsen et al., 2005Berzins et al., 2011; Nakano et al., 2012;Wehr et al., 2013). They also release granzymes and perforin that induce the apoptosis of distressed cells (Novak and Lehuen, 2011), and they activate B lymphocytes by releasing IL-4 (Kitamura et al., 2000).

The capacity of NKT cells to encourage Treg differentiation can partially offset these immune-stimulating effects (Nowak and Stein-Streilein, 2007). NKT cell activity can also be influenced by the competition between sulfatide and a-galactosylceramide for CD1d binding sites on dendritic cells (Kanamori et al., 2012). It is likely that NKT cells have an impact on the incidence and severity of immune-mediated disorders, such as autoimmune hepatitis (Dennert and Aswad, 2006; Cho et al., , 2011; Mattner, 2013), and treatment approaches utilizing glycolipid antigens customized to elicit the intended predominant action are being assessed in human patients with various immune-mediated disorders as well as animal models (Lalazar et al., 2006; Van Kaer et al., 2011; Blumenfeld et al., 2011; Yoshiga et al., 2011; Yang et al., 2012; Mattner, 2013; MontanoLoza and Czaja, 2014).

3.5.5. Gamma Delta Lymphocytes

One gamma chain and one delta chain make up the TCRs of gamma delta lymphocytes, which set them apart from other types of lymphocytes (Hammerich and Tacke, 2014; Montano-Loza and Czaja, 2014). TCRs normally have one alpha chain and one beta chain. Gamma delta lymphocytes have a unique TCR structure that may affect their immunological and inflammatory characteristics. Without antigen priming (innate immune response), gamma delta cells can migrate quickly to tissue damage sites upon recognition of DAMPs (Holtmeier and Kabelitz, 2005). Additionally, class Ib MHC molecules can sensitize them to antigens, leading to the development of immunological memory, or an adaptive immune response (Morita et al., 2000).

According to Hammerich and Tacke (2014), gamma delta cells have the ability to either lyse hepatocytes through the release of cytolytic granules or induce receptor-mediated apoptosis in hepatocytes. By releasing IL-10, they may also suppress the immune system and restrict the growth of the extracellular matrix (Rhodes et al, 2008), decreasing CD8+ cytotoxic T lymphocyte activity (Rhodes et al., , 2008), and inducing hepatic stellate cell receptor-mediated apoptosis (Hammerich et al., 2014). The release of IL-17 and IL-22 may also aid in hepatic regeneration (Rao et al., 2014).

It is unknown how gamma delta lymphocytes function in the development and course of autoimmune hepatitis. There is an increase in gamma delta cells in peripheral blood (Wen et al., 1992) and the liver of individuals suffering from autoimmune hepatitis (Martins et al., , 1996), particularly in the portal regions, however the results are not condition-specific (Kasper et al., 2009). Although their actions are shared by other cell populations and their redundant contributions may be ancillary, supportive, and noncritical, the involvement of gamma delta cells in the immune system and inflammation suggests that they contribute to disease activity.

3.5.6. Regulatory T Lymphocytes

Regulatory T lymphocytes (Tregs) are a specialized subset of T cells that play a critical role in maintaining immune homeostasis and preventing autoimmune diseases. These cells are characterized by the expression of the transcription factor Foxp3, which is crucial for their development and function. Tregs suppress the immune response by inhibiting the activity of effector T cells, dendritic cells, and other immune cells, thereby preventing excessive or inappropriate immune reactions that could damage host tissues. They exert their suppressive functions through various mechanisms, including the secretion of inhibitory cytokines like IL-10 and TGF-β, direct cell-cell contact, and modulation of metabolic pathways. In addition to their role in autoimmunity, Tregs are also involved in controlling inflammation, promoting tissue repair, and maintaining tolerance to commensal microbiota and dietary antigens.

Tregs originate in the thymus as natural Tregs (nTregs) or can be induced in the periphery from conventional CD4+ T cells (induced Tregs or iTregs) under specific conditions. Their development and function are tightly regulated by a network of cytokines, co-stimulatory signals, and transcriptional regulators. Dysregulation of Treg function or number is associated with a variety of immune-mediated diseases, including type 1 diabetes, multiple sclerosis, rheumatoid arthritis, and inflammatory bowel disease. Conversely, Tregs can also be co-opted by tumors to create an immunosuppressive microenvironment, allowing cancer cells to evade immune surveillance.

Research into Tregs has opened up new therapeutic avenues. Enhancing Treg function or numbers holds potential for treating autoimmune and inflammatory diseases, while targeting Tregs to diminish their activity is being explored in cancer immunotherapy. Techniques such as adoptive Treg cell transfer, modulation of Treg-specific pathways, and development of drugs that can selectively expand or inhibit Tregs are under investigation. Furthermore, the manipulation of Tregs in transplantation settings aims to induce tolerance to transplanted organs, reducing the need for long-term immunosuppression.

Overall, regulatory T lymphocytes are indispensable for the fine-tuning of the immune system. Their ability to modulate immune responses makes them a focal point of research, with implications for a wide range of clinical applications from autoimmune disease management to cancer treatment and beyond. Understanding the complex biology of Tregs continues to be a dynamic and evolving field, offering insights that could lead to novel and effective therapies for many challenging medical conditions.

3.6. Molecular Mechanisms of Immune-Mediated Liver Injury

Through molecular mechanisms, cells can migrate to tissue injury sites, interact with one another, cause cell death, encourage tissue repair, or prolong the inflammatory process (Czaja, 2014, 2015b; Montano-Loza and Czaja, 2014). Genetic predispositions may modify homeostatic balance, favor reparative or harmful pathways, and affect the generation of these molecular signals (Czaja, 2008).

3.6.1. Cytokines

Small proteins known as cytokines are released by cells in response to both innate and adaptive immune systems (Peters, 1996; Lucey et al., 1996). They can maintain or increase the activity of the cells from which they are produced in an autocrine manner, and they can stimulate activity in other cells by interacting with particular receptors. Cytokines can have two types of actions: stimulating actions, which amplify or complement the effects of other cytokines, and inhibitory actions, which counteract those effects. The cytokines' net interactive and counter-regulatory effects within the microenvironment control the immune and inflammatory responses. Cytokines are the primary means by which these cells induce tissue damage or facilitate repair, and they are produced and reacted to by each of the cell mediators of liver injury that have been linked to autoimmune liver disease (Montano-Loza and Czaja, 2014; Czaja, 2015b). Individual cells can produce several cytokines, as well as multiples of the same cytokine produced by different cells. The main proinflammatory cytokines are IL-1, IL-6, IL-8, IL-12, IFN-g, and TNF-a. These cytokines make up the type 1 cytokine pathway that is responsible for the clonal expansion of cytotoxic CD8+ T lymphocytes that infiltrate the liver (Lucey et al., 1996; Peters, 1996; Dinarello, 2000; Neurath, 2014). IL-4, IL-10, IL-11, IL-13, and TGF-b are the principal antiinflammatory cytokines, and they constitute the type 2 cytokine pathway involved in the clonal expansion of B lymphocytes into antibody-producing plasma cells (Lucey et al., 1996; Peters, 1996; Dinarello, 2000; Neurath, 2014).

Cytokines of types 1 and 2 are typically counterregulatory. Adapting treatment approaches for various immune-mediated illnesses are predicated on attempting to influence the cytokine environment in a positive way. The use of monoclonal antibodies to TNF-a (infliximab) has shown some preliminary success in treating autoimmune hepatitis (WeilerNormann et al., 2013).

3.6.2. Chemokines

A subclass of cytokines known as chemokines is primarily responsible for controlling the migration of innate and adaptive immune system cells to tissue injury sites (Rollins, 1997; Rossi and Zlotnik, 2000; Czaja, 2014b). At the amino terminus of the chemokine molecule, cysteine (C) residues are conserved, and distinct amino acids (X) divide the conserved motifs (Lee et al., 2009; Takahama and Lei (2012). The type of chemokine is indicated by the arrangement of X amino acids and C residues (C, CC, CXC, and CX3C). The liver's injured cells release chemokines, which act as ligands (L) to draw immune and inflammatory cells to the site of tissue damage that have complementary or cognate receptors (R). The receptors can interact with a variety of ligands linked to immunological and inflammatory responses. At least 50 ligands have been identified for the 19 chemokine receptors that have been identified (Sahin and Wasmuth, 2013). Chemokine ligands and ligand receptors have been linked to the development and maintenance of autoimmune liver disease. They also control the migration of pathogenic inflammatory and immune cells (Lee et al., 2009; Li et al., 2013; Marra & Tacke, 2014; Czaja, 2014b; Landi et al., 2014).

PBC and autoimmune hepatitis both have elevated levels of the chemokines CXCL9 and CXCL10 (Nishioji et al., 2001; Manousou et al,, 2013), and in animal models of autoimmune hepatitis, they have been linked to the severity and course of the disease (Nishioji et al., 2001; Ikeda et al., 2014). Th1 and Th17 lymphocytes are drawn to areas of cell distress and express CXCR3, the cognate receptor of CXCL9 and CXCL10 (Czaja, 2014b; Lee et al., 2009). According to Saeki et al., Tregs can counter the immune response by migrating to the same locations and expressing CXCR3. 2010). Serum levels of CXCL9, CXCL10, and CXCR3 drop with therapy and improvement in disease activity in autoimmune hepatitis and PBC (Manousou et al., 2013; Li et al, 2013) (Table 3.4).

Table 3.3. *Molecular Mechanisms Affecting Immune-Mediated Liver Injury*

Molecular Mechanisms	Features	Significance
Cytokines	Main proinflammatory cytokines (Dinarello, 2000; Neurath, 2014): • IL-1, IL-6, IL-8, IL-12, IFN-γ, and TNF-α Main antiinflammatory cytokines (Dinarello, 2000; Neurath, 2014): • IL-4, IL-10, IL-11, IL-13, and TGF-β	Differentiate immune cells (Peters, 1996; Lucey et al., 1996) Stimulatory and inhibitory actions (Peters, 1996) Modulate inflammatory responses (Peters, 1996) Counter-regulate immune responses (Montano-Loza and Czaja, 2014)
Chemokines	Key chemokines/ligand in AIH (Czaja, 2014b): • CXCL9, CXCL10/CXCR3 Key antifibrotic chemokine/ligand (Karlmark et al., 2010; Aoyama et al., 2010): • CX3CL1 (fractalkine)/CX3CR	Orchestrate cell migrations (Marra and Tacke, 2014; Czaja, 2014b) Increased in AIH and PBC (Nishioji et al., 2001; Manousou et al., 2013) Associated with severity in AIH (Ikeda et al., 2014) Improve with therapy (Li et al., 2013; Manousou et al., 2013)
Receptor-mediated apoptosis (extrinsic)	Cell death receptors activated by ligands (Czaja, 2014d): • Fas/FasL is main death receptor/ligand DISC activate cascade of caspases (Peter and Krammer, 2003) Caspase-3 and caspase-7 cleave DNA (Peter and Krammer, 2003)	Main basis of hepatocyte loss in AIH (Fox et al., 2001) Apoptotic bodies immunogenic (A-Gonzalez et al., 2009; Savill et al., 2002) Apoptotic bodies profibrotic (Canbay et al., 2003b) Self-amplification loop (Canbay et al., 2003a; Czaja, 2014d)
Mitochondrial-induced apoptosis (intrinsic)	ROS increase permeability of MOM (Czaja, 2014d) Cytochrome c efflux forms apoptosome (D'amelio et al., 2008) Procaspase-9 activates caspase cascade (Ekert et al., 2004) Affected by extrinsic path (caspase-8) (Czaja, 2014d)	Second basis of hepatocyte loss in AIH (Fox et al., 2001) Bridged by extrinsic path (Guicciardi and Gores, 2010; Kroemer et al., 2007; Czaja, 2014d) Apoptotic bodies immunogenic (A-Gonzalez et al., 2009; Savill et al., 2002) Apoptotic bodies profibrotic (Canbay et al., 2003b)
Oxidative and nitrosative stress	ROS from hepatocyte mitochondria, P450s (Chambel et al., 2015) NOX4 major pro-ROS liver enzyme (Paik et al., 2014) Glutathione major endogenous antioxidant (Winterbourn, 2008) Nrf2 defends by activating AREs (Nguyen et al., 2003) TGF-β inhibits glutathione synthesis, induces NOX4, inactivates Nrf2, increases ROS (Richter et al., 2015) Aging lowers glutathione, Nrf2 (Suh et al., 2004; Shih and Yen, 2007; Chambel et al., 2015) RNS (nitric oxide, peroxynitrite, nitrotyrosine, nitrosothiols) induce nitrosative stress (Pacher et al., 2007; Squadrito and Pryor, 1998)	ROS damage mitochondria, shorten cell survival, and advance fibrosis (Richter et al., 2015; Paik et al., 2014) Decreased glutathione in cirrhosis (Choi et al., 2014) Increased NO metabolites in AIH (Beyazit et al., 2015a) NO metabolites in severe AIH (Beyazit et al., 2015a) Low vitamin D in AIH (Efe et al., 2014; Beyazit et al., 2015b) Antioxidants improve mortality (Mato et al., 1999) RNS alter protein structure and function and increase in AIH and PBC (Sanz-Cameno et al., 2002; Grattagliano et al., 2014)
Polymorphisms outside MHC	Single nucleotide variations of gene (Czaja, 2008; Cookson et al., 1999; Agarwal et al., 2000, 2007; Hiraide et al., 2005) Diverse and not disease specific (De Boer et al., 2014; Agarwal et al., 2000, 2007; Cookson et al., 1999; Fan et al., 2005b)	May affect phenotype and course (Czaja et al., 1999) Uncertain function and controversial (Czaja, 2015b)

AIH, autoimmune hepatitis; *AREs*, antioxidant response elements in genes; *CXC*, cysteine and amino acid sequence; *DISC*, death inducing signal complex; *IL*, interleukin; *IFN-γ*, interferon-gamma; *MHC*, major histocompatibility complex; *NO*, nitric oxide; *NOX4*, nicotinamide adenine dinucleotide phosphate oxidase 4; *Nfr2*, nuclear factor erythroid 2 related factor 2; *PBC*, primary biliary cholangitis; *RNS*, reactive nitrogen species; *ROS*, reactive oxygen species; *TGF-β*, transforming growth factor-beta; *TNF-α*, tumor necrosis factor-alpha.

Source: L. Dara, et al., 2017, Pathogenesis of Idiosyncratic Drug-induced Liver Injury, yhttp://dx.doi.org/10.1016/B978-0-12-804274-8.00005-9.

Hepatocytes, hepatic stellate cells, and biliary endothelial cells express CX3CL1 (fractalkine) (BourdBoittin et al., 2009; Shimoda & Associates, 2010), with CX3CR1 serving as its cognate receptor (Aoyama et al., 2010). By boosting the expression of the antiapoptotic protein B cell lymphoma-2 (bcl-2) and promoting the survival of inflammatory and immune cells, the CX3CL1/CX3CR1 axis promotes pro- and antiinflammatory responses and may prevent apoptosis (Karlmark et al., 2010). In animal models, the CX3CL1/CX3CR1 axis has been linked to lessened liver fibrosis (Aoyama et al., 2010; Karlmark et al., 2010), potentially through influencing intrahepatic monocyte survival and differentiation (Karlmark et al., 2010).

The interaction between CX3CL1 (fractalkine) and CX3CR1 may also modulate the production of the tissue inhibitor of metalloproteinase-1 and thereby reduce the extracellular matrix (Wasmuth et al., 2008). The production of CX3CL1 and CX3CR1 is increased in chronic liver injury, especially in portal and lobular areas and in regenerating bile ducts (Efsen et al., 2002; Zhang et al., 2011). CCL26 (eotaxin-3), CXCL11, CCL11 (eotaxin 1), CCL20, and CXCL12 (stromal cell-derived factor-1) have also been implicated in the pathogenesis of autoimmune liver disease (Isse et al., 2005; Karlmark et al., 2010; Czaja, 2014b; Landi et al., 2014).

Potential therapeutic targets include ligand receptors and chemokine ligands (Czaja, 2014b). Antibodies that neutralize particular chemokines (monoclonal antibodies to CXCL10, CXCL16, and CCL20), single-domain antibody fragments that bind selectively to their target (nanobodies against CCL2, CCL5, CXCL11, and CXCL12), and synthetic peptides that block receptor activity (inhibitors of CXCR4 binding to CXCL12) are some examples of chemokine-directed therapies that have been tested in animal models and patients with a variety of immune-mediated diseases. The full effect of therapeutic manipulation of the chemoattractant molecules is yet unknown, even though they have a variety of beneficial effects within the homeostatic network.

3.6.3. Receptor-Mediated and Mitochondrial Induced Apoptosis

Apoptosis is the primary cause of hepatocyte loss in autoimmune hepatitis (Fox et al., 2001; Bai and Odin, 2003; Czaja, 2014d). The main route, known as the extrinsic pathway, is receptor-mediated and entails activating death receptors on the hepatocyte membrane. The death receptors that are activated by ligands produced partly by liver-infiltrating CD8+ cytotoxic lymphocytes are Fas (CD95/APO-1), TNF-R1, and TNF-related apoptosis-inducing ligand receptor-1 (TRAIL-R1) and receptor-2 (TRAILR2) (Faubion and Gores, 1999; Guicciardi and Gores, 2010). A death inducing signal complex (DISC) causes the target cell to release caspase-8 and caspase-10, which in turn release caspase-3 and caspase-7 (Peter and Krammer, 2003). Chromosome deoxyribonucleic acid (DNA) cleaves, resulting in cell death.

Liver cell death in autoimmune hepatitis can also occur by a mitochondrial-induced apoptotic pathway (intrinsic pathway) that is triggered mainly by ROS (Kroemer et al., 2007; Czaja, 2014d). ROS generated during the inflammatory response increase the permeability of the MOM (Bai and Odin, 2003; Tsujimoto et al., 2006), and cytochrome c effluxes into the cytoplasm and help form a macromolecular complex (apoptosome) (D'amelio et al., 2008). Procaspase-9 is converted to caspase-9 in the apoptosome, and caspase-9 in turn initiates a cascade of events that results in the activation of the "executioner" caspase-3 and caspase-7 (Rodriguez and Lazebnik, 1999; Ekert et al., 2004; D'amelio et al., 2008). The activation of caspase-8 by the extrinsic apoptotic pathway can also contribute to the activation of the intrinsic apoptotic pathway. Caspase-8 can truncate a proapoptotic protein that can then translocate to the MOM, activate other proapoptotic proteins, and increase the permeability of the MOM (Kroemer et al., 2007; Guicciardi and Gores, 2010; Ma et al., 2013).

Extrinsic and intrinsic pathways of apoptosis both produce free apoptotic bodies, and those that elude macrophages and Kupffer cells can function as neoantigens, extending the immune response by inducing the production of autoantibodies and the adaptive immune response (Savill et al.,2002; A-Gonzalez et al., 2009). ROS, cytokines, and chemokines are released in response to the apoptotic bodies that Kupffer cells absorb (Canbay et al, 2003a,b). Hepatic stellate cells undergo enhanced apoptosis and metamorphose into myofibroblasts. In a self-amplification loop, the myofibroblasts can release ROS, produce extracellular matrix, and encourage hepatocyte apoptosis.

Compared to patients with PBC, individuals with autoimmune hepatitis exhibit higher levels of Fas ligand in their liver tissue and higher expression of the Fas receptor (CD95/APO-1) in their lymphocyte subsets (Fox et al., 2001). In addition, autoimmune hepatitis patients' progenitor cells in their bone marrow have higher levels of apoptotic markers than do healthy individuals (Tsikrikoni et al., 2005). The loss of hepatocytes in autoimmune hepatitis is likely caused by overactive receptor-mediated apoptosis, which also exacerbates hepatic fibrosis (Czaja, 2014d). Since the apoptotic pathways also protect against infection, cancer, and autoimmunity, treatments targeting them have been slow to develop for autoimmune liver disease. Antiapoptotic therapies have the potential to decrease hepatocyte loss while extending the viability of activated immune cells. Treatments that block caspase activity have been tested in both human and experimental diseases, and research on them is highly recommended for autoimmune hepatitis (Czaja, 2014d; D'amelio et al., 2008; Masuoka et al., 2009; Guicciardi and Gores, 2010).

3.6.4. Oxidative Stress

When the production of molecules containing reactive oxygen (superoxide, peroxides, hydroxyl radicals, and singlet oxygen) surpasses the ability of the elimination pathways, oxidative stress results (Richter et al., 2015; Chambel et al., 2015; Czaja, 2016). ROS are primarily byproducts of oxidation reactions that are catalyzed by cytochromes P450. When they build up excessively, they can cause liver cell necrosis, activate hepatic stellate cells, damage mitochondria, induce apoptosis, release proinflammatory cytokines, enhance DNA damage, and promote lipid peroxidation of cell membranes (Samoylenko et al., 2013).

The cytochromes P450 located on the inner membrane of mitochondria are the principal sources of ROS (Danielson, 2002; Meunier et al., 2004; Chambel et al., 2015; Czaja, 2016), but cytochromes P450 within the endoplasmic reticulum also produce ROS (Richter et al., 2015). The oxidation of free fatty acids in peroxisomes is another source of ROS (Paradies et al., 2014). Enzymes implicated in the generation of ROS are the P450 enzymes, peroxisomal oxidases, cyclo-oxygenases, lipo-oxygenases, and nicotinamide adenine dinucleotide phosphate oxidases (NOXs) (Samoylenko et al., 2013). Hepatocytes, Kupffer cells, and hepatic stellate cells that have been stressed or activated are key populations within the liver that generate ROS (Wheeler et al., 2001; Cui et al., 2011; Paik et al., 2014).

The heterodimeric transmembrane enzyme complexes known as NOXs are responsible for transferring electrons produced inside cells to molecules of oxygen outside the cell (Brown and Griendling, 2009; Czaja, 2016). It produces superoxide, which can then change into other ROS like hydrogen peroxide. Different cell types contain different isoforms of NOX, each of which has a unique regulatory subunit. The hepatic fibrosis, oxidative stress, and ROS generation have been most strongly linked to NOX4 (Petry et al., 2006; De Minicis and Brenner, 2007; Paik et al., 2014; Bettaieb et al., 2015). Homeostatic mechanisms involving antioxidants remove the ROS, prevent oxidative damage, and preserve steady-state metabolic activity within the cell. In pathological states, ROS production can be enhanced, and antioxidant protective mechanisms can be deficient (Samoylenko et al., 2013). The main antioxidants that guard against ROS-induced cell damage are glutathione, catalase, superoxide dismutases (SODs), and glutathione peroxidases (Samoylenko et al., 2013) and Czaja (2016). Since glutathione is normally found in large quantities, is widely distributed, and regenerates into glutathione disulfide upon oxidation, it is considered the most significant antioxidant (Winterbourn and Metodiewa, 1994; Winterbourn, 2008). Nuclear factor erythroid 2 related factor 2 (Nrf2) is a transcription factor that constitutes a major defense mechanism against excess ROS (Richter et al., 2015; Chambel et al., 2015; Pall and Levine, 2015). It is bound in the cytoplasm to Kelch-like ECH-associated protein 1 (Keap1), and it is released from Keap1 when ROS are increased (Jain et al., 2008). After translocation to the nucleus and binding to other intranuclear proteins (musculoaponeurotic fibrosarcoma proteins), it promotes the expression of antioxidant response elements (AREs) in genes that encode cytoprotective enzymes (Nguyen et al., 2003). By inhibiting the rate-limiting enzyme glutamate ligase, which is involved in the synthesis of glutathione, TGF-b can subvert the antioxidant defense mechanisms (Arsalane et al., 1997; Czaja, 2016).

TGF-b can also induce NOX4 expression (Boudreau et al., 2012), inhibit the production of SODs, catalase, and glutathione peroxidase (Islam et al., 1997; Michaeloudes et al., 2011), increase the generation of ROS (Sturrock et al., 2006; Carmona-Cuenca et al., 2008), inactivate Nrf2 (Richter et al., 2015), and activate hepatic stellate cells to promote hepatic fibrosis (Proell et al., 2007). Furthermore, ROS can activate TGF-b and replenish its supply in a selfamplification loop by releasing TGF-b from its protein-bound, latent forms (Jobling et al., 2006).

Another process that can impair antioxidant defenses is aging (Czaja, 2016). Reduced glutamate-cysteine ligase activity and glutathione production are linked to aging. In addition, aging raises ROS production, decreases Nrf2 levels, restricts Nrf2's ability to bind to ARE-expressing genes, and is linked to an increased risk of hepatic fibrosis (Suh et al., 2004; Shih and Yen, 2007; Hecker et al., 2009; Thannickal, 2010; Chambel et al., 2015; Richter et al., 2015).

The detrimental impact of ROS derived from NOX on mitochondria and cell survival, as well as their correlation with the progression of hepatic fibrosis (De Minicis and Brenner, 2007; Cui et al., 2011; Paik et al., 2011, 2014) have justified efforts to reduce oxidative stress in diverse chronic liver diseases (Mato et al., 1999; Sanyal et al., 2010; Feld et al., 2011; Esrefoglu, 2012). Glutathione levels are decreased in cirrhosis (Gao and Bataller, 2011; Choi et al., 2014), and ROS levels are increased (Gao and Bataller, 2011; Choi et al., 2014). Metabolites of nitric oxide are more abundant in autoimmune hepatitis than in normal individuals (SanzCameno et al., 2002), and they are associated with severe histological activity (Beyazit et al., 2015a). Antioxidants, such as 25-hydroxy vitamin D, are deficient in autoimmune hepatitis, and this deficiency has been associated with disease severity and fibrosis (Efe et al., 2014; Beyazit et al., 2015b).

Determining the relevant molecular pathways of oxidative stress in autoimmune hepatitis will aid in the identification of site-specific interventions that warrant further investigation (Czaja, 2016). The administration of vitamin A, vitamin K, and B-carotene in particular may have had negative effects. It is noteworthy that meta-analyses have not shown that supplemental antioxidant therapies have been helpful in preventing cancer, cardiovascular diseases, or death (Lee et al., 2001); Bjelakovic et al., 2014; Vrolijk et al.,2015). Any clinical study aiming to understand the mechanisms of oxidative stress must take these uncertainties into account because altering the homeostatic processes that are involved in the maintenance of various cell systems may have far-reaching and unexpected effects.

3.6.5. Nitrosative Stress

Nitrosative stress is caused by the reactive nitrogen-containing molecules nitric oxide, peroxynitrite, nitrosothiols, and nitrotyrosine when they are overproduced or undereliminated (Pryor and Squadrito, 1995; Squadrito and Pryor, 1998; Zhang and Hogg, 2005; Mohiuddin et al., 2006; Pacher et al., 2007; Czaja, 2016). The main intermediate RNS is nitric oxide, which reacts with superoxide to produce peroxynitrite (Pryor and Squadrito, 1995). The conjugation of nitric oxide with thiols and GSH produces nitrosothiols

(Zhang and Hogg, 2005), and the nitration of tyrosine by peroxynitrite and nitrogen dioxide generates nitrotyrosine (Mohiuddin et al., 2006). Oxidative stress and nitrosative stress are interactive. The generation of RNS is in part dependent on the products of oxidative stress, and treatments of oxidative stress have improved manifestations of nitrosative stress (Mani et al., 2006).

Lipid peroxidation and mitochondrial damage can be caused by the potent oxidizing and nitrating agent peroxynitrite (Pryor and Squadrito, 1995; Pacher et al., 2007; Czaja, 2016). Peroxynitrite is a mediator of the oxidation of sulfhydryl groups in both protein and nonprotein substrates. It also nitrates proteins, changing their structure and function, thereby causing posttranslational modifications in proteins (Song et al., 2014). Nitric oxide derivatives are increased in cirrhosis (Albillos et al., 1995); inducible nitric oxide synthase (iNOS), nitrotyrosine, and nitrosothiols are increased in PBC and autoimmune hepatitis (Sanz-Cameno et al., 2002; Grattagliano et al., 2014); and the progression of PBC has been associated with increased levels of nitrosothiols (Grattagliano et al., 2014). The principal modulator of nitrosative stress is thioredoxin, which can suppress the formation of peroxynitrite and cleave nitrosothiols (Zhou et al., 2008). Therapeutic intervention targeting the interactive and counter-regulatory mechanisms of oxidative and nitrosative stress is a promising avenue, and organelle-specific manipulation of critical molecular pathways through management strategies is now achievable (Esrefoglu, 2012; Grattagliano et al., 2014).

3.6.6. Genetic Polymorphisms Outside the Major Histocompatibility Complex

Non-MHC polymorphisms can impact drug metabolism, detoxification mechanisms, cytokine and chemokine production, metabolic processes, immune responses, and reparative processes (Czaja, 2008, 2015b). Genes outside the MHC may impact the clinical phenotype and behavior of the disease, while genes inside the MHC may impact antigen presentation, immune cell differentiation, and disease occurrence (Czaja, 2008, 2015b). Alternative versions of the same gene that differ at a single base pair or locus in the DNA are known as single nucleotide polymorphisms or SNPs. The existence of a polymorphism implies that the variation may have an impact on gene function in disease states.

Diverse SNPs have been described in autoimmune hepatitis, including polymorphisms of the cytotoxic T lymphocyte antigen-4 gene (Agarwal et al., 2000), Fas gene (tumor necrosis factor receptor super-family gene) (Hiraide et al., 2005; Agarwal et al., 2007), tumor necrosis factor-a (TNFA*2) gene (Cookson et al., 1999; Czaja et al., 1999), vitamin D receptor gene (Vogel et al., 2002; Fan et al., 2005a), signal transducer and activator of transcription 4 gene (Migita et al., 2013), TGF-b1 gene (Tang et al., 2012b), and genes of various cytokines (Fan et al., 2005b). Recent genome-wide association studies have implicated a variant of the Scr homology 2 adaptor protein 3 gene and the caspase recruitment domain family member 10 gene in northern European patients with autoimmune hepatitis (De Boer et al., 2014).

These polymorphisms differ amongst ethnic groups, are not disease-specific, and are primarily statistically associated with autoimmune hepatitis (Czaja, 2008, 2015b). Their involvement in the illness is primarily speculative and debatable because the polymorphisms' actual functional differences have not been assessed. SNPs are present in autoimmune hepatitis, though, and as our ability to access the human genome and distinguish genetic variations between diseased and ethnically similar normal populations advances, we should be able to find these variations and determine their significance.

Autoimmune hepatitis is caused by perturbations in an interactive homeostatic network, which are reflected in its occurrence, clinical presentation, and outcome. Failures to dampen the immune response to tissue injury, separate foreign antigens from self-antigens, stop inflammatory and immune cells from infiltrating the liver, disrupt molecular pathways that speed up cell death, and restrict the progression of hepatic fibrosis can all be caused by deficiencies in counterregulatory mechanisms within this network. The inflammatory process may be sustained and prolonged by self-amplification loops based on autocrine stimulation and repetitive activation of pathogenic pathways; additionally, the emergence of autoimmune hepatitis can be facilitated but not determined by a genetic predisposition.

As each individual disruption in the homeostatic network has been thoroughly documented in animal research and cell cultures, they could all play a role in the development of autoimmune hepatitis. A hierarchy of the major disturbances has not yet been established, and these individual disturbances have not yet been included in a well-established comprehensive understanding. Understanding this hierarchy and the other important homeostatic mechanisms that the intervention may disrupt are necessary for developing site-specific therapies that produce safe, desirable, and long-lasting results.

A Closer Look

AIH Management and HCC Risk

Autoimmune hepatitis (AIH) is a chronic inflammatory liver disease characterized by the immune system attacking the liver, leading to hepatitis, fibrosis, and potentially cirrhosis. The management of AIH primarily involves immunosuppressive therapy aimed at achieving and maintaining remission of liver inflammation. Standard treatment typically begins with high-dose corticosteroids, such as prednisone, to quickly control the inflammation. Once remission is achieved, a maintenance regimen is implemented, often combining lower doses of corticosteroids with other immunosuppressive agents like azathioprine to reduce the risk of corticosteroid-related side effects. This combination helps sustain remission and minimize long-term damage to the liver. In some cases, other immunosuppressants such as mycophenolate mofetil, tacrolimus, or cyclosporine may be used, particularly in patients who do not respond to or cannot tolerate standard therapy.

Regular monitoring of liver function tests, immunoglobulin levels, and liver biopsy findings are crucial in managing AIH to assess disease activity and treatment response. The goal is to normalize liver enzymes and histology to prevent progression to cirrhosis. However, even with optimal management, some patients may experience relapses, necessitating adjustments in their therapeutic regimen. Long-term adherence to treatment and follow-up are essential to maintaining remission and monitoring for potential complications.

One of the significant concerns in AIH management is the increased risk of hepatocellular carcinoma (HCC), especially in patients who progress to cirrhosis. Chronic liver inflammation and fibrosis are well-established risk factors for HCC development. The risk of HCC in AIH patients is lower compared to other chronic liver diseases like hepatitis B and C, but it is still significant, particularly in those with advanced fibrosis or cirrhosis. Therefore, surveillance for HCC is a critical component of managing patients with AIH, especially those with cirrhosis.

Surveillance strategies for HCC typically involve regular imaging studies, such as abdominal ultrasound every six months, sometimes supplemented by serum alpha-fetoprotein (AFP) measurements. Early detection of HCC significantly improves the prognosis and expands the therapeutic options available, including surgical resection, liver transplantation, and locoregional therapies such as radiofrequency ablation or transarterial chemoembolization (TACE). In cases where surveillance detects suspicious lesions, further diagnostic workup with more advanced imaging techniques like CT or MRI may be warranted.

Liver transplantation remains a crucial therapeutic option for AIH patients with end-stage liver disease or those who develop HCC that is within the transplant criteria. Transplantation can offer a cure for both liver failure and HCC in eligible patients, although post-transplant immunosuppression must be carefully managed to prevent recurrent AIH in the graft.

The interplay between effective AIH management and HCC risk underscores the importance of a comprehensive, multidisciplinary approach to patient care. This includes hepatologists, pathologists, radiologists, and, when necessary, oncologists and transplant surgeons. Advances in understanding the immunopathogenesis of AIH and the molecular mechanisms underlying HCC are essential for developing more targeted therapies that could improve patient outcomes. Continued research and clinical vigilance are imperative to optimize the management of AIH and mitigate the associated risk of HCC, enhancing the quality of life and survival rates for these patients.

Summary

- Autoimmune hepatitis is a self-perpetuating inflammatory liver disease of unknown cause that is associated with promiscuous humoral and cellular immune responses against homologous self-antigens.
- Autoimmune hepatitis is a life-long and rare liver disease. It is when your body's immune system causes damage to its own healthy liver cells. This leads to inflammation in the liver.
- Reactive oxygen species (ROS) can extend and sustain the loss of hepatocytes and promote fibrosis in another self-amplification loop. Apoptotic bodies can activate Kupffer cells, and activated Kupffer cells can release ROS which may in turn stimulate hepatic stellate cells to transform into myofibroblasts.
- Foreign antigens are selected and presented to naïve CD4+ T helper lymphocytes by class II molecules of the MHC that are expressed on the membrane surface of professional antigen-presenting cells (dendritic cells and macrophages).
- The selection of foreign antigens and the occurrence of autoimmune hepatitis may also be affected by the linkage disequilibrium that can exist between genes of the MHC (epistasis).
- The indigenous antigens that trigger autoimmune hepatitis are unknown, but they are likely to share a common epitope that is also found in self-antigens (molecular mimicry).
- Immune cells migrating to the sites of liver injury can extend and sustain the immune response by unmasking or generating additional antigenic targets (neoantigens) and by expanding the immune response to involve targets of distant homology (epitope spread).
- Human formiminotransferase cyclodeaminase has also been an important antigen in the induction of experimental autoimmune hepatitis when expressed with CYP2D6 in plasmids and administered by immunization.
- Dendritic cells and natural killer (NK) cells are the principal mediators of the innate immune response, and the T helper (Th) lymphocytes (Th1, Th2, and Th17 cells), natural killer T (NKT) cells, gamma delta lymphocytes, and Tregs are the key mediators of the adaptive immune response.
- Chemokines are a subgroup of cytokines that are involved mainly in directing the migration of cells of the innate and adaptive immune systems to sites of tissue injury.

References

1. A-Gonzalez, N., Bensinger, S. J., Hong, C., Beceiro, S., Bradley, M. N., Zelcer, N., et al. (2009). Apoptotic cells promote their own clearance and immune tolerance through activation of the nuclear receptor LXR. *Immunity, 31*(2), 245–258.
2. Abuaf, N., Johanet, C., Chretien, P., Martini, E., Soulier, E., Laperche, S., et al. (1992). Characterization of the liver cytosol antigen type 1 reacting with autoantibodies in chronic active hepatitis. *Hepatology, 16*(4), 892–898.
3. Agarwal, K., Czaja, A. J., & Donaldson, P. T. (2007). A functional Fas promoter polymorphism is associated with a severe phenotype in type 1 autoimmune hepatitis characterized by early development of cirrhosis. *Tissue Antigens, 69*(3), 227–235.

4. Agarwal, K., Czaja, A. J., Jones, D. E., & Donaldson, P. T. (2000). Cytotoxic T lymphocyte antigen-4 (CTLA-4) gene polymorphisms and susceptibility to type 1 autoimmune hepatitis. *Hepatology, 31*(1), 49–53.
5. Aguilera, I., Wichmann, I., Sousa, J. M., Bernardos, A., Franco, E., Garcia-Lozano, J. R., et al. (2001). Antibodies against glutathione S-transferase T1 (GSTT1) in patients with de novo immune hepatitis following liver transplantation. *Clinical and Experimental Immunology, 126*(3), 535–539.
6. Ahonen, P., Myllarniemi, S., Sipila, I., & Perheentupa, J. (1990). Clinical variation of autoimmune polyendocrinopathy-candidiasis-ectodermal dystrophy (APECED) in a series of 68 patients. *New England Journal of Medicine, 322*(26), 1829–1836.
7. Albillos, A., Rossi, I., Cacho, G., Martinez, M. V., Millan, I., Abreu, L., et al. (1995). Enhanced endothelium-dependent vasodilation in patients with cirrhosis. *American Journal of Physiology, 268*(2 Pt 1), G459–G464.
8. Aoki, N., Kido, M., Iwamoto, S., Nishiura, H., Maruoka, R., Tanaka, J., et al. (2011). Dysregulated generation of follicular helper T cells in the spleen triggers fatal autoimmune hepatitis in mice. *Gastroenterology, 140*(4), 1322e1333, –1321–1325.
9. Aoyama, T., Inokuchi, S., Brenner, D. A., & Seki, E. (2010). CX3CL1-CX3CR1 interaction prevents carbon tetrachloride-induced liver inflammation and fibrosis in mice. *Hepatology, 52*(4), 1390–1400.
10. Arenz, M., Meyer Zum Buschenfelde, K. H., & Lohr, H. F. (1998). Limited T cell receptor Vbeta-chain repertoire of liver-infiltrating T cells in autoimmune hepatitis. *Journal of Hepatology, 28*(1), 70–77.
11. Arrenberg, P., Halder, R., Dai, Y., Maricic, I., & Kumar, V. (2010). Oligoclonality and innate-like features in the TCR repertoire of type II NKT cells reactive to a beta-linked self-glycolipid. *Proceedings of the National Academy of Sciences U.S.A., 107*(25), 10984–10989.
12. Arsalane, K., Dubois, C. M., Muanza, T., Begin, R., Boudreau, F., Asselin, C., et al. (1997). Transforming growth factor-beta1 is a potent inhibitor of glutathione synthesis in the lung epithelial cell line A549: Transcriptional effect on the GSH rate-limiting enzyme gamma-glutamylcysteine synthetase. *American Journal of Respiratory Cell and Molecular Biology, 17*(5), 599–607.
13. Bagavant, H., Thompson, C., Ohno, K., Setiady, Y., & Tung, K. S. (2002). Differential effect of neonatal thymectomy on systemic and organ-specific autoimmune disease. *International Immunology, 14*(11), 1397–1406.
14. Bai, J., & Odin, J. A. (2003). Apoptosis and the liver: Relation to autoimmunity and related conditions. *Autoimmunity Reviews, 2*(1), 36–42.
15. Barreira Da Silva, R., & Munz, C. (2011). Natural killer cell activation by dendritic cells: Balancing inhibitory and activating signals. *Cellular and Molecular Life Sciences, 68*(21), 3505–3518.
16. Berzins, S. P., Smyth, M. J., & Baxter, A. G. (2011). Presumed guilty: Natural killer T cell defects and human disease. *Nature Reviews Immunology, 11*(2), 131–142.
17. Beschorner, W. E., Suresch, D. L., Shinozawa, T., Santos, G. W., & Hess, A. D. (1988). Thymic immunopathology after cyclosporine: Effect of irradiation and age on medullary involution and recovery. *Transplant Proceedings, 20*(2), 1072–1078.

18. Bettaieb, A., Jiang, J. X., Sasaki, Y., Chao, T. I., Kiss, Z., Chen, X., et al. (2015). Hepatocyte nicotinamide adenine dinucleotide phosphate reduced oxidase 4 regulates stress signaling, fibrosis, and insulin sensitivity during development of steatohepatitis in mice. *Gastroenterology, 149*(2), 468–480.e410.

19. Bettelli, E., Carrier, Y., Gao, W., Korn, T., Strom, T. B., Oukka, M., et al. (2006). Reciprocal developmental pathways for the generation of pathogenic effector TH17 and regulatory T cells. *Nature, 441*(7090), 235–238.

20. Bettelli, E., Korn, T., Oukka, M., & Kuchroo, V. K. (2008). Induction and effector functions of TH17 cells. *Nature, 453*(7198), 1051–1057.

21. Beyazit, Y., Efe, C., Tanoglu, A., Purnak, T., Sayilir, A., Taskiran, I., et al. (2015a). Nitric oxide is a potential mediator of hepatic inflammation and fibrogenesis in autoimmune hepatitis. *Scandinavian Journal of Gastroenterology, 50*(2), 204–210.

22. Beyazit, Y., Kocak, E., Tanoglu, A., & Kekilli, M. (2015b). Oxidative stress might play a role in low serum vitamin D associated liver fibrosis among patients with autoimmune hepatitis. *Digestive Diseases and Sciences, 60*(5), 1106–1108.

23. Bittencourt, P. L., Goldberg, A. C., Cancado, E. L., Porta, G., Carrilho, F. J., Farias, A. Q., et al. (1999). Genetic heterogeneity in susceptibility to autoimmune hepatitis types 1 and 2. *American Journal of Gastroenterology, 94*(7), 1906–1913.

24. Bjelakovic, G., Nikolova, D., & Gluud, C. (2014). Antioxidant supplements and mortality. *Current Opinion in Clinical Nutrition and Metabolic Care, 17*(1), 40–44.

25. Bjorses, P., Halonen, M., Palvimo, J. J., Kolmer, M., Aaltonen, J., Ellonen, P., et al. (2000). Mutations in the AIRE gene: Effects on subcellular location and transactivation function of the autoimmune polyendocrinopathy-candidiasis-ectodermal dystrophy protein. *American Journal of Human Genetics, 66*(2), 378–392.

26. Blomqvist, M., Rhost, S., Teneberg, S., Lofbom, L., Osterbye, T., Brigl, M., et al. (2009). Multiple tissue-specific isoforms of sulfatide activate CD1d-restricted type II NKT cells. *European Journal of Immunology, 39*(6), 1726–1735.

27. Blumenfeld, H. J., Tohn, R., Haeryfar, S. M., Liu, Y., Savage, P. B., & Delovitch, T. L. (2011). Structure-guided design of an invariant natural killer T cell agonist for optimum protection from type 1 diabetes in non-obese diabetic mice. *Clinical and Experimental Immunology, 166*(1), 121–133.

28. Bogdanos, D. P., Choudhuri, K., & Vergani, D. (2001). Molecular mimicry and autoimmune liver disease: Virtuous intentions, malign consequences. *Liver, 21*(4), 225–232.

29. Boudreau, H. E., Casterline, B. W., Rada, B., Korzeniowska, A., & Leto, T. L. (2012). Nox4 involvement in TGF-beta and SMAD3-driven induction of the epithelial-to-mesenchymal transition and migration of breast epithelial cells. *Free Radical Biology and Medicine, 53*(8), 1489–1499.

30. Bourd-Boittin, K., Basset, L., Bonnier, D., L'helgoualc'h, A., Samson, M., & Theret, N. (2009). CX3CL1/fractalkine shedding by human hepatic stellate cells: Contribution to chronic inflammation in the liver. *Journal of Cellular and Molecular Medicine, 13*(6), 1526–1535.

31. Boyton, R. J., & Altmann, D. M. (2007). Natural killer cells, killer immunoglobulin-like receptors and human leucocyte antigen class I in disease. *Clinical and Experimental Immunology, 149*(1), 1–8.

32. Bridoux-Henno, L., Maggiore, G., Johanet, C., Fabre, M., Vajro, P., Dommergues, J. P., et al. (2004). Features and outcome of autoimmune hepatitis type 2 presenting with isolated positivity for anti-liver cytosol antibody. *Clinical Gastroenterology and Hepatology, 2*(9), 825–830.

33. Brown, D. I., & Griendling, K. K. (2009). Nox proteins in signal transduction. *Free Radical Biology and Medicine, 47*(9), 1239–1253.

34. Brown, J. H., Jardetzky, T. S., Gorga, J. C., Stern, L. J., Urban, R. G., Strominger, J. L., et al. (1993). Three-dimensional structure of the human class II histocompatibility antigen HLA-DR1. *Nature, 364*(6432), 33–39.

35. Brown, J. H., Jardetzky, T., Saper, M. A., Samraoui, B., Bjorkman, P. J., & Wiley, D. C. (1988). A hypothetical model of the foreign antigen binding site of class II histocompatibility molecules. *Nature, 332*(6161), 845–850.

36. Bucy, R. P., Xu, X. Y., Li, J., & Huang, G. (1993). Cyclosporin A-induced autoimmune disease in mice. *Journal of Immunology, 151*(3), 1039–1050.

37. Burnet, F. M. (1960). Theories of immunity. *Perspectives in Biology and Medicine, 3*(4), 447–458.

38. Calcerrada, P., Peluffo, G., & Radi, R. (2011). Nitric oxide-derived oxidants with a focus on peroxynitrite: Molecular targets, cellular responses and therapeutic implications. *Current Pharmaceutical Design, 17*(36), 3905–3932.

39. Canbay, A., Feldstein, A. E., Higuchi, H., Werneburg, N., Grambihler, A., Bronk, S. F., et al. (2003a). Kupffer cell engulfment of apoptotic bodies stimulates death ligand and cytokine expression. *Hepatology, 38*(5), 1188–1198.

40. Canbay, A., Taimr, P., Torok, N., Higuchi, H., Friedman, S., & Gores, G. J. (2003b). Apoptotic body engulfment by a human stellate cell line is profibrogenic. *Laboratory Investigation, 83*(5), 655–663.

41. Carmona-Cuenca, I., Roncero, C., Sancho, P., Caja, L., Fausto, N., Fernández, M., et al. (2008). Upregulation of the NADPH oxidase NOX4 by TGF-beta in hepatocytes is required for its pro-apoptotic activity. *Journal of Hepatology, 49*(6), 965–976.

42. Chambel, S. S., Santos-Gonçalves, A., & Duarte, T. L. (2015). The dual role of Nrf2 in nonalcoholic fatty liver disease: Regulation of antioxidant defenses and hepatic lipid metabolism. *Biomedical Research International, 2015*, 597134.

43. Cho, Y. N., Kee, S. J., Lee, S. J., Seo, S. R., Kim, T. J., Lee, S. S., et al. (2011). Numerical and functional deficiencies of natural killer T cells in systemic lupus erythematosus: Their deficiency related to disease activity. *Rheumatology, 50*(6), 1054–1063.

44. Choi, J., Corder, N. L., Koduru, B., & Wang, Y. (2014). Oxidative stress and hepatic Nox proteins in chronic hepatitis C and hepatocellular carcinoma. *Free Radical Biology and Medicine, 72*, 267–284.

45. Christen, U., & Von Herrath, M. G. (2004). Induction, acceleration or prevention of autoimmunity by molecular mimicry. *Molecular Immunology, 40*(12), 1113–1120.

46. Cookson, S., Constantini, P. K., Clare, M., Underhill, J. A., Bernal, W., Czaja, A. J., et al. (1999). Frequency and nature of cytokine gene polymorphisms in type 1 autoimmune hepatitis. *Hepatology, 30*(4), 851–856.

47. Coquerelle, C., & Moser, M. (2010). DC subsets in positive and negative regulation of immunity. *Immunological Reviews, 234*(1), 317–334.

48. Costa, M., Rodríguez-Sánchez, J. L., Czaja, A. J., & Gelpi, C. (2000). Isolation and characterization of cDNA encoding the antigenic protein of the human tRNP (Ser)Sec complex recognized by autoantibodies from patients with type-1 autoimmune hepatitis. *Clinical and Experimental Immunology, 121*(2), 364–374.

49. Cui, W., Matsuno, K., Iwata, K., Ibi, M., Matsumoto, M., Zhang, J., et al. (2011). NOX1/nicotinamide adenine dinucleotide phosphate, reduced form (NADPH) oxidase promotes proliferation of stellate cells and aggravates liver fibrosis induced by bile duct ligation. *Hepatology, 54*(3), 949–958.

50. Czaja, A. J. (2001). Understanding the pathogenesis of autoimmune hepatitis. *American Journal of Gastroenterology, 96*(5), 1224–1231.

51. Czaja, A. J. (2007). Autoimmune hepatitis. Part A: Pathogenesis. *Expert Review of Gastroenterology & Hepatology, 1*(1), 113–128.

52. Czaja, A. J. (2008). Genetic factors affecting the occurrence, clinical phenotype, and outcome of autoimmune hepatitis. *Clinical Gastroenterology and Hepatology, 6*(4), 379–388.

53. Czaja, A. J. (2009). Special clinical challenges in autoimmune hepatitis: The elderly, males, pregnancy, mild disease, fulminant onset, and nonwhite patients. *Seminars in Liver Disease, 29*(3), 315–330.

54. Czaja, A. J. (2012). Diagnosis, pathogenesis, and treatment of autoimmune hepatitis after liver transplantation. *Digestive Diseases and Sciences, 57*(10), 2248–2266.

55. Czaja, A. J. (2013). Autoimmune hepatitis in diverse ethnic populations and geographical regions. *Expert Review of Gastroenterology & Hepatology, 7*(4), 365–385.

56. Czaja, A. J. (2014a). Hepatic inflammation and progressive liver fibrosis in chronic liver disease. *World Journal of Gastroenterology, 20*(9), 2515–2532.

57. Czaja, A. J. (2014b). Review article: Chemokines as orchestrators of autoimmune hepatitis and potential therapeutic targets. *Alimentary Pharmacology & Therapeutics, 40*(3), 261–279.

58. Czaja, A. J. (2014c). Review article: Prevention and reversal of hepatic fibrosis in autoimmune hepatitis. *Alimentary Pharmacology & Therapeutics, 39*(4), 385–406.

59. Czaja, A. J. (2014d). Targeting apoptosis in autoimmune hepatitis. *Digestive Diseases and Sciences, 59*(12), 2890–2904.

60. Czaja, A. J. (2015a). Adoptive cell transfer in autoimmune hepatitis. *Expert Review of Gastroenterology & Hepatology, 9*(6), 821–836.

61. Czaja, A. J. (2015b). Transitioning from idiopathic to explainable autoimmune hepatitis. *Digestive Diseases and Sciences, 60*(10), 2881–2900.

62. Czaja, A. J. (2016). Nature and implications of oxidative and nitrosative stresses in autoimmune hepatitis. *Digestive Diseases and Sciences, 61*(11), 2784–2803.

63. Czaja, A. J., & Carpenter, H. A. (2006). Distinctive clinical phenotype and treatment outcome of type 1 autoimmune hepatitis in the elderly. *Hepatology, 43*(3), 532–538.

64. Czaja, A. J., & Donaldson, P. T. (2000). Genetic susceptibilities for immune expression and liver cell injury in autoimmune hepatitis. *Immunological Reviews, 174*(1), 250–259.

65. Czaja, A. J., & Manns, M. P. (1995). The validity and importance of subtypes in autoimmune hepatitis: A point of view. *American Journal of Gastroenterology, 90*(8), 1206–1211.

66. Czaja, A. J., Carpenter, H. A., Santrach, P. J., & Moore, S. B. (1993). Significance of HLA DR4 in type 1 autoimmune hepatitis. *Gastroenterology, 105*(6), 1502-1507.

67. Czaja, A. J., Cookson, S., Constantini, P. K., Clare, M., Underhill, J. A., & Donaldson, P. T. (1999). Cytokine polymorphisms associated with clinical features and treatment outcome in type 1 autoimmune hepatitis. *Gastroenterology, 117*(3), 645–652.

68. Czaja, A. J., Doherty, D. G., & Donaldson, P. T. (2002a). Genetic bases of autoimmune hepatitis. *Digestive Diseases and Sciences, 47*(10), 2139–2150.

69. Czaja, A. J., Kruger, M., Santrach, P. J., Moore, S. B., & Manns, M. P. (1997a). Genetic distinctions between types 1 and 2 autoimmune hepatitis. *American Journal of Gastroenterology, 92*(12), 2197–2200.

70. Czaja, A. J., Manns, M. P., & Homburger, H. A. (1992). Frequency and significance of antibodies to liver/kidney microsome type 1 in adults with chronic active hepatitis. *Gastroenterology, 103*(4), 1290–1295.

71. Czaja, A. J., Shums, Z., & Norman, G. L. (2004). Nonstandard antibodies as prognostic markers in autoimmune hepatitis. *Autoimmunity, 37*(3), 195–201.

72. Czaja, A. J., Souto, E. O., Bittencourt, P. L., Cancado, E. L., Porta, G., Goldberg, A. C., et al. (2002b). Clinical distinctions and pathogenic implications of type 1 autoimmune hepatitis in Brazil and the United States. *Journal of Hepatology, 37*(4), 302–308.

73. Czaja, A. J., Strettell, M. D., Thomson, L. J., Santrach, P. J., Moore, S. B., Donaldson, P. T., et al. (1997b). Associations between alleles of the major histocompatibility complex and type 1 autoimmune hepatitis. *Hepatology, 25*(2), 317–323.

74. D'Amelio, M., Tino, E., & Cecconi, F. (2008). The apoptosome: Emerging insights and new potential targets for drug design. *Pharmaceutical Research, 25*(4), 740–751.

75. Da Rocha Junior, L. F., Dantas, A. T., Duarte, A. L., de Melo Rego, M. J., Pitta Ida, R., & Pitta, M. G. (2013). PPARgamma agonists in adaptive immunity: What do immune disorders and their models have to tell us? *PPAR Research, 2013*, 519724.

76. Danielson, P. B. (2002). The cytochrome P450 superfamily: Biochemistry, evolution and drug metabolism in humans. *Current Drug Metabolism, 3*(6), 561–597.

77. Dardalhon, V., Korn, T., Kuchroo, V. K., & Anderson, A. C. (2008). Role of Th1 and Th17 cells in organ-specific autoimmunity. *Journal of Autoimmunity, 31*(3), 252–256.

78. De Boer, Y. S., Van Gerven, N. M., Zwiers, A., Verwer, B. J., Van Hoek, B., Van Erpecum, K. J., et al. (2014). Genome-wide association study identifies variants associated with autoimmune hepatitis type 1. *Gastroenterology, 147*(2), 443–452.

79. De Minicis, S., & Brenner, D. A. (2007). NOX in liver fibrosis. *Archives of Biochemistry and Biophysics, 462*(2), 266–272.

80. Del Prete, G., De Carli, M., Almerigogna, F., Giudizi, M. G., Biagiotti, R., & Romagnani, S. (1993). Human IL-10 is produced by both type 1 helper (Th1) and type 2 helper (Th2) T cell clones and inhibits their antigen-specific proliferation and cytokine production. *Journal of Immunology, 150*(1), 353–360.

81. Dennert, G., & Aswad, F. (2006). The role of NKT cells in animal models of autoimmune hepatitis. *Critical Reviews in Immunology, 26*(5), 453–473.

82. Dessen, A., Lawrence, C. M., Cupo, S., Zaller, D. M., & Wiley, D. C. (1997). X-ray crystal structure of HLA-DR4 (DRA*0101, DRB*10401) complexed with a peptide from human collagen II. *Immunity, 7*(4), 473–481.

83. Dinarello, C. A. (2000). Proinflammatory cytokines. *Chest, 118*(2), 503–508.

84. Djilali-Saiah, I., Renous, R., Caillat-Zucman, S., Debray, D., & Alvarez, F. (2004). Linkage disequilibrium between HLA class II region and autoimmune hepatitis in pediatric patients. *Journal of Hepatology, 40*(6), 904–909.

85. Doherty, D. G., Donaldson, P. T., Underhill, J. A., Farrant, J. M., Duthie, A., Mieli-Vergani, G., et al. (1994). Allelic sequence variation in the HLA class II genes and proteins in patients with autoimmune hepatitis. *Hepatology, 19*(3), 609–615.

86. Doherty, D. G., Penzotti, J. E., Koelle, D. M., Kwok, W. W., Lybrand, T. P., Masewicz, S., et al. (1998). Structural basis of specificity and degeneracy of T cell recognition: Pluriallelic restriction of T cell responses to a peptide antigen involves both specific and promiscuous interactions between the T cell receptor, peptide, and HLA-DR. *Journal of Immunology, 161*(7), 3527–3535.

87. Donaldson, P. T., Doherty, D. G., Hayllar, K. M., McFarlane, I. G., Johnson, P. J., & Williams, R. (1991). Susceptibility to autoimmune chronic active hepatitis: Human leukocyte antigens DR4 and A1-B8-DR3 are independent risk factors. *Hepatology, 13*(4), 701–706.

88. Dustin, M. L., & Shaw, A. S. (1999). Costimulation: Building an immunological synapse. *Science, 283*(5402), 649–650.

89. Efe, C., Kav, T., Aydin, C., Cengiz, M., Imga, N. N., Purnak, T., et al. (2014). Low serum vitamin D levels are associated with severe histological features and poor response to therapy in patients with autoimmune hepatitis. *Digestive Diseases and Sciences, 59*(12), 3035–3042.

90. Efsen, E., Grappone, C., DeFranco, R. M., Milani, S., Romanelli, R. G., Bonacchi, A., et al. (2002). Up-regulated expression of fractalkine and its receptor CX3CR1 during liver injury in humans. *Journal of Hepatology, 37*(1), 39–47.

91. Ehser, J., Holdener, M., Christen, S., Bayer, M., Pfeilschifter, J. M., Hintermann, E., et al. (2013). Molecular mimicry rather than identity breaks T-cell tolerance in the CYP2D6 mouse model for human autoimmune hepatitis. *Journal of Autoimmunity, 42*, 39–49.

92. Ekert, P. G., Read, S. H., Silke, J., Marsden, V. S., Kaufmann, H., Hawkins, C. J., et al. (2004). Apaf-1 and caspase-9 accelerate apoptosis, but do not determine whether factor-deprived or drug-treated cells die. *Journal of Cell Biology, 165*(6), 835–842.

93. Ernst, P. B., Garrison, J. C., & Thompson, L. F. (2010). Much ado about adenosine: Adenosine synthesis and function in regulatory T cell biology. *Journal of Immunology, 185*(4), 1993–1998.

94. Esrefoglu, M. (2012). Oxidative stress and benefits of antioxidant agents in acute and chronic hepatitis. *Hepatitis Monthly, 12*(2), 160–167.

95. Fainboim, L., Canero Velasco, M. C., Marcos, C. Y., Ciocca, M., Roy, A., Theiler, G., et al. (2001). Protracted, but not acute, hepatitis A virus infection is strongly associated with HLA-DRB*1301, a marker for pediatric autoimmune hepatitis. *Hepatology, 33*(6), 1512–1517.

96. Fainboim, L., Marcos, Y., Pando, M., Capucchio, M., Reyes, G. B., Galoppo, C., et al. (1994). Chronic active autoimmune hepatitis in children. Strong association with a particular HLA-DR6 (DRB1*1301) haplotype. *Human Immunology, 41*(2), 146–150.

97. Fan, L. Y., Tu, X. Q., Zhu, Y., Pfeiffer, T., Feltens, R., Stoecker, W., et al. (2005b). Genetic association of cytokines polymorphisms with autoimmune hepatitis and primary biliary cirrhosis in the Chinese. *World Journal of Gastroenterology, 11*(17), 2768–2772.

98. Fan, L., Tu, X., Zhu, Y., Zhou, L., Pfeiffer, T., Feltens, R., et al. (2005a). Genetic association of vitamin D receptor polymorphisms with autoimmune hepatitis and primary biliary cirrhosis in the Chinese. *Journal of Gastroenterology and Hepatology, 20*(2), 249–255.

99. Faubion, W. A., & Gores, G. J. (1999). Death receptors in liver biology and pathobiology. *Hepatology, 29*(1), 1–4.

100. Feld, J. J., Modi, A. A., El-Diwany, R., Rotman, Y., Thomas, E., Ahlenstiel, G., et al. (2011). S-adenosyl methionine improves early viral responses and interferon-stimulated gene induction in hepatitis C nonresponders. *Gastroenterology, 140*(3), 830–839.

101. Fletcher, J. M., Lonergan, R., Costelloe, L., Kinsella, K., Moran, B., O'Farrelly, C., et al. (2009). $CD39^+Foxp3^+$ regulatory T cells suppress pathogenic Th17 cells and are impaired in multiple sclerosis. *Journal of Immunology, 183*(11), 7602–7610.

102. Fontenot, J. D., Gavin, M. A., & Rudensky, A. Y. (2003). Foxp3 programs the development and function of $CD4^+CD25^+$ regulatory T cells. *Nature Immunology, 4*(4), 330–336.

103. Fox, C. K., Furtwaengler, A., Nepomuceno, R. R., Martinez, O. M., & Krams, S. M. (2001). Apoptotic pathways in primary biliary cirrhosis and autoimmune hepatitis. *Liver, 21*(4), 272–279.

104. Ganguly, D., Haak, S., Sisirak, V., & Reizis, B. (2013). The role of dendritic cells in autoimmunity. *Nature Reviews Immunology, 13*(7), 566–577.

105. Gao, B., & Bataller, R. (2011). Alcoholic liver disease: Pathogenesis and new therapeutic targets. *Gastroenterology, 141*(5), 1572–1585.

106. Girardi, E., Maricic, I., Wang, J., Mac, T. T., Iyer, P., Kumar, V., et al. (2012). Type II natural killer T cells use features of both innate-like and conventional T cells to recognize sulfatide self-antigens. *Nature Immunology, 13*(9), 851–856.

107. Godebu, E., Summers-Torres, D., Lin, M. M., Baaten, B. J., & Bradley, L. M. (2008). Polyclonal adaptive regulatory CD4 cells that can reverse type I diabetes become oligoclonal long-term protective memory cells. *Journal of Immunology, 181*(3), 1798–1805.

108. Goldberg, A. C., Bittencourt, P. L., Mougin, B., Cancado, E. L., Porta, G., Carrilho, F., et al. (2001). Analysis of HLA haplotypes in autoimmune hepatitis type 1: Identifying the major susceptibility locus. *Human Immunology, 62*(2), 165–169.

109. Gonzalez, S., Groh, V., & Spies, T. (2006). Immunobiology of human NKG2D and its ligands. *Current Topics in Microbiology and Immunology, 298*, 121–138.

110. Grant, C. R., Liberal, R., Holder, B. S., Cardone, J., Ma, Y., Robson, S. C., et al. (2014). Dysfunctional $CD39^+$ regulatory T cells and aberrant control of T-helper type 17 cells in autoimmune hepatitis. *Hepatology, 59*(3), 1007–1015.

111. Grattagliano, I., Calamita, G., Cocco, T., Wang, D. Q., & Portincasa, P. (2014). Pathogenic role of oxidative and nitrosative stress in primary biliary cirrhosis. *World Journal of Gastroenterology, 20*(21), 5746–5759.

112. Greenfield, E. A., Nguyen, K. A., & Kuchroo, V. K. (1998). CD28/B7 costimulation: A review. *Critical Reviews in Immunology, 18*(4), 389–418.

113. Gregorio, G. V., Portmann, B., Karani, J., Harrison, P., Donaldson, P. T., & Vergani, D. (2001). Autoimmune hepatitis/sclerosing cholangitis overlap syndrome in childhood: A 16-year prospective study. *Hepatology, 33*(3), 544–553.

114. Gregorio, G. V., Portmann, B., Reid, F., Donaldson, P. T., Doherty, D. G., McCartney, M., et al. (1997). Autoimmune hepatitis in childhood: A 20-year experience. *Hepatology, 25*(3), 541–547.

115. Gueguen, M., Yamamoto, A. M., Bernard, O., & Alvarez, F. (1989). Antiliver-kidney microsome antibody type 1 recognizes human cytochrome P450 db1. *Biochemical and Biophysical Research Communications, 159*(2), 542–547.

116. Guicciardi, M. E., & Gores, G. J. (2010). Apoptosis as a mechanism for liver disease progression. *Seminars in Liver Disease, 30*(4), 402–410.

117. Hammerich, L., & Tacke, F. (2014). Role of gamma-delta T cells in liver inflammation and fibrosis. *World Journal of Gastrointestinal Pathophysiology, 5*(2), 107–113.

118. Hammerich, L., Bangen, J. M., Govaere, O., Zimmermann, H. W., Gassler, N., Huss, S., et al. (2014). Chemokine receptor CCR6-dependent accumulation of γδ T cells in injured liver restricts hepatic inflammation and fibrosis. *Hepatology, 59*(2), 630–642.

119. Han, S., Tredger, M., Gregorio, G. V., Mieli-Vergani, G., & Vergani, D. (1995). Anti-liver cytosolic antigen type 1 (LC1) antibodies in childhood autoimmune liver disease. *Hepatology, 21*(1), 58–62.

120. Hanahan, D. (1998). Peripheral-antigen-expressing cells in thymic medulla: Factors in self-tolerance and autoimmunity. *Current Opinion in Immunology, 10*(6), 656–662.

121. Harrington, L. E., Hatton, R. D., Mangan, P. R., Turner, H., Murphy, T. L., Murphy, K. M., et al. (2005). Interleukin 17-producing $CD4^+$ effector T cells develop via a lineage distinct from the T helper type 1 and 2 lineages. *Nature Immunology, 6*(11), 1123–1132.

122. Hecker, L., Vittal, R., Jones, T., Jagirdar, R., Luckhardt, T. R., Horowitz, J. C., et al. (2009). NADPH oxidase-4 mediates myofibroblast activation and fibrogenic responses to lung injury. *Nature Medicine, 15*(10), 1077–1081.

123. Heino, M., Peterson, P., Kudoh, J., Nagamine, K., Lagerstedt, A., Ovod, V., et al. (1999). Autoimmune regulator is expressed in the cells regulating immune tolerance in thymus medulla. *Biochemical and Biophysical Research Communications, 257*(3), 821–825.

124. Hess, A. D., Fischer, A. C., Horwitz, L. R., & Laulis, M. K. (1993). Cyclosporine-induced autoimmunity: Critical role of autoregulation in the prevention of major histocompatibility class II-dependent auto aggression. *Transplant Proceedings, 25*(6), 2811–2813.

125. Hintermann, E., Holdener, M., Bayer, M., Loges, S., Pfeilschifter, J. M., Granier, C., et al. (2011). Epitope spreading of the anti-CYP2D6 antibody response in patients with autoimmune hepatitis and in the CYP2D6 mouse model. *Journal of Autoimmunity, 37*(3), 242–253.

126. Hiraide, A., Imazeki, F., Yokosuka, O., Kanda, T., Kojima, H., Fukai, K., et al. (2005). Fas polymorphisms influence susceptibility to autoimmune hepatitis. *American Journal of Gastroenterology, 100*(6), 1322–1329.

127. Holdener, M., Hintermann, E., Bayer, M., Rhode, A., Rodrigo, E., Hintereder, G., et al. (2008). Breaking tolerance to the natural human liver autoantigen cytochrome P450 2D6 by virus infection. *Journal of Experimental Medicine, 205*(7), 1409–1422.

128. Holdenrieder, S., Eichhorn, P., Beuers, U., Samtleben, W., Stieber, P., Nagel, D., et al. (2007). Soluble NKG2D ligands in hepatic autoimmune diseases and in benign diseases involved in marker metabolism. *Anticancer Research, 27*(4B), 2041–2045.

129. Holtmeier, W., & Kabelitz, D. (2005). γδ T cells link innate and adaptive immune responses. *Chemical Immunology and Allergy, 86*, 151–183.

130. Homberg, J. C., Abuaf, N., Bernard, O., Islam, S., Alvarez, F., Khalil, S. H., et al. (1987). Chronic active hepatitis associated with antiliver/kidney microsome antibody type 1: A second type of "autoimmune" hepatitis. *Hepatology, 7*(6), 1333–1339.

131. Hori, S., Nomura, T., & Sakaguchi, S. (2003). Control of regulatory T cell development by the transcription factor Foxp3. *Science, 299*(5609), 1057–1061.

132. Horwitz, D. A., Zheng, S. G., & Gray, J. D. (2008). Natural and TGF-β-induced $Foxp3^{+}CD4^{+}$ $CD25^{+}$ regulatory T cells are not mirror images of each other. *Trends in Immunology, 29*(9), 429–435.

133. Hubert, F. X., Kinkel, S. A., Davey, G. M., Phipson, B., Mueller, S. N., Liston, A., et al. (2011). Aire regulates the transfer of antigen from mTECs to dendritic cells for induction of thymic tolerance. *Blood, 118*(9), 2462–2472.

134. Hudspeth, K., Pontarini, E., Tentorio, P., Cimino, M., Donadon, M., Torzilli, G., et al. (2013). The role of natural killer cells in autoimmune liver disease: A comprehensive review. *Journal of Autoimmunity, 46*, 55–65.

135. Ikeda, A., Aoki, N., Kido, M., Iwamoto, S., Nishiura, H., Maruoka, R., et al. (2014). Progression of autoimmune hepatitis is mediated by IL-18-producing dendritic cells and hepatic CXCL9 expression in mice. *Hepatology, 60*(1), 224–236.

136. Islam, K. N., Kayanoki, Y., Kaneto, H., Suzuki, K., Asahi, M., Fujii, J., et al. (1997). TGF-β1 triggers oxidative modifications and enhances apoptosis in HIT cells through accumulation of reactive oxygen species by suppression of catalase and glutathione peroxidase. *Free Radical Biology and Medicine, 22*(7), 1007–1017.

137. Isse, K., Harada, K., Zen, Y., Kamihira, T., Shimoda, S., Harada, M., et al. (2005). Fractalkine and CX3CR1 are involved in the recruitment of intraepithelial lymphocytes of intrahepatic bile ducts. *Hepatology, 41*(3), 506–516.

138. Ito, T., Yang, M., Wang, Y. H., Lande, R., Gregorio, J., Perng, O. A., et al. (2007). Plasmacytoid dendritic cells prime IL-10-producing T regulatory cells by inducible costimulator ligand. *Journal of Experimental Medicine, 204*(1), 105–115.

139. Jain, A. K., Mahajan, S., & Jaiswal, A. K. (2008). Phosphorylation and dephosphorylation of tyrosine 141 regulate stability and degradation of INrf2: A novel mechanism in Nrf2 activation. *Journal of Biological Chemistry, 283*(26), 17712–17720.

140. Jobling, M. F., Mott, J. D., Finnegan, M. T., Jurukovski, V., Erickson, A. C., Walian, P. J., et al. (2006). Isoform-specific activation of latent transforming growth factor beta (LTGF-β) by reactive oxygen species. *Radiation Research, 166*(6), 839–848.

141. Kahraman, A., Fingas, C. D., Syn, W. K., Gerken, G., & Canbay, A. (2012). Role of stress-induced NKG2D ligands in liver diseases. *Liver International, 32*(3), 370–382.

142. Kanamori, M., Tasumi, Y., Iyoda, T., Ushida, M., & Inaba, K. (2012). Sulfatide inhibits alpha-galactosylceramide presentation by dendritic cells. *International Immunology, 24*(2), 129–136.

143. Karim, M., Kingsley, C. I., Bushell, A. R., Sawitzki, B. S., & Wood, K. J. (2004). Alloantigen-induced $CD25^{+}CD4^{+}$ regulatory T cells can develop in vivo from $CD25^{-}CD4^{+}$ precursors in a thymus-independent process. *Journal of Immunology, 172*(2), 923–928.

144. Karlmark, K. R., Zimmermann, H. W., Roderburg, C., Gassler, N., Wasmuth, H. E., Luedde, T., et al. (2010). The fractalkine receptor CX (3) CR1 protects against liver fibrosis by controlling differentiation and survival of infiltrating hepatic monocytes. *Hepatology, 52*(5), 1769–1782.

145. Kasper, H. U., Ligum, D., Cucus, J., Stippel, D. L., Dienes, H. P., & Drebber, U. (2009). Liver distribution of γδ-T-cells in patients with chronic hepatitis of different etiology. *APMIS, 117*(9), 779–785.

146. Kerkar, N., Choudhuri, K., Ma, Y., Mahmoud, A., Bogdanos, D. P., Muratori, L., et al. (2003). Cytochrome P4502D6(193–212): A new immunodominant epitope and target of virus/self-cross-reactivity in liver kidney microsomal autoantibody type 1-positive liver disease. *Journal of Immunology, 170*(3), 1481–1489.

147. Kerr, J. F., Cooksley, W. G., Searle, J., Halliday, J. W., Halliday, W. J., Holder, L., et al. (1979). The nature of piecemeal necrosis in chronic active hepatitis. *Lancet, 2*(8141), 827–828.

148. Ki, S. H., Park, O., Zheng, M., Morales-Ibanez, O., Kolls, J. K., Bataller, R., et al. (2010). Interleukin-22 treatment ameliorates alcoholic liver injury in a murine model of chronic-binge ethanol feeding: Role of signal transducer and activator of transcription 3. *Hepatology, 52*(4), 1291–1300.

149. Kido, M., Watanabe, N., Okazaki, T., Akamatsu, T., Tanaka, J., Saga, K., et al. (2008). Fatal autoimmune hepatitis induced by concurrent loss of naturally arising regulatory T cells and PD-1-mediated signaling. *Gastroenterology, 135*(4), 1333–1343.

150. Kirstein, M. M., Metzler, F., Geiger, E., Heinrich, E., Hallensleben, M., Manns, M. P., et al. (2015). Prediction of short- and long-term outcome in patients with autoimmune hepatitis. *Hepatology, 62*(6), 1524–1535.

151. Kitamura, H., Ohta, A., Sekimoto, M., Sato, M., Iwakabe, K., Nakui, M., et al. (2000). α-Galactosylceramide induces early B-cell activation through IL-4 production by NKT cells. *Cell Immunology, 199*(1), 37–42.

152. Korn, T., Bettelli, E., Oukka, M., & Kuchroo, V. K. (2009). IL-17 and Th17 cells. *Annual Review of Immunology, 27*, 485–517.

153. Kroemer, G., Galluzzi, L., & Brenner, C. (2007). Mitochondrial membrane permeabilization in cell death. *Physiological Reviews, 87*(1), 99–163.

154. Kumar, V. (2013). NKT-cell subsets: Promoters and protectors in inflammatory liver disease. *Journal of Hepatology, 59*(3), 618–620.

155. Lalazar, G., Preston, S., Zigmond, E., Ben Yaacov, A., & Ilan, Y. (2006). Glycolipids as immune modulatory tools. *Mini Reviews in Medicinal Chemistry, 6*(12), 1249–1253.

156. Lan, Q., Fan, H., Quesniaux, V., Ryffel, B., Liu, Z., & Zheng, S. G. (2012). Induced $Foxp3^{+}$ regulatory T cells: A potential new weapon to treat autoimmune and inflammatory diseases? *Journal of Molecular Cell Biology, 4*(1), 22–28.

157. Landi, A., Weismuller, T. J., Lankisch, T. O., Santer, D. M., Tyrrell, D. L., Manns, M. P., et al. (2014). Differential serum levels of eosinophilic eotaxins in primary sclerosing cholangitis,

primary biliary cirrhosis, and autoimmune hepatitis. *Journal of Interferon & Cytokine Research, 34*(3), 204–214.

158. Lapierre, P., Djilali-Saiah, I., Vitozzi, S., & Alvarez, F. (2004). A murine model of type 2 autoimmune hepatitis: Xeno immunization with human antigens. *Hepatology, 39*(5), 1066–1074.
159. Lapierre, P., Hajoui, O., Homberg, J. C., & Alvarez, F. (1999). Formiminotransferase cyclodeaminase is an organ-specific autoantigen recognized by sera of patients with autoimmune hepatitis. *Gastroenterology, 116*(3), 643–649.
160. Lee, E. Y., Lee, Z. H., & Song, Y. W. (2009). CXCL10 and autoimmune diseases. *Autoimmunity Reviews, 8*(5), 379–383.
161. Lee, S. H., Oe, T., & Blair, I. A. (2001). Vitamin C-induced decomposition of lipid hydroperoxides to endogenous genotoxins. *Science, 292*(5523), 2083–2086.
162. Lei, Y., & Takahama, Y. (2012). XCL1 and XCR1 in the immune system. *Microbes and Infection, 14*(4), 262–267.
163. Li, Y. L., Liu, N., Zhao, D. T., Li, Z. M., Zhang, H. P., Liu, Y. M., et al. (2013). Investigate circulating levels of chemokines and evaluate the correlation between these chemokines and liver function indicators in autoimmune hepatitis. *Zhonghua Gan Zang Bing Za Zhi, 21*(5), 299–303.
164. Liberal, R., Grant, C. R., Holder, B. S., Ma, Y., Mieli-Vergani, G., Vergani, D., et al. (2012). The impaired immune regulation of autoimmune hepatitis is linked to a defective galectin-9/TIM-3 pathway. *Hepatology, 56*(2), 677–686.
165. Liberal, R., Grant, C. R., Longhi, M. S., Mieli-Vergani, G., & Vergani, D. (2015). Regulatory T cells: Mechanisms of suppression and impairment in autoimmune liver disease. *IUBMB Life, 67*(2), 88–97.
166. Lim, Y. S., Oh, H. B., Choi, S. E., Kwon, O. J., Heo, Y. S., Lee, H. C., et al. (2008). Susceptibility to type 1 autoimmune hepatitis is associated with shared amino acid sequences at positions 70–74 of the HLA-DRB1 molecule. *Journal of Hepatology, 48*(1), 133–139.
167. Linsen, L., Somers, V., & Stinissen, P. (2005). Immunoregulation of autoimmunity by natural killer T cells. *Human Immunology, 66*(12), 1193–1202.
168. Liu, W., Putnam, A. L., Xu-Yu, Z., Szot, G. L., Lee, M. R., Zhu, S., et al. (2006). CD127 expression inversely correlates with FoxP3 and suppressive function of human $CD4^+$ T reg cells. *Journal of Experimental Medicine, 203*(7), 1701–1711.
169. Liu, Y. J. (2005). IPC: Professional type 1 interferon-producing cells and plasmacytoid dendritic cell precursors. *Annual Review of Immunology, 23*, 275–306.
170. Lohr, H., Manns, M., Kyriatsoulis, A., Lohse, A. W., Trautwein, C., Meyer Zum Buschenfelde, K. H., et al. (1991). Clonal analysis of liver infiltrating T cells in patients with LKM-1 antibody-positive autoimmune chronic active hepatitis. *Clinical and Experimental Immunology, 84*(2), 297–302.
171. Lombardi, V. C., & Khaiboullina, S. F. (2014). Plasmacytoid dendritic cells of the gut: Relevance to immunity and pathology. *Clinical Immunology, 153*(2), 165–177.
172. Longhi, M. S., Hussain, M. J., Mitry, R. R., Arora, S. K., Mieli-Vergani, G., Vergani, D., et al. (2006). Functional study of $CD4^+CD25^+$ regulatory T cells in health and autoimmune hepatitis. *Journal of Immunology, 176*(7), 4484–4491.

173. Longhi, M. S., Ma, Y., Bogdanos, D. P., Cheeseman, P., Mieli-Vergani, G., & Vergani, D. (2004). Impairment of $CD4^{+}CD25^{+}$ regulatory T-cells in autoimmune liver disease. *Journal of Hepatology, 41*(1), 31–37.

174. Longhi, M. S., Ma, Y., Mieli-Vergani, G., & Vergani, D. (2012). Regulatory T cells in autoimmune hepatitis. *Journal of Hepatology, 57*(4), 932–933.

175. Longhi, M. S., Ma, Y., Mitry, R. R., Bogdanos, D. P., Heneghan, M., Cheeseman, P., et al. (2005). Effect of $CD4^{+}$ $CD25^{+}$ regulatory T cells on CD8 T-cell function in patients with autoimmune hepatitis. *Journal of Autoimmunity, 25*(1), 63–71.

176. Longhi, M. S., Meda, F., Wang, P., Samyn, M., Mieli-Vergani, G., & Vergani, D. (2008). Expansion and de novo generation of potentially therapeutic regulatory T cells in patients with autoimmune hepatitis. *Hepatology, 47*(2), 581–591.

177. Lucey, D. R., Clerici, M., & Shearer, G. M. (1996). Type 1 and type 2 cytokine dysregulation in human infectious, neoplastic, and inflammatory diseases. *Clinical Microbiology Reviews, 9*(3), 532–562.

178. Ma, S., Hockings, C., Anwari, K., Kratina, T., Fennell, S., Lazarou, M., et al. (2013). Assembly of the Bak apoptotic pore: A critical role for the Bak protein alpha6 helix in the multimerization of homodimers during apoptosis. *Journal of Biological Chemistry, 288*(37), 26027–26038.

179. Ma, Y., Bogdanos, D. P., Hussain, M. J., Underhill, J., Bansal, S., Longhi, M. S., et al. (2006). Polyclonal T-cell responses to cytochrome P450IID6 are associated with disease activity in autoimmune hepatitis type 2. *Gastroenterology, 130*(3), 868–882.

180. Ma, Y., Thomas, M. G., Okamoto, M., Bogdanos, D. P., Nagl, S., Kerkar, N., et al. (2002). Key residues of a major cytochrome P4502D6 epitope are located on the surface of the molecule. *Journal of Immunology, 169*(1), 277–285.

181. Manabe, K., Hibberd, M. L., Donaldson, P. T., Underhill, J. A., Doherty, D. G., Demaine, A. G., et al. (1994). T-cell receptor constant beta germline gene polymorphisms and susceptibility to autoimmune hepatitis. *Gastroenterology, 106*(5), 1321–1325.

182. Mani, A. R., Ippolito, S., Ollosson, R., & Moore, K. P. (2006). Nitration of cardiac proteins is associated with abnormal cardiac chronotropic responses in rats with biliary cirrhosis. *Hepatology, 43*(4), 847–856.

183. Manns, M. P., & Obermayer-Straub, P. (1997). Cytochromes P450 and uridine triphosphate-glucuronosyltransferases: Model autoantigens to study drug-induced, virus-induced, and autoimmune liver disease. *Hepatology, 26*(5), 1054–1066.

184. Manns, M. P., Griffin, K. J., Sullivan, K. F., & Johnson, E. F. (1991). LKM-1 autoantibodies recognize a short linear sequence in P450IID6, a cytochrome P-450 monooxygenase. *Journal of Clinical Investigation, 88*(4), 1370–1378.

185. Manns, M. P., Johnson, E. F., Griffin, K. J., Tan, E. M., & Sullivan, K. F. (1989). Major antigen of liver kidney microsomal autoantibodies in idiopathic autoimmune hepatitis is cytochrome P450db1. *Journal of Clinical Investigation, 83*(3), 1066–1072.

186. Manns, M., Zanger, U., Gerken, G., Sullivan, K. F., Meyer Zum Buschenfelde, K. H., Meyer, U. A., et al. (1990). Patients with type II autoimmune hepatitis express functionally intact cytochrome P-450 db1 that is inhibited by LKM-1 autoantibodies in vitro but not in vivo. *Hepatology, 12*(1), 127–132.

187. Manousou, P., Kolios, G., Drygiannakis, I., Koulentaki, M., Pyrovolaki, K., Voumvouraki, A., et al. (2013). CXCR3 axis in patients with primary biliary cirrhosis: A possible novel mechanism of the effect of ursodeoxycholic acid. *Clinical and Experimental Immunology, 172*(1), 9–15.

188. Marra, F., & Tacke, F. (2014). Roles for chemokines in liver disease. *Gastroenterology, 147*(3), 577–594 e571.

189. Marra, F., Efsen, E., Romanelli, R. G., Caligiuri, A., Pastacaldi, S., Batignani, G., et al. (2000). Ligands of peroxisome proliferator-activated receptor gamma modulate profibrogenic and proinflammatory actions in hepatic stellate cells. *Gastroenterology, 119*(2), 466–478.

190. Martini, E., Abuaf, N., Cavalli, F., Durand, V., Johanet, C., & Homberg, J. C. (1988). Antibody to liver cytosol (anti-LC1) in patients with autoimmune chronic active hepatitis type 2. *Hepatology, 8*(6), 1662–1666.

191. Martins, E. B., Graham, A. K., Chapman, R. W., & Fleming, K. A. (1996). Elevation of gamma delta T lymphocytes in peripheral blood and livers of patients with primary sclerosing cholangitis and other autoimmune liver diseases. *Hepatology, 23*(5), 988–993.

192. Masuoka, H. C., Guicciardi, M. E., & Gores, G. J. (2009). Caspase inhibitors for the treatment of hepatitis C. *Clinical Liver Disease, 13*(3), 467–475.

193. Mato, J. M., Camara, J., Fernandez De Paz, J., Caballeria, L., Coll, S., Caballero, A., et al. (1999). S-adenosylmethionine in alcoholic liver cirrhosis: A randomized, placebo-controlled, double-blind, multicenter clinical trial. *Journal of Hepatology, 30*(6), 1081–1089.

194. Mattner, J. (2013). Natural killer T (NKT) cells in autoimmune hepatitis. *Current Opinion in Immunology, 25*(5), 697–703.

195. Mbongue, J., Nicholas, D., Firek, A., & Langridge, W. (2014). The role of dendritic cells in tissue-specific autoimmunity. *Journal of Immunology Research, 2014*, 857143.

196. Meunier, B., De Visser, S. P., & Shaik, S. (2004). Mechanism of oxidation reactions catalyzed by cytochrome P450 enzymes. *Chemical Reviews, 104*(9), 3947–3980.

197. Michaeloudes, C., Sukkar, M. B., Khorasani, N. M., Bhavsar, P. K., & Chung, K. F. (2011). TGF-beta regulates Nox4, MnSOD, and catalase expression, and IL-6 release in airway smooth muscle cells. *American Journal of Physiology–Lung Cellular and Molecular Physiology, 300*(2), L295–L304.

198. Migita, K., Nakamura, M., Abiru, S., Jiuchi, Y., Nagaoka, S., Komori, A., et al. (2013). Association of STAT4 polymorphisms with susceptibility to type-1 autoimmune hepatitis in the Japanese population. *PLoS One, 8*(7), e71382.

199. Miller, J. F., Morahan, G., Slattery, R., & Allison, J. (1990). Transgenic models of T-cell self-tolerance and autoimmunity. *Immunological Reviews, 118*(1), 21–35

200. Mohiuddin, I., Chai, H., Lin, P. H., Lumsden, A. B., Yao, Q., & Chen, C. (2006). Nitro tyrosine and chloropyrazine: Clinical significance and biological functions in the vascular system. *Journal of Surgical Research, 133*(2), 143–149.

201. Montano-Loza, A. J., & Czaja, A. J. (2014). Cell mediators of autoimmune hepatitis and their therapeutic implications. *Digestive Diseases and Sciences, 60*(6), 1528–1542.

202. Moretta, A., Sivori, S., Vitale, M., Pende, D., Morelli, L., Augugliaro, R., et al. (1995). Existence of both inhibitory (p58) and activatory (p50) receptors for HLA-C molecules in human natural killer cells. *Journal of Experimental Medicine, 182*(3), 875–884.

203. Morita, C. T., Mariuzza, R. A., & Brenner, M. B. (2000). Antigen recognition by human gamma delta T cells: Pattern recognition by the adaptive immune system. *Springer Seminars in Immunopathology, 22*(2), 191–217.

204. Muratori, L., Cataleta, M., Muratori, P., Lenzi, M., & Bianchi, F. B. (1998). Liver/kidney microsomal antibody type 1 and liver cytosol antibody type 1 concentrations in type 2 autoimmune hepatitis. *Gut, 42*(5), 721–726.

205. Muratori, L., Cataleta, M., Muratori, P., Manotti, P., Lenzi, M., Cassani, F., et al. (1995). Detection of anti-liver cytosol antibody type 1 (anti-LC1) by immunodiffusion, counter immunoelectrophoresis, and immunoblotting: Comparison of different techniques. *Journal of Immunological Methods, 187*(2), 259–264.

206. Muratori, L., Sztul, E., Muratori, P., Gao, Y., Ripalti, A., Ponti, C., et al. (2001). Distinct epitopes on formiminotransferase cyclodeaminase induce autoimmune liver cytosol antibody type 1. *Hepatology, 34*(3), 494–501.

207. Muratori, P., Lalanne, C., Fabbri, A., Cassani, F., Lenzi, M., & Muratori, L. (2015). Type 1 and type 2 autoimmune hepatitis in adults share the same clinical phenotype. *Alimentary Pharmacology & Therapeutics, 41*(12), 1281–1287.

208. Nakano, M., Saeki, C., Takahashi, H., Homma, S., Tajiri, H., & Zeniya, M. (2012). Activated natural killer T cells producing interferon-gamma elicit promoting activity to murine dendritic cell-based autoimmune hepatic inflammation. *Clinical and Experimental Immunology, 170*(2), 274–282.

209. Neurath, M. F. (2014). Cytokines in inflammatory bowel disease. *Nature Reviews Immunology, 14*(5), 329–342.

210. Nguyen, T. L., Sullivan, N. L., Ebel, M., Teague, R. M., & Dipaolo, R. J. (2011). Antigen-specific TGF-beta-induced regulatory T cells secrete chemokines, regulate T cell trafficking, and suppress ongoing autoimmunity. *Journal of Immunology, 187*(4), 1745–1753.

211. Nguyen, T., Sherratt, P. J., & Pickett, C. B. (2003). Regulatory mechanisms controlling gene expression mediated by the antioxidant response element. *Annual Review of Pharmacology and Toxicology, 43*, 233–260.

212. Nishioji, K., Okanoue, T., Itoh, Y., Narumi, S., Sakamoto, M., Nakamura, H., et al. (2001). Increase of chemokine interferon-inducible protein-10 (IP-10) in the serum of patients with autoimmune liver diseases and increase of its mRNA expression in hepatocytes. *Clinical and Experimental Immunology, 123*(2), 271–279.

213. Novak, J., & Lehuen, A. (2011). Mechanism of regulation of autoimmunity by iNKT cells. *Cytokine, 53*(3), 263–270.

214. Nowak, M., & Stein-Streilein, J. (2007). Invariant NKT cells and tolerance. *International Reviews of Immunology, 26*(2), 95–119.

215. Oikonomou, K. G., Zachou, K., & Dalekos, G. N. (2011). Alpha-actinin: A multidisciplinary protein with important role in B-cell driven autoimmunity. *Autoimmunity Reviews, 10*(7), 389–396.

216. Opelz, G., Vogten, A. J., Summerskill, W. H., Schalm, S. W., & Terasaki, P. I. (1977). HLA determinants in chronic active liver disease: Possible relation of HLA-Dw3 to prognosis. *Tissue Antigens, 9*(1), 36–40.

217. Pacher, P., Beckman, J. S., & Liaudet, L. (2007). Nitric oxide and peroxynitrite in health and disease. *Physiological Reviews, 87*(1), 315–424.

218. Paik, Y. H., Iwaisako, K., Seki, E., Inokuchi, S., Schnabl, B., Osterreicher, C. H., et al. (2011). The nicotinamide adenine dinucleotide phosphate oxidase (NOX) homologues NOX_1 and NOX_2/gp91(phox) mediate hepatic fibrosis in mice. *Hepatology, 53*(5), 1730–1741.

219. Paik, Y. H., Kim, J., Aoyama, T., De Minicis, S., Bataller, R., & Brenner, D. A. (2014). Role of NADPH oxidases in liver fibrosis. *Antioxidants & Redox Signaling, 20*(18), 2854–2872.

220. Pall, M. L., & Levine, S. (2015). Nrf2, a master regulator of detoxification and also antioxidant, anti-inflammatory and other cytoprotective mechanisms, is raised by health promoting factors. *Sheng Li Xue Bao, 67*(1), 1–18.

221. Pando, M., Larriba, J., Fernandez, G. C., Fainboim, H., Ciocca, M., Ramonet, M., et al. (1999). Pediatric and adult forms of type I autoimmune hepatitis in Argentina: Evidence for differential genetic predisposition. *Hepatology, 30*(6), 1374–1380.

222. Paradies, G., Paradies, V., Ruggiero, F. M., & Petrosillo, G. (2014). Oxidative stress, cardiolipin, and mitochondrial dysfunction in nonalcoholic fatty liver disease. *World Journal of Gastroenterology, 20*(40), 14205–14218.

223. Peiseler, M., Sebode, M., Franke, B., Wortmann, F., Schwinge, D., Quaas, A., et al. (2012a). FOXP3+ regulatory T cells in autoimmune hepatitis are fully functional and not reduced in frequency. *Journal of Hepatology, 57*(1), 125–132.

224. Peiseler, M., Sebode, M., Schramm, C., & Herkel, J. (2012b). Reply to: "Regulatory T cells in autoimmune hepatitis". *Journal of Hepatology, 57*(5), 933–934.

225. Peter, M. E., & Krammer, P. H. (2003). The CD95 (APO-1/Fas) DISC and beyond. *Cell Death & Differentiation, 10*(1), 26–35.

226. Peters, M. (1996). Actions of cytokines on the immune response and viral interactions: An overview. *Hepatology, 23*(4), 909–916.

227. Petry, A., Djordjevic, T., Weitnauer, M., Kietzmann, T., & Hess, J. (2006). NOX2 and NOX4 mediate proliferative response in endothelial cells. *Antioxidants & Redox Signaling, 8*(11–12), 1473–1484.

228. Pitkanen, J., Doucas, V., Sternsdorf, T., Nakajima, T., Aratani, S., Jensen, K., et al. (2000). The autoimmune regulator protein has transcriptional transactivating properties and interacts with the common coactivator CREB-binding protein. *Journal of Biological Chemistry, 275*(22), 16802–16809.

229. Preuss, B., Berg, C., Dengjel, J., Stevanovic, S., & Klein, R. (2012). Relevance of the inner mitochondrial membrane enzyme F1F0-ATPase as an autoantigen in autoimmune liver disorders. *Liver International, 32*(2), 249–257.

230. Proell, V., Carmona-Cuenca, I., Murillo, M. M., Huber, H., Fabregat, I., & Mikulits, W. (2007). TGF-beta dependent regulation of oxygen radicals during trans differentiation of activated hepatic stellate cells to myofibroblast cells. *Comparative Hepatology, 6*, 1.

231. Pryor, W. A., & Squadrito, G. L. (1995). The chemistry of peroxynitrite: A product from the reaction of nitric oxide with superoxide. *American Journal of Physiology, 268*(6 Pt 1), L699–L722.

232. Qiu, D. K., & Ma, X. (2003). Relationship between human leukocyte antigen DRB1 and autoimmune hepatitis type I in Chinese patients. *Journal of Gastroenterology and Hepatology, 18*(1), 63–67.

233. Radi, R., Beckman, J. S., Bush, K. M., & Freeman, B. A. (1991). Peroxynitrite oxidation of sulfhydryls: The cytotoxic potential of superoxide and nitric oxide. *Journal of Biological Chemistry, 266*(7), 4244–4250.

234. Rao, R., Graffeo, C. S., Gulati, R., Jamal, M., Narayan, S., Zambirinis, C. P., et al. (2014). Interleukin 17-producing gamma delta T cells promote hepatic regeneration in mice. *Gastroenterology, 147*(2), 473–484.e472.

235. Rhodes, K. A., Andrew, E. M., Newton, D. J., Tramonti, D., & Carding, S. R. (2008). A subset of IL-10-producing gamma delta T cells protect the liver from Listeria-elicited, CD8+ T cell-mediated injury. *European Journal of Immunology, 38*(8), 2274–2283.

236. Richter, K., Konzack, A., Pihlajaniemi, T., Heljasvaara, R., & Kietzmann, T. (2015). Redox-fibrosis: Impact of TGF-beta1 on ROS generators, mediators, and functional consequences. *Redox Biology, 6*, 344–352.

237. Rodriguez-Manzanet, R., Dekruyff, R. H., Kuchroo, V. K., & Umetsu, D. T. (2009). The costimulatory role of TIM molecules. *Immunological Reviews, 229*(1), 259–270.

238. Rodriguez, J., & Lazebnik, Y. (1999). Caspase-9 and APAF-1 form an active holoenzyme. *Genes & Development, 13*(24), 3179–3184.

239. Rollins, B. J. (1997). Chemokines. *Blood, 90*(3), 909–928.

240. Rossi, D., & Zlotnik, A. (2000). The biology of chemokines and their receptors. *Annual Review of Immunology, 18*, 217–242.

241. Saeki, C., Nakano, M., Takahashi, H., Saito, S., Homma, S., Tajiri, H., et al. (2010). Accumulation of functional regulatory T cells in actively inflamed liver in mouse dendritic cell-based autoimmune hepatic inflammation. *Clinical Immunology, 135*(1), 156–166.

242. Sahin, H., & Wasmuth, H. E. (2013). Chemokines in tissue fibrosis. *Biochimica et Biophysica Acta, 1832*(7), 1041–1048.

243. Samoylenko, A., Hossain, J. A., Mennerich, D., Kellokumpu, S., Hiltunen, J. K., & Kietzmann, T. (2013). Nutritional countermeasures targeting reactive oxygen species in cancer: From mechanisms to biomarkers and clinical evidence. *Antioxidants & Redox Signaling, 19*(19), 2157–2196.

244. Sanyal, A. J., Chalasani, N., Kowdley, K. V., McCullough, A., Diehl, A. M., Bass, N. M., et al. (2010). Pioglitazone, vitamin E, or placebo for nonalcoholic steatohepatitis. *New England Journal of Medicine, 362*(18), 1675–1685.

245. Sanz-Cameno, P., Medina, J., Garcia-Buey, L., Garcia-Sanchez, A., Borque, M. J., Martin-Vilchez, S., et al. (2002). Enhanced intrahepatic inducible nitric oxide synthase expression and nitro tyrosine accumulation in primary biliary cirrhosis and autoimmune hepatitis. *Journal of Hepatology, 37*(6), 723–729.

246. Savill, J., Dransfield, I., Gregory, C., & Haslett, C. (2002). A blast from the past: Clearance of apoptotic cells regulates immune responses. *Nature Reviews Immunology, 2*(12), 965–975.

247. Schreuder, G. M., Hurley, C. K., Marsh, S. G., Lau, M., Maiers, M., Kollman, C., et al. (2001). The HLA dictionary 2001: A summary of HLA-A, -B, -C, -DRB1/3/4/5, -DQB1 alleles and

their association with serologically defined HLA-A, -B, -C, -DR, and -DQ antigens. *Human Immunology, 62*(8), 826–849.

248. Seki, T., Kiyosawa, K., Inoko, H., & Ota, M. (1990). Association of autoimmune hepatitis with HLA-Bw54 and DR4 in Japanese patients. *Hepatology, 12*(6), 1300–1304.
249. Seki, T., Ota, M., Furuta, S., Fukushima, H., Kondo, T., Hino, K., et al. (1992). HLA class II molecules and autoimmune hepatitis susceptibility in Japanese patients. *Gastroenterology, 103*(3), 1041–1047.
250. Shih, P. H., & Yen, G. C. (2007). Differential expressions of antioxidant status in aging rats: The role of transcriptional factor Nrf2 and MAPK signaling pathway. *Biogerontology, 8*(1), 71–80.
251. Shimoda, S., Harada, K., Niiro, H., Taketomi, A., Maehara, Y., Tsuneyama, K., et al. (2010). CX3CL1 (fractalkine): A signpost for biliary inflammation in primary biliary cirrhosis. *Hepatology, 51*(2), 567–575.
252. Shimoda, S., Hisamoto, S., Harada, K., Iwasaka, S., Chong, Y., Nakamura, M., et al. (2015). Natural killer cells regulate T cell immune responses in primary biliary cirrhosis. *Hepatology, 62*(6), 1817–1827.
253. Shklovskaya, E., & Fazekas De St Groth, B. (2007). Balancing tolerance and immunity: The role of dendritic cell and T cell subsets. *Methods in Molecular Biology, 380*, 25–46.
254. Song, B. J., Akbar, M., Abdelmegeed, M. A., Byun, K., Lee, B., Yoon, S. K., et al. (2014). Mitochondrial dysfunction and tissue injury by alcohol, high fat, nonalcoholic substances and pathological conditions through post-translational protein modifications. *Redox Biology, 3*, 109–123.
255. Squadrito, G. L., & Pryor, W. A. (1998). Oxidative chemistry of nitric oxide: The roles of superoxide, peroxynitrite, and carbon dioxide. *Free Radical Biology and Medicine, 25*(4), 392–403.
256. Stern, L. J., Brown, J. H., Jardetzky, T. S., Gorga, J. C., Urban, R. G., Strominger, J. L., et al. (1994). Crystal structure of the human class II MHC protein HLA-DR1 complexed with an influenza virus peptide. *Nature, 368*(6468), 215–221.
257. Strettell, M. D., Donaldson, P. T., Thomson, L. J., Santrach, P. J., Moore, S. B., Czaja, A. J., et al. (1997). Allelic basis for HLA-encoded susceptibility to type 1 autoimmune hepatitis. *Gastroenterology, 112*(6), 2028–2035.
258. Sturrock, A., Cahill, B., Norman, K., Huecksteadt, T. P., Hill, K., Sanders, K., et al. (2006). Transforming growth factor-beta1 induces Nox4 NAD(P)H oxidase and reactive oxygen species-dependent proliferation in human pulmonary artery smooth muscle cells. *American Journal of Physiology–Lung Cellular and Molecular Physiology, 290*(3), L661–L673.
259. Subleski, J. J., Jiang, Q., Weiss, J. M., & Wiltrout, R. H. (2011). The split personality of NKT cells in malignancy, autoimmune, and allergic disorders. *Immunotherapy, 3*(11), 1167–1184.
260. Suh, J. H., Shenvi, S. V., Dixon, B. M., Liu, H., Jaiswal, A. K., Liu, R. M., et al. (2004). Decline in transcriptional activity of Nrf2 causes age-related loss of glutathione synthesis, which is reversible with lipoic acid. *Proceedings of the National Academy of Sciences U.S.A., 101*(10), 3381–3386.
261. Sun, J. C., Beilke, J. N., & Lanier, L. L. (2009). Adaptive immune features of natural killer cells. *Nature, 457*(7229), 557–561.

262. Swain, M. G. (2010). Natural killer T cells within the liver: Conductors of the hepatic immune orchestra. *Digestive Diseases, 28*(1), 7–13.

263. Takeshita, L. Y., Gonzalez-Galarza, F. F., Dos Santos, E. J., Maia, M. H., Rahman, M. M., Zain, S. M., et al. (2013). A database for curating the associations between killer cell immunoglobulin-like receptors and diseases in worldwide populations. *Database (Oxford), 2013,* bat021.

264. Tang, D., Kang, R., Coyne, C. B., Zeh, H. J., & Lotze, M. T. (2012a). PAMPs and DAMPs: Signal 0s that spur autophagy and immunity. *Immunological Reviews, 249*(1), 158–175.

265. Tang, J., Zhou, C., Zhang, Z. J., & Zheng, S. S. (2012b). Association of polymorphisms in non-classic MHC genes with susceptibility to autoimmune hepatitis. *Hepatobiliary & Pancreatic Diseases International, 11*(2), 125–131.

266. Thannickal, V. J. (2010). Aging, antagonistic pleiotropy, and fibrotic disease. *International Journal of Biochemistry & Cell Biology, 42*(9), 1398–1400.

267. Toussirot, E., Auge, B., Tiberghien, P., Chabod, J., & Cedoz, J. P. (1999). HLA-DRB1 alleles and shared amino acid sequences in disease susceptibility and severity in patients from eastern France with rheumatoid arthritis. *Journal of Rheumatology, 26*(6), 1446–1451.

268. Tran, G. T., Hodgkinson, S. J., Carter, N. M., Verma, N. D., Plain, K. M., Boyd, R., et al. (2012). IL-5 promotes induction of antigen-specific CD4+CD25+ T regulatory cells that suppress autoimmunity. *Blood, 119*(18), 4441–4450.

269. Tsikrikoni, A., Kyriakou, D. S., Rigopoulou, E. I., Alexandrakis, M. G., Zachou, K., Passam, F., et al. (2005). Markers of cell activation and apoptosis in bone marrow mononuclear cells of patients with autoimmune hepatitis type 1 and primary biliary cirrhosis. *Journal of Hepatology, 42*(3), 393–399.

270. Tsujimoto, Y., Nakagawa, T., & Shimizu, S. (2006). Mitochondrial membrane permeability transition and cell death. *Biochimica et Biophysica Acta, 1757*(11), 1297–1300.

271. Uhrberg, M., Valiante, N. M., Shum, B. P., Shilling, H. G., Lienert-Weidenbach, K., Corliss, B., et al. (1997). Human diversity in killer cell inhibitory receptor genes. *Immunity, 7*(5), 753–763.

272. Van Gerven, N. M., De Boer, Y. S., Zwiers, A., Verwer, B. J., Drenth, J. P., Van Hoek, B., et al. (2015). HLA-DRB1*03:01 and HLA-DRB1*04:01 modify the presentation and outcome in autoimmune hepatitis type 1. *Genes & Immunity, 16*(4), 247–252.

273. Van Kaer, L., Parekh, V. V., & Wu, L. (2011). Invariant NK T cells: Potential for immunotherapeutic targeting with glycolipid antigens. *Immunotherapy, 3*(1), 59–75.

274. Vazquez-Garcia, M. N., Alaez, C., Olivo, A., Debaz, H., Perez-Luque, E., Burguete, A., et al. (1998). MHC class II sequences of susceptibility and protection in Mexicans with autoimmune hepatitis. *Journal of Hepatology, 28*(6), 985–990.

275. Vergani, D., Choudhuri, K., Bogdanos, D. P., & Mieli-Vergani, G. (2002). Pathogenesis of autoimmune hepatitis. *Clinical Liver Disease, 6*(3), 727–737.

276. Vergani, D., Mieli-Vergani, G., Mondelli, M., Portmann, B., & Eddleston, A. L. (1987). Immunoglobulin on the surface of isolated hepatocytes is associated with antibody-dependent cell-mediated cytotoxicity and liver damage. *Liver, 7*(5), 307–315.

277. Vivier, E., Raulet, D. H., Moretta, A., Caligiuri, M. A., Zitvogel, L., Lanier, L. L., et al. (2011). Innate or adaptive immunity? The example of natural killer cells. *Science, 331*(6013), 44–49.

278. Vogel, A., Liermann, H., Harms, A., Strassburg, C. P., Manns, M. P., & Obermayer-Straub, P. (2001). Autoimmune regulator AIRE: Evidence for genetic differences between autoimmune hepatitis and hepatitis as part of the autoimmune polyglandular syndrome type 1. *Hepatology, 33*(5), 1047–1052.

279. Vogel, A., Strassburg, C. P., & Manns, M. P. (2002). Genetic association of vitamin D receptor polymorphisms with primary biliary cirrhosis and autoimmune hepatitis. *Hepatology, 35*(1), 126–131.

280. Vrolijk, M. F., Opperhuizen, A., Jansen, E. H., Godschalk, R. W., Van Schooten, F. J., Bast, A., et al. (2015). The shifting perception on antioxidants: The case of vitamin E and beta-carotene. *Redox Biology, 4*, 272–278.

281. Wang, J., Ioan-Facsinay, A., Van Der Voort, E. I., Huizinga, T. W., & Toes, R. E. (2007). Transient expression of FOXP3 in human activated nonregulatory CD4+ T cells. *European Journal of Immunology, 37*(1), 129–138.

282. Wasmuth, H. E., Zaldivar, M. M., Berres, M. L., Werth, A., Scholten, D., Hillebrandt, S., et al. (2008). The fractalkine receptor CX3CR1 is involved in liver fibrosis due to chronic hepatitis C infection. *Journal of Hepatology, 48*(2), 208–215.

283. Watanabe, Y., Kawakami, H., Kawamoto, H., Ikemoto, Y., Masuda, K., Takezaki, E., et al. (1987). Effect of neonatal thymectomy on experimental autoimmune hepatitis in mice. *Clinical & Experimental Immunology, 67*(1), 105–113.

284. Wehr, A., Baeck, C., Heymann, F., Niemietz, P. M., Hammerich, L., Martin, C., et al. (2013). Chemokine receptor CXCR6-dependent hepatic NK T cell accumulation promotes inflammation and liver fibrosis. *Journal of Immunology, 190*(10), 5226–5236.

285. Weiler-Normann, C., Schramm, C., Quaas, A., Wiegard, C., Glaubke, C., Pannicke, N., et al. (2013). Infliximab as a rescue treatment in difficult-to-treat autoimmune hepatitis. *Journal of Hepatology, 58*(3), 529–534.

286. Wen, L., Peakman, M., Mieli-Vergani, G., & Vergani, D. (1992). Elevation of activated gamma delta T cell receptor bearing T lymphocytes in patients with autoimmune chronic liver disease. *Clinical & Experimental Immunology, 89*(1), 78–82.

287. Wheeler, M. D., Kono, H., Yin, M., Nakagami, M., Uesugi, T., Arteel, G. E., et al. (2001). The role of Kupffer cell oxidant production in early ethanol-induced liver disease. *Free Radical Biology and Medicine, 31*(12), 1544–1549.

288. Winterbourn, C. C. (2008). Reconciling the chemistry and biology of reactive oxygen species. *Nature Chemical Biology, 4*(5), 278–286.

289. Winterbourn, C. C., & Metodiewa, D. (1994). The reaction of superoxide with reduced glutathione. *Archives of Biochemistry and Biophysics, 314*(2), 284–290.

290. Wright, G. P., Notley, C. A., Xue, S. A., Bendle, G. M., Holler, A., Schumacher, T. N., et al. (2009). Adoptive therapy with redirected primary regulatory T cells results in antigen-specific suppression of arthritis. *Proceedings of the National Academy of Sciences U.S.A., 106*(47), 19078–19083.

291. Wu, L., & Van Kaer, L. (2011). Natural killer T cells in health and disease. *Frontiers in Bioscience (Scholar Edition), 3*, 236–251.

292. Yang, J. Q., Kim, P. J., & Singh, R. R. (2012). Brief treatment with iNKT cell ligand alpha-galactosylceramide confers a long-term protection against lupus. *Journal of Clinical Immunology, 32*(1), 106–113.

293. Yokosawa, S., Yoshizawa, K., Ota, M., Katsuyama, Y., Kawa, S., Ichijo, T., et al. (2007). A genome-wide DNA microsatellite association study of Japanese patients with autoimmune hepatitis type 1. *Hepatology, 45*(2), 384–390.

294. Yoshiga, Y., Goto, D., Segawa, S., Horikoshi, M., Hayashi, T., Matsumoto, I., et al. (2011). Activation of natural killer T cells by alpha-carba-GalCer (RCAI-56), a novel synthetic glycolipid ligand, suppresses murine collagen-induced arthritis. *Clinical & Experimental Immunology, 164*(2), 236–247.

295. Yoshizawa, K., Ota, M., Katsuyama, Y., Ichijo, T., Matsumoto, A., Tanaka, E., et al. (2005). Genetic analysis of the HLA region of Japanese patients with type 1 autoimmune hepatitis. *Journal of Hepatology, 42*(4), 578–584.

296. Zeissig, S., & Blumberg, R. S. (2012). Primary immunodeficiency associated with defects in CD1 and CD1-restricted T cells. *Annals of the New York Academy of Sciences, 1250*(1), 14–24.

297. Zhan, S. S., Jiang, J. X., Wu, J., Halsted, C., Friedman, S. L., Zern, M. A., et al. (2006). Phagocytosis of apoptotic bodies by hepatic stellate cells induces NADPH oxidase and is associated with liver fibrosis in vivo. *Hepatology, 43*(2), 435–443.

298. Zhang, W., Ono, Y., Miyamura, Y., Bowlus, C. L., Gershwin, M. E., & Maverakis, E. (2011). T cell clonal expansions detected in patients with primary biliary cirrhosis express CX3CR1. *Journal of Autoimmunity, 37*(1), 71–78.

299. Zhang, Y., & Hogg, N. (2005). S-Nitrosothiols: Cellular formation and transport. *Free Radical Biology and Medicine, 38*(6), 831–838.

300. Zhao, L., Tang, Y., You, Z., Wang, Q., Liang, S., Han, X., et al. (2011). Interleukin-17 contributes to the pathogenesis of autoimmune hepatitis through inducing hepatic interleukin-6 expression. *PLoS One, 6*(5), e18909.

301. Zhou, J., Eleni, C., Spyrou, G., & Brune, B. (2008). The mitochondrial thioredoxin system regulates nitric oxide-induced HIF-1α protein. *Free Radical Biology and Medicine, 44*(1), 91–98.

302. Zolfino, T., Heneghan, M. A., Norris, S., Harrison, P. M., Portmann, B. C., & McFarlane, I. G. (2002). Characteristics of autoimmune hepatitis in patients who are not of European Caucasoid ethnic origin. *Gut, 50*(5), 713–717.

Chapter

AMEBIC LIVER ABSCESS

4

Contents

Introduction

It has long been believed that one of the main parasitic causes of death in humans is invasive amebiasis, which is caused by the protozoan *Entamoeba histolytica* (Walsh, 1986). Associated with a notable morbidity and mortality rate, amebic liver abscess (ALA) is the most prevalent extraintestinal manifestation of this infection. Considering that liver lesions can be detected clinically, in a lab, or through postmortem investigations, the prevalence of ALA is a valid indicator of amebic infection rates (Espinosa-Cantellano and Martínez-Palomo, 2000; Martínez-Palomo and EspinosaCantellano, 2004, 2005).

Orientation and Directional Terms

Term	Definition	Illustration
Amebic liver abscess (ALA)	Amebic liver abscess is the most common extra-intestinal manifestation of the protozoan, Entamoeba histolytica. The life cycle involves consumption of fecally contaminated food and water, that reaches and penetrates the small intestine to enter the mesenteric vessels and finally the liver.	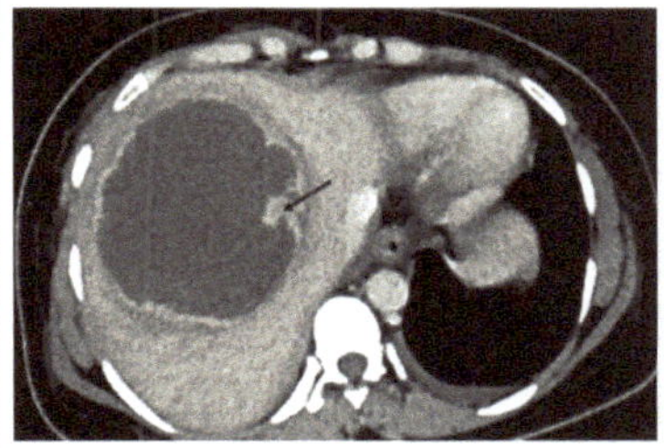
Indirect hemagglutination (IHA)	An indirect hemagglutination (IHA) test using sonicated extract as the antigen was developed for the detection of antibodies to Clostridium chauvoei.	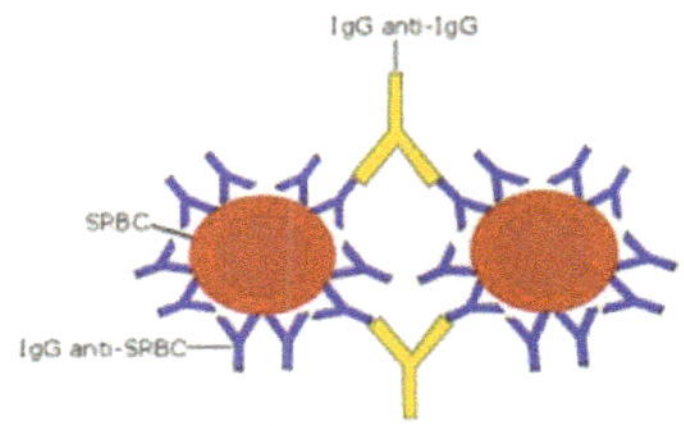
Vagus nerve (VN)	The vagus nerve serves as the body's superhighway, carrying information between the brain and the internal organs and controlling the body's response in times of rest and relaxation.	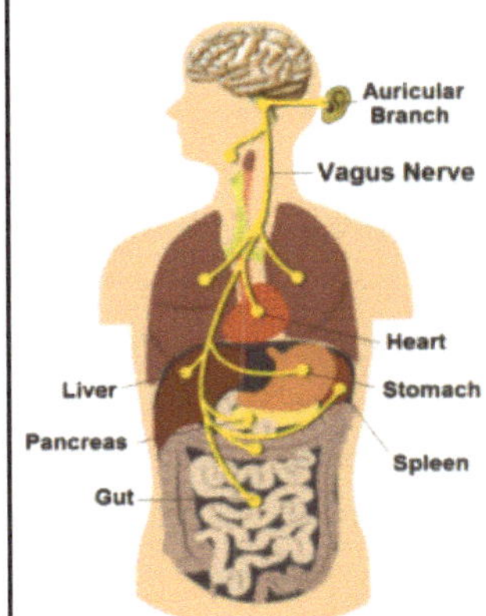
Superoxide dismutase (SOD)	Superoxide dismutase is an enzyme that alternately catalyzes the dismutation of the superoxide anion radical into normal molecular oxygen and hydrogen peroxide. Superoxide is produced as a by-product of oxygen metabolism and, if not regulated, causes many types of cell damage.	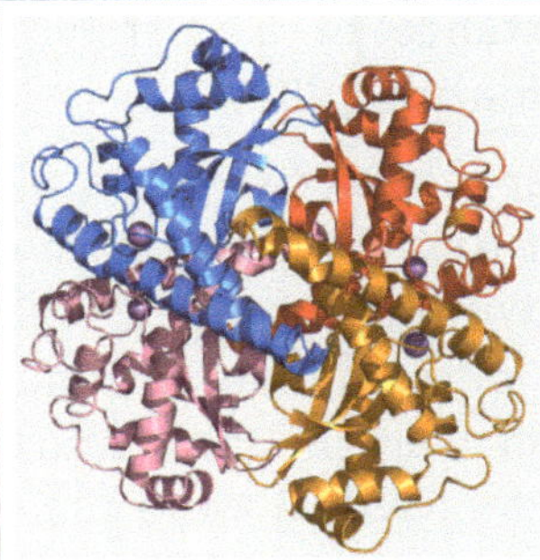

4.1. Prevalence of Amebic Liver Abscess

The absence of more recent data has created the false impression that invasive amebiasis is no longer a significant health issue in developing nations, despite the fact that rough estimates of the geographic distribution and prevalence of ALAs have been produced in the past (Walsh, 1986; Wells and Arguedas, 2004). As a result, amebiasis is still a disease that is ignored by international health agencies.

Researchers have carried out a bibliographical analysis of clinical cases of ALA that have been published between 2011 and 2015 in order to gain insight into the condition's prevalence. The findings unequivocally show that ALA is still a prevalent clinical consequence of amebiasis infection in Latin American, Asian, and African nations; this is especially the case for low-income, illiterate populations with high alcoholism indexes. Treatment-wise, there has been an unexpected trend in recent years to frequently use percutaneous drainage of the ALA contents in addition to metronidazole or its derivatives. This is likely because the majority of cases are hospitalized on surgical grounds. Mortality rates exceed 10% in certain settings, and no fatal cases are reported in other series. There have been no clinical suggestions of resistance of *E. histolytica* infections to metronidazole.

Over the last five years, GTR has treated 61 cases of ALA in the Mexican state of San Luis Potosí, with no fatalities. 75% of the patients needed percutaneous drainage, the majority of whom were in their fourth decade of life and 80% of whom were male. Two cases had abscess contents greater than 500 mL, but aspirated volumes were typically less than 300 mL (Tsutsumi et al., 2015).

A particularly high incidence of ALA on a regional level was reported in the province of Hué in Central Vietnam where 2031 patients were treated between 1990 and 1998. Significant observations of this study were: (1) the substantial higher incidence of this condition in males, not due to a higher rate of infection with *E. histolytica*; (2) a direct correlation of ALA cases with population density, and (3) the annual number of cases was rather constant, suggesting a stable epidemiological situation (Blessmann et al., 2002).

4.2. Clinical Manifestations

The migration of *E. histolytica* trophozoites from the colon to the liver through the portal circulation causes ALA. It is unknown how long it takes for damage to the hepatic parenchyma to occur after the large intestine's mucosa is penetrated. Only one-third of cases of hepatic abscess have amebic colitis, as confirmed by clinical observations and numerous autopsies. Although amebic hepatic abscesses can present with a variety of signs and symptoms, they typically begin suddenly and cause pain that radiates to the right hypochondrium, right shoulder, and right scapular region. When breathing deeply, coughing, or walking on the right foot, the pain usually gets worse. A pleuritic-type pain and an irritative cough, occasionally productive, are the symptoms of an abscess localized to the right lobe. Upper left lobe abscesses can cause epigastric pain, which can also occasionally progress to dyspnea and sometimes spread to the base of the neck and one or both shoulders. An abrupt increase in pain that is concentrated in the precordial area is highly suggestive of pericardial space penetration by the abscess.

The cause of this complication, cardiac tamponade, is almost always fatal. If the abscess is located close to the diaphragm, it may puncture the pleura, resulting in empyema or pleurisy. Pus may be vomited if the bronchi become involved, which would improve the patient's condition. There may be the formation of an abscess and pulmonary consolidation if the lung is affected. The abscess can spread to nearby organs and the peritoneal cavity when it is situated in the inferior portion of the liver (Sepúlveda & Treviño, 1986).

Every patient with ALA has a fever of 38 to 40 degrees Celsius. The patient frequently experiences chills and excessive perspiration at night and in the afternoon. Anorexia, nausea, vomiting, diarrhea (with or without blood), and dysentery are additional symptoms. Hepatomegaly, or painful hepatic dysfunction, is the primary physical indicator of ALA. Fist percussion and digital pressure frequently cause excruciating pain in the liver area. When the liver is palpated, it is smooth and soft, as opposed to the rough, irregular liver found in patients with cirrhosis and hepatocarcinoma. Eight percent of patients who respond well to treatment have jaundice. Multiple abscesses should be suspected in cases of severe jaundice. Hepatic coma and ascites are uncommon, but the prognosis is bad for those who experience them (Sepúlveda & Treviño, 1986).

4.3. Pathology

Based on a significant number of autopsies, the pathology of human hepatic amebiasis has been thoroughly described (Pérez-Tamayo, 1986). From a macroscopic perspective, an amebic abscess is a clearly defined region where the liver parenchyma is entirely replaced by creamy-colored necrotic material. Typically, this area is encircled by a rim of crowded liver tissue. The necrotic material is often thick and slightly mucinous, but it can also be firm, soft, or semifluid. While the more solid phase of the necrotic area adheres to the cavity's inner surface, the fluid portion of the necrotic area is typically located in the center. There are numerous exceptions to the general rule that smaller abscesses are denser than larger ones. The necrotic material takes on a reddish-brown shade when combined with blood, which typically occurs following paracentesis.

ALAs can range widely in size from tiny lesions to massive masses of necrotic material that can replace almost 90% of the organ. These abscesses typically have a diameter of 5 to 15 cm according to autopsy material. The right lobe is the preferred location for ALAs, and they are more often single than multiple. Statistics on these two characteristics differ depending on the data source. Large and multiple abscesses are typically reported in autopsy series, whereas small and single abscesses predominate in clinically diagnosed and successfully treated series.

Rarely does an amebic hepatic abscess' microscopic appearance warrant the term "abscess.." Typically, the lesion is composed of granular eosinophilic necrotic material with nuclear debris and few or no polymorphonuclear (PMN) leukocytes. Amebas are typically located on the outside of the lesion, rarely within the necrotic material itself. Under a microscope, it is difficult to see the clearly defined macroscopically separation between the abscess and the uninvolved parenchyma. The liver cell plates next to the lesion appear thin and disorganized due to fibrosis; the compression caused by the expanding abscess is quite noticeable. Even in large abscesses that undoubtedly involve large blood vessels, hemorrhage is not seen. The absence of PMN leukocytes is notable, particularly in large lesions; amebic necrosis of the liver might be a more appropriate term to describe the condition than "abscess," though this is not always the case. Three paths may be taken by ALA: dispersal, rupture, or healing. Many patients with amebic liver abscesses recover with appropriate care (Table 4.1). The healing process is not well documented, but sonography and computerized axial tomography (CAT) scans show that the abscess is rapidly shrinking with little sign of collapse, based on the amount of fluid obtained during paracentesis. This has been explained as the outcome of liver parenchyma regeneration. In certain patients, the only thing visible is a tiny patch of subcapsular fibrous tissue that extends into the surrounding parenchyma in the form of thin stellate prolongations.

Table 4.1. *Amebic Liver Abscess (ALA), Reports 2011–15*

Country	Number of ALA	Comments	References
India	82	Catheter drainage of large abscesses	Gupta et al. (2011)
India	67	Use of touchdown rRNA PCR reaction for diagnosis	Singh et al. (2011)
Saudi Arabia	19	Patient from India or travelers to India. Mortality 10.8%	Albenmousa et al. (2011)
USA	848	Mostly Hispanics; mortality 0.8%. Percutaneous drainage 48%	Congly et al. (2011)
Bangladesh	250	Most do not require invasive treatment. Follow-up by sonography	Debnath et al. (2012)
Mexico	40	No deaths; 60% responded to medical treatment alone	Sánchez-Aguilar et al. (2012)
France	90	ALA similar in European and foreign-born patients. No fatal cases	Cordel et al. (2013)
Bangladesh	30	Detailed clinical presentation, mostly male patients	Hoque et al. (2014)
Bangladesh	90	Analysis of sociodemographic determinants: Poverty, illiteracy, alcohol	Alam et al. (2014)
India	110	Use of sonography and percutaneous drainage	Jha et al. (2015)
India	114	Pharmacological treatment 45%. Mortality 3.5%	Chaudhary et al. (2016)
Mexico	61	Average one ALA a month. Percutaneous drainage 75%. No fatal cases	Tsutsumi et al. (2015)

Source. A. Martı´nez-Palomo, et al., Amebic Liver Abscess, http://dx.doi.org/10.1016/B978-0-12-804274-8.00013-8.

4.4. Experimental Hepatic Amebiasis

Human studies on the initial phases of hepatic amebic invasion are lacking. When *E. histolytica* trophozoites are injected into the portal vein of experimental animals, the result is multiple liver foci of infection with neutrophil accumulation surrounding the parasites, followed by focal necrosis and granulomatous infiltration (Tsutsumi et al., 1984). CD38 most likely acts as a mediator of neutrophil accumulation (Estrada-Figueroa et al., 2011). Granulomas eventually turn necrotic and merge with necrotic tissue, taking up increasing amounts of the liver as lesions enlarge. Hepatocytes in proximity to the initial lesions undergo necrotic degeneration, although there is seldom evidence of direct hepatocyte-ameba interaction. Large areas of liquefied necrotic material encircled by a thin, fibrous-appearing capsule may eventually make up the lesions (Tsutsumi et al., 1984).

Large numbers of PMN leukocytes are recruited around amebas invading the liver parenchyma, as demonstrated by electron microscopy observations (Tsutsumi & Martínez Palomo, 1988).

These leukocytes lyse, most likely as a result of the trophozoites' contact-mediated damage. Moreover, eosinophils and macrophages were drawn to the sites of inflammation. When tested, the majority of trophozoites persisted despite coming into contact with PMNs or eosinophils that were degranulating. Furthermore, during the early phases of the parasite-induced focal necrosis, there is no direct interaction between amebas and liver parenchymal cells, thereby bolstering the theory that hepatic damage could be indirectly caused by inflammatory cell lysis.

The idea that host immune responses are a major factor in the liver pathology caused by *E. histolytica* infection is supported by reports using a mouse model of ALA. According to the study's findings, Kupffer cells and inflammatory monocytes—rather than neutrophils—are most likely the immune populations that cause tissue destruction, with TNFa serving as a crucial cytokine mediator (Helk et al., 2013).

4.5. Humoral Response

The amount of time that elapses between an *E. histolytica* infection and the onset of local antibody responses is still unknown. Indirect hemagglutination (IHA) revealed copreantibodies in 80% of amebic dysentery patients; however, this percentage dropped to 55% three weeks following the acute episode. This was accompanied by an increase in serum antibodies, indicating that in patients with invasive intestinal amebiasis, a brief and transitory local secretory response precedes the development of systemic antibodies and initiates the humoral immune response. As early as one week after the onset of symptoms in both humans and experimental animal models, circulating antibodies to *E. histolytica*, predominantly IgG class, can be found. The levels of circulating antibodies in humans do not correspond with the severity of the disease, in contrast to findings in animals. According to Knobloch and Mannweiler (1983), high antibody titers typically arise early in the course of the illness and continue even after invasive amebiasis is cured. The sensitivity of the test being used determines the rate at which antibody levels decrease after treatment. When invasive amebic episodes occur more than three years ago and there is no evidence of recurrent infection, the extremely sensitive methods of IHA or ELISA can identify antibodies (reviewed in Kretschmer, 1986).

Many studies have been conducted on the detrimental effects of antiamebic antibodies on trophozoites cultured in vitro. The cytotoxic effect of amebae on cultured cell lines and the process of erythrophagocytosis by *E. histolytica* can be inhibited by immune sera. Immune serum causes trophozoites to lyse quickly at high concentrations (reviewed in Kretschmer, 1986). Amebae may, in certain situations, withstand exposure to antibodies, which appears to contradict these findings. Immune serum incubation causes surface-bound antigens to quickly redistribute to the uroid; the caps that form can then be released or endocytosed. Actin and myosin are involved in a sliding mechanism that drives this pH and temperature-dependent process that is controlled by myosin light chain kinase and calmodulin (Espinosa-Cantellano and Martínez-Palomo, 1994). After shedding the antibody-antigen complexes, the parasite seems to come out unscathed.

As evidenced by the finding that experimental animals depleted of cobra venom factor are noticeably more likely to develop ALA than normal animals, complement may also play a role in limiting amebiasis. Furthermore, cobra venom factor reduces complement-sensitive strain lysis when added to normal human serum. Furthermore, even in the absence of antibodies, amebae can activate complement via both the classical and alternative pathways. In vitro, this activation is fatal to long-term cultured *E. histolytica* strains that have partially lost their virulence, as well as to the noninvasive *Entamoeba dispar*. A mechanism for avoiding complement lysis has been developed by some amebae, as evidenced by the fact that fresh isolates from patients with colitis or ALAs are resistant to complement-mediated lysis and that axenic *E. histolytica* trophozoites may develop complement resistance when repeatedly treated with human serum (Calderón and Tovar, 1986).

When considered collectively, these data imply that even though the host mounts a quick humoral immune response in response to an invasion by *E. histolytica* , the parasite has effective evasion mechanisms, such as complement resistance and the ability to cap and shed surface proteins. Thus, antibodies are thought to be ineffective against *E. histolytica* . This view is further reinforced by the finding that patients with invasive amebiasis had high antibody levels, and that individuals with elevated antibody titers had high rates of reinfection.

4.6. Cellular Response

Systemic cell-mediated immunity has been verified in vitro by lymphokine, blastogenic response, leukocyte adherence inhibition, and lymphocytotoxic assays, as well as in vivo by delayed hypersensitivity skin reactions. However, in the early stages of the disease, many patients do not respond to delayed skin tests using amebic antigens, presumably because they are in a specific state of nonresponsiveness. In vitro tests that demonstrate a temporary inability to produce macrophage inhibition factor and a decrease in lymphocyte cytotoxicity in patients with untreated hepatic amebiasis in the early stages have both identified this unresponsiveness (reviewed in Kretschmer, 1986). Consequently, tissue invasion by *E. histolytica* is correlated with and requires a certain level of T cell suppression due to suppressor T cell induction or selection. T cell-mediated suppression may contribute to invasive amebiasis, as evidenced by the association between malnourishment and ALA in more than 90% of clinical and autopsy cases as well as the markedly elevated HLA-DR3 antigen levels in Mexican ALA patients (Kretschmer, 1986).

Cell-mediated immunity against invasive amebiasis is not rendered ineffective by the presence of an early transient energy state. In fact, the low rate of recurrences of ALAs in humans—0.04% versus 0.2% ALA per initial infection per year calculated in Mexico City—may be due to a state of cell-mediated immunity (Kretschmer, 1986). The protection seen in cases of resolved invasive amebiasis appears to be caused by Th1-driven immune responses (García-Zepeda et al., 2007). However, the idea of permanent immunity against recurrent liver abscess was refuted by a 2013 study of ALA cases in Vietnam (Blessmann et al., 2002).

4.7. Diagnosis

Amebic abscess should always be suspected in patients with spiking fever, weight loss, upper right quadrant or epigastrium abdominal pain, and liver area tenderness in endemic areas or when there is a history of travel to such places. An elevated right diaphragm (observable on a chest X-ray), leukocytosis, and a high alkaline phosphatase level all point to the possibility of a hepatic abscess. CAT scans or ultrasonography are used to confirm the diagnosis. The latter is the most accurate way to diagnose hepatic abscesses, especially if they are small, and it is very helpful in differentiating them from other liver focal lesions. However, due to its non-invasiveness, affordability, and ease of use, ultrasonography is the recommended imaging method for ALA detection (Treviño-García Manzo and Sepúlveda, 1986; Kimura et al, 1997). Furthermore, the analysis of ALA aspirates is being accomplished with success using polymerase chain reaction tests (Fotedar et al., 2007). Antiamebic antibody serological tests are positive in >90% of patients with ALAs and c. 75% of patients with invasive colonic amebiasis.

4.8. Chemotherapy

The morbidity and death rates of amebiasis have significantly decreased as a result of the use of amebicides in patient treatment. Luminal, tissue, and mixed amebicides are the three categories into which antiamebic medications can be divided. Diiodohydroxyquinoline (650 mg orally three times daily for twenty days), diloxanide furoate (500 mg orally three times daily for ten days), and paromomycin (500 mg orally three times daily for five to ten days) are the most commonly used amebicides with luminal action. These days, tissue amebicides are rarely employed.

Metronidazole and the nitroimidazole derivatives tinidazole and ornidazole are amebicides that are effective in both tissues and the intestinal lumen. These medications have the benefit of being administered orally and having the highest therapeutic efficacy, in addition to being active in tissues and the intestinal lumen. They are fairly well tolerated, and although they have been shown to have a carcinogenic effect in rodents and the potential to cause mutagenicity in bacteria, no such effect has been found in humans. Despite a few uncomfortable but manageable side effects, they are therefore the preferred medications for treating invasive amebiasis. Those with invasive intestinal amebiasis receive 500–800 mg of metronidazole orally three times a day for five days, while those with liver abscesses receive it for five to ten days. Oral administration of 2g of ornidazole or tinidazole once daily for 1–3 days is recommended. To obtain additional information regarding amebiasis chemotherapy, please read Martínez-Palomo and Ruíz-Palacios (1990).

It has been shown that in over 85% of cases, pharmacologic therapy alone is sufficient (Wells and Arguedas, 2004). Medication resistance does not exist in amebiasis. The few reports of treatment failure pertain to cases that were advanced and treatment was given too late, with the amebic abscess replacing the majority of the liver parenchyma. Drug sensitivity was confirmed in every instance by in vitro investigations using newly isolated pathogenic amebae and asymptomatic carriers, as well as axenically cultured pathogenic amebae (Burchard and Mirelman, 1988).

4.9. Surgical Treatment

The management of amebic disease-related liver lesions has changed significantly over time. The incorrect belief that the treatment of a hepatic abscess should be approached like that of any other suppurating lesion and that "pus" should be removed surgically right away led to the previous misuse of surgery, including aspiration. But unlike the latter lesion, the hepatic abscess is primarily composed of necrotic material created during the liquefaction process; only 2% of them are bacterially contaminated, usually as a consequence of surgical intervention or the abscess opening up to the outside world (Guarner, 1986).

When metronidazole was first available for use in 1970, there was a significant decrease in the number of surgical procedures performed, which also led to a significant drop in mortality. A prospective investigation was done by Guarner et al., compared the benefits of a conservative versus a surgical approach for the management of amebic hepatic abscess in 1974. According to the study's findings, surgical drainage should only be used in cases where there is a perforation and abscesses that do not improve with medication treatment should be aspirated (Guarner, 1986; Esquivel López et al., 1979). However, as previously mentioned, there is an unexpected propensity to treat hepatic amebiasis by percutaneous drainage of the ALA contents; this is likely due to the fact that the majority of cases are admitted to hospitals for surgery (Tsutsumi et al., 2015). Whether intestinal, hepatic, or cutaneous, one of the most remarkable characteristics of invasive amebiasis is that, with proper care, amebic lesions heal without leaving any scars. This peculiarity of the disease's pathology appears to have no known explanation.

4.10. Vaccination

There are primarily two sets of observations that support the existence of acquired immunity against amebiasis. First, it is commonly known that ALA recurrences are extremely rare. The prevalence of amebic liver abscesses per year in the general population is 0.1–0.2%; however, estimates from the early 1970s in Mexico City showed that 0.04% of patients who recovered from an ALA had recurrences during a 7-year follow-up period (reviewed in Kretschmer, 1986). No recent data are available. The second set of data in favor of acquired immunity comes from research on laboratory animals that, following either spontaneous or induced recovery, are resistant to amebic hepatic reinvasion.

Additionally, there is evidence that invasive amebiasis does not cause immunity to develop. Amebic hepatic abscess recurrence was reported in a Vietnamese study (Blessmann et al., 2002). For example, the idea of effective acquired protective immunity is called into question by the rise in morbidity and mortality caused by *E. histolytica* with advancing age. Furthermore, it has been noted that not all antibodies offer protection; for example, passive immunization against intrahepatic challenge with *E. histolytica* using purified antiamebic immunoglobulins has been shown to be ineffective (Campos-Rodríguez et al., 1995). Despite significant efforts, there is currently insufficient scientific proof to support the eventual efficacy of the antiamebic vaccine.

4.11. Role of Cytokines and Reactive Oxygen Species in the Amebic Liver Abscess Produced by Entamoeba histolytica

Despite the fact that *E. histolytica* is known to be the etiological agent of human amebiasis and despite the disease's significant impact on public health, especially in developing nations, many aspects of the host-parasite relationship remain unclear. However, recent developments in the understanding of the host response to infection, intriguing reports on the genetic analysis of the parasite with knowledge of several virulence factors, and the use of in vitro, in vivo, and ex vivo models for producing experimental intestinal and hepatic amebiasis have all contributed to a better understanding of the various mechanisms that occur during the pathogenesis of the amebiasis.

4.11.1. Human Amebiasis

An estimated 500 million cases of human amebiasis are caused by the primary and most common cause each year, with the nonpathogenic *Entamoeba dispar* accounting for at least 90 p% of these infections. However, according to Ackers and Mirelman (2006), the remaining infections are linked to *E. histolytica* and are thought to be responsible for 40,000–100,000 fatalities per year.

The large intestine is the primary organ affected by the intestinal infectious disease amebiasis; nevertheless, *E. histolytica* can cause harm to almost any type of human tissue. The most prevalent, well-defined clinical condition is called ulcerative colitis of the amebix. Formally known as an amebic liver abscess (ALA), large necrotic areas of the liver are a characteristic of the most common extraintestinal lesion, hepatic amebiasis (Brandt and Tamayo, 1970). Macroscopically, ALA is a well-defined region where necrotic material with a creamy consistency and yellowish color has completely replaced the liver parenchyma (Martinez-Palomo et al, 1985; Martinez-Palomo, 1987). Under a microscope, trophozoites are found near the seemingly normal parenchyma on the edge of the necrotic material; amebas may include ingested erythrocytes or cell debris. Although the degree of inflammation varies, certain regions exhibit high levels of persistent inflammation.

4.11.2. Life Cycle of Entamoeba histolytica

The two primary stages of the *E. histolytica* life cycle are trophozoites and cysts. The cycle starts when mature cysts (resistant, infectious phase) are consumed. These cysts can withstand the stomach's acidic pH and expel themselves in the terminal ileum. Trophozoites, also known as ameba (invasive phase, motile form), enter the large intestine and begin to colonize it. The ameba re-starts the cycle when it responds to unknown stimuli by changing morphologically and biochemically. These changes result in the formation of cysts, which are then removed in the feces and spread to other hosts through the consumption of contaminated food or water (EspinosaCantellano and Martinez-Palomo, 2000).

4.11.3. Virulence Factors

Host-parasite interactions start signaling processes in both cells, which aids in the infection. Understanding microbial pathogenicity requires an understanding of these interactions, which take place between the pathogen and the surface of the host cell. Adhesins, which are molecules involved in the virulence of the parasites, are visible on the heterogeneous and biochemical complex of the microbial surface. The primary target of the immune responses is adhesins. *E. histolytica* offers a variety of immune-evasion techniques, such as the use of cysteine proteases, which are involved in tissue invasion and destruction. E histolytica can damage tissue by interacting with the extracellular matrix (ECM) of intestinal or hepatic cells. In this situation, the ameba may move by releasing pseudopods and may cling to the extracellular matrix (ECM) through particular receptors; most research has used the parasite's lectin galactose-N-acetylgalactosamine (Gal/GalNac) and the target cells' glycoproteins (Petri et al., 2002). In *E. histolytica* trophozoites, a number of cysteine proteases from the membrane or secreted by the parasite that break down host proteins have been identified; the majority of research has concentrated on CP1 and CP5. Depending on the ameba strain and the culture conditions, over 50 genes can encode for cysteine proteinases, which are expressed in various ways (Loftus et al., 2005; Hall & Loftus, 2005) (Figure 4.1).

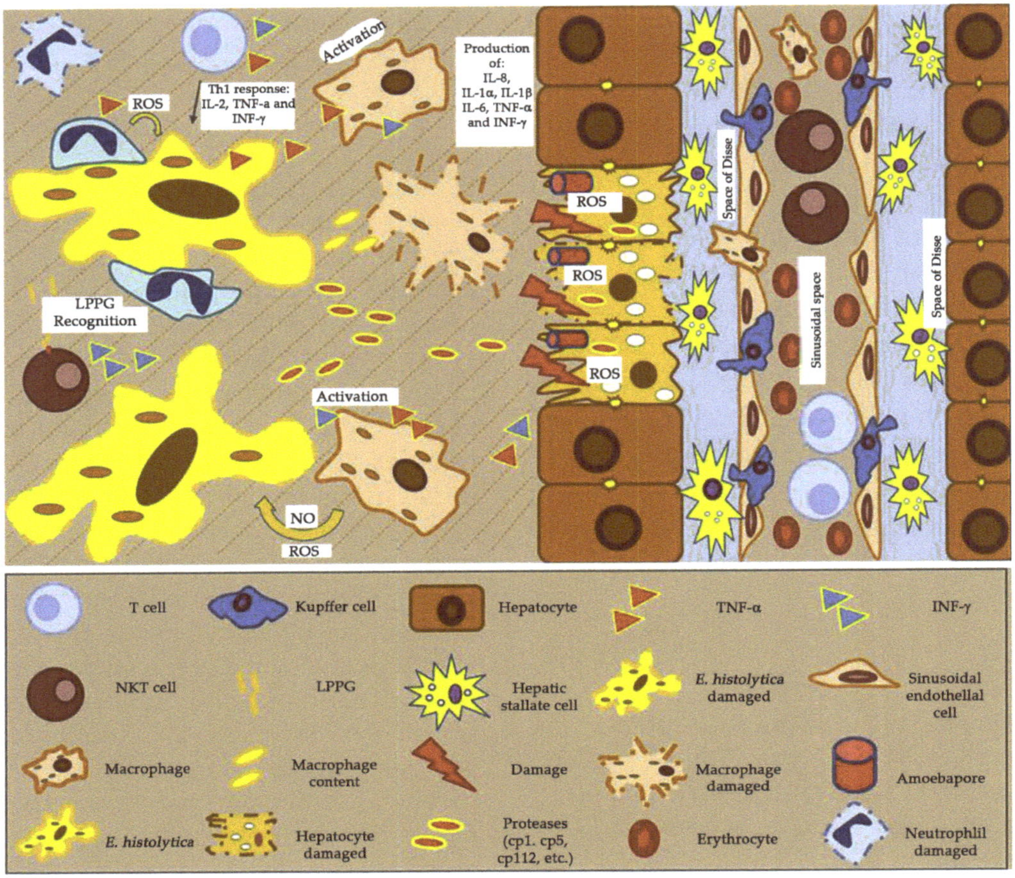

Figure 4.1. *Schematic representation of cytokines, nitric oxide, and reactive oxygen species production during amebic liver abscess (ALA) development. Entamoeba histolytica trophozoites in the liver tissue produce an inflammatory reaction mainly composed of neutrophils and macrophages; therefore, the cytokines, reactive oxygen species (ROS), and nitric oxide (NO) produced by the inflammation leads to the progression of the ALA.*

Source: A. Martı´nez-Palomo, et al., Amebic Liver Abscess, http://dx.doi.org/10.1016/B978-0-12-804274-8.00013-8.

Numerous compounds have been identified as virulent components in amebiasis. Little peptides known as ameba pores have the ability to lyse cells and may be involved in the destruction of immune host cells, hepatocytes, and intestinal cells. Amebas can lyse host cells and trigger apoptosis in those cells. According to Stanley and Reed (2001), one significant factor causing tissue damage caused by inflammatory cell lysis is the host response.

4.11.4. Animal Models of Amebiasis

The understanding of this significant human disease has been greatly advanced by the use of in vivo animal models. Nevertheless, no animal model exists that can replicate the complete cycle of human amebiasis. Therefore, either intestinal or hepatic models have been used in the majority of in vivo studies of experimental amebiasis. Understanding many facets of the molecular and cell biology, immunology, and physiopathology of amebic ulcer and ALA development has been made possible by the use of susceptible and resistant rodents.

- *Experimental Amebic Liver Abscess:* The hamster was the first animal to be used successfully to treat hepatic amebiasis. Large amebic abscesses were created when various authors injected *E. histolytica* axenic trophozoites directly into the hepatic lobe or through the portal vein. In 1984, a study on the histopathology of liver damage from its early stages to chronic liver damage was published. The amebas were injected via the portal vein in this iconic work. It was suggested that inflammatory cell lysis contributes to the hepatic lesion after the authors showed that the ameba caused liver damage. The gerbil is another highly susceptible rodent in ALA; the lesions it produces are similar to those of hamsters, but the liver damage in gerbils progresses more slowly and they die over a longer period of time due to the less virulent behavior of *E. histolytica E. histolytica* trophozoites. The gerbils' inflammatory response also revealed amebas near the hepatocytes, but it is still similar to the hamster's inflammatory response linked to trophozoites. These factors lead some researchers to believe that this rodent is more akin to humans (Tsutsumi and Shibayama, 2006) (Figure 4.2).

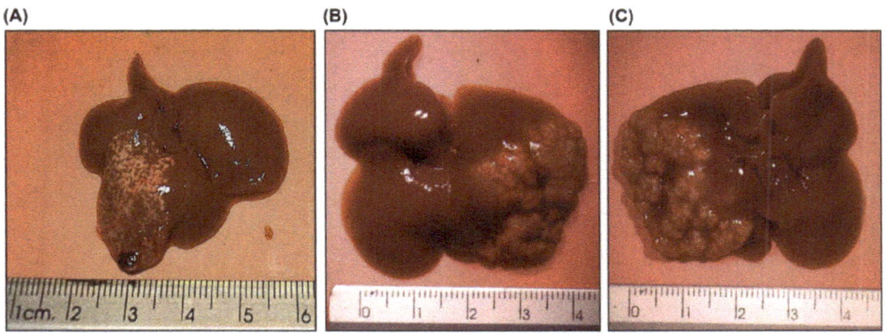

Figure 4.2. *Macroscopic aspect of amebic liver abscess (ALA) in hamster. Amebas were inoculated by the portal vein with 1 106 trophozoites of Entamoeba histolytica strain HM1:IMSS. (A) 12 h post-intraportal inoculation. We can observe multiple white-pink point lesions on the diaphragmatic face. (B and C) ALA at 7 days post-infection (diaphragmatic and visceral face, respectively). Whitish lesions are covering the entire lobule.*

Source. A. Martı´nez-Palomo, et al., Amebic Liver Abscess, http://dx.doi.org/10.1016/B978–0-12–804274–8.00013–8.

4.12. Role of Cytokines in the Amebic Liver Abscess

E. histolytica has the ability to penetrate the intestinal wall and spread to other organs, including the brain, liver, and lungs. Several pathogenic and immunological responses are triggered in both the parasite and the host during the development of ALA. Although in vitro research has shown that *E. histolytica* induces the secretion of cytokines in human cells, the host maintains the equilibrium between pro- and anti-inflammatory cytokines (Eckmann et al., 1995; Salata et al., 1987). There have been numerous reports of experimental ALA studies that address the host response. In both positive and negative contexts, the significance of inflammation and the function of cytokines have regulatory ramifications (BekkerMendez et al., Helk et al., 2006; Denis and Chadee, 1989; Campbell & Chadee, 1997a. 2013). The precise regulatory pathways governing the various cytokines are still not fully understood, though. Several animal models, including gerbils, mice, and hamsters, have been used to explain this phenomenon (Campbell & Chadee, 1997a; Shibayama et al., 1997; Lotter et al, 2006; Pacheco-Yepez et al.,2011; Shibayama and Tsutsumi, 2006). According to these studies, neutrophils and macrophages make up the majority of the inflammatory response, and cytokine modulation has a direct impact on the migration and activation of this cellular response (Campbell and Chadee, 1997b).

The hamster model is commonly used for studying ALA evolution due to its similarity to ALA in humans. However, a sophisticated artificial mouse model has also been utilized in specific circumstances, providing valuable insights into the molecular network of cytokines during ALA progression (Cieslak et al., 1992). Recent research has revealed the presence and localization of various cytokines such as TNF-a, INF-g, IL-1b, IL-8, and IL-10 in liver lesions of hamsters infected with amebas. The production of these cytokines was found to be associated with the presence of PMN and macrophages at different stages of ALA development (Pacheco-Yepez et al., 2011). Cytokines have been extensively studied for their indirect amebicidal effects on *E.histolytica*, and Th1-driven responses may play a role in protective immunity against resolved amebiasis (Campbell and Chadee, 1997a; Garcia-Zepeda et al., 2007).

The hamster model is commonly used for studying ALA evolution due to its similarity to ALA in humans. However, a sophisticated artificial mouse model has also been utilized in specific circumstances, providing valuable insights into the molecular network of cytokines during ALA progression (Cieslak et al., 1992). Recent research has revealed the presence and localization of various cytokines such as TNF-a, INF-g, IL-1b, IL-8, and IL-10 in liver lesions of hamsters infected with amebas. The production of these cytokines was found to be associated with the presence of PMN and macrophages at different stages of ALA development (Pacheco-Yepez et al., 2011). Cytokines have been extensively studied for their indirect amebicidal effects on *E.histolytica*, and Th1-driven responses may play a role in protective immunity against resolved amebiasis (Campbell and Chadee, 1997a; Garcia-Zepeda et al., 2007).

During the infection, epithelial and stromal cells are stimulated by live trophozoites and amebic products to increase the expression of chemokines, such as IL-8, GROa, and GM-CSF, and pro-inflammatory cytokines, such as IL-1a, IL-1b, and IL-6 that provoke polymorphonuclear infiltration, plasma cells, lymphocytes, eosinophils, and macrophages (Eckmann et al., 1995). The expression and production of TNF-a and IL-8 have also been observed by the hepatocytes during ALA evolution (Pacheco-Yepez et al., 2011) (Figure 4.3).

After reaching the infection site, neutrophils move into the infected tissue; this migration is linked to the production of IL8 (Kolaczkowska and Kubes, 2013). The hepatocytes' generation of IL-8 may be connected to the neutrophils' entry into the hepatic parenchyma. Furthermore, it has been documented that TNF-a and IFN-g are necessary for neutrophil activation (Segal, 2005;

Kolaczkowska and Kubes, 2013). It has been demonstrated that TNF-a and IFN-g-activated neutrophils exhibited amebicidal effects in vitro through H_2O_2-dependent mechanisms (Denis and Chadee, 1989; Guerrant et al., 1981); in contrast, nonactivated neutrophils are killed by *E. histolytica* (Guerrant et al., 1981). Similarly, amebicidal effect has been observed by neutrophils activated by IL-4 (Garcia-Zepeda et al., 2007).

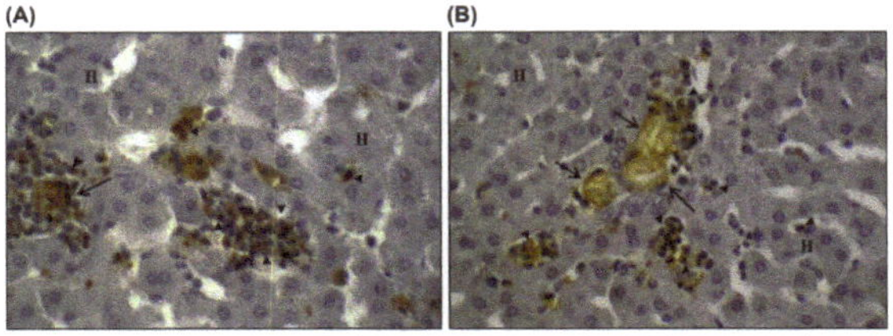

Figure 4.3. *Immunohistochemistry of cytokines in amebic liver abscess 1 h after portal inoculation. (A) TNF-a, the liver parenchyma (H) presents two foci of inflammatory reaction positive to peroxidase (arrow-heads). Ameba are also present (arrow). (B) INF-g, amebas are inside a branch of a portal vein (arrows); inflammatory cells are also present and are positive to the label (arrow-heads).*

Source. A. Martı´nez-Palomo, et al., Amebic Liver Abscess, http://dx.doi.org/10.1016/B978-0-12-804274-8.00013-8.

In vitro ALA experiments, however, have examined the function of liver-resident macrophages or Kupffer cells (KCs); the findings point to a potential protective function for these cells. For these cells to kill the trophozoites, IFN-g had to activate them (Ghadirian and Denis, 1992a,b; Ghadirian and Salimi, 1993; Salimi and Ghadirian, 1993). Some in vitro results showed that TNF-a induces nitric oxide (NO) production by macrophages, which is cytotoxic to *E. histolytica* (Wang et al., 1992). Interestingly in a gerbil model, liver granuloma macrophages were refractive to IFN-g, do not produce inflammatory cytokines, and are unable to eliminate *E. histolytica* trophozoites (Denis and Chadee, 1988). In addition, the authors report that macrophages at sites distant to liver lesions are unaffected; part of this phenomenon has been associated with prostaglandin E2 (PGE2) production by *E. histolytica* (Denis & Chadee, 1988; Wang et al., 1994; Dey et al., 2003). Purified Gal/GalNac induces stable TNF-a production in naive murine macrophages in vitro (Seguin et al., 1995). TNF-a plays a complex role in amebiasis; the overproduction of this cytokine promotes an amebicidal effect, but low levels allow amebic granulomas (Campbell & Chadee, 1997b). Moreover, naive macrophages exposed to soluble amebic products and then stimulated with IFN-g showed a decrease in TNF-a mRNA expression. The TGF-b produced by macrophages, as well as IL-4 and IL-10 produced by T cells, have inhibitory effects on macrophage functions and Th1- type T cells. The stimulation of a Th2-type response during ALA would likely suppress macrophage-mediated control of the infection (Campbell and Chadee, 1997b; GarciaZepeda et al., 2007).

T and B cells, NK cells, DCs, and natural killer T (NKT) cells make up the liver lymphocyte population (Racanelli and Rehermann, 2006). It has been reported that NKT and NK cells regulate cytokines by producing IFN-g, which adjusts macrophage activation to release TNF-a during ALA production (Lotter et al., 2009). Extracted lipopeptidophosphoglycan (LPPG) from E. NKT cells recognizE. *histolytica* via CD1d, TLR2, and TLR4; recognition via Toll receptors triggered the production of protective INF-g and did not trigger Th2 responses, preventing the mouse from developing ALA (Lotter et al., 2009). The levels of IL-2 in gerbils appear to be reduced during the acute phase of ALA; in contrast, high levels of IL-2 and low levels of IL-4 and TNF-a expression are linked to later stages of infection and resistance to re-infection. Since IL-2 is crucial for T cell activation and proliferation, the development may be linked to the cytokine's suppression (Campbell et al., 1999). Moreover, reduced IL-6 cytokine production—which has been linked to lymphocytes exposed to *E. coli* 220 kDa lectin—may promote the development of ALA. histolytica (Zepeda-García et al., 2007). Furthermore, T cells seem to be hyporesponsive during amebic infection, promoting Th2 responses and suppressing Th1 during ALA due to amebic antigens (Talamas-Rohana et al., 1995). Tregs have been linked to the regulatory development of ALA, but further research is needed to fully understand this finding (Mortimer and Chadee, 2010).

A significant further consequence of cytokine regulation during ALA development may be directly linked to systemic cytokine regulation; in these kinds of investigations, splenectomy, vagus nerve excision, or gender involvement have all been investigated. Research has been done on the spleen's function in hepatic amebiasis in hamsters (Ghadirian and Meerovitch, 1981a). The findings showed that, in comparison to hamsters with splenectomy, animals without splenectomy had a significant reduction in the size of ALA and a reduction in the ameba's dissemination to other organs. As a result, the authors concluded that ALA control requires a cellular immune response, specifically lymphocytic cells (Ghadirian and Meerovitch, 1981b). Currently, there are conflicting findings about lymphocytic cells. It is important to thoroughly research the function of the spleen in hepatic amebiasis. The authors show that, in the absence of the vagus nerve (VN), increases in the production of IL-1b, IL-8, TNF-a, and IL-6 are correlated with neutrophil and macrophage activation in a vagotomy hamster model from 6 hours to 7 days. Because the liver is innervated by both sympathetic and parasympathetic nerves, this study has a direct relationship with the cholinergic system. The cholinergic system modulates the production of IFN-g, TNF-a, and IL-10 (Friedman and Tordoff, 1994; Sánchez-Áleman et al., 2015). At the liver parenchyma level, there was an increase in neutrophils and macrophages positive for nuclear factor transcription (NFkB) during the evolution of ALA in the absence of the VN. Ultimately, the scientists concluded that tissue damage is caused by dysregulation of inflammatory responses (IR), which is regulated by NFkB during the development of ALA (Sánchez-Áleman et al., 2015).

In terms of sexual dimorphism, males are more likely to have ALA disease, and the male-to-female ratio varies based on age, ranging from 2:1 to 7:1. Studies conducted in 2006 using immunocompetent C57BL/6 mice offer some insights into why male mice are more susceptible than female mice. The researchers discovered that during the early stages of abscess development, male and female mice produce cytokines, such as IFN-g and IL-4, very differently from one another. Male mice were found to have high concentrations of IL-4-producing cells in their spleens, while female mice had higher levels of IFN-g-positive lymphocytes (Lotter et al., 2006). The authors propose that gender-specific variations in early cytokine production, at least partially mediated by NKT cells in response are responsible for the sexual dimorphism in the regulation of ALA liver infection caused by *E.histolytica*.

4.13. Reactive Oxygen Species in the Pathogenesis of the Amebic Liver Abscess

The production of excessive reactive metabolites of molecular oxygen (O_2), such as superoxide anions (O_2), hydrogen peroxide (H_2O_2), or the hydroxyl radical (OH), is the cause of reactive oxygen species (ROS) and oxidative stress. Because it can produce more reactive agents like the OH radical, the O_2 radical has the potential to be toxic. Damage to cells is caused by an imbalance between oxidants and antioxidants, which is known as oxidative stress. The antioxidant defense and repair mechanisms of the cell, which eliminate molecules that cause tissue damage, allow it to withstand oxidative stress (Ha et al., 2010). Disproportions in these systems may be caused by an excess of oxidant species or a deficiency of antioxidant capacity brought on by modifications in their production. ROS have the potential to harm cells if these species are not properly regulated. When ROS act on proteins, they inactivate the sulfhydryl group and prevent protein synthesis; when they act on DNA, nitrogenous bases in nucleic acids are hydroxylated; when they act on lipids, they cause lipid peroxidation, which damages the fatty acids. Changes in ROS also affect the expression of genes, cell adhesion, metabolism, cell cycle, and ultimately, cell death. According to Ha et al.,(2010) oxidative stress has been linked to long-term liver injury damage.

4.13.1. Amebic Liver Abscess and Free Radical Production

The oxygen metabolites are the effector molecules in this activity, and amebic liver abscesses involve an inflammatory immune response in both the acute and chronic stages of the hepatic lesion. A weak immune response in susceptible people or experimental animal models permits amebic liver damage (Stanley, 2001; Tsutsumi et al., , 1984), but animals or people who are resistant have an effective innate immune response that can get rid of the parasite (Seydel & Co. 1997; Velazquez et al.,, 1998; Jarillo-Luna et al., 2002). Nitric oxide (NO) and reactive oxygen species (ROS), two harmful molecules that either cause or cure ALA, are present in the inflammatory response of both susceptible and resistant models. According to some reports, neutrophils and macrophages produce reactive oxygen species (ROS) that harm *E. histolytica* trophozoites (Murray et al., 1986. 1981).

Early works studied the in vitro susceptibility of amebas to the oxygen intermediates O_2, H_2O_2, and OH; amebas exposed to H_2O_2 were susceptible to damage, and when peroxidase and halide were added to the system, an increase in H_2O_2 levels was observed and the killing of trophozoites occurs, showing the amebic susceptibility to this oxygen intermediate (Murray et al., 1981). Later, Ghadirian et al., (1986) analyzed the direct effect of H_2O_2 and hypochlorite on the viability of virulent and nonvirulent strains of *E. histolytica*. Virulent amebas incubated with H_2O_2 presented lower susceptibility than non-virulent amebas to the H_2O_2 effect. The effect of H_2O_2 was confirmed by trophozoites co-incubated with H_2O_2 and catalase; the latter reduced the toxic effect of the H_2O_2 in the ameba.

4.13.2. Reactive Oxygen Species: Superoxide, Peroxide, and Hypochlorous Acid

The transmembrane and cytosolic subunits of the large NADPH-oxidase complex assemble at the phagosomal and plasma membranes during an "oxidative burst" that activated neutrophils go through. They then transfer electrons to molecular oxygen to produce superoxide (O_2). Superoxide is quickly transformed into hydrogen peroxide (H_2O_2), which is then the substrate of MPO to form hypochlorous acid (HOCl), either spontaneously or through catalysis by superoxide dismutase (SOD). According to Hampton et al., HOCl is the most bactericidal oxidant in neutrophils. 1998; Mayer-Scholl et al,2004, Segal, 2005, Nathan, 2006, Urban et al., 2006). Since *E. histolytica* is sensitive to H_2O_2, numerous investigations have shown that this molecule is a crucial oxygen derivative that kills ameba (Choi et al., 2005; Ghadirian et al., 1986; Ghosh et al.,2010; Murray and others. 1981).

Recently, Ghosh et al., (2010) investigated apoptotic markers in the strain 200:NIH subjected to different concentrations (0.5, 1.0, 1.5, and 2.0 mM) of H_2O_2 for different periods of times. The results showed that *E. histolytica E. histolytica* presented morphological features similar to an apoptotic phenotype, suggesting apoptosis-like cell death when exposed to 2.0 mM of H_2O_2 treatment.

When H_2O_2 was applied to the ameba, *E. histolytica* displayed DNA fragmentation, phosphatidyl serine externalization, and an increase in endogenous ROS levels. On the other hand, in a different study, trophozoites of a virulent strain of *E. histolytica* HM1:IMSS were exposed to 1 mM hydrogen peroxide, which resulted in cell stress but little death (Vicente et al., , 2009); the amebas were co-incubated with nitrosative and oxidative species, and the whole genome expression profile was examined using an oligonucleotide microarray. In the virulent *E. histolytica* HM1:IMSS strain, the authors showed that H_2O_2 (286 genes regulated) and NO (1036 genes regulated) significantly modulated gene expression, enabling the ameba to adapt to oxidative and nitrosative stresses. Moran et al., (2002) investigated the oxidative burst function of peripheral mononuclear cells in a patient who experienced recurrent episodes of amebic cell damage. The findings revealed impaired production of reactive oxygen species (ROS) by the mononuclear phagocytes, suggesting a potential role for ROS in this process.

4.13.3. Inflammation Produces Oxidative Molecules Against Entamoeba histolytica

The immune system produces oxidative and nitrosative species in reaction to the ameba during *E. histolytica* invasion. Numerous studies demonstrated that oxidative molecules like superoxide and peroxide are harmed by neutrophils in *E. histolytica*. Following activation, neutrophils and macrophages produce reduced oxygen species through the respiratory burst, including the molecules superoxide (O_2) and hydrogen peroxide (H_2O_2). (Nathan, 2006; Segal, 2005). *E. histolytica* is destroyed by H_2O_2, an oxygen product (Denis and Chadee, 1989; Ghadirian et al, 1986), as well as cytokines (TNF-a and IFN-g) and phorbol myristate acetate (PMA) give macrophages a high level of amebicidal activity that is correlated with an H_2O_2-dependent mechanism (Denis and Chadee, 1989). The authors incubated the amebas in the presence or absence of an inhibitor of reactive oxygen intermediates (ROI) to corroborate the involvement of this oxidative molecule with macrophages in ameba damage. Catalase inhibited ameba destruction by 45%, indicating that H2O2 is involved in the macrophage-mediated killing of *E. histolytica* trophozoites (Denis and Chadee, 1989). In order to fully comprehend how the ameba affects the respiratory burst of macrophages, Lin et al., showed that amebic proteins control the activity of this oxidative molecule by pretreating peritoneal macrophages with crude and soluble proteins from *E. histolytica* and causing increased O_2 and H_2O_2 release in response to PMA (1993). Amebas were incubated with sodium nitroprusside, sodium nitrite, and sodium nitrate in order to examine their effects on *E. histolytica* apoptosis; the death of trophozoites was completed after 24 hours. The parasites vanished in less than six hours after being injected into the hamster liver after having previously been incubated with these substances, indicating the liver's incapacity to support life (Ramos et al., 2007). According to another unpublished data, researchers analyzed the release of ROS in situ and the total antioxidant status (TAS) in the hepatic parenchyma distant from ALA at different times post-intraportal inoculation with *E. histolytica* trophozoites; other groups of hamsters were inoculated with the same inoculum and treated with an antioxidant, Corabion. The lipoperoxidation in ALA was analyzed by measurement of thiobarbituric acid reactive substances (TBARs) and compared with hamsters that were orally administered with the antioxidant Corabion (200 mg/kg). The TAS was measured by generating the 2,20 -azinobis (3-ethylbenzothiazoline-6-sulfonic acid) (ABTS) radical cation by spectrophotometric assay at 600 nm of absorbance. The mmol/mg of total protein and the TAS levels were the same. The animals treated with corabion and inoculated with trophozoites differed significantly from the hamsters inoculated with amebas. In contrast to the animals inoculated with amebas and treated with corabion, which had lower TBAR values, the hamsters inoculated with *E. histolytica* exhibited significantly higher levels of TBARs at different points in the evolution of ALA (12 and 48 hours). Compared to hamsters inoculated with amebas and treated with corabion, animals inoculated with amebas had a lower level of TAS. In contrast, a nonenzymatic antioxidant preserves the antioxidant defenses that maintain a low release of ROS and may prevent ALA evolution in the animals inoculated with amebas and treated with corabion. This is because the livers of the animals inoculated with *E histolityca* had a weaker antioxidant system and a higher degree of oxidative stress (Figure 4.4).

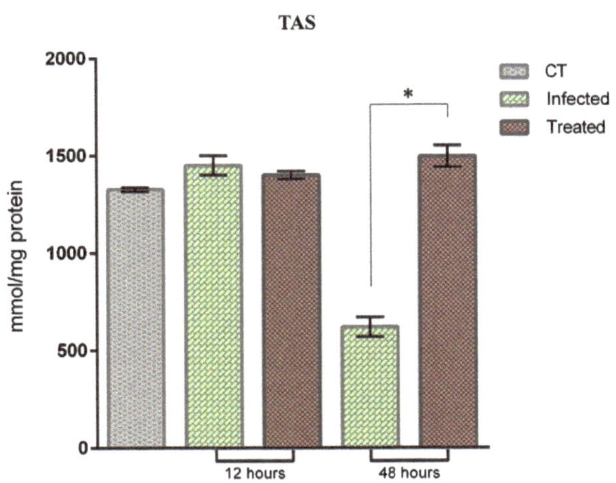

Figure 4.4. *The TAS (total antioxidant capacity) was quantified in samples distant from the amebic liver abscess (ALA) at different times post-intraportal inoculation. The hamsters were inoculated with 1×10^6 trophozoites of Entamoeba histolytica (infected group) and the second group of hamsters were treated with 200 mg/kg of Corabion for 5 days with oral administration and were then challenged with 1×10^6 trophozoites (treated group). The animals were sacrificed at 12 and 48 h postinoculation. At 12 h of ALA, Corabion did not produce an important effect over TAS levels. At 48 h of ALA evolution, TAS decreased importantly in the infected group compared with the treated animals (*p < .005).*

Source. A. Martı´nez-Palomo, et al., Amebic Liver Abscess, http://dx.doi.org/10.1016/B978-0-12-804274-8.00013-8.

4.13.4. Entamoeba histolytica Defense Against Reactive Oxygen Species

Because oxygen causes ROS to be produced, oxygen is bad for amebas. *E. histolytica* has therefore evolved defense mechanisms to fend off these oxygen derivatives. Compared to non-virulent amebas, virulent amebas have been shown to be more resistant to H_2O_2 (Ghadirian et al., 1986). Amebic proteins prevent peritoneal macrophages from causing the respiratory burst (ROI: H_2O_2, O2, OH), indicating the function of *E. histolytica* proteins in controlling defense immune mechanisms (Lin et al., 1993). Spleen macrophages can release large amounts of H_2O_2 when certain cytokines, like TNF-a and IFN-g, are present, but this decreases the amebicidal activity. Comparing virulent and non-virulent *E. histolytica* revealed that the former were more susceptible to O_2, while the latter had a greater capacity to decrease O_2 and exhibited greater resistance to H_2O_2. These two mechanisms are associated with the ameba's resistance to ROS (Ramos-Martinez et al., 2009). Three antioxidant-producing enzymes are found in the trophozoites of *E. histolytica* : (1) iron superoxide dismutase (Fe-SOD), which catalyzes the conversion of superoxide to O_2 and H_2O_2. The cultivation of amebic strains under different culture conditions showed that in the presence of superoxide radical anions or ferrous iron chelators there is a considerable increase in the activity and protein concentration of *E. histolytica* Fe-SOD enzyme (Bruchhaus and Tannich, 1994; Murray et al., 1981), demonstrating the role of ameba Fe-SOD in the protection from toxic oxygen metabolites. (2) NADPH: flavin oxidoreductase, which catalyzes the reduction of O_2 to H_2O_2, as well as of the reduction of disulfides such as 50 50 -dithiobis-(2-nitrobenzoic acid) (DTNB) and cysteine (Bruchhaus et al., 1998) and (3) a peroxiredoxin described in the nucleotide sequence of cDNA by Torian et al., (1990), is the major peroxidase against oxidative stress by decomposing H_2O_2; peroxynitrites use hydrogens provided by thioredoxin reductase, and NADPH (Flores et al., 1993; Bruchhaus et al., 1997; Wood et al., 2003). In this manner, the site of hepatic lesions, where a highly oxygenrich microenvironment exists, the amebic peroxiredoxin blocks the H_2O_2 production, facilitating the survival of the ameba in the host (Bera et al., 2006; Bruchhaus et al., 1998). Immunization of gerbils with recombinant peroxiredoxin protects against ALA development and reduces the size of ALA (Soong et al., 1995). Previous reports showed that the *E. histolytica* genome contains genes encoding enzymes involved in the detoxification of ROS, including peroxiredoxin, rubrerythrin, and SOD. Peroxiredoxin (29 kDa) constitutes an important defense against oxidative stress; it is induced by a high-oxygen environment (Akbar et al., 2004).

This enzyme facilitates the amebic invasion by detoxifying H2O2, which adds to *E. histolytica* virulence. The overexpression of the peroxiredoxin gene in a high-oxygen environment inhibits the harmful production of H_2O_2, promoting the survival of *E. histolytica* (Akbar et al., 2004). The authors report a 55% inhibition of eh29 expression, a lower viability in 29 kDa downregulated amebas, and an important decrease in cytopathic and cytotoxic activities when peroxiredoxin gene expression is inhibited by an antisense RNA strategy, which leads to ROS accumulation (Sen et al., 2007). Furthermore, abscess sizes were smaller in hamsters inoculated with 29 kDa downregulated trophozoites than in the control group (only in the HM1:IMSS strain). The authors come to the conclusion that the ameba's ability to survive in the presence of ROS is significantly influenced by the 29 kDa protein of *E. histolytica* (Sen et al., 2007) (Figure 4.5).

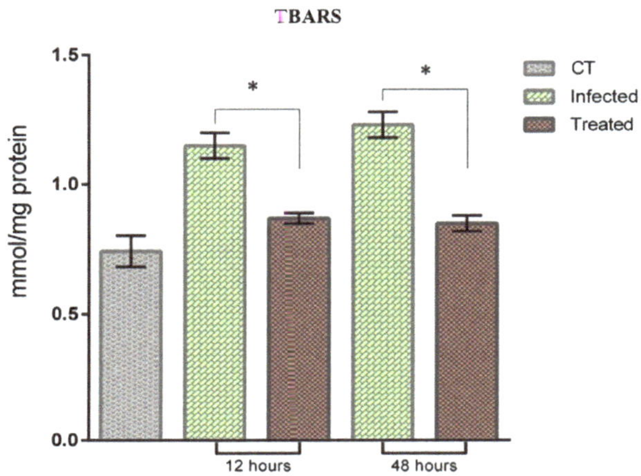

Figure 4.5. *Levels of thiobarbituric acid reactive substances (TBARs) (measured by thiobarbituric acid reactive) were analyzed in samples distant from the amebic liver abscess. The animals were inoculated through the portal vein with 1×10^6 trophozoites of Entamoeba histolytica (infected group), and the other group of hamsters was treated with 200 mg/kg of Corabion (antioxidant compound) for 5 days by oral administration and then were challenged with 1×10^6 trophozoites (treated group). The hamsters were sacrificed at 12 and 48 h postintraportal inoculation. We observed that the treated group presented a decrement in the levels of TBARs (<0.9 nmol/mg protein) during ALA evolution compared to the infected and untreated groups (*p < .005).*

Source. A. Martı´nez-Palomo, et al., Amebic Liver Abscess, http://dx.doi.org/10.1016/B978-0-12-804274-8.00013-8.

Two hypothetical proteins that have been shown to increase parasite survival when the ameba is exposed to exogenous hydrogen peroxide have been identified in recent studies, indicating that trophozoites mount a defense against host oxidative stress (Rastew et al., 2012). The parasite's ability to withstand oxidative stress is facilitated by the *E. histolytica* stress-induced adhesion factor (EhSIAF) and elevated protein levels of phospholipid transporting Ptype ATPase/flippase (EhPTPA) (Rastew et al., 2012). By activating ERK1/2 and Src tyrosine kinases, which are mediated by ROS, *E. histolytica* trophozoites induce neutrophil apoptosis (Sim et al., 2010).

4.13.5. Role of Nitric Oxide in Amebic Liver Abscess

Several studies have mentioned that chronic inflammation contributes to liver abscess formation, and the effector mechanisms of this inflammation with amebicidal activity are developed by NO and ROS (Ramos et al., 2007; Olivos-Garcia et al., 2009; SantiRocca et al., 2009; Pacheco-Yepez et al., 2014;). Some reports have shown that ROS and NO are produced by neutrophils and mononuclear cells from different rodents with ALA (Seydel et al., 2000; Jarillo-Luna et al., 2002; Ramos-Martinez et al., 2009), and these oxygen species lyse *E. histolytica* trophozoites (Wang et al., 1994). Early studies explored the effect of NO produced by activated macrophages as a defense mechanism against *E. histolytica* (Wang et al., 1994). Macrophages isolated from the peritoneum and spleen stimulated with IFN-g and LPS kill *E. histolytica* trophozoites related to the production of high levels of NO, showing that NO is the main cytotoxic molecule produced by macrophages against *E. histolytica*. Furthermore, NCX972, a molecule obtained by adding an NO moiety to metronidazole, releases NO and enhances the killing of *E. histolytica* trophozoites; treatment with NCX972 results in significant inhibitory activity (Sannella et al., 2003).

The role of NO has been studied in immunocompetent mice; ALA was induced, and the resistance mechanisms against invasive amebiasis were explored (Seydel et al., 2000). In iNOS knockout mice, the animals produced larger amebic liver lesions compared with the control SCID mice, showing that iNOS/ mice are more susceptible to developing ALA and that iNOS is necessary for the control of ALA in immunocompetent mice. The authors concluded that NO produced by the inflammatory reaction plays a significant role in protection against ALA development in mice (Seydel et al., 2000). These results are in agreement with the observations by Jarillo-Luna et al., (2002), showing that neutrophils and macrophages from Balb/c and C3H/HeJ mice were highly positive to iNOS and presented increased serum production of NO, demonstrating the amebicidal activity of this molecule. The amebic target for the NO molecule was explored by Siman-Tov and Ankri (2003), and the results showed that amebic cysteine proteinases and alcohol dehydrogenase 2 were inhibited by S-nitroso-glutathione, an NO donor that limits the survival of the parasite (SimanTov & Ankri, 2003). Recently, in identifying *E. histolytica* proteins susceptible to S-nitrosylation, the authors detected 142 S-nitrosylated proteins that are involved in various metabolic processes, such as glycolysis, gluconeogenesis, protein transport, and adherence via Gal/ GalNac lectin. The S-nitrosylated cysteine residues in the carbohydrate recognition domain (CRD) of the lectin impairs its function and contributes to the inhibition of the ameba to the target cells by NO (Hertz et al., 2014).

Although the anti-amebic role of NO in in-vitro and in-vivo has been extensively studied in a susceptible model (hamster), NO did not appear to be relevant in the ALA resolution.

Increasing serum NO levels correlated with the ALA size. In addition, NO and nitric oxide synthase (NOS) were detected in the necrotic and inflammatory hepatic areas; however, the presence of these molecules does not participate in the elimination of *E. histolytica* in the liver parenchyma (Pacheco-Yépez et al., 2001).

4.13.6. Entamoeba histolytica Modulates Nitric Oxide Activity

The ameba has the capacity to regulate the effect of NO. Previous studies showed that *E. histolytica* and amebic proteins decreased the inducible NOS gene expression. Macrophages from ALA were defective in killing *E. histolytica* trophozoites, which correlated with low NO levels and reduced iNOS mRNA expression; the authors suggest that ameba might modulate NO production, resulting in protection from NO cytotoxic activity (Wang et al., 1994). In addition, soluble ameba proteins inhibit NO production by bone marrow-derived macrophages and affect the cytotoxic activity of these mononuclear leukocytes by the modulation of iNOS mRNA expression and NO production, allowing for amebic survival (Wang et al., 1994). The competitive consumption of L-arginine (NO synthase substrate) by *E. histolytica* arginase has also been associated with the blockade of NO production by macrophages (Elnekave et al., 2003). The parasite acts over macrophages from ALA inducing dysfunction through iNOS and NO, and this modulation contributes to the survival of *E. histolytica* in the liver. On the other hand, the ameba displays the monocyte locomotion inhibitor factor (MLIF) that inhibits the production of NO by human leukocytes, and the diminished production of this molecule avoids the damage of *E. histolytica* by monocytes and neutrophils (Rico et al., 2003).

In spite of the abundant information regarding the mechanism of the production of the different profiles of cytokines and ROS produced by an important inflammatory reaction present in the intestine or the liver, several in vitro and in vivo studies have shown that this environment is critical in ALA development. Moreover, virulent amebas activate and express genes in response to the stress produced by the inflammation, which are essential for the invasive process and the consequent liver damage. Recent information regarding ALA production by *E. histolytica* has focused on the apoptosis of hepatocytes, which is probably regulated by pro-inflammatory cytokines and other molecules, such as ROS and NO. A better knowledge of the regulation of these molecules is necessary to have a clearer understanding of the physiopathology of amebiasis.

A Closer Look

Pyogenic Liver Abscess

A pyogenic liver abscess is a pus-filled cavity within the liver resulting from a bacterial infection. It is a serious medical condition that can lead to significant morbidity and mortality if not promptly diagnosed and treated. The condition can arise from various sources of infection, including intra-abdominal infections such as appendicitis, diverticulitis, or biliary tract disease like cholangitis and cholecystitis. It can also result from hematogenous spread from systemic infections, direct extension from adjacent infected organs, or trauma.

The most common causative organisms of pyogenic liver abscesses include bacteria such as *Escherichia coli*, *Klebsiella pneumoniae*, and *Streptococcus* species. These pathogens can reach the liver through the portal vein, hepatic artery, or direct extension from a contiguous infection. In some cases, the infection may be polymicrobial, involving multiple bacterial species.

Clinically, patients with a pyogenic liver abscess typically present with nonspecific symptoms that can include fever, chills, right upper quadrant abdominal pain, and jaundice. These symptoms can be accompanied by malaise, anorexia, weight loss, and nausea. Physical examination may reveal hepatomegaly and tenderness over the liver. Laboratory findings often show elevated white blood cell counts, elevated liver enzymes, and abnormal liver function tests.

Diagnosis of a pyogenic liver abscess is primarily made through imaging studies. Ultrasound and computed tomography (CT) scans are the most commonly used modalities, with CT providing more detailed information about the size, number, and location of abscesses. Magnetic resonance imaging (MRI) can also be utilized but is less commonly performed. Blood cultures are essential for identifying the causative organisms and guiding antibiotic therapy. In some cases, aspiration of the abscess under imaging guidance may be performed to obtain pus for culture and to relieve the abscess.

Treatment of pyogenic liver abscess involves a combination of antibiotic therapy and drainage of the abscess. Broad-spectrum antibiotics are typically initiated empirically and then tailored based on culture results. Percutaneous drainage, guided by ultrasound or CT, is the preferred method for draining the abscess. This minimally invasive procedure involves inserting a needle or catheter into the abscess cavity to remove pus. In some cases, surgical drainage may be required, particularly if the abscess is large, multiloculated, or associated with complications such as rupture or failure of percutaneous drainage.

The prognosis for patients with pyogenic liver abscesses has improved significantly with advances in diagnostic imaging, antibiotic therapy, and minimally invasive drainage techniques.

However, the condition still carries a risk of serious complications, including sepsis, metastatic infections, and liver failure, particularly if diagnosis and treatment are delayed. Therefore, early recognition and prompt management are crucial for improving outcomes.

Preventive measures for pyogenic liver abscesses focus on managing risk factors and underlying conditions that predispose individuals to liver infections. This includes appropriate treatment of intra-abdominal infections, careful management of biliary tract diseases, and prompt attention to systemic infections. In healthcare settings, maintaining aseptic techniques during procedures that could introduce bacteria into the bloodstream or liver is also important. Overall, a high index of suspicion, timely diagnosis, and appropriate therapeutic interventions are key to effectively managing pyogenic liver abscess and reducing associated morbidity and mortality.

Summary

- Amebic liver abscess is a collection of pus in the liver in response to an intestinal parasite called *Entamoeba histolytica*.
- This parasite causes amebiasis, an intestinal infection that is also called amebic dysentery. After an infection has occurred, the parasite may be carried by the bloodstream from the intestines to the liver.
- Amebic liver abscess involves an inflammatory immune response in the acute and chronic stages of the hepatic lesion, and the oxygen metabolites are the effector molecules in this activity.
- Antibiotics such as metronidazole (Flagyl) or tinidazole (Tindamax) are the usual treatment for liver abscesses. A medicine such as paromomycin or diloxanide must also be taken to get rid of all the ameba in the intestine and to prevent the disease from coming back. This treatment can usually wait until after the abscess has been treated.
- The humoral immune response, also known as antibody-mediated immunity, is part of the adaptive immune system. The immune system is what protects an organism from disease, and is activated when antigens, any sort of substance that triggers an immune response, are found in the body. Once these antigens are detected, B cell lymphocytes, a type of white blood cell, undergo a differentiation process that creates memory B cells and effector B cells.
- Evidence of systemic cell-mediated immunity has been confirmed in vivo through delayed hypersensitivity skin reactions, and in vitro through lymphokine, blastogenic response, leukocyte adherence inhibition, and lymphocytotoxic assays.
- Host-parasite interactions contribute to the infection by initiating signaling events in both cells. These interactions involve the pathogen and the host cell surface, and this step is critical in the understanding of microbial pathogenicity.
- Reactive oxygen species (ROS) and oxidative stress are results of aerobic metabolism that produces excessive reactive metabolites of molecular oxygen (O_2) that comprise superoxide anions (O_2), hydrogen peroxide (H_2O_2), or the hydroxyl radical (OH).

References

1. Ackers, J. P., & Mirelman, D. (2006). Progress in research on *Entamoeba histolytica* pathogenesis. *Current Opinion in Microbiology, 9*(4), 367–373.
2. Akbar, M. A., Chatterjee, N. S., Sen, P., Debnath, A., Pal, A., Bera, T., et al. (2004). Genes induced by a high-oxygen environment in *Entamoeba histolytica*. *Molecular and Biochemical Parasitology, 133*(2), 187–196.
3. Alam, F., Abdus Salam, M., Hassan, P., Mahmood, I., Kabir, M., & Haque, R. (2014). Amebic liver abscess in northern region of Bangladesh; sociodemographic determinants and clinical outcomes. *BMC Research Notes, 7*, 625.

4. Albenmousa, A., Sanai, F. M., Singhai, A., Babatin, M. A., Al Zanbagi, A. A., Al-Otaibi, M. M., et al. (2011). Liver abscess presentation and management in Saudi Arabia and the United Kingdom. *Annals of Saudi Medicine, 31*(5), 528–532.
5. Bekker-Mendez, V. C., Perez-Castillo, V. L., Rico-Rosillo, M. G., Perez-Rodriguez, M., Arellano-Blanco, J., Kretschmer-Schmid, R. R., et al. (2006). Downregulation of selected cytokines in amebiasis. *Archives of Medical Research, 37*(5), 556–558.
6. Bera, T., Nandi, N., Sudhahar, D., Akbar, M. A., Sen, A., & Das, P. (2006). Preliminary evidence on existence of trans plasma membrane electron transport in *Entamoeba histolytica* trophozoites: A key mechanism for maintaining optimal redox balance. *Journal of Bioenergetics and Bio membranes, 38*(5), 299–308.
7. Blessmann, J., Van Linh, P., Anh Ton Nu, P., Duong Thi, H., Muller-Myhsok, B., Buss, H., et al. (2002). Epidemiology of amebiasis in a region of high incidence of amebic liver abscess in central Vietnam. *American Journal of Tropical Medicine and Hygiene, 66*(5), 578–583.
8. Brandt, H., & Tamayo, R. P. (1970). Pathology of human amebiasis. *Human Pathology, 1*(4), 351–385.
9. Bruchhaus, I., & Tannich, E. (1994). Induction of the iron-containing superoxide dismutase in *Entamoeba histolytica* by a superoxide anion-generating system or by iron chelation. *Molecular and Biochemical Parasitology, 67*(3), 281–288.
10. Bruchhaus, I., Richter, S., & Tannich, E. (1997). Removal of hydrogen peroxide by the 29 kDa protein of *Entamoeba histolytica*. *Biochemical Journal, 326*(3), 785–789.
11. Bruchhaus, I., Richter, S., & Tannich, E. (1998). Recombinant expression and biochemical characterization of an NADPH oxidoreductase from *Entamoeba histolytica*. *Biochemical Journal, 330*(4), 1217–1221.
12. Burchard, G. D., & Mirelman, D. (1988). *Entamoeba histolytica*: Virulence potential and sensitivity to metronidazole and emetine of four isolates possessing nonpathogenic zymodemes. *Experimental Parasitology, 66*(3), 231–242.
13. Calderón, J., & Tovar, R. (1986). Loss of susceptibility to complement lysis in *Entamoeba histolytica* HM1 by treatment with human serum. *Immunology, 58*(3), 467–471.
14. Campbell, D., & Chadee, K. (1997a). Interleukin (IL)-2, IL-4, and tumor necrosis factor-alpha responses during *Entamoeba histolytica* liver abscess development in gerbils. *Journal of Infectious Diseases, 175*(5), 1176–1183.
15. Campbell, D., & Chadee, K. (1997b). Survival strategies of *Entamoeba histolytica*: Modulation of cell-mediated immune responses. *Parasitol. Today, 13*(6), 184–190.
16. Campbell, D., Gaucher, D., & Chadee, K. (1999). Serum from *Entamoeba histolytica*-infected gerbils selectively suppress T cell proliferation by inhibiting interleukin-2 production. *Journal of Infectious Diseases, 179*(6), 1495–1501.
17. Campos-Rodríguez, R., Shibayama-Salas, M., Pacheco-Yépez, J., Martínez-Palomo, A., & Tsutsumi, V. (1995). Passive immunization during experimental amebic liver-abscess development. *Parasitology Research, 81*(1), 86–88.
18. Chaudhary, S., Noor, M. T., Jain, S., Kumar, R., & Thakur, B. S. (2016). Amoebic liver abscess: A report from central India. *Tropical Doctor, 46*(1), 12–15.

19. Choi, M. H., Sajed, D., Poole, L., Hirata, K., Herdman, S., Torian, B. E., et al. (2005). An unusual surface peroxiredoxin protects invasive *Entamoeba histolytica* from oxidant attack. *Molecular and Biochemical Parasitology, 143*(1), 80–89.

20. Cieslak, P. R., Virgin, H. W., & Stanley Jr., S. L. (1992). A severe combined immunodeficient (SCID) mouse model for infection with *Entamoeba histolytica*. *Journal of Experimental Medicine, 176*(6), 1605–1609.

21. Congly, S. E., Shaheen, A. A., Medding, L., Kaplan, G. G., & Myers, R. P. (2011). Amoebic liver abscess in the USA: A population-based study of incidence, temporal trends, and mortality. *Liver International, 31*(8), 1191–1198.

22. Cordel, H., Prendki, V., Madec, Y., Houze, S., Paris, L., Bourée, P., et al. (2013). Imported amoebic liver abscess in France. *PLoS Neglected Tropical Diseases, 7*(7), e2333.

23. Debnath, M. R., Debnath, C. R., Rahman, S. I., & Mahmuduzzaman, M. (2012). Ultrasonographic evaluation of morphologic pattern of amoebic liver abscess. *Mymensingh Medical Journal, 21*(4), 583–587.

24. Denis, M., & Chadee, K. (1988). In vitro and in vivo studies of macrophage functions in amebiasis. *Infection and Immunity, 56*(11), 3126–3131.

25. Denis, M., & Chadee, K. (1989). Cytokine activation of murine macrophages for in vitro killing of *Entamoeba histolytica* trophozoites. *Infection and Immunity, 57*(5), 1750–1756.

26. Dey, I., Keller, K., Belley, A., & Chadee, K. (2003). Identification and characterization of a cyclooxygenase-like enzyme from *Entamoeba histolytica*. *Proceedings of the National Academy of Sciences of the United States of America, 100*(24), 13561–13566.

27. Eckmann, L., Reed, S. L., Smith, J. R., & Kagnoff, M. F. (1995). *Entamoeba histolytica* trophozoites induce an inflammatory cytokine response by cultured human cells through the paracrine action of cytolytically released interleukin-1 alpha. *Journal of Clinical Investigation, 96*(3), 1269–1279.

28. Elnekave, K., Siman-Tov, R., & Ankri, S. (2003). Consumption of L-arginine mediated by *Entamoeba histolytica* L-arginase (EhArg) inhibits amoebicidal activity and nitric oxide production by activated macrophages. *Parasite Immunology, 25*(12), 597–608.

29. Espinosa-Cantellano, M., & Martínez-Palomo, A. (1994). *Entamoeba histolytica*: Mechanism of surface receptor capping. *Experimental Parasitology, 79*(4), 424–435.

30. Espinosa-Cantellano, M., & Martínez-Palomo, A. (2000). Pathogenesis of intestinal amebiasis: From molecules to disease. *Clinical Microbiology Reviews, 13*(3), 318–331.

31. Esquivel López, A., González Espínola, G., García Garduño, J. R., & Guarner Dalias, V. (1979). Various considerations in the treatment of amebic liver abscess. *Revista de Gastroenterología de México, 44*(1), 51–56.

32. Estrada-Figueroa, L. A., Ramírez-Jiménez, Y., Osorio-Trujillo, C., Shibayama, M., Navarro-García, F., García-Tovar, C., & Talamás-Rohana, P. (2011). Absence of CD38 delays arrival of neutrophils to the liver and innate immune response development during hepatic amoebiasis by *Entamoeba histolytica*. *Parasite Immunology, 33*(11), 661–668.

33. Flores, B. M., Batzer, M. A., Stein, M. A., Petersen, C., Diedrich, D. L., & Torian, B. E. (1993). Structural analysis and demonstration of the 29 kDa antigen of pathogenic *Entamoeba*

histolytica as the major accessible free thiol-containing surface protein. *Molecular Microbiology, 7*(5), 755–763.

34. Fotedar, R., Stark, D., Beebe, N., Marriott, D., Ellis, J., & Harkness, J. (2007). Laboratory diagnostic techniques for *Entamoeba* species. *Clinical Microbiology Reviews, 20*(3), 511–532.
35. Garcia-Zepeda, E. A., Rojas-Lopez, A., Esquivel-Velazquez, M., & Ostoa-Saloma, P. (2007). Regulation of the inflammatory immune response by the cytokine/chemokine network in amoebiasis. *Parasite Immunology, 29*(12), 679–684.
36. Ghadirian, E., & Denis, M. (1992a). In vivo activation of macrophages by IFN-gamma to kill *Entamoeba histolytica* trophozoites in vitro. *Parasite Immunology, 14*(5), 397–404.
37. Ghadirian, E., & Denis, M. (1992b). *Entamoeba histolytica* extract and interferon-gamma activation of macrophage-mediated amoebicidal function. *Immunobiology, 185*(1), 1–10.
38. Ghadirian, E., & Meerovitch, E. (1981a). Effect of splenectomy on the size of amoebic liver abscesses and metastatic foci in hamsters. *Infection and Immunity, 31*(2), 571–573.
39. Ghadirian, E., & Meerovitch, E. (1981b). Effect of immunosuppression on the size and metastasis of amoebic liver abscesses in hamsters. *Parasite Immunology, 3*(4), 329–338.
40. Ghadirian, E., & Salimi, A. (1993). In vitro effect of recombinant interferon gamma in combination with LPS on amoebicidal activity of murine Kupffer cells. *Immunobiology, 188*(3), 203–219.
41. Ghadirian, E., Somerfield, S. D., & Kongshavn, P. A. (1986). Susceptibility of *Entamoeba histolytica* to oxidants. *Infection and Immunity, 51*(1), 263–267.
42. Ghosh, A. S., Dutta, S., & Raha, S. (2010). Hydrogen peroxide-induced apoptosis-like cell death in *Entamoeba histolytica*. *Parasitology International, 59*(2), 166–172.
43. Guarner, V. (1986). Treatment of amebiasis. In A. Martínez-Palomo (Ed.), *Amebiasis* (pp. 189–212). Elsevier.
44. Guerrant, R. L., Brush, J., Ravdin, J. I., Sullivan, J. A., & Mandell, G. L. (1981). Interaction between *Entamoeba histolytica* and human polymorphonuclear neutrophils. *Journal of Infectious Diseases, 143*(1), 83–93.
45. Gupta, S. S., Singh, O., Sabharwal, G., & Hastin, A. (2011). Catheter drainage versus needle aspiration in management of large (>10 cm diameter) amoebic liver abscesses. *ANZ Journal of Surgery, 81*(8), 547–551.
46. Ha, H. L., Shin, H. J., Feitelson, M. A., & Yu, D. Y. (2010). Oxidative stress and antioxidants in hepatic pathogenesis. *World Journal of Gastroenterology, 16*(48), 6035–6043.
47. Hampton, M. B., Kettle, A. J., & Winterbourn, C. C. (1998). Inside the neutrophil phagosome: Oxidants, myeloperoxidase, and bacterial killing. *Blood, 92*(9), 3007–3017.
48. Helk, E., Bernin, H., Ernst, T., Ittrich, H., Jacobs, T., Heeren, J., Tacke, F., Tannich, E., & Lotter, H. (2013). TNFα-mediated liver destruction by Kupffer cells and Ly6Chi monocytes during *Entamoeba histolytica* infection. *PLoS Pathogens, 9*(5), e1003096. https://doi.org/10.1371/journal.ppat.1003096.
49. Hertz, R., Ben Lulu, S., Shahi, P., Trebicz-Geffen, M., Benhar, M., & Ankri, S. (2014). Proteomic identification of S-nitrosylated proteins in the parasite *Entamoeba histolytica* by resin-assisted capture: Insights into the regulation of the Gal/GalNAc lectin by nitric oxide. *PLoS One, 9*(7), e91518.

50. Hoque, M. L., Uddin, M. S., Saker, A. R., & Uddi, M. K. (2014). Common presentation of amebic liver abscess: A study in a tertiary care hospital in Bangladesh. *Mymensingh Medical Journal, 23*(4), 724–729.

51. Jarillo-Luna, R. A., Campos-Rodriguez, R., & Tsutsumi, V. (2002). *Entamoeba histolytica*: Immunohistochemical study of hepatic amoebiasis in mouse. Neutrophils and nitric oxide as possible factors of resistance. *Experimental Parasitology, 101*(1), 40–56.

52. Jha, A. K., Das, A., Chowdhury, F., Biswas, M. R., Prasad, S. K., & Chattopadhyay, S. (2015). Clinicopathological study and management of liver abscess in a tertiary care center. *Journal of Natural Science, Biology, and Medicine, 6*(1), 71–75.

53. Kimura, K., Stoopen, M., Reeder, M. M., & Moncada, R. (1997). Amebiasis: Modern diagnostic imaging with pathological and clinical correlation. *Seminars in Roentgenology, 32*(4), 250–275.

54. Knobloch, J., & Mannweiler, E. (1983). Development and persistence of antibodies to *Entamoeba histolytica* in patients with amebic liver abscess: Analysis of 216 cases. *American Journal of Tropical Medicine and Hygiene, 32*(4), 727–732.

55. Kolaczkowska, E., & Kubes, P. (2013). Neutrophil recruitment and function in health and inflammation. *Nature Reviews Immunology, 13*(3), 159–175.

56. Kretschmer, R. (1986). In A. Martínez-Palomo (Ed.), *Amebiasis* (pp. 95–168). Elsevier.

57. Lin, J. Y., Keller, K., & Chadee, K. (1993). *Entamoeba histolytica* proteins modulate the respiratory burst potential by murine macrophages. *Immunology, 78*(2), 291–297.

58. Loftus, B. J., & Hall, N. (2005). Entamoeba: Still more to be learned from the genome. *Trends in Parasitology, 21*(9), 453.

59. Loftus, B., Anderson, I., Davies, R., Alsmark, U. C., Samuelson, J., Amedeo, P., et al. (2005). The genome of the protist parasite *Entamoeba histolytica*. *Nature, 433*(7028), 865–868.

60. Lotter, H., Gonzalez-Roldan, N., Lindner, B., Winau, F., Isibasi, A., Moreno-Lafont, M., et al. (2009). Natural killer T cells activated by a lipopeptidophosphoglycan from *Entamoeba histolytica* are critically important to control amebic liver abscess. *PLoS Pathogens, 5*(5), e1000434.

61. Lotter, H., Jacobs, T., Gaworski, I., & Tannich, E. (2006). Sexual dimorphism in the control of amebic liver abscess in a mouse model of disease. *Infection and Immunity, 74*(1), 118–124.

62. Martínez-Palomo, A. (1987). The pathogenesis of amoebiasis. *Parasitol. Today, 3*(4), 111–118.

63. Martínez-Palomo, A., & Espinosa-Cantellano, M. (2004). Amebiasis and other protozoan infections. In J. Cohen & W. G. Powerly (Eds.), *Infectious Diseases* (2nd ed., pp. 1567–1571). Elsevier.

64. Martínez-Palomo, A., & Espinosa-Cantellano, M. (2005). Amoebiasis. In F. E. G. Cox, D. Wakelin, & D. D. Despommier (Eds.), *Topley & Wilson's Microbiology and Microbial Infections* (10th ed., pp. 200–217). Arnold.

65. Martínez-Palomo, A., & Ruíz-Palacios, G. (1990). Amebiasis. In K. S. Warren & A. A. F. Mahmoud (Eds.), *Tropical and Geographical Medicine* (2nd ed., pp. 327–344). McGraw-Hill.

66. Martínez-Palomo, A., Gonzalez-Robles, A., Chavez, B., Orozco, E., Fernández-Castelo, S., & Cervantes, A. (1985). Structural bases of the cytolytic mechanisms of *Entamoeba histolytica*. *Journal of Protozoology, 32*(2), 166–175.

67. Mayer-Scholl, A., Averhoff, P., & Zychlinsky, A. (2004). How do neutrophils and pathogens interact? *Current Opinion in Microbiology, 7*(1), 62–66.

68. Moran, P., Rico, G., Ramiro, M., Olvera, H., Ramos, F., Gonzalez, E., et al. (2002). Defective production of reactive oxygen intermediates (ROI) in a patient with recurrent amebic liver abscess. *American Journal of Tropical Medicine and Hygiene, 67*(6), 632–635.

69. Mortimer, L., & Chadee, K. (2010). The immunopathogenesis of *Entamoeba histolytica*. *Experimental Parasitology, 126*(4), 366–380.

70. Murray, H. W., Aley, S. B., & Scott, W. A. (1981). Susceptibility of *Entamoeba histolytica* to oxygen intermediates. *Molecular and Biochemical Parasitology, 3*(4), 381–391.

71. Nathan, C. (2006). Neutrophils and immunity: Challenges and opportunities. *Nature Reviews Immunology, 6*(3), 173–182.

72. Olivos-Garcia, A., Saavedra, E., Ramos-Martinez, E., Nequiz, M., & Pérez-Tamayo, R. (2009). Molecular nature of virulence in *Entamoeba histolytica*. *Infection, Genetics and Evolution, 9*(6), 1033–1037.

73. Pacheco-Yépez, J., Campos-Rodriguez, R., Shibayama, M., Ventura-Juarez, J., Serrano-Luna, J., & Tsutsumi, V. (2001). *Entamoeba histolytica*: Production of nitric oxide and in situ activity of NADPH diaphorase in amebic liver abscess of hamsters. *Parasitology Research, 87*(1), 49–56.

74. Pacheco-Yépez, J., Galván-Moroyoqui, J. M., Meza, I., Tsutsumi, V., & Shibayama, M. (2011). Expression of cytokines and their regulation during amoebic liver abscess development. *Parasite Immunology, 33*(1), 56–64.

75. Pacheco-Yépez, J., Jarillo-Luna, R. A., Gutiérrez-Meza, M., Abarca-Rojano, E., Larsen, B. A., & Campos-Rodriguez, R. (2014). Peroxynitrite and peroxiredoxin in the pathogenesis of experimental amebic liver abscess. *Biomedical Research International, 2014*, 324230.

76. Pérez-Tamayo, R. (1986). Pathology of amebiasis. In A. Martínez-Palomo (Ed.), *Amebiasis* (pp. 45–94). Elsevier.

77. Petri Jr., W. A., Haque, R., & Mann, B. J. (2002). The bittersweet interface of parasite and host: Lectin-carbohydrate interactions during human invasion by the parasite *Entamoeba histolytica*. *Annual Review of Microbiology, 56*, 39–64.

78. Racanelli, V., & Rehermann, B. (2006). The liver as an immunological organ. *Hepatology, 43*(2), S54–S62.

79. Ramos-Martinez, E., Olivos-Garcia, A., Saavedra, E., Nequiz, M., Sanchez, E. C., Tello, E., et al. (2009). *Entamoeba histolytica*: Oxygen resistance and virulence. *International Journal for Parasitology, 39*(7), 693–702.

80. Ramos, E., Olivos-Garcia, A., Nequiz, M., Saavedra, E., Tello, E., & Saralegui, A. (2007). *Entamoeba histolytica*: Apoptosis induced in vitro by nitric oxide species. *Experimental Parasitology, 116*(3), 257–265.

81. Rastew, E., Vicente, J. B., & Singh, U. (2012). Oxidative stress resistance genes contribute to the pathogenic potential of the anaerobic protozoan parasite *Entamoeba histolytica*. *International Journal for Parasitology, 42*(11), 1007–1015.

82. Rico, G., Leandro, E., Rojas, S., Gimenez, J. A., & Kretschmer, R. R. (2003). The monocyte locomotion inhibitory factor produced by *Entamoeba histolytica* inhibits induced nitric oxide production in human leukocytes. *Parasitology Research, 90*(4), 264–267.

83. Salata, R. A., Murray, H. W., Rubin, B. Y., & Ravdin, J. I. (1987). The role of gamma interferon in the generation of human macrophages cytotoxic for *Entamoeba histolytica* trophozoites. *American Journal of Tropical Medicine and Hygiene, 37*(1), 72–78.

84. Salimi, A., & Ghadirian, E. (1993). Effect of recombinant tumor necrosis factor alpha on in vitro amoebicidal activity of murine Kupffer cells. *Microbial Pathogenesis, 14*(4), 261–274.

85. Sánchez-Aguilar, M., Morán-Mendoza, O., Herrera-Hernández, M. F., Hernández-Sierra, J. F., Mandeville, P. B., Tapia-Pérez, J. H., et al. (2012). Prognostic indications of the failure to treat amoebic liver abscesses. *Pathogens and Global Health, 106*(4), 232–237.

86. Sánchez-Áleman, E., Quintanar-Stephano, A., Escobedo, G., Campos-Esparza, M. D. R., Campos-Rodriguez, R., & Ventura-Juarez, J. (2015). Vagotomy induces deregulation of the inflammatory response during the development of amoebic liver abscess in hamsters. *Neuroimmunomodulation, 22*(3), 166–180.

87. Sannella, A., Gradoni, L., Persichini, T., Ongini, E., & Venturini, G. (2003). Intracellular release of nitric oxide by NCX 972, an NO-releasing metronidazole, enhances in vitro killing of *Entamoeba histolytica*. *Antimicrobial Agents and Chemotherapy, 47*(7), 2303–2306.

88. Santi-Rocca, J., Rigothier, M. C., & Guillen, N. (2009). Host-microbe interactions and defense mechanisms in the development of amoebic liver abscesses. *Clinical Microbiology Reviews, 22*(1), 65–75.

89. Segal, A. W. (2005). How neutrophils kill microbes. *Annual Review of Immunology, 23*, 197–223.

90. Seguin, R., Mann, B. J., Keller, K., & Chadee, K. (1995). Identification of the galactose-adherence lectin epitopes of *Entamoeba histolytica* that stimulate tumor necrosis factor-alpha production by macrophages. *Proceedings of the National Academy of Sciences USA, 92*(26), 12175–12179.

91. Sen, A., Chatterjee, N. S., Akbar, M. A., Nandi, N., & Das, P. (2007). The 29-kilodalton thiol-dependent peroxidase of *Entamoeba histolytica* is a factor involved in pathogenesis and survival of the parasite during oxidative stress. *Eukaryotic Cell, 6*(4), 664–673.

92. Sepúlveda, B., & Treviño García-Manzo, N. (1986). Clinical manifestations and diagnosis of amebiasis. In A. Martínez-Palomo (Ed.), *Amebiasis* (pp. 169–188). Elsevier.

93. Seydel, K. B., Smith, S. J., & Stanley Jr., S. L. (2000). Innate immunity to amebic liver abscess is dependent on gamma interferon and nitric oxide in a murine model of disease. *Infection and Immunity, 68*(1), 400–402.

94. Seydel, K. B., Zhang, T., & Stanley Jr., S. L. (1997). Neutrophils play a critical role in early resistance to amebic liver abscesses in severe combined immunodeficient mice. *Infection and Immunity, 65*(10), 3951–3953.

95. Shibayama, M., Navarro-Garcia, F., Lopez-Revilla, R., Martínez-Palomo, A., & Tsutsumi, V. (1997). In vivo and in vitro experimental intestinal amebiasis in Mongolian gerbils (*Meriones unguiculatus*). *Parasitology Research, 83*(3), 170–176.

96. Sim, S., Yu, J. R., Lee, Y. A., & Shin, M. H. (2010). Involvement of Src family tyrosine kinase in apoptosis of human neutrophils induced by protozoan parasite *Entamoeba histolytica*. *Korean Journal of Parasitology, 48*(4), 285–290.

97. Siman-Tov, R., & Ankri, S. (2003). Nitric oxide inhibits cysteine proteinases and alcohol dehydrogenase 2 of *Entamoeba histolytica*. *Parasitology Research, 89*(3), 146–149.

98. Singh, P., Mirdha, B. R., Ahuja, V., & Singh, S. (2011). Evaluation of small-subunit rRNA touchdown polymerase chain reaction for direct detection of *Entamoeba histolytica* in human pus samples from patients with amoebic liver abscess. *Indian Journal of Medical Microbiology, 29*(2), 141–146.

99. Soong, C. J., Torian, B. E., Abd-Alla, M. D., Jackson, T. F., Gatharim, V., & Ravdin, J. I. (1995). Protection of gerbils from amebic liver abscess by immunization with recombinant *Entamoeba histolytica* 29-kilodalton antigen. *Infection and Immunity, 63*(2), 472–477.

100. Stanley Jr., S. L., & Reed, S. L. (2001). Microbes and microbial toxins: Paradigms for microbial-mucosal interactions. VI. *Entamoeba histolytica*: Parasite-host interactions. *American Journal of Physiology–Gastrointestinal and Liver Physiology, 280*(5), G1049–G1054.

101. Stanley, S. L. (2001). Pathophysiology of amoebiasis. *Trends in Parasitology, 17*(6), 280–285.

102. Talamas-Rohana, P., Schlie-Guzman, M. A., Hernandez-Ramirez, V. I., & Rosales-Encina, J. L. (1995). T-cell suppression and selective in vivo activation of TH2 subpopulation by the *Entamoeba histolytica* 220-kilodalton lectin. *Infection and Immunity, 63*(10), 3953–3958.

103. Tordoff, M. G., & Friedman, M. I. (1994). Altered hepatic metabolic response to carbohydrate loads in rats with hepatic branch vagotomy or cholinergic blockade. *Journal of the Autonomic Nervous System, 47*(3), 255–261.

104. Torian, B. E., Flores, B. M., Stroeher, V. L., Hagen, F. S., & Stamm, W. E. (1990). cDNA sequence analysis of a 29-kDa cysteine-rich surface antigen of pathogenic *Entamoeba histolytica*. *Proceedings of the National Academy of Sciences USA, 87*(16), 6358–6362.

105. Tsutsumi, R., Vázquez-González, R., Gaitán-Gaona, F. I., Bravo-González, R., Jesús-Romero, O., Blanda-Martínez, C., et al. (2015). Report of 66 cases of amebic liver abscess admitted in a public hospital in Mexico: Comparative analysis with cases reported at the seminar on Amebiasis (1970–80). In *XVII International Seminar on Amebiasis*, Campeche, Mexico.

106. Tsutsumi, V., & Martínez-Palomo, A. (1988). Inflammatory reaction in experimental hepatic amebiasis. *American Journal of Pathology, 130*(1), 112–119.

107. Tsutsumi, V., & Shibayama, M. (2006). Experimental amebiasis: A selected review of some in vivo models. *Archives of Medical Research, 37*(2), 210–220.

108. Tsutsumi, V., Mena-López, R., Anaya-Velázquez, F., & Martínez-Palomo, A. (1984). Cellular bases of experimental amebic liver abscess formation. *American Journal of Pathology, 117*(1), 81–91.

109. Urban, C. F., Lourido, S., & Zychlinsky, A. (2006). How do microbes evade neutrophil killing? *Cellular Microbiology, 8*(11), 1687–1696.

110. Velazquez, C., Shibayama-Salas, M., Aguirre-Garcia, J., Tsutsumi, V., & Calderon, J. (1998). Role of neutrophils in innate resistance to *Entamoeba histolytica* liver infection in mice. *Parasitology Immunology, 20*(5), 255–262.

111. Vicente, J. B., Ehrenkaufer, G. M., Saraiva, L. M., Teixeira, M., & Singh, U. (2009). *Entamoeba histolytica* modulates a complex repertoire of novel genes in response to oxidative and nitrosative stresses: Implications for amebic pathogenesis. *Cellular Microbiology, 11*(1), 51–69.

112. Walsh, J. A. (1986). Problems in recognition and diagnosis of amebiasis: Estimation of the global magnitude of morbidity and mortality. *Reviews of Infectious Diseases, 8*(2), 228–238.

113. Wang, W., Keller, K., & Chadee, K. (1992). Modulation of tumor necrosis factor production by macrophages in *Entamoeba histolytica* infection. *Infection and Immunity, 60*(8), 3169–3174.

114. Wang, W., Keller, K., & Chadee, K. (1994). *Entamoeba histolytica* modulates the nitric oxide synthase gene and nitric oxide production by macrophages for cytotoxicity against amoebae and tumor cells. *Immunology, 83*(4), 601–610.

115. Wells, C. D., & Arguedas, M. (2004). Amebic liver abscess. *Southern Medical Journal, 97*(6), 673–680.

116. Wood, Z. A., Poole, L. B., & Karplus, P. A. (2003). Peroxiredoxin evolution and the regulation of hydrogen peroxide signaling. *Science, 300*(5619), 650–653.

Chapter

5

PATHOGENESIS OF IDIOSYNCRATIC DRUG-INDUCED LIVER INJURY AND LIVER REGENERATION

Contents

Introduction

The primary cause of acute liver failure (ALF) in the US is drug-induced liver injury (DILI), which is a significant cause of liver damage. Actually, DILI accounts for over half of all ALF cases in the US, with acetaminophen being the primary cause (Lee, 2003; Reuben et al., 2010). Additionally, DILI is the main cause of clinical drug development failures, regulatory actions against developing drugs, indication restrictions, and market withdrawals (Watkins and Seeff, 2006; Chen et al., 2013). The two types of DILI are idiosyncratic and direct hepatotoxicity. While some medications can cause predictable, dose-dependent, and direct hepatotoxicity, such as aspirin, acetaminophen, and chemotherapy agents, the majority of drug-induced liver injury cases are unique. Only a small percentage of those exposed experience idiosyncratic drug-induced liver injury (IDILI), which is unpredictable and has a lengthy latency. A range of clinical signs and symptoms are indicative of hepatotoxicity, including cholestatic liver injury, sinusoidal obstruction syndrome, hepatitis, nodular regenerative hyperplasia, and steatohepatitis. The R ratio, which divides phenotypically IDILI into cholestatic and multiple of the upper limit of normal (ULN) categories, determines the distribution of alanine transaminase (ALT) over alkaline phosphatase. <2), hepatocellular (> 5), as well as mixed (2–5) patterns of damage. In general, DILI is an exclusion diagnosis, meaning that common liver disorders like autoimmune hepatitis (AIH), circulatory dysfunction, heart failure, ischemic hepatitis, viral hepatitis, biliary tract disease, and sepsis need to be ruled out. Given the exclusion of all other possible factors, a high index of suspicion regarding drug toxicity, appropriate dosing timing, and congruence between the injury's characteristics and the drug's signature (if available), there is a high likelihood of an IDILI event. Even though they are less frequent, allergic symptoms like rash, fever, and eosinophilia can be beneficial. If there are any signs of centrilobular necrosis, granulomas, or eosinophilic infiltrates, a liver biopsy may be beneficial. IDILI is still difficult to diagnose since there is no particular test to establish causation, and liver biopsies are frequently inconclusive. Additionally, IDILI is a complicated multifactorial illness that is still poorly understood. Risk factors linked to the development of IDILI have been identified over the last ten years using sizable patient cohorts.

The hapten/prohapten hypothesis is expanded upon in the current IDILI hypothesis. According to the suggested model, a drug is changed into a "reactive metabolite," which in some people with susceptible HLA haplotypes can trigger the adaptive immune system by acting as a neoantigen or through molecular mimicry. In hepatocytes, the reactive metabolite can induce cellular stress and trigger stress response pathways, such as mitochondrial stress and the endoplasmic reticulum (ER). Hepatotoxicity cannot be fully explained by the human leukocyte antigen (HLA) polymorphism alone because IDILI is uncommon and the majority of HLA haplotypes linked to toxicity are fairly common in the general population. As a result, not every person with the susceptible HLA shows signs of severe liver damage after taking the medication. Many reactive metabolites are normally produced in the liver during metabolism, but the liver microenvironment—which includes Kupffer cells, sinusoidal cells, and regulatory T cells—induces an immune tolerance state that either reverses or prevents toxicity, a process known as adaptation. Therefore, a failure to adapt may be a further or concurrent requirement for the development of IDILI. This chapter will cover the pathophysiology of IDILI, host genetic and adaptive immune factors, and drug characteristics that affect hepatotoxicity susceptibility.

Orientation and Directional Terms

Term	Definition	Illustration
Drug-Induced Liver Injury (DILI)	DILI, drug and herbal & dietary supplement-induced liver injury, DHILI, drug induced liver failure, DILF, drug induced hepatitis, or drug induced hepatotoxicity.	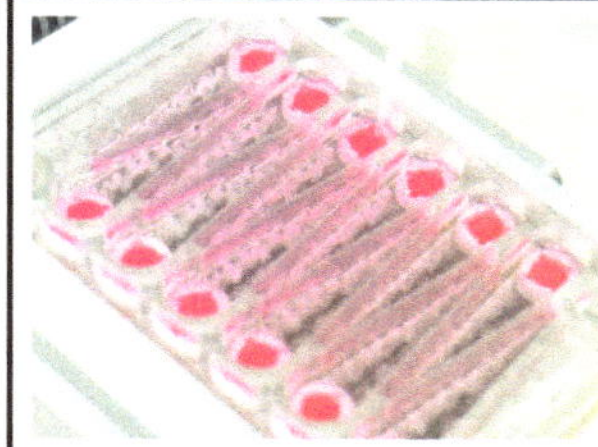
Alanine transaminase (ALT)	The alanine aminotransferase (ALT) test is a blood test that checks for liver damage. ALT used to be called serum glutamic-pyruvic transaminase (SGPT).	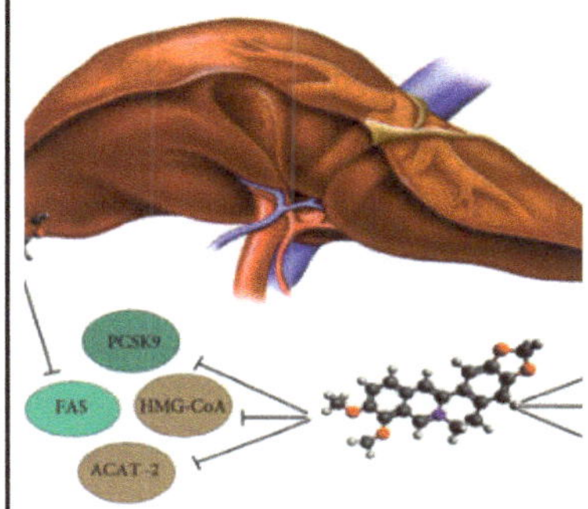
Glutathione S-transferases (GST)	GST is a multifunctional enzyme, involved in detoxification processes. This role is achieved by catalytic conjugation of glutathione with a large number of electrophilic toxins and carcinogens. In mammals, GST is found in all tissues and organs.	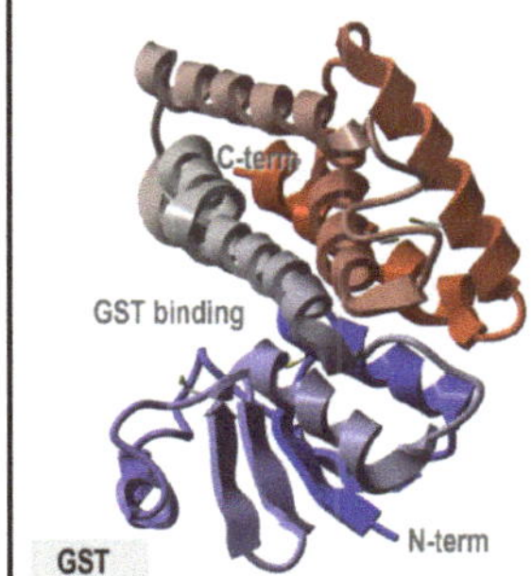
Organic anion-transporting polypeptides (OATPs)	Members of the solute carrier organic anion transporting polypeptide (OATPs) family function as transporters for a large variety of amphipathic organic anions including endogenous metabolites and clinical drugs, such as bile salts, steroids, thyroid hormones, statins, antibiotics, antivirals, and anticancer drugs.	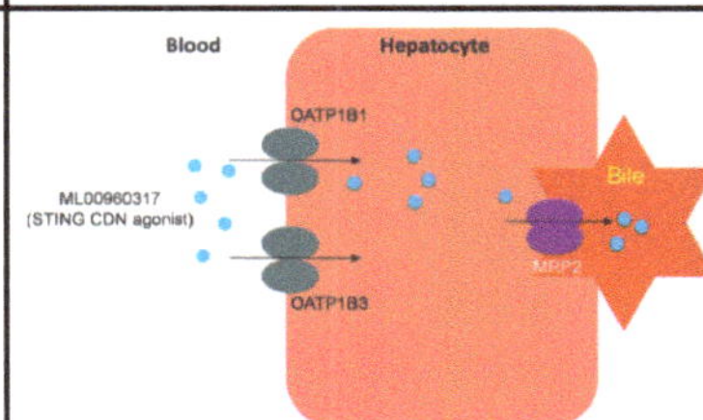

5.1. Epidemiology of Idiosyncratic Drug-Induced Liver Injury

The epidemiology of IDILI remains poorly understood due to limited reporting and surveillance systems, as well as the absence of a standardized diagnostic method (Chen et al., 2013). IDILI, a rare but serious adverse reaction to pharmaceutical and herbal medications, has been reported to have an incidence of 13.9 per 100,000 in the French population and 19.1 per 100,000 in Iceland (Sgro et al., 2002; Bjornsson et al., 2013). Despite its low frequency, IDILI is the second leading cause of acute liver failure in the United States (13%), surpassed only by DILI caused by acetaminophen (40%) (Ostapowicz et al., 2002). The significance of IDILI is highlighted by the fact that nearly 1 in 10 patients with hepatocellular IDILI die or require a liver transplant within 6 months of onset, and 20% experience persistent liver damage at 6 months, decreasing slightly at 12 months (Fontana et al., 2014, 2015).

In an attempt to gather and thoroughly characterize cases of clinically apparent DILI and comprehend underlying susceptibility factors and mechanisms of injury, the National Institutes of Health established the Drug-induced Liver Injury Network (DILIN) to gather cases of IDILI (Hoofnagle, 2004). We now have a much better understanding of the epidemiology, patient characteristics, and prognostic markers of IDILI thanks to DILIN and many international multicenter networks in Europe and Asia (Spain, Iceland, the United Kingdom, Japan, China, and Korea) (Bjornsson et al., 2013; Andrade et al., , 2005; Takikawa et al.,; Molokhia and McKeigue, 2006. 2009). Some commonalities among the DILI cohorts are the gender distribution (with a preference for females), the subjects' median age, and the percentage of patients (42–58%) who present with acute hepatocellular injury (Fontana, 2014). The primary agents implicated in IDILI cases are antibiotics, followed by agents pertaining to the central nervous system. Antibiotics, antineoplastics, and phenytoin have been identified as the main causes of hepatotoxicity in hospitalized patients receiving intravenous medication (Ghabril et al., 2013). Interestingly, the percentage of hepatotoxicity from dietary and herbal supplements as the causes of IDILI has increased dramatically in the past few years, in addition to traditional pharmaceuticals (Navarro et al., 2014). Some phenotypic characteristics are concerning for increased risk of death or need for transplant, regardless of drug class. According to Hy's law, an elevated total bilirubin level (ULN) and a serum ALT equal to or greater than five times the ULN are known to indicate a poor prognosis.

Multiple hepatotoxicity registries have confirmed that hepatocellular injury and jaundice are the highest prognostic markers of an unfavorable outcome (Andrade et al., 2005; Bjornsson and Olsson, 2005). For instance, the Spanish DILI registry found that patients with hepatocellular jaundice had an 11.7% chance of death or need for a liver transplant (Andrade et al., 2005). These registries also conducted long-term follow-up studies on patients after their initial DILI event. In Iceland, it was observed that the development of clinically significant liver disease after surviving an IDILI event was rare after 10 years (Bjornsson and Davidsdottir, 2009). However, 22% of patients, all females, in this population developed autoimmune hepatitis (Bjornsson & Davidsdottir, 2009). In the Spanish registry, after a 20-month follow-up, 5.7% of total cases were found to have persistent liver injury, with the cholestatic and mixed phenotypes being more likely to lead to chronicity compared to those with an initial hepatocellular pattern of injury (Andrade et al., 2006, 2008).

5.2. Factors Contributing to the Development of Idiosyncratic Drug-Induced Liver Injury

In contrast to traditional direct-acting hepatotoxins like acetaminophen or chemotherapy drugs, IDILI exhibits variability in its latency and is mainly dose-independent above a threshold dose (Dara et al., 2015). The precise etiology of IDILI is complex and involves host and drug-related variables, including age, gender, drug metabolism, transport, and factors influencing the adaptive immune response (genetic polymorphisms in HLA molecules). IDILI has been linked to specific drug characteristics like dosage and lipophilicity (Chen et al., 2013). Indeed, a threshold level of exposure is required because drugs that are taken at a high dose (greater than 100 mg/day) and that have a calculated octanol-water partition coefficient (log P > 3) that makes them lipophilic have a higher positive predictive value for inducing toxicity than a dose alone (Kaplowitz, 2013).

The ability of a drug to cause mitochondrial stress is another intriguing characteristic linked to toxicity. Porceddu et al., (2012) used isolated mouse liver mitochondria in culture to report a significant correlation between medications that cause IDILI and the loss of mitochondrial integrity. They created a high throughput technique for screening mitochondrial toxicity using isolated mouse liver mitochondria by employing readouts such as cytochrome c release, membrane permeabilization (swelling), collapse of membrane potential, and changes in respiration caused by succinate or malate/glutamate. They examined 124 chemical compounds, 37 of which had no known hepatotoxicity and 87 of which had been shown in the literature to cause DILI. Remarkably, the possibility of causing mitochondrial toxicity had a high positive predictive value of 82–89% and a sensitivity of 92–94% for a hepatotoxic result (Porceddu et al., 2012). The fact that IDILI only happens in a small percentage of people exposed to a particular drug indicates that individual host factors play a major role in the harmful outcome, even though drug factors are still a crucial area of research for toxicity.

5.3. Individual Host Factors

5.3.1. Age

Many host factors have been linked to liver injury, although it is nearly impossible to predict a person's risk of developing toxicity with a particular drug based on our current understanding of IDILI. Age and gender, for instance, are well-known risk factors for the toxicity of particular medications. Aspirin and valproic acid are nearly exclusively linked to Reye's syndrome and DILI in early life, but isoniazid (INH) hepatotoxicity is known to rise with age (Larrey, 1999, 2002; Jinjuvadia et al., 2007; Nolan et al). Actually, patients over 50 have a five-fold higher incidence of hepatotoxicity from INH than patients under 35 (Fountain et al., 2005). Hepatotoxicity from amoxicillin and clavulanic acid is also associated with older age. It's interesting to note that age influences the phenotypic injury profile of amoxicillin/clavulanic acid, with older age linked to cholestatic/mixed type of damage and younger age associated with hepatocellular damage (Lucena et al., 2006). Since growing older does not dramatically change drug metabolism, it is unclear how age affects the development of IDILI (Herrlinger and Klotz, 2001). Age might affect the adaptive immune response instead of changing how drugs are metabolized. Naturally, as people age, they take more medications, and polypharmacy is more common.

5.3.2. Gender

Numerous studies have shown that women are more likely to develop drug-induced liver injury (DILI), although this risk may vary depending on the specific drug. While some research, such as the Spanish DILI registry by Lucena et al., (2009), has not found a significant overall association between female sex and increased incidence of DILI, women have been linked to specific patterns of liver injury, severe liver failure, and poorer outcomes. Studies have reported a higher risk of toxicity in women for drugs like halothane, flucloxacillin, INH, nitrofurantoin, chlorpromazine, macrolides, and diclofenac (Larrey, 2002; De Abajo et al., 2004; Bell and Chalasani, 2009; Chalasani and Bjornsson, 2010).

5.3.3. Hepatic Metabolism

The parent drug typically forms a reactive metabolite that can covalently bind intracellular proteins and cause cellular stress as the initial stage of an IDILI event. Since reactive metabolites are assumed to trigger the first stage of toxicity, CYP polymorphisms have been investigated for correlations with toxicity. Individual variations in CYP activity are significant. Although it hasn't been verified, CYP2C9 polymorphisms have been linked to diclofenac toxicity (Aithal et al., 2000); Scordo et al. , 2001) and the Spanish DILIN registry has not shown any discernible correlations with CYP2C9 and CYP2C19 polymorphisms (Pachkoria et al., 2007). Hepatotoxicity from INH has been linked to CYP2E1 polymorphisms (Huang et al., 2003). Humans express N-acetyl transferase (NAT)1 and NAT2, which are involved in the detoxifying process of N-acetylation in drug metabolism. Numerous studies have examined the connection between NAT2 gene polymorphisms and DILI brought on by INH (Metushi et al., 2014). INH hepatotoxicity is more likely to develop in people with low NAT2 activity due to the formation of hazardous intermediary metabolites (Musch et al., 1982; Urban and others. 2014). Consequently, slow acetylators have a higher incidence of IDILI, suggesting that NAT activity modulates susceptibility to INH hepatotoxicity (Pande et al.,1996; Wong et al , 2000; Huang et al.,2003). Another risk factor for sulfonamide toxicity is slow acetylation (Rieder et al., 1991).

Variations in the detoxifying enzymes manganese superoxide dismutase (MnSOD) and glutathione S-transferases (GST) have also been considered as risk factors for IDILI. People with GSTT and GSTM1 null genotypes in the Spanish DILIN database had a markedly increased risk of DILI; this association was particularly strong for nonsteroidal anti-inflammatory drug IDILI and antibiotic-associated IDILI (Lucena et al., 2008). The MnSOD C allele and the GSTM1 null genotype were linked to an increased risk of hepatotoxicity from antituberculosis drugs in a Taiwanese study that examined 115 patients with DILI (Huang et al., 2007). The nicotinamide adenine dinucleotide phosphate:quinone oxidoreductase, however, did not show any correlation (Huang et al., 2007). Diclofenac toxicity has also been linked to polymorphisms in the genes that code for the phase 1 and phase 2 enzymes in the diclofenac pathway. A UK study found that mutations in the transporter multidrug resistance-associated protein 2 (MRP2), CYP2C8, and uridine glucuronosyl transferase 2B7 (UGT2B7) predispose to the formation and accumulation of reactive diclofenac metabolites and are linked to toxicity (Daly et al., 2007). When comparing patients who took diclofenac but did not have liver damage or healthy controls, those with at least one UGT2B7 mutant allele had a significantly higher odds ratio (OR) of diclofenac IDILI (Daly et al., 2007).

5.4. Expression and Polymorphisms of Hepatocyte Transporters

A cholestatic or mixed phenotype of liver injury is present in nearly half (46%) of all DILI cases (Chalasani et al., 2015). With sinusoidal/basolateral, apical, and highly polarized membranes, hepatocytes are cells with a distinct repertoire of transmembrane proteins and transporters. For the majority of medications that are processed in the liver to diffuse across the cell membrane, active or assisted transport is necessary (Bohan & Boyer, 2002; Pauli-Magnus & Meier, 2006). Following absorption, medications go through conjugation/esterification procedures like glucuronidation and sulfation as well as oxidation, hydroxylation, and other reactions mediated by the cytochrome P450 system (phase I). to increase in water solubility (phase II). The section on hepatic metabolism goes into further detail about how polymorphisms in the Cyps can result in extremely reactive and toxic metabolites, even though these processes are intended to be detoxifying steps. Then, these reactive substances may prevent the uptake, transport, and secretion of bile acids as well as canalicular efflux. Excretion into bile is the rate-limiting step in the clearance of lipophilic drugs (Padda et al., 2011). The transcriptional and posttranscriptional levels of hepatocellular transport regulation are highly sensitive, enabling adaptations to alterations in the bile salt pool (Trauner et al., 1998; Pauli-Magnus & Meier, 2006).

The major basolateral transporters include the sodium-dependent (sodium taurocholate cotransporting peptide) and independent (superfamily of organic anion-transporting polypeptides (OATPs) and OATs) basolateral transporters that are involved in the uptake of conjugated and unconjugated bile salts, bromosulfophthalein, neutral steroids, steroid sulfates and glucuronides, and selected organic cations (Pauli-Magnus & Meier, 2006). Many drugs are substrates of OATPs and can therefore theoretically bind to, inhibit, or interfere with transport functions. Drug substrates for OATPs include drugs such as fexofenadine, opioids, digoxin, pravastatin, rifampin, enalapril, and methotrexate. In addition, the OATPs take up phalloidin, microcystins and amanita toxin (Hagenbuch and Stieger, 2013). Oatp1b2 knockout mice are resistant to uptake and therefore toxicity from phalloidin and microcystin (Lu et al., 2008). Glibenclamide is an example of a drug known to inhibit OATPs (1B1 and 1B3) (Hagenbuch and Stieger, 2013). The basolateral membrane of the hepatocytes is the location for (ATP)-dependent efflux pumps belonging to the superfamily of multidrug resistanceassociated proteins (MRPs or ATP-binding cassette subfamily C (ABCC), which transport organic anions and play a role in efflux of conjugated drug metabolites, nucleoside analog drugs (zidovudine, lamivudine, stavudine), and methotrexate and 6-metacaptopurine (Borst et al., 2000; PauliMagnus and Meier, 2006; Boyer, 2013).

The bile salt export pump (BSEP) and multidrug resistance (MDRs) are found on the hepatocyte's canalicular membrane, and the ABC transporter family makes up the apical/canalicular transporters. Furthermore, the apical membrane is home to MRP2 (ABCC2), the ABC half transporters, such as breast cancer resistance protein, and the cholesterol flippase ABCG5 and ABCG8. Studies conducted in vitro with isolated canalicular membrane vesicles from the livers of rats and humans have shown that medications like calcineurin inhibitors can prevent leukotriene C4 and ATP-dependent bile salt transport. Endothelin antagonist bosentan, cyclosporin A, rifamycin, sulindac, glibenclamide, and troglitazone can cause cholestatic liver toxicity, inhibit BSEP, and prevent bile salt excretion (Fattinger et al., 2001; Kostrubsky et al., 2001; Seeff & Watkins, 2006).

Interestingly, in rat models, certain medications like diclofenac and estrogen conjugates secreted into the canaliculus via Mrp2 transinhibite Bsep from the canalicular side, while cyclosporine, rifampin, and bosentan cis-inhibit the Bsep transporter (Seitz et al., 1998; Huang et al,2000). Another illustration is how cyclosporine reduces bile salt-independent bile flow in rats by blocking Mrp2 and glutathione synthesis, which causes cholestatic DILI (Bramow et al., 2001). As a substrate of MDR1, cyclosporin can affect membrane fluidity and the ABC proteins through competitive inhibition, which prevents bilirubin transport (Padda et al., 2011). Studies on Mrp2 deficient Wistar rats show that bile transporters eliminate troglitazone, indicating that canalicular elimination through Mrp2 may play a significant role in the pathophysiology of troglitazone-induced cholestasis (Kostrubsky et al., 2001). A genetic predisposition or polymorphism in the transporters can cause drugs to inhibit or interfere with these transport mechanisms, which can result in cholestatic liver injury. For instance, polymorphisms in any one of these transporters may alter their expression, protein structure, and drug binding, which may lead to cholestasis and liver damage. Variations in MDR1 may also be linked to elevated plasma drug concentrations (Brinkmann and Eichelbaum, 2001). There are polymorphisms that cause MRP2, BSEP, and MDR1 expression to decrease (Padda et al., 2011).

Considerable individual and ethnic variety exist in the expression of OATPs as well as canalicular ABC transport proteins with many haplotypes leading to decreased expression (Tirona et al., 2001; Meier et al., 2006; Lang et al., 2006). Mutations in BSEP and MDR3 have been associated with DILI (Lang et al., 2007). Mutations in MRP2 (as well as glucuronide transferase and Cyp2C8) have been associated with diclofenac DILI (Daly et al., 2007). Many drugs that cause cholestatic forms of DILI have been shown to inhibit BSEP (Bohme et al., 1994; Fattinger et al., 2001; Funk et al., 2001; Hirano et al., 2006). Dawson et al., investigated the effect of 85 compounds (known hepatotoxins and nonhepatotoxic drugs) on the inhibition of rat and human BSEP using membrane vesicles from insect cells expressing the transporters. Drugs that cause cholestatic or mixed-type DILI were more likely to inhibit BSEP (60–64%) compared to drugs that cause hepatocellular injury (27%) or no DILI (38%) (Dawson et al., 2012). Therefore, the inhibition of BSEP correlates with drugs that exhibit a cholestatic phenotype of DILI. BSEP effectively secretes bile acids across the canalicular membrane against a steep concentration gradient, the accumulation of bile acids due to inhibition of BSEP can result in accumulation in liver cells resulting in cellular stress, inflammation, and susceptibility to innate and adaptive immune killing (Wang et al., 2011). When hydrophobic bile acids (glycine conjugates of dihydroxy bile acids) build up, they are especially harmful to hepatocytes (Malhi et al., 2010; Luedde et al., 2014). The induction of cell death by encouraging death receptor-mediated apoptosis by upregulating expression and trafficking of FAS and TNF-related apoptosis-inducing ligand to the cell membrane is one likely mechanism of hepatocyte toxicity in this case (Higuchi et al., 2004; Sodeman et al., 2000; Faubion et al., 1999). Even in the absence of ligand binding, the accumulation of death receptors leads to oligomerization and the activation of death pathways via caspase-8. It is outside the purview of this chapter to examine in detail the various liver cell trans-membrane transporters, their regulation, roles, and connections to drug transport and cholestatic DILI; for further reading, please see the following sources.

5.5. Adaptive Immune System

Effectively identifying inciting drugs and tracking patients to better understand IDILI phenotypes are the goals of the DILI registries. It is still difficult to identify patients who are more vulnerable to this erratic type of liver damage. There is a definite correlation between drug toxicity and immunity. Certain drugs, like minocycline or nitrofurantoin, can mimic or induce autoimmune hepatitis, and certain types of DILI, like halothane, dihydralazine, and anticonvulsants, are clearly associated with an immune allergic phenotype with rash and eosinophilia (Liu & Kaplowitz, 2002). Other noteworthy medications that may cause an immuno-allergic phenotype and elevated eosinophil counts include ciprofloxacin, cefazolin, and trimethoprim/sulfamethoxazole (Chalasani et al., 2015).

IDILI has also been linked to severe allergic skin reactions with poor prognoses, such as toxic epidermal necrosis (10) and Stevens Johnson syndrome (SJS) (Chalasani et al., 2015). Furthermore, the idea that host immune factors contribute to IDILI is supported by the fact that medications or drug-protein adducts from IDILI compounds can activate peripheral blood lymphocytes (lymphocyte stimulation test) (Tsutsui et al., 2013). Due to the uncommon nature of IDILI, a genetic predisposition has been considered an essential host factor, and as such, it has been the main focus of numerous consortia that have amassed sizable patient databases. Numerous DILI registries have carried out genetic research to find polymorphisms that could account for some people's predisposition to experience drug-induced liver damage while the majority of the exposed population does not. Numerous HLA correlations have been linked to different medications, suggesting that adaptive immunity may play a part. The majority of the detected HLA polymorphisms, however, are rather widespread in the general population and as a result, have a low risk of developing IDILI. Consequently, susceptibility must be influenced by additional contributing factors. Defective immune tolerance, or the liver's remarkable ability to adapt to foreign antigens, has been proposed as a major contributing factor to the development of IDILI (Uetrecht & Kaplowitz, 2015). The failure of adaptive immune responses in the liver. Circumstantial evidence suggests a potential mechanism, despite the lack of a direct causal relationship. Examples of this include the discovery of IL-10 polymorphisms in patients with diclofenac DILI and, more recently, animal models of defective adaptation leading to IDILI-like features in mice (Dara et al., 2015). A summary of the evidence supporting the adaptive immune system's role in the pathophysiology of IDILI will be provided in the discussion that follows.

5.6. Genetic Variations and Polymorphisms in Human Leukocyte Antigen

It has long been believed that the unique characteristics of the majority of drug reactions point to a genetic susceptibility to hepatotoxicity. It has been amply shown that a number of HLA polymorphisms are connected to IDILI (Table 5.1) (Kurosaki et al., 2000; Hirata et al., 2008; Xu et al., 2015; Phillips et al., 2013; Spraggs et al., 2011; Chen et al., 2015; Sharma et al., 2002; Daly et al., 2009; Hautekeete et al., 1999; Kindmark et al., 2008; Lucena et al., 2011). In a genome-wide association study examining patients with flucloxacillin toxicity, one of the earliest instances of such associations was found, where the HLAB*57:01 allele was linked to a hazard ratio of 100 for toxicity (Daly et al., 2009). Flucloxacillin can activate $CD8^+$ T cells in drug-naïve individuals with the HLA-B*57:01 allele, indicating a strong association between the allele and the resulting harmful phenotype. Peripheral blood mononuclear cells of patients with flucloxacillin DILI show immune activation with reexposure to the drug (Monshi et al., 2013; Wuillemin et al., 2013; Urban et al., 2014). Another illustration of a significant connection between these genetic variations and unique adverse reactions is the heightened susceptibility to amoxicillin-clavulanate toxicity among patients possessing DRB1*15:01-DQB1*06:02 and HLA-A*02:01 haplotypes (Hautekeete et al., 1999; O'donohue et al., 2000; Kindmark et al., 2008; Lucena et al., 2011).

Table 5.1. *Idiosyncratic Drug-induced Liver Injury (IDILI) Drugs and Their Known Human Leukocyte Antigen (HLA) Polymorphism Associations*

Drug	Phenotype	HLA	Comments	References
Amoxicillin –clavulanate	Spectrum cholestatic to hepatocellular	A*02:01 B*18:01 DRB1*1501 DGB1*0602 DRB1*07	DRB1*07 protective, PSC ?Halothane ?Nitrofurantoin	Hautekeete et al. (1999) Gastroenterology, Lucena et al. (2011) Gastroenterology, Kindmark et al. (2008) Pharmacogenomics J.
Anti-tuberculosis (TB) drugs	Hepatocellular and mixed	DQB1*02:01 DQA1*01:02 DQB1*05:02	HLA-DQA1*01:02 is protective DRB1*01, DRB1*03, and DRB1*07 associated in bivariate analysis	Sharma et al. (2002) Am. J. Respir. Crit. Care Med., Chen et al. (2015) J. Clin. Pharm. Ther.
Fenofibrate	Cholestatic	A*33:01	Association seen with cholestatic DILI cases	Aithal (2015) American Association for the Study of Liver Disease (AASLD) Abstr. 225
Flucloxacillin	Cholestatic	B*57:01 DRB1*07:01 DQB1*03:03 DRB1*15	Associated with Abacavir rash DRB1*15 is associated with reduced risk	Daly et al. (2009) Nat. Genet.
Lapatinib	Hepatocellular and mixed (delayed)	DQA1*02:01 DQB1*02:02 DRB1*07:01	Associated with ximelagatran	Spraggs et al. (2011) J. Clin. Oncol.
Lumiracoxib	Hepatocellular (delayed)	DRB1*15:01 DQB1*06:02 DRB5*01:01 DQA1*01:02	Associated with amoxicillin–clavulanate multiple sclerosis	Singer et al. (2010) Nat. Genet.
Minocyclin	Hepatocellular	HLA B*35:02		Urban (2015) AASLD Abstr. 1930
Nevirapine	Hepatocellular	DRB*01:02	Low CD4 protective	Phillips et al. (2013) J. Acquir. Immune Defic. Syndr.
Pazopanib	Hepatocellular	B*57:01	Weak association	Xu et al. (2015). Clin. Cancer Res.
Ticlopidine	Cholestatic	A*33:03 A*33:01	Japanese	Hirata et al. (2008) Pharmacogenomics J.
Tiopronin	Cholestatic	A*33		Kurosaki et al. (2000) Dig. Dis. Sci.
Terbinafine	Mixed	A*33:01	Cholestatic fenofibrate and ticlopidine	Aithal (2015) AASLD Abstr. 225
Ximelagatran	Hepatocellular	DRB1*0701 DQA1*0201	Associated with AIH 2 and ? TB meds and Caucasians	Kindmark et al. (2008) Pharmacogenomics J.

Source: L. Dara, et al., Pathogenesis of Idiosyncratic Drug-induced Liver Injury, http://dx.doi.org/10.1016/B978-0-12-804274-8.00005-9 C.

An immunological response can be triggered by ximelagatran, an anticoagulant that was taken off the market due to hepatotoxicity reports (Kindmark et al., 2008). Table 5.1 contains a list of additional medications with HLA associations. The immunological response's underlying mechanisms remain unclear despite the fact that HLA restriction has been widely accepted for years. The hapteneprohapten hypothesis, the altered peptide repertoire hypothesis, and the pharmacological interaction hypothesis (p-i hypothesis) are the three main mechanisms that have been proposed for T-cell activation and aberrant adaptive immune responses. According to the hapten/prohapten hypothesis, some medications produce reactive metabolites when they go through phase I (Cyp450) detoxification. These reactive compounds are probably formed due to a combination of drug properties and individual metabolic differences. After that, the reactive metabolite covalently attaches itself to intracellular proteins, creating adducts that cause organellar stress. When this adduct, or neo-antigen, is presented by antigen-presenting cells (APC), some individuals who are genetically susceptible and have a compromised ability to elicit adequate compensatory immune tolerance may interpret it as foreign and mount an immune response. HLA variations that have a higher affinity for neoantigens cause T cells to present the neoantigen more intensely, activating T cells and ultimately causing hepatocyte death through immunological means, which causes liver damage (Grove & Aithal, 2015). Innate immunity can also be activated by haptenization, at least in vitro (Megherbi et al., 2009). Other mechanisms of HLA-restricted immune responses due to aberrant antigen presentation by APCs have been proposed in addition to the hapten hypothesis for immune activation (Grove & Aithal, 2015). Furthermore, because a given protein contains multiple binding sites, one would expect several potential hapten peptides to interact with multiple HLA alleles after processing; however, the hapten hypothesis falls short in explaining why only a few HLA associations have been observed for any given drug. As a result, many propose different mechanisms than the happened hypothesis. The activation of the adaptive immune system is thought to be influenced by interactions between covalent and noncovalent proteins and APC binding groves. According to the "pharmacological interaction hypothesis," medications can interact noncovalently with MHC molecules or T-cell receptors to activate T cells without the need for an antigenic peptide (Pichler, 2002).

This theory was created to explain the characteristics of drug-responsive T-cell clones that were unable to process drugs and were metabolically inactive. According to the p-i hypothesis, medications may also interact with pre-bound peptides on MHC molecules to stimulate T cells. Grove and Aithal (2015) argue that, given the enormous diversity of MHC molecules, it is not surprising to find a T-cell receptor or MHC molecule that can bind the drug with sufficient affinity, since many drugs are engineered to interact with receptors. One instance of the p-i hypothesis's potential clinical applicability is with ximelagatran DILI. The hapten hypothesis is unlikely to be relevant to ximelagatran's mode of toxicity because it does not covalently bind proteins to form neo-antigens. The p-i hypothesis, however, may be a potential mechanism for immune activation and DILI because in vitro research has demonstrated a direct inhibition of peptide binding to HLA DRB1*0701 (Grove & Aithal, 2015). There are two different ways that flucloxacillin can stimulate T cells (Wuillemin et al., 2013). Wuillemin along with others showed this by isolating untreated individuals with HLB*57:01 positive and negative haplotypes and using them to generate flucloxacillin-reacting T cells in order to study the mechanisms of T-cell activation. The covalent binding of flucloxacillin, which makes it resistant to washing, and its dependence on proteasomal processing for stable presentation on different HLA molecules point to a possible hapten mechanism. Flucloxacillin, on the other hand, was shown in a labile manner in individuals who tested positive for HLAB*57:01; this was independent of proteasomal processing and immediate T-cell clone activation, indicating a pi-based stimulation of T cells that is specific to this HLA haplotype (Wuillemin et al., 2013).

The hepatotoxicity seen in people with the susceptible haplotype may be caused by this p-i type interaction; however, it is crucial to remember that these studies were conducted in healthy volunteers and have not yet been replicated in patients with flucloxacillin DILI. Abacavir IDILI and carbamazepine-induced SJS have both been linked to direct drug presentation to an HLA (Wei et al., 2012; Ostrov et al.,2012). The nucleoside analog abacavir, which is used as an antiviral treatment for

HIV, causes immunological-mediated drug-induced lymphopenia (IDILI), which has also been limited to HLAB*57:01 (Hackett & Dairkee, 1991; Rauch et al., 2006). Abacavir can bind the F pocket of HLAB*57:01 thereby altering the repertoire of self-peptide ligands that are bound and presented (Ostrov et al., 2012). This model has been dubbed, the altered peptide repertoire model and suggests that small molecules can noncovalently occupy the sites of peptide binding grooves of MHC proteins leading to an alteration of the specificities of the MHC-peptide binding and resulting in erroneous presentation of self-peptides that are different to those normally recognized by that MHC (Bharadwaj et al., 2012; Illing et al., 2012). This is proposed to be the central mechanism of abacavir hypersensitivity, as normally tolerated peptides appear to become immunogenic in the presence of abacavir binding to HLAB*57:01 (Illing et al., 2012). This may account for IDILI seen with many small molecules capable of fitting in the MHC groove, though further studies are needed.

5.7. Defective Adaptation

Immune tolerance to dietary and exogenous antigens is induced in large part by the liver microenvironment. Diversion of portal flow from the liver eliminates the protective effect of portal administration of 1-chloro 2,4-dinitrobenzene before cutaneous injection, suggesting that the liver plays a role in immune processing of antigens and in promoting both systemic and local immune tolerance (Dumont & Cantor, 1967; Callery et al., , 1989). One key characteristic of idiosyncratic DILI is that minor injuries (e.g., ALT < 3 upper limit of normal) is far more common than severe injury (Hy's law & ALF), and mild injury typically goes away even when the medication is continued. Known as clinical adaptation, this phenomenon should not be confused with other types of biochemical adaptive responses (e.g., cellular stress responses, such as the activation of the mitogen activated protein kinase pathway, ER and mitochondrial unfolded protein responses (Dara et al., 2015).

The idiosyncratic nature of the injury has made it irreproducible, which has hindered the discovery of IDILI's mechanistic pathways. Recently, by modifying immune tolerance pathways, two separate labs were able to effectively create animal models of IDILI (Chakraborty et al., 2015; Metushi et al., 2015). Casitas Blineage lymphoma (Cbl-b1) is an E3 ubiquitin ligase and a central player in the immune-checkpoint. Cbl-b1 is expressed in all leukocytes and regulates immune activation in T cells, B cells, NK cells, and different myeloid cells (Lutz-Nicoladoni et al., 2015). Cbl-b1 suppresses immune activation through antigen or pattern recognition molecules and induces a state of immune tolerance. Using mice deficient in Cbl-b1 or programmed cell death protein 1 (PD-1) a.k.a. CD 279, another immune checkpoint protein that prevents T-cell activation and promotes self-tolerance, Metushi et al., (2015) were able to induce an IDILI-like type of injury with the drug. Mice knockout for either Cbl-b1 or PD-1 knockout mice exhibited liver injury with amodiaquine greater than that of wild-type mice. Interestingly, despite the initial insult, the injury resolved with continuation of amodiaquine suggesting a form of adaptation and dampening of the immune response. The authors hypothesized that other immune checkpoint mechanisms are at play and interference with additional pathways is necessary to circumvent adaptation and induce persistent and more severe toxicity. By blocking cytotoxic T-lymphocyteassociate protein 4 (CTLA4), a key inducer of immune tolerance, using an anti-CTLA4 antibody in PD-1$^{-/-}$ mice prior to amodiaquine they demonstrated a more histologically severe injury with greater ALT elevation, and this did not resolve with continuous exposure to the drug (Dara et al., 2015; Metushi et al., 2015). By depleting $CD8^+$ T cells in this model they were able to prevent the liver injury, indicating that the immune injury was mediated by cytotoxic CD8+ T lymphocytes (Mak and Uetrecht, 2015b; Uetrecht and Kaplowitz, 2015). The same group reproduced similar findings with two common IDILI drugs, INH (antituberculosis) and nevirapine (nonnucleoside reverse transcriptase inhibitor for HIV). In both instances, blocking immune checkpoints with multiple mechanisms by treatment of $PD1^{-/-}$ mice with CTLA4 antibody prior to administration of INH or nevirapine resulted unmasked mild liver injury, whereas administration of the drug alone had no significant effect (Mak & Uetrecht, 2015a).

Since the combination of PD-1 knockout and CTLA4 inhibition was required to overcome or break the immune tolerance, this work illustrates the numerous redundancies built into ensuring an immune-tolerant state in the liver. Even with these models, the injury still resolves. Adaptation may still result from additional immune tolerance-promoting factors. Given that numerous drug, host, and immune factors must coincide for the toxicity event to occur, this may also help to explain why clinically overt IDILI is relatively uncommon (Dara et al., 2015). Amodiaquine, INH, and nevirapine—all of the medications used in these studies—are metabolized to haptens, which covalently bind to liver proteins and appear to trigger an immune response in a way that is HLA unrestricted. However, this immune response is quickly offset by tolerogenic mechanisms, which either limit adaptive immune injury or encourage a "clinical adaptation" in which the injury resolves despite the medication being taken continuously.

Reexposure to halothane in humans frequently results in a drug allergy-induced liver injury that manifests as eosinophilia and rash. Chakraborty et al (2015), investigated the effects of halothane on allergic hepatitis in mice whose immune systems were weakened by the loss of myeloid-derived suppressor cells. To make the mice more sensitive to the drug, halothane was given to them twice, separated by 14 days. Following each dosage, normal mice experienced an acute direct toxicity that quickly subsided (adaptation). The authors targeted these cells to overcome immune tolerance because intraperitoneal halothane induced the infiltration of leukocytes in the liver, a significant proportion of which were CD11b and Gr1high positive and had an immune suppressive effect on T cells ($CD4^+$ and $CD8^+$ in a dose dependent manner) (Chakraborty et al., 2015). Mice were given Gr1 antibody, which led to the depletion of the $CD11b{+}Gr1^{high}$ immune-suppressor cells, in order to investigate the functional significance of these cells. Nine days after the second dose of halothane challenge, this results in worsened liver damage. After the initial episodes of hepatitis resolved, the immune target, the hapten-drug metabolite, continued to exist, which allowed for a rebound in injury when the tolerance was broken. In response to halothane and its metabolite, mice treated with anti-Gr1 displayed increased T-cell response, delayed severe inflammation, and necrosis (Chakraborty et al., 2015). Interestingly, unlike the amodiaquine model (which was $CD8^+$ T cell dependent), in this model the response to halothane was abrogated only by anti-CD4 antibody. In this case, antibody-dependent cytotoxicity was the mechanism responsible for liver damage.

The significance of immune tolerance in guarding against IDILI is deftly illustrated by these two models, which target immune checkpoints and immune modulating and suppressor cells. The liver's ability to withstand immune responses was altered in both animal models to produce an IDILI phenotype, although distinct tolerance pathways were targeted in each study. This also shows that the drugs used in these studies showed different signatures of injury, even though a common concept was manipulated to replicate an IDILI model. For instance, halothane causes eosinophilia, a symptom that amodiaquine DILI does not exhibit. It's interesting to note that depletion of $CD4^+$ T-cells eliminated the toxic phenotype in halothane DILI, while depletion of $CD8^+$ T cells did the same in the amodiaquine model (Dara et al., 2015); Kaplowitz and Uetrecht, 2015). This might be because the pathophysiology of IDILI varies depending on the drug—that is, T-cell cytotoxicity versus antibody dependence. Furthermore, these two different models show that immune tolerance regulation is complex and involves several different pathways. Tolerance is also dynamic in regulating the length of the injury in the amodiaquine and halothane models, its actual occurrence in the INH and nevirapine models, and the severity of the initial injury in the long latency amodiaquine model.

Despite these recent advances in proof of principle for the potential role of immune tolerance, the exact underlying mechanism of defective clinical adaptation even in those individuals with HLA risk and how it results in IDILI remains unknown. However, many interesting associations are apparent, such as the frequency of IDILI with antibiotics (9 out of the top 10 agents causing IDILI in the DILIN database are antimicrobials) (Chalasani et al., 2015). LPS from gut accompanies ingested food antigens and has been shown to have immune-tolerogenic properties. Supporting this hypothesis are observations that mice unresponsive to LPS (C3H/HeJ) lack tolerance to dietary antigens (Kiyono et al., 1982). Low levels of gut derived LPS constantly stimulates immune cells and antigen presenting cells in the liver, in particular Kupffer cells (KC) and sinusoidal endothelial cells (LSECs). This results in the secretion of immune suppressive cytokines such as IL-10, TGF-b, TNF-a, and prostaglandins expressed by either KC or LSECs (constitutively or in response to LPS), leading to downregulation of leukocyte adhesion to LSECs, expansion of regulatory T cells (Tregs), and abrogation of T-cell activation that contributes to the immune-tolerant environment in the liver (Dieter et al., 1987; ; Rieder et al., 1990; Bissell et al., 1995; Knolle et al., 1995, 1999, 1998). Given the evidence for the tolerogenic properties of LPS on antigen presentation and cytokine secretion, it is intriguing to hypothesize that the antibiotic effects on gut microflora and changes in LPS exposure may contribute to defective adaptation (Dara et al., 2015). The changes in gut microbiota may also have effects on the phenotypes and functions of regulatory immune cells in the liver immune system, for example, KC polarization (pro- or antiinflammatory), Treg expansion/frequency, hepatic stellate cells, etc. Furthermore, it is important to point out that the microbiome can influence drug toxicity and the liver not only by the tolerogenic properties of LPS but also by affecting drug metabolism (Clayton et al., 2009).

IDILI has also investigated the function of cytokines in the development of immune tolerance. An important immunomodulatory cytokine, IL-10 prevents T-cell activation that is specific to an antigen. According to Aidal et al., IL-10 polymorphisms have been linked to diclofenac DILI susceptibility. 2004). All patients with DILI in this small cohort receiving diclofenac had positive serum adducts for the medication, and a strong correlation was found in polymorphisms leading to low IL-10 (OR of 2.8), indicating an immune-mediated role for toxicity and bolstering the theory that immunological tolerance loss may be a contributing factor to the disease process (Aithal et al., 2004). Further evidence that IL-10 plays a significant role comes from the Spanish DILIN, which found a link between poor patient outcomes and IL-10 polymorphisms that result in lower IL-10 levels

(Pachkoria et al., 2008). As IL-10 has strong anti-inflammatory properties, it acts directly on macrophages, lowering their levels of IL-8, interferon-g, and IL-12 while also preventing T-cell activation (De Vries, 1995). This results in the induction of immune tolerance. The main effector cytokine through which Tregs inhibit both the innate and adaptive immune responses is IL-10. In certain patients, therefore, decreased, ineffective IL-10 could be a proxy for a state of impaired clinical adaptation. We must underline that while these correlations are interesting and offer hints about the potential involvement of poor adaptation in IDILI, there isn't any concrete evidence linking them to causality.

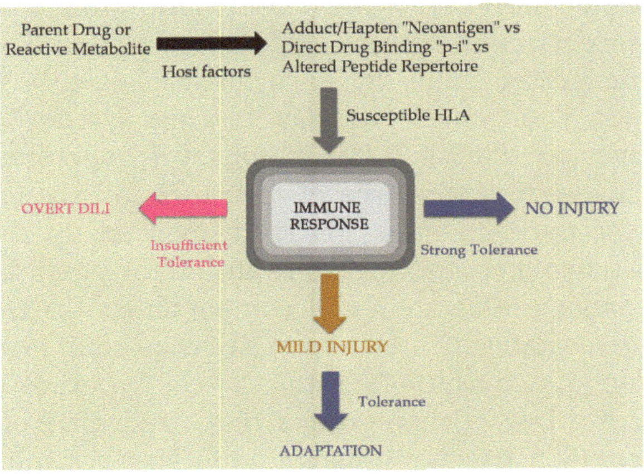

Figure 5.1. *The pathogenesis of idiosyncratic drug-induced liver injury (IDILI): Drugs or their metabolites can activate the adaptive immune system in individuals with susceptible human leukocyte antigen (HLA) haplotypes. Once the immune system is activated the majority of patients with the susceptible HLA will exhibit no injury due to strong tolerance and a minority will develop mild injury followed by adaptation with continuation of the drug. A minority of the susceptible individuals (less than 10%) will develop clinically significant and overt DILI.*

Sourc:. L. Dara, et al., Pathogenesis of Idiosyncratic Drug-induced Liver Injury, http://dx.doi.org/10.1016/B978-0-12-804274-8.00005-9 C.

IDILI is an uncommon disorder for which there is no single known cause. Instead, IDILI is the outcome of a complicated interaction between the host's immune system and substances that may be immunogenic.

A "threshold exposure level" that is dictated by the drug's dosage, lipophilicity, and host's metabolic capacity must be exceeded for the drug exposure to occur. A toxic and electrophilic drug metabolite may be exposed to a sufficient degree by a host due to factors like age, gender, or polymorphisms in phase I detoxifying enzymes or drug transporters, which can trigger an immune response (Figure 5.1).

Hepatocytes exposed to parent drugs or reactive metabolites may trigger a range of stress responses and adaptive mechanisms. These responses may alter the susceptibility of hepatocytes to immune-mediated apoptosis or serve as danger signals for the innate and adaptive immune systems. On the other hand, the majority of patients exposed to these metabolites experience mild abnormalities that are temporary and go away with further exposure (clinical adaptation). When exposed to these extremely immunogenic substances, some people with polymorphisms in their HLA molecules may experience overt clinical IDILI. The hapten/prohapten hypothesis, the pharmacologic interaction hypothesis, and the altered peptide repertoire hypothesis—all of which have been thoroughly covered previously—have been advanced as the three main theories to explain HLA-restricted adaptive immune activation. The majority of people with susceptible HLA genotypes do not develop IDILI when exposed to many drug types that cause IDILI, despite obvious HLA restrictions. This suggests that additional mechanisms in adaptive immunity contribute to mild or severe IDILI. The inability to adapt clinically owing to a malfunctioning immune checkpoint and insufficient immune tolerance could be one such instance. With a wide range of variables that can affect the different outcomes in IDILI, such as no injury, mild injury, very severe injury, or clinical adaptation and its failure, a very complex picture eventually becomes apparent. The infrequency of clinically significant and severe IDILI may be explained by this intricate interaction.

5.8. Liver Regeneration

It is remarkable that the liver can regenerate from a wide range of liver injuries. The concept of liver regeneration dates back several decades, to the myth of Prometheus in classical Greek mythology. Because of its anatomical location and the portal vein that supplies blood derived from the gut that is rich in nutrients, the liver is exposed to a variety of toxic and biologic substances. Moreover, the liver is impacted by genetic and metabolic disorders as well as hepatotropic viruses (Bird et al., 2008). Because of its distinct microstructure and environment, the liver has evolved to meet the demands placed upon it. In fact, compensatory proliferation of liver cells allows restoration of original liver mass in less than 2 weeks when there is a loss of liver mass, for example, after 70% partial tissue removal in mice (Riehle et al.,2011; Kang et al., 2012). The liver's regenerative process is extremely intricate and involves activating various cell types according to the type and severity of the injury, as well as numerous intricate signaling pathways that interact with one another (Fausto et al., 2006; Riehle et al., 2011). After injury, the liver mass is restored primarily by two mechanisms: either transdifferentiation from facultative stem cells, or hepatic progenitor cells (HPCs) (a stem celledependent mechanism), or self-replication of already-existing individual cell types (a stem celleindependent mechanism) (Stanger and Yanger, 2011; Miyajima et al., 2014). The relative importance of the two mechanisms' contributions to liver repopulation has not received enough attention, despite the fact that they are not totally mutually exclusive.

5.8.1. Normal Turnover (Homeostasis) of the Liver

A healthy liver is a dormant organ. This indicates that the mature hepatocytes are not cycling and that their turnover happens gradually over a few months (Fausto et al, 2006; Riehle et al., 2011; Miyajima et al,.2014). Indeed, 200–400 days have been estimated to be the lifespan of hepatocytes (McDonald, 1961). According to the widely held belief, the proliferation of mature hepatocytes sustains liver cell mass in normal, nonpathological circumstances, suggesting that a stem/progenitor cell compartment is not necessary for liver maintenance in these circumstances. However, a potent and unexpected study by Furuyama et al., (2011) used the genetic lineage tracing system. It revealed that CK7-/Sox9$^+$ biliary (progenitor) cells were the source of nutrition for normal liver parenchyma. This study backed up the notion of hepatocyte migration and the potential existence of a stem cell compartment for the homeostatic maintenance of a normal adult liver, also known as the "streaming liver hypothesis" of the liver. Other groups that used different genetic tracing systems found different results, contrary to this study (Carpentier et al, 2011; Malato et al., 2011; Español-Suñer et al., 2012; Yanger et al., 2013) and there was no evidence of a label-negative, nonhepatocytic lineage cell (including biliary epithelial cells) contributing to the parenchyma's upkeep (Malato et al., 2011; Yanger et al., 2013) indicating that the growth of hepatocytes could sustain the mass of liver cells and they could act as real stem cells.

A fascinating new study by Wang et al., cast doubt once more on the idea that the liver cell mass is maintained by the proliferation of the mature hepatocytes already present who discovered a self-renewing axin-2+ (Wnt-responsive gene) cell population in the pericentral region, or zone 3, of the liver of unharmed mice (Wang et al., 2015). These diploid pericentral cells differ from mature hepatocytes, which are primarily polyploid, in that they express the early liver progenitor marker Tbx3. It is noteworthy that these cells have the potential to differentiate into polyploid hepatocytes that are Tbx3-negative and can replenish up to 40% of the liver mass during homeostatic renewal outside of the pericentral zone (Wang et al., 2015).

This study, which looks into chromosome complement, Wang et al., somehow confirms our prior understanding of the "streaming liver hypothesis" while also raising new questions about normal liver turnover, such as how pericentral hepatocytes differ from periportal hepatocytes discovered that the chromosomes of many pericentral hepatocytes are normal. On the other hand, the majority of hepatocytes have multiple copies of every chromosome, which causes chromosomal imbalances during division and renders them unsuitable for liver repopulation (Duncan et al., 2010). Next, given that pericentral hepatocytes are known to divide a little bit more quickly than other hepatocytes under normal circumstances, we can hypothesize that, under normal, nonpathological circumstances, hepatocytes in the central zone are a better candidate for liver regeneration (Magami et al., 2002; Zaret, 2015. Since zone 3 of the hepatic lobule is located far from the portal area, it is a more protected area of the liver and may therefore be a more desirable location for cells involved in normal hepatic aging. Furthermore, according to Zaret (2015) & Wang et al., (2015), these hepatocytes are the only ones affected by Wnt signals that are generated by the endothelial cells lining the central vein. When combined, these findings demonstrate that pericentral hepatocytes—which are descended from diploid Axin2+ cells that can self-renew—have the ability to behave like true stem cells when they are in a niche that is close by. In this way, there is currently disagreement over the relative roles played by various epithelial cells in maintaining normal liver homeostasis.

5.8.2. Liver Regeneration After Partial Hepatectomy

Because there is no necrosis, which results in the infiltration of macrophages and other cells and complicates the analysis of the biochemistry of the regenerative process, and because the remaining liver is undamaged, the partial hepatectomy (PH) model offers an excellent opportunity to study the proliferative capability of the existing normal hepatocytes physiologically. Following PH, quiescent hepatocytes replace the removed portion of the liver by entering the cell cycle. The remaining hepatocytes replicate in tightly synchronized rounds to restore the original hepatic mass in approximately 6–8 weeks in humans. Fine pieces by Weglarz and colleagues demonstrated the cell-autonomous timing of the hepatocytes' entry into DNA synthesis. When mouse hepatocytes were transplanted into a rat liver along with two-thirds PH, researchers discovered that although both transplanted and surrounding rat hepatocytes divided at the same time—24 hours—the transplanted mouse hepatocytes divided a little later (at 40 h) than the surrounding rat hepatocytes . As the authors (Weglarz & Sandgren, 2000) concluded, these observations demonstrate that factors intrinsic to the hepatocyte must regulate the timing of entry into DNA synthesis and suggest that locally or distantly produced cytokines or growth factors may have a permissive but not an instructive role in progression to S phase (DNA synthesis). Furthermore, with respect to the time course of proliferating hepatocytes in different zones, labeling studies have been observed three peeks of DNA synthesis after PH initiating in zone 1 and propagating to zone 2 and 3, respectively (Wu et al., 2011). Although cholangiocytes start to proliferate almost as early as hepatocytes, nonparenchymal cells initiate DNA synthesis a few hours behind of that for hepatocytes with Kupffer cells and stellate cells first (peaking at 48–72 h in rat) and sinusoidal endothelial cells (SECs) later (peaking at 96 h in rat) (Riehle et al., 2011; Kang et al., 2012). Age is also an important determinant of both timing and the magnitude of the response; in older animals the process is longer and more protracted and the number of proliferating hepatocyte is decreased.

After photoaging, the most significant pathway for regeneration is thought to be stem cell-independent self-replication of the various cell types that are already present. Despite this, recent research has suggested that HPCs may play a role in liver regeneration following PH. According to recent research by Diehl's group, PH causes wild-type (WT) mice's livers to accumulate fibroblast growth factor (FGF)-inducible 14 (Fn14) cells. Loss of Fn14 signaling also led to liver failure and impaired proper liver regeneration after PH, indicating that Fn14+ progenitors are necessary for liver regeneration after PH (Karaca et al., 2014). To solve this problem, more research employing lineage tracing techniques (genetically labeling Fn14+ cells and tracking their post-PH fate) is required.

5.8.3. Molecular Mechanisms of Liver Regeneration After Partial Hepatectomy

During a PH event, multiple growth, metabolic, and cytokine factors regulate the regenerating liver simultaneously. Tumor necrosis factor-alpha (TNF-a) and interleukin (IL)-6, which are produced by Kupffer cells and stellate cells in response to innate immunity components C3a, C5a, and gut-derived lipopolysaccharide, prime hepatocytes to respond to growth factors such as epidermal growth factor (EGF) and hepatocyte growth factor (HGF). There are only two known "complete mitogens" for hepatocytes: EGFR ligands and HGF. To activate the tyrosine receptor kinase MET, HGF binds to its multifunctional receptor. HGF acts on hepatocytes in a biphasic endocrine and paracrine manner following PH (Figure 5.2).

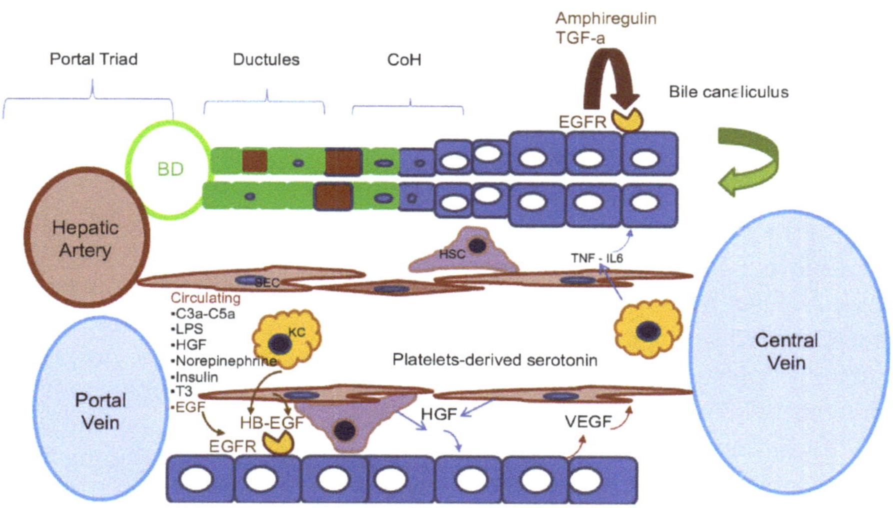

Figure 5.2. *Cells and signals regulating liver regeneration.*

Source: https://www.sciencedirect.com/science/article/abs/pii/B9780128042748000072

Matrix, the endocrine action of HGF, is thought to be the source of the first round of HGF/MET signaling. After HGF's paracrine action on hepatocytes, stellate cells and endothelial cells generate new HGF (Kang et al., 2012). Ligands for the EGFR that are critical for survival following PH include: (1) heparin-binding EGF-like growth factor (HB-EGF), which is produced by Kupffer cells and SECs and acts in an autocrine manner to promote hepatocyte proliferation; and (2) amphiregulin and transforming growth factor-alpha (TGF-a), which are produced by hepatocytes (Kiso et al., , 1995) (paracrine manner); and (3) EGF, which is secreted by the duodenum's Brunner's glands and salivary glands (Olsen et al., 1988) in an endocrine way. Additional auxiliary mitogens consist of insulin, bile acids, serotonin, leptin, estrogens, triodothronine, FGF1 and 2, Notch and jagged, platelet-derived growth factor, vascular endothelial growth factor, and norepinephrine (Mao et al., 2014). Combination signals from the aforementioned elements cause the cell cycle progression of hepatocytes, which in turn triggers DNA synthesis and, as was previously stated, hepatocyte proliferation.

Analyzing mouse liver after 70% PH, Ochoa et al., (2010) demonstrated that PH could induce the production of Hedgehog (Hh) ligands and activate Hh signaling in liver cells. Both hepatocytes and bile ductular cells expressed Hh-target genes, and inhibition of Hh signaling by cyclopamine caused significant inhibition of cell proliferation at 48 h postoperation and 98% mortality during the first 3 days after PH, despite no difference in liver histology and serum aminotransferases levels in surviving cyclopamine-treated mice and controls, suggesting that Hh activation is critical for liver regeneration after PH. Furthermore, adding cyclopamine to cultures of regenerating hepatocytes from 24 to 48 h post-PH resulted in reduced Hh signaling and hepatocyte proliferation. Considering the fact that mature hepatocytes are not responsive to Hh, these observations are somehow surprising and further work is needed to elucidate the mechanisms behind these results. Anyway, one potential explanation could be the involvement of HPCs in regeneration after PH and their response to Hh ligands. This is supported by the observation that expression of various progenitor markers, such as AFP, Fn14, and keratin (K)19 was increased following PH and that inhibiting Hh signaling by cyclopamine also reduced mRNA and/or protein expression of those progenitor markers (Ochoa et al., 2010). As previously mentioned, Diehl's group has also shown that liver regeneration also depends upon Fn14+ progenitors after PH (Karaca et al., 2014)

5.8.4. Liver Regeneration After Different Models of Hepatic Injury

Hepatocytes play a role in liver regeneration following mild to moderate liver damage. Although there is some degree of uncertainty regarding the clinical significance of this regenerative pathway in cases of acute or chronic liver failure, stem cell-dependent mechanisms of liver regeneration will account for the repopulation of the damaged liver when the regenerative capability of the existing mature hepatocytes is compromised, for example, in different models of moderate to severe acute and chronic (toxic) liver damage. Although it is widely acknowledged that ductular reactions (DRs) are the mechanism underlying this form of liver regeneration, there is still debate regarding the cell types and their source in histologically observed DRs. In fact, the damaged liver appears to be very malleable in terms of the cell of origin for regeneration, and various cell types can act as HPCs to mediate DRs and repopulate the liver based on the species, type, nature, and degree of the damage. This will enable the interpretation of numerous contradictory reports about the source of the repopulating HPCs (Hindley et al., 2014).

5.8.5. Nomenclature and Niche of Hepatic Progenitor Cells

In the healthy human liver, HPCs, also known as "oval cells" in rodents, are found in the bile ductules and the canals of Hering (CoH), which are situated in the periportal parenchyma and the portal tract (Roskams et al., 2004). These cells are also known as "ductular hepatocytes," "intermediate hepatobiliary cells," and "atypical ductular reactive cells." They express markers belonging to the hepatocyte lineage (K8, K18, C-met, and albumin) as well as the biliary epithelial cell lineage (K7, K19, K14, and A6 [rodents]). They can differentiate into cholangiocytes or hepatocytes, depending on which type of epithelial cell—hepatocyte versus bile duct epithelial cell—is most damaged (Xiao et al., 2003).

Most people agree that oval cells originate from precursors of oval cells in the bile duct epithelium. Label-retaining studies found small label-retaining epithelial cells [5-bromo-20-deoxyuridine (BrdU)] in the portal and periportal areas of mice livers where a sublethal dose of acetaminophen was administered coincident with BrdU provide strong evidence for the existence of the HPCs niche in the portale parenchymal interface (Kuwahara et al., 2008). Lineage-tracing studies in a mouse model of oval cell-mediated liver injury fed a methionine- and choline-deficient diet supplemented with 0.15% methionine have further supported the existence of the HPC niche in the portal-periportal area by demonstrating a continuous cell supply from the Sox9-expressing progenitor zone within the portal area (Furuyama et al., 2011). Furthermore Carpentier et al., (2011) demonstrated quite elegantly that in mouse models of 3,5-diethoxycarbonyl-1,4-dihydro-collidine (DDC) or CDE injury, HPCs originate from the progeny of the ductal plate cells. Recent methods for lineage tracing have produced some contradictory findings, though. On the one hand, biliary cells were the main precursors of DRs in a number of experimental and genetic liver injury models (Jörs et al, 2015) in line with earlier research. However, research has demonstrated that hepatocytes, not cholangiocytes, are the primary source of new ductules generated in response to specific chronic liver damage (DDC diet), which has led to the controversy surrounding the origins of hepatocyte-derived macrophages (HPCs) (Sekiya & Suzuki, 2014). This discussion will be further enriched by the idea of hepatocytes' biliary metaplasia in response to injury (Yanger et al., 2013; Tarlow et al., 2014).

5.8.6. Hepatic Progenitor Cells Activation in Human Liver Diseases

Humans with a wide range of liver diseases, where there is some degree of hepatocyte loss and damage along with poor regeneration of the remaining hepatocytes and/or bile duct epithelial cells, have been found to have proliferation of HPCs (Katoonizadeh et al., 2006, 2010; Fausto et al., 2006); Nobili et al.,; Roskams, 2003. 2012). We have previously demonstrated that extensive HPC activation requires a threshold of 50% loss of hepatocytes, which is associated with a significant decrease in the proliferative activity of the remaining mature hepatocytes (Katoonizadeh et al., 2006). Since surviving patients had significantly less HPC activation and more hepatocyte proliferation than either the transplanted or deceased patients, this activation occurred early in the disease course (within 1 week) and was a sign of severity of acute liver disease (Katoonizadeh et al., 2006), indicating the role that hepatocyte proliferation plays in patient survival. High HPC activation was also noted in patients with decompensated alcoholic cirrhosis; there was no difference in the level of activation between those patients who experienced an acute exacerbation of the underlying cirrhosis and a less favorable prognosis. While the quantity of proliferating hepatocytes was relatively low in both groups, HPCs were similarly highly activated (Katoonizadeh et al., 2010).

5.8.7. Oval Cells/Hepatic Progenitor Cells Contribution to Liver Regeneration

Numerous rodent models of toxic liver damage are linked to a broad accumulation of oval cells and varying degrees of functionality. There is currently debate over these cells' actual role in the recovery of liver mass. Indeed, different groups have found conflicting results using different genetic lineage tracing approaches in a wide range of liver injury models. Suñer Español et al (2012), used transgenic mice with inducible OPN-Cre and HNF1b-Cre to demonstrate a minor (up to 2.5%) oval cell contribution to hepatocytes only in the CDE-induced injury model; this contribution was not seen in the CCL4, DDC, or PH models. Similar results were also obtained by Rodrigo-Torres et al., (2014). Forbes group in an elegant recent study showed that transplantation of CD45-CD31-Ter119-EpCAM+CD24+CD133+ population of HPCs in a AhCre^{+} Mdm2$^{flox/flox}$ adult mouse resulted in hepatocytes and biliary epithelia regeneration, highlighting the in vivo lineage potency for this population of HPCs (Lu et al., 2015).

On the other hand, in various models of liver injury, other groups examined the fate of hepatocytes rather than oval cells using either Mx1-Cre mice or infection by adeno-associated viruses (AAV). They discovered that hepatocytes were the source of newly formed hepatocytes and that oval cells did not contribute to the pool of hepatocytes (Tanimizu et al., 2014; Schaub et al.,2014). Moreover, certain researchers have demonstrated that hepatocytes are capable of transdifferentiating into biliary epithelial cells and then back into hepatocytes (Tarlow et al., 2014; Yanger et al., 2014;Yimlamai et al., 2014). The variations observed among those studies may be partially explained by the utilization of disparate injury models and techniques to track the destiny of distinct cells. For instance, using AAV-based models results in a recombination efficiency that is much higher than regular transgenic lineage tracing (up to 99% versus as low as 7% in Sox9-CreER mouse lines).

Numerous liver diseases have been linked to the proliferation of HPCs. Since it is challenging to use cell tracking techniques to investigate the functional role of those adult putative progenitor cells in humans, the clinical significance of such activation/proliferation to liver repopulation remains unclear. Despite this, there are indications that HPCs may play a part in liver repopulation; however, it is unclear how much. Yoon and companions. (2011) observed a gradual telomere shortening from DRs to epithelial cell adhesion molecule (EpCAM) hepatocytes and to EpCAM hepatocytes in their study on liver biopsies of patients with hepatitis B- and C-induced cirrhosis. This suggests that EpCAM-positive hepatocytes are derived from slow-cycling cells of the DRs, offering direct evidence for a lineage link between HPCs of DRs and mature hepatocytes. Additional indirect evidence of a connection between DRs' HPCs and regenerative nodules in human cirrhosis includes studies that have employed mitochondrial DNA mutations as clonal markers to track cell lineages (Lin et al., 2010). In addition, sequential histological observations of the native liver in patients who underwent auxiliary partial orthotopic liver transplantation for acute liver failure showed full regeneration of the liver from resident HPCs/ductular hepatocytes (Oldhafer et al., 1993; Bismuth et al., 1995; Fujita et al., 2000). Furthermore, three-dimensional reconstruction of CK19 positive DRs in massive necrosis caused by acetaminophen, suggests that these reactions are proliferations of the cells lining the CoH and ductules and some hepatocytes seem to be originated from those cells (Theise et al., 1999). Similar (three dimensional structure) findings were also observed in patients with chronic hepatitis B and C, autoimmune hepatitis, and fatty liver diseases (Falkowski et al., 2003; Clouston et al., 2005; Richardson et al., 2007). Taken together, aforementioned studies show that in severe acute and chronic liver disease, HPCs are capable of producing new hepatocytes, but its significance still needs to be defined.

5.8.8. Signaling Pathways Regulating Hepatic Progenitor Cells Activation and Differentiation

The key factor governing the HPCs' capacity for self-renewal, maintenance, and differentiation appears to be the interaction between various niche components. This interaction, which can decide the fate and differentiation pathways of HPCs, is in some ways characterized by a unique microenvironment developed in response to a particular liver damage. Thus, the kind and severity of liver disease may have an impact on how well HPCs respond to and take part in liver regeneration (Scadden, 2006; Bird et al., 2008). Depending on the type and extent of the injury, various cell types in the injured liver, including cholangiocytes, hepatocytes, hepatic stellate cells (HSCs)/myofibroblasts (MFs), endothelial cells, macrophages, and other inflammatory cells, may interact with HPCs and with one another (Katoonizadeh & Poustchi, 2014; Katoonizadeh et al., 2014). The majority of what we currently know about this topic comes from studying liver injury in animals and seeing oval cell activation and differentiation. According to these models, macrophages and lymphocytes play a crucial role in inducing and starting a regenerative response (Strick-Marchand et al., 2008). The findings that in chronic viral hepatitis, HPCs are encircled by inflammatory infiltrate and that there is a correlation between the activation and localization of HPCs and the degree and location of the inflammatory infiltrate (Libbrecht et al., 2000).

Furthermore, studies have demonstrated a strong correlation between the activation of hepatic progenitor cells (HPCs) and the severity of liver disease in both animals and humans (Roskams et al., 1998; Lowes et al., 1999; Katoonizadeh et al., 2006). This suggests that inflammatory cells, cytokines, growth factors, and chemotactic factors play a crucial role in the expansion of oval cells/HPCs during liver injury. Research has also highlighted the involvement of various proinflammatory cytokines from the TNF superfamily, such as TNF-alpha, IL-6, lymphotoxins, and oncostatin M, in the activation of HPCs (Knight & Yeoh, 2005; Streetz et al., 2003; Fausto et al., 2006; Znoyko et al., 2005). Additionally, regulatory molecules like leukemia inhibitory factor, interferon gamma (IFN-g), chemokine stromal cell-derived factor 1 (SDF-1), TNF-like weak inducer of apoptosis (TWEAK), as well as components of Hh and Wnt signaling pathways, have been identified as key players in this process (Terada et al., 2003; Sicklick et al., 2006; Tirnitz-Parker et al., 2010).

5.8.9. TWEAK/FN14 Signaling

The effects of various TNF family members on HPCs vary (Knight and Yeoh, 2005). TWEAK is a significant member of this family. TWEAK is now regarded as a crucial regulator for HPCs. It has been demonstrated that TWEAK only affects HPCs and not mature hepatocytes, in contrast to the other members of the TNF superfamily (Jakubowski et al., 2005; Kuramitsu et al., 2013). It is mostly produced by macrophages, T lymphocytes, and monocytes. It directly promotes the proliferation of HPCs by binding to its particular receptor, Fn14 (Kuramitsu et al., 2013). The TWEAK receptor

(Fn14) is typically expressed by epithelial and mesenchymal cells. Its expression is relatively low in a healthy liver, but it is overexpressed in many chronic human liver diseases, such as viral hepatitis and (non)alcoholic cirrhosis, as well as in liver injury after DDC treatment or after PH in murine models (Jakubowski et al., 2005; Tirnitz-Parker et al., 2010; Karaca et al., 2015). It has been demonstrated that exogenous TWEAK administration significantly increases the quantity of periportal oval cells (Bird et al., 2013). Furthermore, activation of oval cells was markedly decreased after TWEAK/Fn14 axis inhibition via the use of an anti-TWEAK antibody or Fn14-null mice (Jakubowski et al., 2005), indicating a possible involvement of the TWEAK/Fn14 axis in the proliferation of oval cells and PHCs.

It is also important to take into account the fact that some MFs and activated HSCs express the TWEAK receptor (Kuramitsu et al., 2013), indicating a possible part for TWEAK in the coregulation of liver fibrosis and HPC activation. In fibrotic mice undergoing PH, some groups demonstrated an oval-cell-driven fibrogenic response by using recombinant TWEAK to stimulate oval cell expansion (Kuramitsu et al., 2013). But it's possible that TWEAK influences MFs in a complementary way to induce fibrosis (Chen et al., 2012). According to Novoyatleva et al, there is an elevation of TWEAK and its receptor in tissue injury models that feature fibrosis. 2013, Son and others. 2013, as well as Ucero et al, 2013. TWEAK/Fn14 pathway deficient mice exposed to models of injury and fibrosis demonstrated decreased fibroblast proliferation, a-SMA, collagen gene expression, and extracellular matrix (ECM) deposition in a model of cardiac fibrosis (Novoyatleva et al., 2015). These findings further support the fibrogenic effect of TWEAK. (2013). The interactions between lymphotoxin-b producing HPCs and lymphotoxin-b receptor-expressing HSCs could also be a possibility. These cells can indirectly mediate fibrogenesis by expressing intercellular adhesion molecule 1, also known as CD54, by HSCs and regulated on activation, which is the expression and secreted product of normal T cells and also known as CCL5 (Ruddell et al., 2009).

5.8.10. Fibroblast Growth Factor 7

The family of growth factors known as FGFs has a variety of functions during development and adulthood. They play a variety of biological roles in different organs, such as morphogenesis, angiogenesis, and stem cell system regulation (Turner & Grose, 2010). FGF7, a member of the FGF family, is an essential HPC regulator. In the livers of mouse models and the serum of patients suffering from acute liver failure, its expression was concurrently induced with oval cells/HPCs response (Takase et al., 2013). Since it can cause oval cells and HPCs to activate de novo, it is especially significant. Indeed, hepatic dysfunction was lessened by transgenic expression of FGF7 in vivo, which also induced the development of cells resembling HPCs. When a toxin caused hepatic injury, FGF7-deficient mice showed noticeably reduced HPC expansion and increased mortality (Takase et al., 2013). FGF7-deficient mice did not exhibit HPC activation even after long-term liver injury, in contrast to Fn14-deficient mice (Tirnitz-Parker et al., 2010; Takase et al., 2013), indicating a more direct involvement of FGF7 than Fn14 in the regulation of HPCs.

5.8.11. Stromal-Cell-Derived Factor 1

Additionally, it has been demonstrated that chemokine SDF-1 is upregulated in human chronic liver diseases and oval celle-inducing rodent injury, though there is some debate regarding the cells that produce it (Terada et al., 2003; Mavier et al., 2004, Hatch et al., 2002). It attaches itself to its receptor, CXCR4, and performs a number of functions, one of which is attracting bone marrow (BM) cells to the injured liver. Oval cells were shown to migrate along an SDF-1a gradient in vitro chemotaxis assays. This implies that the SDF-1a/CXCR4 interaction may be a mechanism through which the oval cell compartment is activated, potentially attracting a second wave of stem cells from BM to the injured liver (Hatch et al., 2002). Numerous cell types, such as inflammatory cells, bone marrow stem cells (BMSCs), and HPCs, express CXCR4 (Hatch et al., 2002; Terada and colleagues (2003); Mavier et al,2004). SDF-1 draws inflammatory cells that express TWEAK and are $CXCR4^+$ (Ginès et al., 2011; Hatch et al., 2002).

5.8.12. Hedgehog Signaling

Because it can influence stem cell behavior in those responsive tissues, hh signaling plays a role in the proliferation and maintenance of a number of adult tissues. When Hh ligands—the Sonic, Indian, and Desert hedgehogs—bind to their transmembrane receptor patched (PTC), glioblastoma (Gli) family transcription factors are nuclear localized and the signaling pathway is activated. Numerous target genes, including a few that are part of the Hh signaling pathway itself, are activated by nuclear Gli. A growing body of research indicates that Hh signaling inhibits the apoptosis of several types of liver cells, including HSCs and HPCs (Omenetti et al., 2007, 2011; Sicklick et al., 2006). Research has shown that the oval cell compartment expresses both the Hh receptor and Hh ligands concurrently (Sicklick et al., 2006). Furthermore, research on patients with primary biliary cirrhosis (PBC) and alcoholic steatohepatitis has demonstrated that HPCs and the HSCs that surround them can both produce and react to Hh ligands (Jung et al., 2007, 2008), indicating that autocrine and/or paracrine Hh signaling is responsible for oval cells'/HPCs' lifelong viability. In fact, as mature hepatocytes die, they release Hh ligands that stimulate the growth of progenitors and MFs as a means of retaliation (Jung et al., 2010) because HPCs are Hh-responsive cells, which allows them to live in an environment rich in Hh ligands, in contrast to mature hepatocytes (Sicklick et al., 2006). In this sense, progenitor cells and dying hepatocytes are linked by the Hh pathway (Jung et al., 2010). The same as fibrogenic effect of TWEAK, the Hh ligands can also stimulate epithelial to mesenchymal transition in cells of DRs (Omenetti et al., 2008), which together with the Hh-dependent induction of MFs genes and its consequent enhancement of the proliferative activity of MF-HSCs (Sicklick et al., 2005) will result in promotion of hepatic fibrosis, a phenomenon which is accompanied by different types of chronic liver injury.

5.8.13. WNT and Notch Signaling

In many organs, the Wnt and Notch signaling pathways play a crucial role in regulating stem cell maintenance and differentiation. In various liver injury models where oval cells and HPC proliferation have been observed, expression of multiple Wnt/Notch family genes has been discovered (Apte et al., 2008; Yang et al., 2008; Spee et al., 2010; Boulter et al., 2012), suggesting the involvement of those pathways in oval cells/HPCs proliferation.

The Wnt/beta-catenin signaling pathway may have a major role in the expansion of HPCs in both hepatocytic (hepatitis C cirrhosis) and cholangiocytic (PBC) human liver diseases, according to our previous study that examined the gene expression of laser microdissected HPCs and their niche in these conditions. The results showed high expression of Wnt components in both hepatitis C-induced cirrhosis and PBC. Unlike parenchymal diseases, HPCs in PBC exhibited a high level of Notch signaling activation, suggesting that the Notch signaling pathway is involved in the HPCs' decision to belong to the cholangiocytic lineage (congruent with findings from animal experiments). In order to identify contributing cell types and to better explore the mechanism underlying

Notch inhibition in hepatocytic diseases, Boulter et al., (2012) discovered that proper delineation of bipotential HPCs fate (hepatocellular versus biliary) depends on injury-specific HPCs niche changes. Periportal a-SMAepositive MFs that express Jagged-1 and produce collagen matrix are more prevalent in human biliary liver damage, which is commonly seen in PBC and primary sclerosing cholangitis. When mouse and human biliary liver diseases occur, oval cells/HPCs express the receptors Notch-1 or Notch-2, respectively, which are triggered by their interaction with the ligand Jagged-1 (Boulter et al., 2012; Spee et al., 2010) (Figure 5.3).

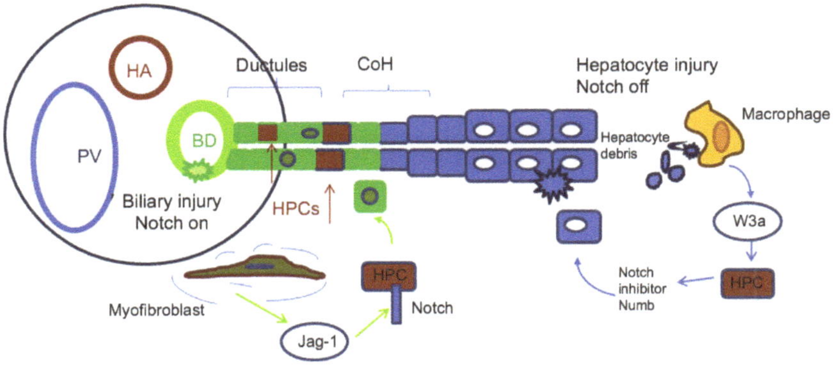

Figure 5.3. *Cartoon showing how hepatic progenitor cells (HPCs), located in the Canals of Hering (CoH) and bile ductules, supply different lineage cells depending on the type of liver damage.*

Source: L. A. Katoonizadeh, Liver Regeneration, http://dx.doi.org/10.1016/B978-0-12-804274-8.00007-2.

The Notch-signaling pathway is triggered by Notch/Jagged interactions, which results in the downstream expression of Notch target genes. Nonetheless, during the hepatocytic differentiation of HPCs, the Notch pathway is severely inhibited. There is an increase in infiltrating macrophages in the periportal areas of parenchymal (hepatocytic) diseases in both humans and rodents (Lorenzini et al., 2010; Spee et al., 2010; Boulter et al., 2012). In reaction to the phagocytosis of apoptotic hepatocytes and other biological debris, macrophages express Wnt3a. Macrophages secreting Wnt3a cause surrounding oval cells to express Numb, an inhibitor of the Notch pathway that is activated by b-catenin and suppresses the transcription of Notch target genes, thereby inhibiting biliary differentiation (Boulter et al., 2012). Intestinal stem cells have also been shown to exhibit this cross-talk between Notch and Wnt in the fate determination of stem/progenitor cells. Tian et al, (2015) showed that derepression of the Wnt signaling pathway caused by Notch blockade disrupts the function of intestinal stem cells. Remarkably, Zhu et al, (2014) demonstrated that Notch blockade is essential for determining the fate of hepatocytic cells by improving hepatocytic differentiation of induced multipotent progenitor cells at the expense of biliary differentiation.

5.8.14. Contribution of Bone Marrow Cells to Liver Regeneration

Because of their potential for great plasticity, BMSCs can differentiate into a variety of cell types, including cells that resemble hepatocytes. BM's role in liver regeneration has been documented by numerous researchers. It has been demonstrated that BMSCs can mobilize into the liver following liver damage in both humans and rodents (Fujii et al., 2002; Zocco et al., 2011).

The primary function of BM-derived cells is to support the liver's nonparenchymal cells that are regenerating; they appear to have little effect on the regeneration of epithelial cells. Fujii et al., In their study, lethally irradiated mice were engrafted with bone marrow cells from a transgenic donor that expressed green fluorescent protein (GFP) in combination with PH four weeks later. The results revealed that nearly 12% of the nonparenchymal cells were GFP-positive, of which 70% were endothelial cells and 30% were Kupffer cells. Regenerating livers did not contain GFP-expressing hepatocytes or cholangiocytes (Fujii et al., 2002).

BMSCs being the origin of at least a proportion of liver sinusoidal endothelial cells (LSECs) were also shown by other studies. These newly BM-derived endothelial cells produce a variety of growth factors such as HGF, EGF, and TGF-a, all of which promote liver regeneration (Taniguchi et al., 2006). Contribution of BMderived LSECs to liver regeneration after PH in rats is even more than resident LSECs because they are a major source of newly synthesized HGF (Wang et al., 2012). In addition to endothelial cells, a proportion of hepatic Kupffer cells and HSCs/MFs are BM-derived (Abe et al., 2003; Forbes et al., 2004; Russo et al., 2006; Higashiyama et al., 2007), suggesting the implication of BM cells in hepatic inflammation, regeneration, fibrosis, and ECM remodeling. Cell fusion does not seem to be the mechanism by which this contribution to the regeneration of nonparenchymal liver cells occurs. Using various animal models of liver injury, several groups have looked into the potential of transplanted BM stem cells to repopulate the liver (directly through transdifferentiation to hepatocytes, or indirectly through the production of oval cells) (Petersen et al., 1999; Alison et al., 2000; Wagers et al., 2002; Vassilopoulos et al., 2003; Christ & Dollinger, 2011). When combined, these studies' findings show that the rate of newly stem cell-derived hepatocytes is extremely low, and it is unclear what the biologic relevance of these cells is in the absence of a selective growth advantage for stem cells—which has only been seen in fumarylacetoacetate hydrolase-deficient mice (FAH-/- mice) thus far. Furthermore, distinct results can be seen in terms of the quantity and mode of newly generated hepatocytes, contingent upon the origin and phenotype of the isolated/transplanted stem cellerich populations as well as the model and species of liver injury. Specifically, in the injured liver, BM mesenchymal stem cells do not contribute significantly to the growth of new hepatocytes. On the other hand, by secreting a variety of chemokines, cytokines, and growth factors that have trophic and/or paracrine effects, such as stimulation of revascularization and regeneration of endogenous parenchymal cells, the transplantation of BM mesenchymal stem cells somehow encourages the recipient's liver to heal itself (Caplan & Dennis, 2006; Parekkadan et al., 2007a,b).

In humans, although donor-derived hepatocytes have been observed in archival liver biopsies (Kleeberger et al., 2002), the lack of molecular data has made it difficult to find the mechanism regulating their hepatocytic differentiation from BMSCs, if any (Wu et al., 2003), and therefore, their biological and clinical relevance still remain to be clarified.

A Closer Look

The Spectrum of Drug-Induced Liver Injury

Drug-induced liver injury (DILI) represents a significant clinical challenge due to its complex and often unpredictable nature, encompassing a wide spectrum of liver damage caused by pharmaceutical agents. DILI can manifest in various forms, ranging from mild, transient elevations in liver enzymes to severe liver failure requiring transplantation. The pathogenesis of DILI is multifactorial, involving direct hepatotoxic effects, immune-mediated mechanisms, and idiosyncratic reactions that are not dose-dependent and often difficult to predict. Commonly implicated drugs include acetaminophen, antibiotics (such as amoxicillin-clavulanate), antiepileptics, and nonsteroidal anti-inflammatory drugs (NSAIDs), each contributing to the spectrum of liver injury through different mechanisms.

Acetaminophen, for instance, is notorious for its dose-dependent hepatotoxicity, primarily when taken in overdose. It leads to the formation of a toxic metabolite, N-acetyl-p-benzoquinone imine (NAPQI), which depletes glutathione and causes oxidative stress and cellular damage in the liver. This type of injury is characterized by centrilobular necrosis and can rapidly progress to acute liver failure if not promptly managed. In contrast, idiosyncratic DILI, often seen with antibiotics and antiepileptics, occurs unpredictably and is not related to the drug dose. The mechanisms are varied, involving immune-mediated responses or metabolic idiosyncrasies that trigger hepatocyte injury or cholestasis.

Clinically, DILI presents with a wide range of symptoms, from asymptomatic elevations in liver enzymes detected incidentally to severe jaundice, coagulopathy, and hepatic encephalopathy. The diagnostic approach to DILI involves a thorough patient history, including detailed medication use, exclusion of other causes of liver disease, and assessment of the pattern of liver enzyme abnormalities. Hepatocellular injury is indicated by elevated alanine aminotransferase (ALT) levels, cholestatic injury by elevated alkaline phosphatase (ALP) levels, and mixed patterns by increases in both enzymes. The Roussel Uclaf Causality Assessment Method (RUCAM) is a commonly used tool to assess the likelihood of DILI, considering factors such as the timing of drug intake, exclusion of other causes, and the course of liver injury upon drug withdrawal or re-administration.

Management of DILI primarily involves discontinuing the offending drug and providing supportive care. In cases of acetaminophen toxicity, N-acetylcysteine (NAC) is the antidote of choice, offering significant benefits when administered early. For other types of DILI, treatment is largely supportive, focusing on monitoring liver function and managing complications. In severe cases, particularly with fulminant liver failure, liver transplantation may be necessary. Preventive strategies emphasize cautious prescribing practices, routine monitoring of liver function tests in high-risk drugs, and patient education regarding the signs and symptoms of liver injury.

Research into DILI is ongoing, with efforts to identify genetic and environmental risk factors that predispose individuals to this condition. Pharmacogenomics holds promise in predicting susceptibility to DILI by identifying genetic variants associated with drug metabolism and immune responses. Additionally, advancements in biomarker discovery aim to improve the early detection and differentiation of DILI from other liver diseases. Understanding the spectrum of DILI, its mechanisms, clinical presentation, and management strategies is crucial for minimizing its impact and improving patient outcomes.

Summary

- Drug-induced liver injury (DILI) and herbal-induced liver injury (HILI) are well-recognized and symptomatically can mimic both acute and chronic liver diseases.
- The chance of developing drug-induced liver injury increases with age. We don't know exactly why this happens. It could be because of changes in your body as you get older. Or because older people tend to take more medicines and so there is more chance that one of those medicines will cause a problem.
- Drug-induced liver injury with predominant elevations in aminotransferase levels (hepatocellular pattern) in those who develop jaundice has a mortality of approximately 10% (Hy's law).
- N-Acetylcysteine should be considered for patients with nonacetaminophen drug-induced acute liver failure because it has been shown to improve transplant-free mortality in a randomized controlled trial.
- DILI is a broad term applied to any injury to the liver by prescribed medication, over-the-counter medication, herb, or dietary supplement manifesting as a spectrum from asymptomatic liver test elevations to ALF.
- Genetic variations have been explored as possible risk factors for DILI. An impressive number of amoxicillin/clavulanate DILI cases (n=201) were subjected to a genomewide associated study that demonstrated that human leukocyte antigen (HLA)-I and HLA-II genotypes conferred susceptibility.
- The epidemiology of idiosyncratic DILI has become clearer with the addition of the Iceland study, demonstrating a crude annual incidence of 19 per 100,000 inhabitants. Idiosyncratic DILI is a serious problem, accounting for approximately 10% of the ALF cases in the United States.
- Liver regeneration is the process by which the liver is able to replace damaged or lost liver tissue. The liver is the only visceral organ with the capacity to regenerate. The liver can regenerate after partial hepatectomy or injury due to hepatotoxic agents such as certain medications, toxins, or chemicals.
- Liver regeneration following partial hepatectomy is a very complex and well-coordinated phenomenon. It involves all types of mature liver cells. The process includes growth factors involved in signaling cascades, cytokines, matrix remodeling, and several feedback reactions of stimulation and inhibition of growth-related signals.
- The liver is a critical organ that is responsible for many different homeostatic functions that help support metabolism, immunity, digestion, detoxification, and carbohydrates and vitamin storage. The detoxification function of the liver exposes the organ to many chemicals, which can induce hepatocyte injury and death.

References

1. Abe, S., Lauby, G., Boyer, C., Rennard, S., & Sharp, J. (2003). Transplanted BM and BM side population cells contribute progeny to the lung and liver in irradiated mice. *Cytotherapy, 5*(6), 523–533.
2. Aithal, G. P., Day, C. P., Leathart, J. B., & Daly, A. K. (2000). Relationship of polymorphism in CYP2C9 to genetic susceptibility to diclofenac-induced hepatitis. *Pharmacogenetics, 10*(6), 511–518.
3. Aithal, G. P., Ramsay, L., Daly, A. K., Sonchit, N., Leathart, J. B., Alexander, G., Kenna, J. G., Caldwell, J., & Day, C. P. (2004). Hepatic adducts, circulating antibodies, and cytokine polymorphisms in patients with diclofenac hepatotoxicity. *Hepatology, 39*(6), 1430–1440.
4. Alison, M. R., Poulsom, R., Jeffery, R., Dhillon, A. P., Quaglia, A., Jacob, J., et al. (2000). Cell differentiation: Hepatocytes from nonhepatic adult stem cells. *Nature, 406*(6791), 257.
5. Andrade, R. J., Lopez-Ortega, S., Lopez-Vega, M. C., Robles, M., Cueto, I., & Lucena, M. I. (2008). Idiosyncratic drug hepatotoxicity: A 2008 update. *Expert Review of Clinical Pharmacology, 1*(2), 261–276.
6. Andrade, R. J., Lucena, M. I., Fernandez, M. C., Pelaez, G., Pachkoria, K., Garcia-Ruiz, E., Garcia-Munoz, B., Gonzalez-Grande, R., Pizarro, A., Duran, J. A., Jimenez, M., Rodrigo, L., Romero-Gomez, M., Navarro, J. M., Planas, R., Costa, J., Borras, A., Soler, A., Salmeron, J., & Spanish Group For The Study Of Drug-Induced Liver, D. (2005). Drug-induced liver injury: An analysis of 461 incidences submitted to the Spanish registry over a 10-year period. *Gastroenterology, 129*(3), 512–521.
7. Andrade, R. J., Lucena, M. I., Kaplowitz, N., Garcia-Munoz, B., Borraz, Y., Pachkoria, K., Garcia-Cortes, M., Fernandez, M. C., Pelaez, G., Rodrigo, L., Duran, J. A., Costa, J., Planas, R., Barriocanal, A., Guarner, C., Romero-Gomez, M., Munoz-Yague, T., Salmeron, J., & Hidalgo, R. (2006). Outcome of acute idiosyncratic drug-induced liver injury: Long-term follow-up in a hepatotoxicity registry. *Hepatology, 44*(6), 1581–1588.
8. Apte, U., Thompson, M. D., Cui, S., Liu, B., Cieply, B., & Monga, S. P. (2008). Wnt/β-catenin signaling mediates oval cell response in rodents. *Hepatology, 47*(1), 288–295.
9. Bell, L. N., & Chalasani, N. (2009). Epidemiology of idiosyncratic drug-induced liver injury. *Seminars in Liver Disease, 29*(4), 337–347.
10. Bharadwaj, M., Illing, P., Theodossis, A., Purcell, A. W., Rossjohn, J., & Mccluskey, J. (2012). Drug hypersensitivity and human leukocyte antigens of the major histocompatibility complex. *Annual Review of Pharmacology and Toxicology, 52*, 401–431.
11. Bird, T. G., Lorenzini, S., & Forbes, S. J. (2008). Activation of stem cells in hepatic diseases. *Cell and Tissue Research, 331*(2), 283–300.
12. Bird, T. G., Lu, W. Y., Boulter, L., Gordon-Keylock, S., Ridgway, R. A., Williams, M. J., et al. (2013). Bone marrow injection stimulates hepatic ductular reactions in the absence of injury via macrophage-mediated TWEAK signaling. *Proceedings of the National Academy of Sciences USA, 110*(16), 6542–6547.
13. Bismuth, H., Samuel, D., Castaing, D., Adam, R., Saliba, F., Johann, M., et al. (1995). Orthotopic liver transplantation in fulminant and sub fulminant hepatitis. The Paul Brousse experience. *Annals of Surgery, 222*(2), 109–120.

14. Bissell, D. M., Wang, S. S., Jarnagin, W. R., & Roll, F. J. (1995). Cell-specific expression of transforming growth factor-beta in rat liver: Evidence for autocrine regulation of hepatocyte proliferation. *Journal of Clinical Investigation, 96*(1), 447–455.

15. Bjornsson, E. S., Bergmann, O. M., Bjornsson, H. K., Kvaran, R. B., & Olafsson, S. (2013). Incidence, presentation, and outcomes in patients with drug-induced liver injury in the general population of Iceland. *Gastroenterology, 144*(5), 1419–1425, 1425.e1–3; quiz e19–20.

16. Bjornsson, E., & Davidsdottir, L. (2009). The long-term follow-up after idiosyncratic drug-induced liver injury with jaundice. *Journal of Hepatology, 50*(3), 511–517.

17. Bjornsson, E., & Olsson, R. (2005). Outcome and prognostic markers in severe drug-induced liver disease. *Hepatology, 42*(2), 481–489.

18. Bohan, A., & Boyer, J. L. (2002). Mechanisms of hepatic transport of drugs: Implications for cholestatic drug reactions. *Seminars in Liver Disease, 22*(2), 123–136.

19. Bohme, M., Muller, M., Leier, I., Jedlitschky, G., & Keppler, D. (1994). Cholestasis caused by inhibition of the adenosine triphosphate-dependent bile salt transport in rat liver. *Gastroenterology, 107*(1), 255–265.

20. Borst, P., Evers, R., Kool, M., & Wijnholds, J. (2000). A family of drug transporters: The multidrug resistance-associated proteins. *Journal of the National Cancer Institute, 92*(16), 1295–1302.

21. Boulter, L., Govaere, O., Bird, T. G., Radulescu, S., Ramachandran, P., Pellicoro, A., et al. (2012). Macrophage-derived Wnt opposes Notch signaling to specify hepatic progenitor cell fate in chronic liver disease. *Nature Medicine, 18*(3), 572–579.

22. Boyer, J. L. (2013). Bile formation and secretion. *Comprehensive Physiology, 3*(1), 1035–1078.

23. Bramow, S., Ott, P., Thomsen Nielsen, F., Bangert, K., Tygstrup, N., & Dalhoff, K. (2001). Cholestasis and regulation of genes related to drug metabolism and biliary transport in rat liver following treatment with cyclosporine A and sirolimus (Rapamycin). *Pharmacology & Toxicology, 89*(3), 133–139.

24. Brinkmann, U., & Eichelbaum, M. (2001). Polymorphisms in the ABC drug transporter gene MDR1. *Pharmacogenomics Journal, 1*(2), 59–64.

25. Callery, M. P., Kamei, T., & Flye, M. W. (1989). The effect of portacaval shunt on delayed-hypersensitivity responses following antigen feeding. *Journal of Surgical Research, 46*(4), 391–394.

26. Cantor, H. M., & Dumont, A. E. (1967). Hepatic suppression of sensitization to antigen absorbed into the portal system. *Nature, 215*(5096), 744–745.

27. Caplan, A. I., & Dennis, J. E. (2006). Mesenchymal stem cells as trophic mediators. *Journal of Cellular Biochemistry, 98*(5), 1076–1084.

28. Carpentier, R., Suñer, R. E., Van Hul, N., Kopp, J. L., Beaudry, J. B., Cordi, S., et al. (2011). Embryonic ductal plate cells give rise to cholangiocytes, periportal hepatocytes, and adult liver progenitor cells. *Gastroenterology, 141*(4), 1432–1438.e4.

29. Chakraborty, M., Fullerton, A. M., Semple, K., Chea, L. S., Proctor, W. R., Bourdi, M., Kleiner, D. E., Zeng, X., Ryan, P. M., Dagur, P. K., Berkson, J. D., Reilly, T. P., & Pohl, L. R. (2015). Drug-induced allergic hepatitis developed in mice when myeloid-derived suppressor cells were depleted prior to halothane treatment. *Hepatology, 62*(4), 1061–1070.

30. Chalasani, N., Bonkovsky, H. L., Fontana, R., Lee, W., Stolz, A., Talwalkar, J., Reddy, K. R., Watkins, P. B., Navarro, V., Barnhart, H., Gu, J., Serrano, J., & United States Drug-induced Liver Injury Network. (2015). Features and outcomes of 899 patients with drug-induced liver injury: The DILIN prospective study. *Gastroenterology, 148*(1), 1340–1352.e7.

31. Chen, H. N., Wang, D. J., Ren, M. Y., Wang, Q. L., & Sui, S. J. (2012). TWEAK/Fn14 promotes the proliferation and collagen synthesis of rat cardiac fibroblasts via the NF-κB pathway. *Molecular Biology Reports, 39*(8), 8231–8241.

32. Chen, M., Borlak, J., & Tong, W. (2013). High lipophilicity and high daily dose of oral medications are associated with significant risk for drug-induced liver injury. *Hepatology, 58*(2), 388–396.

33. Chen, R., Zhang, Y., Tang, S., Lv, X., Wu, S., Sun, F., Xia, Y., & Zhan, S. Y. (2015). The association between HLA-DQB1 polymorphism and antituberculosis drug-induced liver injury: A case-control study. *Journal of Clinical Pharmacy and Therapeutics, 40*(1), 110–115.

34. Christ, B., & Dollinger, M. M. (2011). The generation of hepatocytes from mesenchymal stem cells and engraftment into the liver. *Current Opinion in Organ Transplantation, 16*(1), 69–75.

35. Clayton, T. A., Baker, D., Lindon, J. C., Everett, J. R., & Nicholson, J. K. (2009). Pharmacometabolomic identification of a significant host-microbiome metabolic interaction affecting human drug metabolism. *Proceedings of the National Academy of Sciences USA, 106*(29), 14728–14733.

36. Clouston, A. D., Powell, E. E., Walsh, M. J., Richardson, M. M., Demetris, A. J., & Jonsson, J. R. (2005). Fibrosis correlates with a ductular reaction in hepatitis C: Roles of impaired replication, progenitor cells, and steatosis. *Hepatology, 41*(4), 809–818.

37. Dairkee, S. H., & Hackett, A. J. (1991). Differential retention of rhodamine 123 by breast carcinoma and normal human mammary tissue. *Breast Cancer Research and Treatment, 18*(1), 57–61.

38. Daly, A. K., Aithal, G. P., Leathart, J. B., Swainsbury, R. A., Dang, T. S., & Day, C. P. (2007). Genetic susceptibility to diclofenac-induced hepatotoxicity: Contribution of UGT2B7, CYP2C8, and ABCC2 genotypes. *Gastroenterology, 132*(1), 272–281.

39. Daly, A. K., Donaldson, P. T., Bhatnagar, P., Shen, Y., Pe'er, I., Floratos, A., Daly, M. J., Goldstein, D. B., John, S., Nelson, M. R., Graham, J., Park, B. K., Dillon, J. F., Bernal, W., Cordell, H. J., Pirmohamed, M., Aithal, G. P., Day, C. P., Study, D., & International Serious Adverse Events Consortium. (2009). HLA-B*5701 genotype is a major determinant of drug-induced liver injury due to flucloxacillin. *Nature Genetics, 41*(7), 816–819.

40. Dara, L., Liu, Z. X., & Kaplowitz, N. (2015). Mechanisms of adaptation and progression in idiosyncratic drug-induced liver injury: Clinical implications. *Liver International, 36*(2), 154–163.

41. Dawson, S., Stahl, S., Paul, N., Barber, J., & Kenna, J. G. (2012). In vitro inhibition of the bile salt export pump correlates with risk of cholestatic drug-induced liver injury in humans. *Drug Metabolism and Disposition, 40*(1), 130–138.

42. De Abajo, F. J., Montero, D., Madurga, M., & Garcia Rodriguez, L. A. (2004). Acute and clinically relevant drug-induced liver injury: A population-based case-control study. *British Journal of Clinical Pharmacology, 58*(1), 71–80.

43. De Vries, J. E. (1995). Immunosuppressive and anti-inflammatory properties of interleukin 10. *Annals of Medicine, 27*(5), 537–541.

44. Dieter, P., Schulze-Specking, A., Karck, U., & Decker, K. (1987). Prostaglandin release but not superoxide production by rat Kupffer cells stimulated in vitro depends on Na^+/H^+ exchange. *European Journal of Biochemistry, 170*(2), 201–206.

45. Duncan, A. W., Taylor, M. H., Hickey, R. D., Newell, A. E. H., Lenzi, M. L., Olson, S. B., et al. (2010). The ploidy conveyor of mature hepatocytes as a source of genetic variation. *Nature, 467*(7312), 707–710.

46. Españole-Suñer, R., Carpentier, R., Van Hul, N., Legry, V., Achouri, Y., Cordi, S., et al. (2012). Liver progenitor cells yield functional hepatocytes in response to chronic liver injury in mice. *Gastroenterology, 143*(6), 1564–1575.e7.

47. Falkowski, O., An, H. J., Ianus, I. A., Chiriboga, L., Yee, H., West, A. B., et al. (2003). Regeneration of hepatocyte 'buds' in cirrhosis from intrabiliary stem cells. *Journal of Hepatology, 39*(3), 357–364.

48. Fattinger, K., Funk, C., Pantze, M., Weber, C., Reichen, J., Stieger, B., & Meier, P. J. (2001). The endothelin antagonist bosentan inhibits the canalicular bile salt export pump: A potential mechanism for hepatic adverse reactions. *Clinical Pharmacology & Therapeutics, 69*(3), 223–231.

49. Faubion, W. A., Guicciardi, M. E., Miyoshi, H., Bronk, S. F., Roberts, P. J., Svingen, P. A., Kaufmann, S. H., & Gores, G. J. (1999). Toxic bile salts induce rodent hepatocyte apoptosis via direct activation of Fas. *Journal of Clinical Investigation, 103*(1), 137–145.

50. Fausto, N., Campbell, J. S., & Riehle, K. J. (2006). Liver regeneration. *Hepatology, 43*(2 Suppl 1), S45–S53.

51. Fontana, R. J. (2014). Pathogenesis of idiosyncratic drug-induced liver injury and clinical perspectives. *Gastroenterology, 146*(5), 914–928.

52. Fontana, R. J., Hayashi, P. H., Barnhart, H., Kleiner, D. E., Reddy, K. R., Chalasani, N., Lee, W. M., Stolz, A., Phillips, T., Serrano, J., & Watkins, P. B. (2015). Persistent liver biochemistry abnormalities are more common in older patients and those with cholestatic drug-induced liver injury. *American Journal of Gastroenterology, 110*(10), 1450–1459.

53. Fontana, R. J., Hayashi, P. H., Gu, J., Reddy, K. R., Barnhart, H., Watkins, P. B., Serrano, J., Lee, W. M., Chalasani, N., Stolz, A., Davern, T., Talwakar, J. A., & Drug-Induced Liver Injury Network. (2014). Idiosyncratic drug-induced liver injury is associated with substantial morbidity and mortality within 6 months from onset. *Gastroenterology, 147*(1), 96–108.e4.

54. Forbes, S. J., Russo, F. P., Rey, V., Burra, P., Rugge, M., Wright, N. A., et al. (2004). A significant proportion of myofibroblasts are of bone marrow origin in human liver fibrosis. *Gastroenterology, 126*(4), 955–963.

55. Fountain, F. F., Tolley, E., Chrisman, C. R., & Self, T. H. (2005). Isoniazid hepatotoxicity associated with treatment of latent tuberculosis infection: A 7-year evaluation from a public health tuberculosis clinic. *Chest, 128*(1), 116–123.

56. Fujii, H., Hirose, T., Oe, S., Yasuchika, K., Azuma, H., Fujikawa, T., et al. (2002). Contribution of bone marrow cells to liver regeneration after partial hepatectomy in mice. *Journal of Hepatology, 36*(5), 653–659.

57. Fujita, M., Furukawa, H., Hattori, M., Todo, S., Ishida, Y., & Nagashima, K. (2000). Sequential observation of liver cell regeneration after massive hepatic necrosis in auxiliary partial orthotopic liver transplantation. *Modern Pathology, 13*(2), 152–157.

58. Funk, C., Pantze, M., Jehle, L., Ponelle, C., Scheuermann, G., Lazendic, M., & Gasser, R. (2001). Troglitazone-induced intrahepatic cholestasis by an interference with the hepatobiliary export of bile acids in male and female rats: Correlation with the gender difference in troglitazone sulfate formation and the inhibition of the canalicular bile salt export pump (Bsep) by troglitazone and troglitazone sulfate. *Toxicology, 167*(2), 83–98.

59. Furuyama, K., Kawaguchi, Y., Akiyama, H., Horiguchi, M., Kodama, S., Kuhara, T., et al. (2011). Continuous cell supply from a Sox9-expressing progenitor zone in adult liver, exocrine pancreas, and intestine. *Nature Genetics, 43*(1), 34–41.

60. Ghabril, M., Fontana, R., Rockey, D., Jiezhun, G., & Chalasani, N. (2013). Drug-induced liver injury caused by intravenously administered medications: The Drug-induced liver injury network experience. *Journal of Clinical Gastroenterology, 47*(6), 553–558.

61. Ginès, P., Kamath, P., & Arroyo, V. (2011). Stem cells and chronic liver failure: Potential new therapeutics. In *Chronic Liver Failure: Mechanisms and Management* (pp. 305–316). Humana Press.

62. Grove, J. I., & Aithal, G. P. (2015). Human leukocyte antigen genetic risk factors of drug-induced liver toxicology. *Expert Opinion on Drug Metabolism & Toxicology, 11*(3), 395–409.

63. Hagenbuch, B., & Stieger, B. (2013). The SLCO (former SLC21) superfamily of transporters. *Molecular Aspects of Medicine, 34*(2), 396–412.

64. Hatch, H. M., Zheng, D., Jorgensen, M. L., & Petersen, B. E. (2002). SDF-1α/CXCR4: A mechanism for hepatic oval cell activation and bone marrow stem cell recruitment to the injured liver of rats. *Cloning and Stem Cells, 4*(4), 339–351.

65. Hautekeete, M. L., Horsmans, Y., Van Waeyenberge, C., Demanet, C., Henrion, J., Verbist, L., Brenard, R., Sempoux, C., Michielsen, P. P., Yap, P. S., Rahier, J., & Geubel, A. P. (1999). HLA association of amoxicillin-clavulanate-induced hepatitis. *Gastroenterology, 117*(5), 1181–1186.

66. Herrlinger, C., & Klotz, U. (2001). Drug metabolism and drug interactions in the elderly. *Best Practice & Research Clinical Gastroenterology, 15*(6), 897–918.

67. Higashiyama, R., Inagaki, Y., Hong, Y. Y., Kushida, M., Nakao, S., Niioka, M., et al. (2007). Bone marrow-derived cells express matrix metalloproteinases and contribute to regression of liver fibrosis in mice. *Hepatology, 45*(1), 213–222.

68. Higuchi, H., Grambihler, A., Canbay, A., Bronk, S. F., & Gores, G. J. (2004). Bile acids up-regulate death receptor 5/TRAIL-receptor 2 expression via a c-Jun N-terminal kinase-dependent pathway involving Sp1. *Journal of Biological Chemistry, 279*(1), 51–60.

69. Hindley, C. J., Mastrogiovanni, G., & Huch, M. (2014). The plastic liver: Differentiated cells, stem cells, every cell? *Journal of Clinical Investigation, 124*(11), 5099–5102.

70. Hirano, H., Kurata, A., Onishi, Y., Sakurai, A., Saito, H., Nakagawa, H., Tarui, S., Kanamori, Y., Kitajima, M., & Ishikawa, T. (2006). High-speed screening and QSAR analysis of human ATP-binding cassette transporter ABCB11 (bile salt export pump) to predict drug-induced intrahepatic cholestasis. *Molecular Pharmaceutics, 3*(2), 252–265.

71. Hirata, K., Takagi, H., Yamamoto, M., Matsumoto, T., Nishiya, T., Mori, K., Shimizu, S., Masumoto, H., & Okutani, Y. (2008). Ticlopidine-induced hepatotoxicity is associated with specific human leukocyte antigen genomic subtypes in Japanese patients: A preliminary case-control study. *Pharmacogenomics Journal, 8*(1), 29–33.

72. Hoofnagle, J. H. (2004). Drug-induced liver injury network (DILIN). *Hepatology, 40*(4), 773.

73. Huang, L., Smit, J. W., Meijer, D. K., & Vore, M. (2000). Mrp2 is essential for estradiol-17β (β-D-glucuronide)-induced cholestasis in rats. *Hepatology, 32*(1), 66–72.

74. Huang, Y. S., Chern, H. D., Su, W. J., Wu, J. C., Chang, S. C., Chiang, C. H., Chang, F. Y., & Lee, S. D. (2003). Cytochrome P450 2E1 genotype and the susceptibility to antituberculosis drug-induced hepatitis. *Hepatology, 37*(4), 924–930.

75. Huang, Y. S., Su, W. J., Huang, Y. H., Chen, C. Y., Chang, F. Y., Lin, H. C., & Lee, S. D. (2007). Genetic polymorphisms of manganese superoxide dismutase, NAD(P)H oxidoreductase, glutathione S-transferase M1 and T1, and the susceptibility to drug-induced liver injury. *Journal of Hepatology, 47*(1), 128–134.

76. Illing, P. T., Vivian, J. P., Dudek, N. L., Kostenko, L., Chen, Z., Bharadwaj, M., Miles, J. J., Kjer-Nielsen, L., Gras, S., Williamson, N. A., Burrows, S. R., Purcell, A. W., Rossjohn, J., & McCluskey, J. (2012). Immune self-reactivity triggered by drug-modified HLA-peptide repertoire. *Nature, 486*(7404), 554–558.

77. Jakubowski, A., Ambrose, C., Parr, M., Lincecum, J. M., Wang, M. Z., Zheng, T. S., et al. (2005). TWEAK induces liver progenitor cell proliferation. *Journal of Clinical Investigation, 115*(9), 2330–2340.

78. Jinjuvadia, K., Kwan, W., & Fontana, R. J. (2007). Searching for a needle in a haystack: Use of ICD-9-CM codes in drug-induced liver injury. *American Journal of Gastroenterology, 102*(11), 2437–2443.

79. Jörs, S., Jeliazkova, P., Ringelhan, M., Thalhammer, J., Dürl, S., Ferrer, J., et al. (2015). Lineage fate of ductular reactions in liver injury and carcinogenesis. *Journal of Clinical Investigation, 125*(6), 2445–2457.

80. Jung, Y., Brown, K. D., Witek, R. P., Omenetti, A., Yang, L., Vandongen, M., et al. (2008). Accumulation of hedgehog-responsive progenitors parallels alcoholic liver disease severity in mice and humans. *Gastroenterology, 134*(6), 1532–1543.

81. Jung, Y., McCall, S. J., Li, Y. X., & Diehl, A. M. (2007). Bile ductules and stromal cells express hedgehog ligands and/or hedgehog target genes in primary biliary cirrhosis. *Hepatology, 45*(5), 1091–1096.

82. Jung, Y., Witek, R. P., Syn, W. K., Choi, S. S., Omenetti, A., Premont, R., et al. (2010). Signals from dying hepatocytes trigger growth of liver progenitors. *Gut, 59*(5), 655–665.

83. Kang, L. I., Mars, W. M., & Michalopoulos, G. K. (2012). Signals and cells involved in regulating liver regeneration. *Cells, 1*(4), 1261–1292.

84. Kaplowitz, N. (2013). Avoiding idiosyncratic DILI: Two is better than one. *Hepatology, 58*(1), 15–17.

85. Karaca, G., Swiderska-Syn, M., Xie, G., Syn, W. K., Krüger, L., Machado, M. V., et al. (2014). TWEAK/Fn14 signaling is required for liver regeneration after partial hepatectomy in mice. *PLoS One, 9*(10), e83987.

86. Karaca, G., Xie, G., Moylan, C., Swiderska-Syn, M., Guy, C. D., Krüger, L., et al. (2015). Role of Fn14 in acute alcoholic steatohepatitis in mice. *American Journal of Physiology - Gastrointestinal and Liver Physiology, 308*(3), G325–G334.

87. Katoonizadeh, A., & Poustchi, H. (2014). Adult hepatic progenitor cell niche: How it affects the progenitor cell fate. *Middle East Journal of Digestive Diseases, 6*(2), 57–64.

88. Katoonizadeh, A., Laleman, W., Verslype, C., Wilmer, A., Maleux, G., Roskams, T., et al. (2010). Early features of acute-on-chronic alcoholic liver failure: A prospective cohort study. *Gut, 59*(11), 1561–1569.

89. Katoonizadeh, A., Nevens, F., Verslype, C., Pirenne, J., & Roskams, T. (2006). Liver regeneration in acute severe liver impairment: A clinicopathological correlation study. *Liver International, 26*(10), 1225–1233.

90. Katoonizadeh, A., Poustchi, H., & Malekzadeh, R. (2014). Hepatic progenitor cells in liver regeneration: Current advances and clinical perspectives. *Liver International, 34*(10), 1464–1472.

91. Kindmark, A., Jawaid, A., Harbron, C. G., Barratt, B. J., Bengtsson, O. F., Andersson, T. B., Carlsson, S., Cederbrant, K. E., Gibson, N. J., Armstrong, M., Lagerstrom-Fermer, M. E., Dellsen, A., Brown, E. M., Thornton, M., Dukes, C., Jenkins, S. C., Firth, M. A., Harrod, G. O., Pinel, T. H., Billing-Clason, S. M., Cardon, L. R., & March, R. E. (2008). Genome-wide pharmacogenetic investigation of a hepatic adverse event without clinical signs of immunopathology suggests an underlying immune pathogenesis. *Pharmacogenomics Journal, 8*(3), 186–195.

92. Kiso, S., Kawata, S., Tamura, S., Higashiyama, S., Ito, N., Tsushima, H., et al. (1995). Role of heparin-binding epidermal growth factor-like growth factor as a hepatotrophic factor in rat liver regeneration after partial hepatectomy. *Hepatology, 22*(5), 1584–1590.

93. Kiyono, H., McGhee, J. R., Wannemuehler, M. J., & Michalek, S. M. (1982). Lack of oral tolerance in C3H/HeJ mice. *Journal of Experimental Medicine, 155*(2), 605–610.

94. Kleeberger, W., Rothämel, T., Glöckner, S., Flemming, P., Lehmann, U., & Kreipe, H. (2002). High frequency of epithelial chimerism in liver transplants demonstrated by microdissection and STR-analysis. *Hepatology, 35*(1), 110–116.

95. Knight, B., & Yeoh, G. C. (2005). TNF/LTa double knockout mice display abnormal inflammatory and regenerative responses to acute and chronic liver injury. *Cell and Tissue Research, 319*(1), 61–70.

96. Knolle, P. A., Germann, T., Treichel, U., Uhrig, A., Schmitt, E., Hegenbarth, S., Lohse, A. W., & Gerken, G. (1999). Endotoxin downregulates T cell activation by antigen-presenting liver sinusoidal endothelial cells. *Journal of Immunology, 162*(3), 1401–1407.

97. Knolle, P. A., Uhrig, A., Protzer, U., Trippler, M., Duchmann, R., Meyer Zum Buschenfelde, K. H., & Gerken, G. (1998). Interleukin-10 expression is autoregulated at the transcriptional level in human and murine Kupffer cells. *Hepatology, 27*(1), 93–99.

98. Knolle, P., Schlaak, J., Uhrig, A., Kempf, P., Meyer Zum Buschenfelde, K. H., & Gerken, G. (1995). Human Kupffer cells secrete IL-10 in response to lipopolysaccharide (LPS) challenge. *Journal of Hepatology, 22*(2), 226–229.

99. Kostrubsky, V. E., Vore, M., Kindt, E., Burleigh, J., Rogers, K., Peter, G., Altrogge, D., & Sinz, M. W. (2001). The effect of troglitazone biliary excretion on metabolite distribution and cholestasis in transporter-deficient rats. *Drug Metabolism and Disposition, 29*(12), 1561–1566.

100. Kuramitsu, K., Sverdlov, D. Y., Liu, S. B., Csizmadia, E., Burkly, L., Schuppan, D., et al. (2013). Failure of fibrotic liver regeneration in mice is linked to a severe fibro genic response driven by hepatic progenitor cell activation. *American Journal of Pathology, 183*(1), 182–194.

101. Kurosaki, M., Takagi, H., & Mori, M. (2000). HLA-A33/B44/DR6 is highly related to intrahepatic cholestasis induced by tiopronin. *Digestive Diseases and Sciences, 45*(6), 1103–1108.

102. Kuwahara, R., Kofman, A. V., Landis, C. S., Swenson, E. S., Barendswaard, E., & Theise, N. D. (2008). The hepatic stem cell niche: Identification by label-retaining cell assay. *Hepatology, 47*(6), 1994–2002.

103. Lang, C., Meier, Y., Stieger, B., Beuers, U., Lang, T., Kerb, R., Kullak-Ublick, G. A., Meier, P. J., & Pauli-Magnus, C. (2007). Mutations and polymorphisms in the bile salt export pump and the multidrug resistance protein 3 associated with drug-induced liver injury. *Pharmacogenetics and Genomics, 17*(1), 47–60.

104. Lang, T., Haberl, M., Jung, D., Drescher, A., Schlagenhaufer, R., Keil, A., Mornhinweg, E., Stieger, B., Kullak-Ublick, G. A., & Kerb, R. (2006). Genetic variability, haplotype structures, and ethnic diversity of hepatic transporters MDR3 (ABCB4) and bile salt export pump (ABCB11). *Drug Metabolism and Disposition, 34*(9), 1582–1599.

105. Larrey, D. (2002). Epidemiology and individual susceptibility to adverse drug reactions affecting the liver. *Seminars in Liver Disease, 22*(2), 145–155.

106. Lee, W. M. (2003). Drug-induced hepatotoxicity. *New England Journal of Medicine, 349*(5), 474–485.

107. Libbrecht, L., Desmet, V., Van Damme, B., & Roskams, T. (2000). Deep intralobular extension of human hepatic 'progenitor cells' correlates with parenchymal inflammation in chronic viral hepatitis: Can 'progenitor cells' migrate? *Journal of Pathology, 192*(3), 373–378.

108. Lin, W. R., Lim, S. N., McDonald, S. A., Graham, T., Wright, V. L., Peplow, C. L., et al. (2010). The histogenesis of regenerative nodules in human liver cirrhosis. *Hepatology, 51*(3), 1017–1026.

109. Liu, Z. X., & Kaplowitz, N. (2002). Immune-mediated drug-induced liver disease. *Clinical Liver Disease, 6*(4), 755–774.

110. Lorenzini, S., Bird, T. G., Boulter, L., Bellamy, C., Samuel, K., Aucott, R., et al. (2010). Characterization of a stereotypical cellular and extracellular adult liver progenitor cell niche in rodents and diseased human liver. *Gut, 59*(5), 645–654.

111. Lowes, K. N., Brennan, B. A., Yeoh, G. C., & Olynyk, J. K. (1999). Oval cell numbers in human chronic liver diseases are directly related to disease severity. *American Journal of Pathology, 154*(2), 537–541.

112. Lu, H., Choudhuri, S., Ogura, K., Csanaky, I. L., Lei, X., Cheng, X., Song, P. Z., & Klaassen, C. D. (2008). Characterization of organic anion transporting polypeptide 1b2-null mice: Essential role in hepatic uptake/toxicity of phalloidin and microcystin-LR. *Toxicological Sciences, 103*(1), 35–45.

113. Lu, W. Y., Bird, T. G., Boulter, L., Tsuchiya, A., Cole, A. M., Hay, T., et al. (2015). Hepatic progenitor cells of biliary origin with liver repopulation capacity. *Nature Cell Biology, 17*(7), 971–983.

114. Lucena, M. I., Andrade, R. J., Fernandez, M. C., Pachkoria, K., Pelaez, G., Duran, J. A., Villar, M., Rodrigo, L., Romero-Gomez, M., Planas, R., Barriocanal, A., Costa, J., Guarner, C., Blanco, S., Navarro, J. M., Pons, F., Castiella, A., Avila, S., & Spanish Group for The Study of Drug-Induced Liver Injury. (2006). Determinants of the clinical expression of amoxicillin-clavulanate hepatotoxicity: A prospective series from Spain. *Hepatology, 44*(4), 850–856.

115. Lucena, M. I., Andrade, R. J., Kaplowitz, N., Garcia-Cortes, M., Fernandez, M. C., Romero-Gomez, M., Bruguera, M., Hallal, H., Robles-Diaz, M., Rodriguez-Gonzalez, J. F., Navarro, J. M., Salmeron, J., Martinez-Odriozola, P., Perez-Alvarez, R., Borraz, Y., Hidalgo, R., & Spanish Group for the Study of Drug-Induced Liver Injury. (2009). Phenotypic characterization of idiosyncratic drug-induced liver injury: The influence of age and sex. *Hepatology, 49*(6), 2001–2009.

116. Lucena, M. I., Andrade, R. J., Martinez, C., Ulzurrun, E., Garcia-Martin, E., Borraz, Y., Fernandez, M. C., Romero-Gomez, M., Castiella, A., Planas, R., Costa, J., Anzola, S., Agundez, J. A., & Spanish Group for the Study of Drug-Induced Liver Injury. (2008). Glutathione S-transferase m1 and t1 null genotypes increase susceptibility to idiosyncratic drug-induced liver injury. *Hepatology, 48*(2), 588–596.

117. Lucena, M. I., Molokhia, M., Shen, Y., Urban, T. J., Aithal, G. P., Andrade, R. J., Day, C. P., Ruiz-Cabello, F., Donaldson, P. T., Stephens, C., Pirmohamed, M., Romero-Gomez, M., Navarro, J. M., Fontana, R. J., Miller, M., Groome, M., Bondon-Guitton, E., Conforti, A., Stricker, B. H., Carvajal, A., Ibanez, L., Yue, Q. Y., Eichelbaum, M., Floratos, A., Pe'er, I., Daly, M. J., Goldstein, D. B., Dillon, J. F., Nelson, M. R., Watkins, P. B., Daly, A. K., Spanish Drug-Induced Liver Injury Network, & Eudragene, Dilin, Diligen, International Study. (2011). Susceptibility to amoxicillin-clavulanate-induced liver injury is influenced by multiple HLA class I and II alleles. *Gastroenterology, 141*(1), 338–347.

118. Luedde, T., Kaplowitz, N., & Schwabe, R. F. (2014). Cell death and cell death responses in liver disease: Mechanisms and clinical relevance. *Gastroenterology, 147*(4), 765–783.e4.

119. Lutz-Nicoladoni, C., Wolf, D., & Sopper, S. (2015). Modulation of immune cell functions by the E3 ligase Cbl-b. *Frontiers in Oncology, 5*, 58.

120. Magami, Y., Azuma, T., Inokuchi, H., Kokuno, S., Moriyasu, F., & Kawai, K. (2002). Cell proliferation and renewal of normal hepatocytes and bile duct cells in adult mouse liver. *Liver, 22*(6), 419–425.

121. Mak, A., & Uetrecht, J. (2015a). The combination of anti-CTLA-4 and PD1−/− mice unmasks the potential of isoniazid and nevirapine to cause liver injury. *Chemical Research in Toxicology, 28*(8), 1567–1573.

122. Mak, A., & Uetrecht, J. (2015b). The role of CD8 T cells in amodiaquine-induced liver injury in PD1−/− mice cotreated with anti-CTLA-4. *Chemical Research in Toxicology, 28*(8), 1567–1573.

123. Malato, Y., Naqvi, S., Schürmann, N., Ng, R., Wang, B., Zape, J., et al. (2011). Fate tracing of mature hepatocytes in mouse liver homeostasis and regeneration. *Journal of Clinical Investigation, 121*(12), 4850–4860.

124. Malhi, H., Guicciardi, M. E., & Gores, G. J. (2010). Hepatocyte death: A clear and present danger. *Physiological Reviews, 90*(4), 1165–1194.

125. Mao, S. A., Glorioso, J. M., & Nyberg, S. L. (2014). Liver regeneration. *Translational Research: The Journal of Laboratory and Clinical Medicine, 163*(5), 352–362.

126. Mavier, P., Martin, N., Couchie, D., Préaux, A. M., Laperche, Y., & Zafrani, E. S. (2004). Expression of stromal cell-derived factor-1 and of its receptor CXCR4 in liver regeneration from oval cells in rat. *American Journal of Pathology, 165*(6), 1969–1977.

127. McDonald, R. (1961). Lifespan of liver cells. *Archives of Internal Medicine, 107*(1), 79–87.

128. Megherbi, R., Kiorpelidou, E., Foster, B., Rowe, C., Naisbitt, D. J., Goldring, C. E., & Park, B. K. (2009). Role of protein haptenation in triggering maturation events in the dendritic cell surrogate cell line THP-1. *Toxicology and Applied Pharmacology, 238*(2), 120–132.

129. Meier, Y., Pauli-Magnus, C., Zanger, U. M., Klein, K., Schaeffeler, E., Nussler, A. K., Nussler, N., Eichelbaum, M., Meier, P. J., & Stieger, B. (2006). Interindividual variability of canalicular ATP-binding-cassette (ABC)-transporter expression in human liver. *Hepatology, 44*(1), 62–74.

130. Metushi, I. G., Hayes, M. A., & Uetrecht, J. (2015). Treatment of PD-1(–/–) mice with amodiaquine and anti-CTLA4 leads to liver injury similar to idiosyncratic liver injury in patients. *Hepatology, 61*(4), 1332–1342.

131. Metushi, I. G., Sanders, C., Acute Liver Study Group, Lee, W. M., & Uetrecht, J. (2014). Detection of anti-isoniazid and anti-cytochrome P450 antibodies in patients with isoniazid-induced liver failure. *Hepatology, 59*(3), 1084–1093.

132. Miyajima, A., Tanaka, M., & Itoh, T. (2014). Stem/progenitor cells in liver development, homeostasis, regeneration, and reprogramming. *Cell Stem Cell, 14*(5), 561–574.

133. Molokhia, M., & McKeigue, P. (2006). EUDRAGENE: European collaboration to establish a case-control DNA collection for studying the genetic basis of adverse drug reactions. *Pharmacogenomics, 7*(4), 633–638.

134. Monshi, M. M., Faulkner, L., Gibson, A., Jenkins, R. E., Farrell, J., Earnshaw, C. J., Alfirevic, A., Cederbrant, K., Daly, A. K., French, N., Pirmohamed, M., Park, B. K., & Naisbitt, D. J. (2013). Human leukocyte antigen (HLA)-B*57:01-restricted activation of drug-specific T cells provides the immunological basis for flucloxacillin-induced liver injury. *Hepatology, 57*(2), 727–739.

135. Musch, E., Eichelbaum, M., Wang, J. K., Von Sassen, W., Castro-Parra, M., & Dengler, H. J. (1982). Incidence of hepatotoxic side effects during antituberculous therapy (INH, RMP, EMB) in relation to the acetylator phenotype. *Klinische Wochenschrift, 60*(9), 513–519.

136. Navarro, V. J., Barnhart, H., Bonkovsky, H. L., Davern, T., Fontana, R. J., Grant, L., Reddy, K. R., Seeff, L. B., Serrano, J., Sherker, A. H., Stolz, A., Talwalkar, J., Vega, M., & Vuppalanchi, R. (2014). Liver injury from herbals and dietary supplements in the US Drug-Induced Liver Injury Network. *Hepatology, 60*(4), 1399–1408.

137. Nobili, V., Carpino, G., Alisi, A., Franchitto, A., Alpini, G., De Vito, R., et al. (2012). Hepatic progenitor cells activation, fibrosis, and adipokines production in pediatric nonalcoholic fatty liver disease. *Hepatology, 56*(5), 2142–2153.

138. Nolan, C. M., Goldberg, S. V., & Buskin, S. E. (1999). Hepatotoxicity associated with isoniazid preventive therapy: A 7-year survey from a public health tuberculosis clinic. *JAMA, 281*(10), 1014–1018.

139. Novoyatleva, T., Schymura, Y., Janssen, W., Strobl, F., Swiercz, J. M., Patra, C., et al. (2013). Deletion of Fn14 receptor protects from right heart fibrosis and dysfunction. *Basic Research in Cardiology, 108*(5), 1–13.

140. O'Donohue, J., Oien, K. A., Donaldson, P., Underhill, J., Clare, M., Macsween, R. N., & Mills, P. R. (2000). Co-amoxiclav jaundice: Clinical and histological features and HLA class II association. *Gut, 47*(5), 717–720.

141. Ochoa, B., Syn, W. K., Delgado, I., Karaca, G. F., Jung, Y., Wang, J., et al. (2010). Hedgehog signaling is critical for normal liver regeneration after partial hepatectomy in mice. *Hepatology, 51*(5), 1712–1723.

142. Oldhafer, K., Gubernatis, G., Schlitt, H. J., Rodeck, B., Böker, K., & Pichlmayr, R. (1993). Auxiliary partial orthotopic liver transplantation for acute liver failure: The Hannover experience. *Clinical Transplants*, 181–187.

143. Olsen, P. S., Boesby, S., Kirkegaard, P., Therkelsen, K., Almdal, T., Poulsen, S. S., et al. (1988). Influence of epidermal growth factor on liver regeneration after partial hepatectomy in rats. *Hepatology, 8*(4), 992–996.

144. Omenetti, A., Choi, S., Michelotti, G., & Diehl, A. M. (2011). Hedgehog signaling in the liver. *Journal of Hepatology, 54*(2), 366–373.

145. Omenetti, A., Porrello, A., Jung, Y., Yang, L., Popov, Y., Choi, S. S., et al. (2008). Hedgehog signaling regulates epithelial-mesenchymal transition during biliary fibrosis in rodents and humans. *Journal of Clinical Investigation, 118*(10), 3331.

146. Omenetti, A., Yang, L., Li, Y. X., McCall, S. J., Jung, Y., Sicklick, J. K., et al. (2007). Hedgehog-mediated mesenchymal-epithelial interactions modulate hepatic response to bile duct ligation. *Laboratory Investigation, 87*(5), 499–514.

147. Ostapowicz, G., Fontana, R. J., Schiodt, F. V., Larson, A., Davern, T. J., Han, S. H., McCashland, T. M., Shakil, A. O., Hay, J. E., Hynan, L., Crippin, J. S., Blei, A. T., Samuel, G., Reisch, J., Lee, W. M., & the U.S. Acute Liver Failure Study Group. (2002). Results of a prospective study of acute liver failure at 17 tertiary care centers in the United States. *Annals of Internal Medicine, 137*(12), 947–954.

148. Ostrov, D. A., Grant, B. J., Pompeu, Y. A., Sidney, J., Harndahl, M., Southwood, S., Oseroff, C., Lu, S., Jakoncic, J., De Oliveira, C. A., Yang, L., Mei, H., Shi, L., Shabanowitz, J., English, A. M., Wriston, A., Lucas, A., Phillips, E., Mallal, S., Grey, H. M., Sette, A., Hunt, D. F., Buus, S., & Peters, B. (2012). Drug hypersensitivity caused by alteration of the MHC-presented self-peptide repertoire. *Proceedings of the National Academy of Sciences U.S.A., 109*(25), 9959–9964.

149. Pachkoria, K., Lucena, M. I., Crespo, E., Ruiz-Cabello, F., López-Ortega, S., Fernández, M. A., Romero-Gómez, M., Madrazo, A., Durán, J. A., De Dios, A. M., Borraz, Y., Navarro, J. M., Andrade, R. J., & the Spanish Group for the Study of Drug-Induced Liver Injury. (2008). Analysis of IL-10, IL-4 and TNF-alpha polymorphisms in drug-induced liver injury (DILI) and its outcome. *Journal of Hepatology, 49*(1), 107–114.

150. Pachkoria, K., Lucena, M. I., Ruiz-Cabello, F., Crespo, E., Cabello, M. R., Andrade, R. J., & the Spanish Group for the Study of Drug-Induced Liver Injury. (2007). Genetic polymorphisms of CYP2C9 and CYP2C19 are not related to drug-induced idiosyncratic liver injury (DILI). *British Journal of Pharmacology, 150*(6), 808–815.

151. Padda, M. S., Sanchez, M., Akhtar, A. J., & Boyer, J. L. (2011). Drug-induced cholestasis. *Hepatology, 53*(4), 1377–1387.

152. Pande, J. N., Singh, S. P., Khilnani, G. C., Khilnani, S., & Tandon, R. K. (1996). Risk factors for hepatotoxicity from antituberculosis drugs: A case-control study. *Thorax, 51*(2), 132–136.

153. Parekkadan, B., Van Poll, D., Megeed, Z., Kobayashi, N., Tilles, A. W., Berthiaume, F., et al. (2007a). Immunomodulation of activated hepatic stellate cells by mesenchymal stem cells. *Biochemical and Biophysical Research Communications, 363*(1), 247–252.

154. Parekkadan, B., Van Poll, D., Suganuma, K., Carter, E. A., Berthiaume, F., Tilles, A. W., et al. (2007b). Mesenchymal stem cell-derived molecules reverse fulminant hepatic failure. *PLoS One, 2*(9), e941.

155. Pauli-Magnus, C., & Meier, P. J. (2006). Hepatobiliary transporters and drug-induced cholestasis. *Hepatology, 44*(4), 778–787.

156. Petersen, B., Bowen, W., Patrene, K., Mars, W., Sullivan, A., Murase, N., et al. (1999). Bone marrow as a potential source of hepatic oval cells. *Science, 284*(5417), 1168–1170.

157. Phillips, E., Bartlett, J. A., Sanne, I., Lederman, M. M., Hinkle, J., Rousseau, F., Dunn, D., Pavlos, R., James, I., Mallal, S. A., & Haas, D. W. (2013). Associations between HLA-DRB1*0102, HLA-B*5801, and hepatotoxicity during initiation of nevirapine-containing regimens in South Africa. *Journal of Acquired Immune Deficiency Syndromes, 62*(1), e55–e57.

158. Pichler, W. J. (2002). Pharmacological interaction of drugs with antigen-specific immune receptors: The p-I concepts. *Current Opinion in Allergy and Clinical Immunology, 2*(4), 301–305.

159. Porceddu, M., Buron, N., Roussel, C., Labbe, G., Fromenty, B., & Borgne-Sanchez, A. (2012). Prediction of liver injury induced by chemicals in humans with a multiparametric assay on isolated mouse liver mitochondria. *Toxicological Sciences, 129*(2), 332–345.

160. Rauch, A., Nolan, D., Martin, A., McKinnon, E., Almeida, C., & Mallal, S. (2006). Prospective genetic screening decreases the incidence of abacavir hypersensitivity reactions in the Western Australian HIV cohort study. *Clinical Infectious Diseases, 43*(1), 99–102.

161. Reuben, A., Koch, D. G., & Lee, W. M. (2010). Drug-induced acute liver failure: Results of a US multicenter, prospective study. *Hepatology, 52*(6), 2065–2076.

162. Richardson, M. M., Jonsson, J. R., Powell, E. E., Brunt, E. M., Neuschwander-Tetri, B. A., Bhathal, P. S., et al. (2007). Progressive fibrosis in nonalcoholic steatohepatitis: Association with altered regeneration and a ductular reaction. *Gastroenterology, 133*(1), 80–90.

163. Rieder, M. J., Shear, N. H., Kanee, A., Tang, B. K., & Spielberg, S. P. (1991). Prominence of slow acetylator phenotype among patients with sulfonamide hypersensitivity reactions. *Clinical Pharmacology & Therapeutics, 49*(1), 13–17.

164. Riehle, K. J., Dan, Y. Y., Campbell, J. S., & Fausto, N. (2011). New concepts in liver regeneration. *Journal of Gastroenterology and Hepatology, 26*(2), 203–212.

165. Rodrigo-Torres, D., Affò, S., Coll, M., Morales-Ibáñez, O., Millán, C., Blaya, D., et al. (2014). The biliary epithelium gives rise to liver progenitor cells. *Hepatology, 60*(4), 1367–1377.

166. Roskams, T. (2003). Progenitor cell involvement in cirrhotic human liver diseases: From controversy to consensus. *Journal of Hepatology, 39*(3), 431–434.

167. Roskams, T. A., Theise, N. D., Balabaud, C., Bhagat, G., Bhathal, P. S., Bioulac-Sage, P., et al. (2004). Nomenclature of the finer branches of the biliary tree: Canals, ductules, and ductular reactions in human livers. *Hepatology, 39*(6), 1739–1745.

168. Roskams, T., De Vos, R., Van Eyken, P., Miyazaki, H., Van Damme, B., & Desmet, V. (1998). Hepatic OV-6 expression in human liver disease and rat experiments: Evidence for hepatic progenitor cells in man. *Journal of Hepatology, 29*(3), 455–463.

169. Ruddell, R. G., Knight, B., Tirnitz-Parker, J. E., Akhurst, B., Summerville, L., Subramaniam, V. N., et al. (2009). Lymphotoxin-b receptor signaling regulates hepatic stellate cell function and wound healing in a murine model of chronic liver injury. *Hepatology, 49*(1), 227–239.

170. Russo, F. P., Alison, M. R., Bigger, B. W., Amofah, E., Florou, A., Amin, F., et al. (2006). The bone marrow functionally contributes to liver fibrosis. *Gastroenterology, 130*(6), 1807–1821.

171. Scadden, D. T. (2006). The stem-cell niche as an entity of action. *Nature, 441*(7097), 1075–1079.

172. Schaub, J. R., Malato, Y., Gormond, C., & Willenbring, H. (2014). Evidence against a stem cell origin of new hepatocytes in a common mouse model of chronic liver injury. *Cell Reports, 8*(4), 933–939.

173. Scordo, M. G., Aklillu, E., Yasar, U., Dahl, M. L., Spina, E., & Ingelman-Sundberg, M. (2001). Genetic polymorphism of cytochrome P450 2C9 in a Caucasian and a Black African population. *British Journal of Clinical Pharmacology, 52*(4), 447–450.

174. Seitz, S., Kretz-Rommel, A., Oude Elferink, R. P., & Boelsterli, U. A. (1998). Selective protein adduct formation of diclofenac glucuronide is critically dependent on the rat canalicular conjugate export pump (Mrp2). *Chemical Research in Toxicology, 11*(5), 513–519.

175. Sekiya, S., & Suzuki, A. (2014). Hepatocytes, rather than cholangiocytes, can be the major source of primitive ductulus in the chronically injured mouse liver. *American Journal of Pathology, 184*(6), 1468–1478.

176. Sgro, C., Clinard, F., Ouazir, K., Chanay, H., Allard, C., Guilleminet, C., Lenoir, C., Lemoine, A., & Hillon, P. (2002). Incidence of drug-induced hepatic injuries: A French population-based study. *Hepatology, 36*(2), 451–455.

177. Sharma, S. K., Balamurugan, A., Saha, P. K., Pandey, R. M., & Mehra, N. K. (2002). Evaluation of clinical and immunogenetic risk factors for the development of hepatotoxicity during antituberculosis treatment. *American Journal of Respiratory and Critical Care Medicine, 166*(7), 916–919.

178. Sicklick, J. K., Li, Y. X., Choi, S. S., Qi, Y., Chen, W., Bustamante, M., et al. (2005). Role for hedgehog signaling in hepatic stellate cell activation and viability. *Laboratory Investigation, 85*(11), 1368–1380.

179. Sicklick, J. K., Li, Y. X., Melhem, A., Schmelzer, E., Zdanowicz, M., Huang, J., et al. (2006). Hedgehog signaling maintains resident hepatic progenitors throughout life. *Journal of Physiology-Gastrointestinal and Liver Physiology, 290*(5), G859–G870.

180. Singer, J. B., Lewitzky, S., Leroy, E., Yang, F., Zhao, X., Klickstein, L., et al. (2010). A genome-wide study identifies HLA alleles associated with lumiracoxib-related liver injury. *Nature Genetics, 42*(8), 711–714.

181. Sodeman, T., Bronk, S. F., Roberts, P. J., Miyoshi, H., & Gores, G. J. (2000). Bile salts mediate hepatocyte apoptosis by increasing cell surface trafficking of Fas. *American Journal of Physiology-Gastrointestinal and Liver Physiology, 278*(6), G992–G999.

182. Son, A., Oshio, T., Kawamura, Y., Hagiwara, T., Yamazaki, M., Inagaki-Ohara, K., et al. (2013). TWEAK/Fn14 pathway promotes a T helper 2-type chronic colitis with fibrosis in mice. *Mucosal Immunology, 6*(6), 1131–1142.

183. Spee, B., Carpino, G., Schotanus, B. A., Katoonizadeh, A., Vander Borght, S., Gaudio, E., et al. (2010). Characterization of the liver progenitor cell niche in liver diseases: Potential involvement of Wnt and Notch signaling. *Gut, 59*(2), 247–257.

184. Spraggs, C. F., Budde, L. R., Briley, L. P., Bing, N., Cox, C. J., King, K. S., Whittaker, J. C., Mooser, V. E., Preston, A. J., Stein, S. H., & Cardon, L. R. (2011). HLA-DQA1*02:01 is a major risk factor for lapatinib-induced hepatotoxicity in women with advanced breast cancer. *Journal of Clinical Oncology, 29*(6), 667–673.

185. Streetz, K. L., Tacke, F., Leifeld, L., Wüstefeld, T., Graw, A., Klein, C., et al. (2003). Interleukin 6/gp130-dependent pathways are protective during chronic liver diseases. *Hepatology, 38*(1), 218–229.

186. Strick-Marchand, H., Masse, G. X., Weiss, M. C., & Di Santo, J. P. (2008). Lymphocytes support oval cell-dependent liver regeneration. *Journal of Immunology, 181*(4), 2764–2771.

187. Takase, H. M., Itoh, T., Ino, S., Wang, T., Koji, T., Akira, S., et al. (2013). FGF7 is a functional niche signal required for stimulation of adult liver progenitor cells that support liver regeneration. *Genes & Development, 27*(2), 169–181.

188. Takikawa, H., Murata, Y., Horiike, N., Fukui, H., & Onji, M. (2009). Drug-induced liver injury in Japan: An analysis of 1676 cases between 1997 and 2006. *Hepatology Research, 39*(5), 427–431.

189. Taniguchi, E., Kin, M., Torimura, T., Nakamura, T., Kumemura, H., Hanada, S., et al. (2006). Endothelial progenitor cell transplantation improves the survival following liver injury in mice. *Gastroenterology, 130*(2), 521–531.

190. Tanimizu, N., Nishikawa, Y., Ichinohe, N., Akiyama, H., & Mitaka, T. (2014). SRY HMG box protein 9-positive (Sox9+) epithelial cell adhesion molecule-negative (EpCAM) biphenotypic cells derived from hepatocytes are involved in mouse liver regeneration. *Journal of Biological Chemistry, 289*(11), 7589–7598.

191. Tarlow, B. D., Pelz, C., Naugler, W. E., Wakefield, L., Wilson, E. M., Finegold, M. J., et al. (2014). Bipotential adult liver progenitors are derived from chronically injured mature hepatocytes. *Cell Stem Cell, 15*(5), 605–618.

192. Terada, R., Yamamoto, K., Hakoda, T., Shimada, N., Okano, N., Baba, N., et al. (2003). Stromal cell-derived factor-1 from biliary epithelial cells recruits CXCR4-positive cells: Implications for inflammatory liver diseases. *Laboratory Investigation, 83*(5), 665–672.

193. Theise, N. D., Saxena, R., Portmann, B. C., Thung, S. N., Yee, H., Chiriboga, L., et al. (1999). The canals of Hering and hepatic stem cells in humans. *Hepatology, 30*(6), 1425–1433.

194. Tian, H., Biehs, B., Chiu, C., Siebel, C. W., Wu, Y., Costa, M., et al. (2015). Opposing activities of Notch and Wnt signaling regulate intestinal stem cells and gut homeostasis. *Cell Reports, 11*(1), 33–42.

195. Tirnitz-Parker, J. E. E., Viebahn, C. S., Jakubowski, A., Klopcic, B. R., Olynyk, J. K., Yeoh, G. C. T., et al. (2010). Tumor necrosis factor-like weak inducer of apoptosis is a mitogen for liver progenitor cells. *Hepatology, 52*(1), 291–302.

196. Tirona, R. G., Leake, B. F., Merino, G., & Kim, R. B. (2001). Polymorphisms in OATP-C: Identification of multiple allelic variants associated with altered transport activity among European- and African-Americans. *Journal of Biological Chemistry, 276*(42), 35669–35675.

197. Trauner, M., Meier, P. J., & Boyer, J. L. (1998). Molecular pathogenesis of cholestasis. *New England Journal of Medicine, 339*(18), 1217–1227.

198. Tsutsui, H., Terano, Y., Sakagami, C., Hasegawa, I., Mizoguchi, Y., & Morisawa, S. (1992). Drug-specific T cells derived from patients with drug-induced allergic hepatitis. *Journal of Immunology, 149*(2), 706–716.

199. Turner, N., & Grose, R. (2010). Fibroblast growth factor signaling: From development to cancer. *Nature Reviews Cancer, 10*(2), 116–129.

200. Ucero, A. C., Benito-Martín, A., Fuentes-Calvo, I., Santamaría, B., Blanco, J., López-Novoa, J. M., et al. (2013). TNF-related weak inducer of apoptosis (TWEAK) promotes kidney fibrosis and Ras-dependent proliferation of cultured renal fibroblasts. *Biochimica et Biophysica Acta–Molecular Basis of Disease, 1832*(10), 1744–1755.

201. Uetrecht, J., & Kaplowitz, N. (2015). Inhibition of immune tolerance unmasks drug-induced allergic hepatitis. *Hepatology, 62*(2), 346–348.

202. Urban, T. J., Daly, A. K., & Aithal, G. P. (2014). Genetic basis of drug-induced liver injury: Present and future. *Seminars in Liver Disease, 34*(2), 123–133.

203. Vassilopoulos, G., Wang, P. R., & Russell, D. W. (2003). Transplanted bone marrow regenerates liver by cell fusion. *Nature, 422*(6929), 901–904.

204. Wagers, A. J., Sherwood, R. I., Christensen, J. L., & Weissman, I. L. (2002). Little evidence for developmental plasticity of adult hematopoietic stem cells. *Science, 297*(5587), 2256–2259.

205. Wang, B., Zhao, L., Fish, M., Logan, C. Y., & Nusse, R. (2015). Self-renewing diploid Axin2+ cells fuel homeostatic renewal of the liver. *Nature, 524*(7565), 180–185.

206. Wang, L., Wang, X., Xie, G., Wang, L., Hill, C. K., & Deleve, L. D. (2012). Liver sinusoidal endothelial cell progenitor cells promote liver regeneration in rats. *Journal of Clinical Investigation, 122*(4), 1567–1573.

207. Wang, R., Sheps, J. A., & Ling, V. (2011). ABC transporters, bile acids, and inflammatory stress in liver cancer. *Current Pharmaceutical Biotechnology, 12*(5), 636–646.

208. Watkins, P. B., & Seeff, L. B. (2006). Drug-induced liver injury: Summary of a single topic clinical research conference. *Hepatology, 43*(3), 618–631.

209. Weglarz, T. C., & Sandgren, E. P. (2000). Timing of hepatocyte entry into DNA synthesis after partial hepatectomy is cell autonomous. *Proceedings of the National Academy of Sciences U.S.A., 97*(23), 12595–12600.

210. Weglarz, T. C., Degen, J. L., & Sandgren, E. P. (2000). Hepatocyte transplantation into diseased mouse liver: Kinetics of parenchymal repopulation and identification of the proliferative capacity of tetraploid and octaploid hepatocytes. *American Journal of Pathology, 157*(6), 1963–1974.

211. Wei, C. Y., Chung, W. H., Huang, H. W., Chen, Y. T., & Hung, S. I. (2012). Direct interaction between HLA-B and carbamazepine activates T cells in patients with Stevens-Johnson syndrome. *Journal of Allergy and Clinical Immunology, 129*(6), 1562–1569.e5.

212. Wong, W. M., Wu, P. C., Yuen, M. F., Cheng, C. C., Yew, W. W., Wong, P. C., Tam, C. M., Leung, C. C., & Lai, C. L. (2000). Antituberculosis drug-related liver dysfunction in chronic hepatitis B infection. *Hepatology, 31*(1), 201–206.

213. Wu, T., Cieply, K., Nalesnik, M. A., Randhawa, P. S., Sonzogni, A., Bellamy, C., et al. (2003). Minimal evidence of trans differentiation from recipient bone marrow to parenchymal cells in regenerating and long-surviving human allografts. *American Journal of Transplantation, 3*(9), 1173–1181.

214. Wu, Y., Guo, F., Liu, J., Xiao, X., Huang, L., & He, D. (2011). Triple labeling with three thymidine analogs reveals a well-orchestrated regulation of hepatocyte proliferation during liver regeneration. *Hepatology Research, 41*(12), 1230–1239.

215. Wuillemin, N., Adam, J., Fontana, S., Krahenbuhl, S., Pichler, W. J., & Yerly, D. (2013). HLA haplotype determines hapten or p-i T cell reactivity to flucloxacillin. *Journal of Immunology, 190*(10), 4956–4964.

216. Xiao, J. C., Ruck, P., Adam, A., Wang, T. X., & Kaiserling, E. (2003). Small epithelial cells in human liver cirrhosis exhibit features of hepatic stem-like cells: Immunohistochemical, electron microscopic and immunoelectron microscopic findings. *Histopathology, 42*(2), 141–149.

217. Xu, C. F., Johnson, T., Wang, X., Carpenter, C., Graves, A., Warren, L., Xue, Z., King, K. S., Fraser, D. J., Stinnett, S., Briley, L. P., Mitrica, I., Spraggs, C. F., Nelson, M. R., Tada, H., Du Bois, A., Powles, T., Kaplowitz, N., & Pandite, L. N. (2015). HLA-B*57:01 confers susceptibility to Pazopanib-associated liver injury in patients with cancer. *Clinical Cancer Research, 22*(12), 2964–2972.

218. Yang, W., Yan, H. X., Chen, L., Liu, Q., He, Y. Q., Yu, L. X., et al. (2008). Wnt/β-catenin signaling contributes to activation of normal and tumorigenic liver progenitor cells. *Cancer Research, 68*(11), 4287–4295.

219. Yanger, K., & Stanger, B. Z. (2011). Facultative stem cells in liver and pancreas: Fact and fancy. *Developmental Dynamics, 240*(5), 521–529.

220. Yanger, K., Knigin, D., Zong, Y., Maggs, L., Gu, G., Akiyama, H., et al. (2014). Adult hepatocytes are generated by self-duplication rather than stem cell differentiation. *Cell Stem Cell, 15*(3), 340–349.

221. Yanger, K., Zong, Y., Maggs, L. R., Shapira, S. N., Maddipati, R., Aiello, N. M., et al. (2013). Robust cellular reprogramming occurs spontaneously during liver regeneration. *Genes & Development, 27*(7), 719–724.

222. Yimlamai, D., Christodoulou, C., Galli, G. G., Yanger, K., Pepe-Mooney, B., Gurung, B., et al. (2014). Hippo pathway activity influences liver cell fate. *Cell, 157*(6), 1324–1338.

223. Yoon, S. M., Gerasimidou, D., Kuwahara, R., Hytiroglou, P., Yoo, J. E., Park, Y. N., et al. (2011). Epithelial cell adhesion molecule (EpCAM) marks hepatocytes newly derived from stem/progenitor cells in humans. *Hepatology, 53*(3), 964–973.

224. Zaret, K. S. (2015). Regenerative biology: Maintaining liver mass. *Nature, 524*(7565), 165–166.

225. Zhu, S., Rezvani, M., Harbell, J., Mattis, A. N., Wolfe, A. R., Benet, L. Z., et al. (2014). Mouse liver repopulation with hepatocytes generated from human fibroblasts. *Nature, 508*(7496), 93–97.

226. Znoyko, I., Sohara, N., Spicer, S. S., Trojanowska, M., & Reuben, A. (2005). Expression of oncostatin M and its receptors in normal and cirrhotic human liver. *Journal of Hepatology, 43*(6), 893–900.

227. Zocco, M. A., Piscaglia, A. C., Giuliante, F., Arena, V., Novi, M., Rinninella, E., et al. (2011). CD133+ stem cell mobilization after partial hepatectomy depends on resection extent and underlying disease. *Digestive and Liver Disease, 43*(2), 147–154.

Chapter

THE PATHOPHYSIOLOGY OF ALCOHOLIC LIVER DISEASE

6

Contents

Introduction

Alcoholic liver disease (ALD) has a very complex pathophysiology because it develops gradually over many years, involving multiple mechanisms of liver injury that ultimately lead to liver failure. Steatosis is the first step in the sequence of various pathophysiological mechanisms of liver injury. This is followed by inflammatory changes brought on by oxidative stress secondary to the production of free radicals by Cytochrome P450 2E1 (CYP2E1), as well as cytokines and chemokines that activate the complement and inflammasome systems. Concurrently, nuclear factor kB (NFkB) expression is activated downstream by the toll-like receptor (TLR) signaling mechanism in response to lipopolysaccharides (LPS) produced by a leaky gut, which stimulates the innate immune system. When excessive blood alcohol levels (BALs) are maintained or binge drinking occurs, epigenetic modifications are set off.

Later, balloon cell degeneration arises from the accumulation of misfolded proteins in the cytoplasm of the enlarged hepatocytes due to the breakdown of the hepatocellular protein quality control complex system. Mallory-Denk bodies (MDBs) are the final product of the misfolded proteins aggregating. In response to transforming growth factor beta (TGFb) produced by macrophages, hepatocellular injury triggers stellate cell activation (HSC) that causes pericellular fibrosis. Ultimately, liver hypoxic changes result from the extension of liver fibrosis into cirrhosis, which is brought on by a reduction in sinusoidal blood flow. Many cell cycle inhibitors, such as p21, p27, p15, p16, and TGFb, are overexpressed, which leads to cell cycle arrest. Liver failure is ultimately the result of a confluence of factors including liver cell loss, senescence, and absence of regeneration. The loss of liver cells as a result of the division of liver cells into bile ductules exacerbates the lack of regeneration. Because the HSC adjacent to the metaplastic ductules are activated to form the stromal support for the newly formed ductules, this causes periportal fibrosis when the liver cell bile duct transition occurs.

Orientation and Directional Terms

Term	Definition	Illustration
Lipopolysaccharides (LPS)	Lipopolysaccharides (LPS) are important outer membrane components of gram-negative bacteria. They are large amphipathic glycoconjugates that typically consist of a lipid domain (hydrophobic) attached to a core oligosaccharide and a distal polysaccharide.	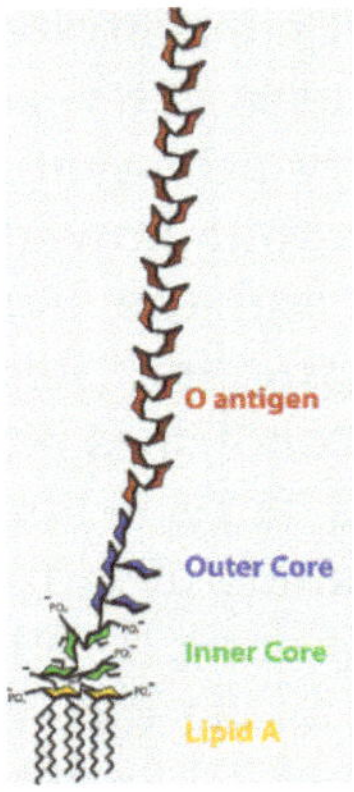
Blood alcohol levels (BALs)	Blood Alcohol Level (BAL) is the amount of alcohol present in your blood as you drink. It's calculated by determining how many milligrams of alcohol are present in 100 milliliters of blood.	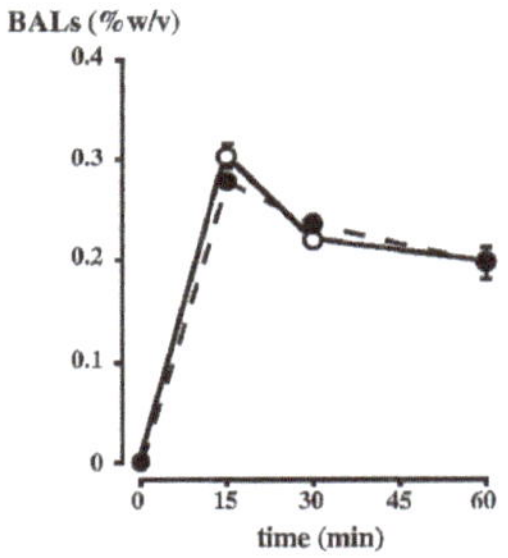
Mallory-Denk bodies (MDBs)	Mallory-Denk bodies (MDBs) is an inclusion found in the cytoplasm of liver cells. Mallory bodies are damaged intermediate filaments within the liver cells.	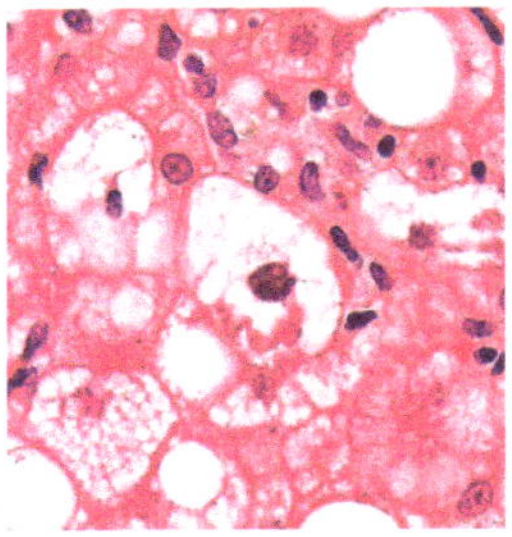
Immunohistochemistry (IHC)	Immunohistochemistry (IHC) is a powerful technique that exploits the specific binding between an antibody and antigen to detect and localize specific antigens in cells and tissue, most commonly detected and examined with the light microscope.	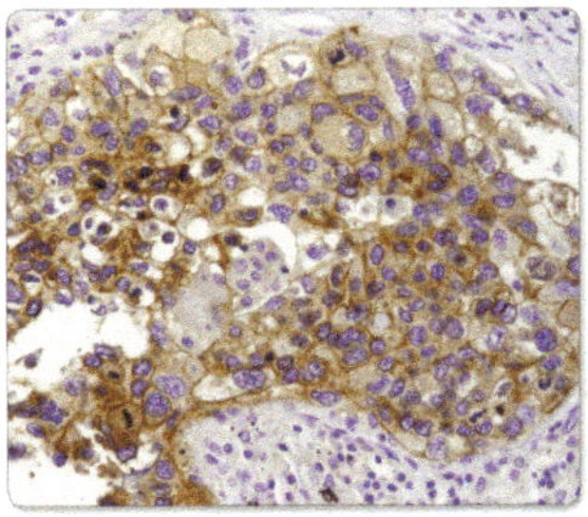

6.1. Steatosis

Numerous studies on the mechanism of alcohol-induced steatosis have been conducted over the years. Here, we'll concentrate on how alcohol consumption causes fatty acid oxidation to decrease and fatty acid synthesis to increase. We'll also talk about how it increases lipid droplet storage and the liver secretes very low-density lipoproteins (Resineci and Casey, 2012). Dietary alcohol does not induce steatosis if only saturated fatty acids are included in the diet, so the kinds of fatty acids consumed are crucial (Nanji et al., 1989a,b). Ethanol can induce steatosis in the diet with only a small amount of unsaturated fatty acids, like linoleic acid (Nanji and French, 1989).

The oxidation of ethanol produces acetaldehyde, which stimulates the synthesis of sterol regulatory element-binding transcription factor 1 (SREBP-1c), increasing the synthesis of fatty acids in liver cells (You et al., 2002). A number of hepatic transcriptional regulators, such as AMP-activated kinase (AMPK) Y, lipid, Ib [, sterol regulatory elementbinding protein 1 (SREBP) [, peroxisome proliferatore activated receptor-g (PPARg) Y, ACC [, peroxisome proliferatoreactivated receptor gamma coactivator-1a (PGC-1a) Y, and nuclear transcription adiponectin Y, and NFkB [. The effect of ethanol on these regulators is triggered by its inhibition of sirtuin 1 (SIRT1). SIRT is a deacetylase whose activity is reliant on the coactivator NADP. The metabolism of ethanol lowers NADP levels. SIRT1 deregulation of lipogenesis, fatty acid b-oxidation, lipoprotein uptake and secretion, and overexpression of proinflammatory cytokines in the liver governs the pathways of liver lipid metabolism, the inflammatory response, and alcohol-induced fatty liver in rodents and humans (You et al., 2015).

Quite the opposite changes were seen when the rat ethanol intragastric tube feeding model was used, where a high BAL was maintained. In this model, feeding naringin or resveratrol prevented the overexpression of SIRT1 in the liver, which was overexpressed several times over control levels. Moreover, there was a multifold overexpression of SIRT3, which naringin did not stop but resveratrol did. PGC-1a overexpression was significantly elevated by ethanol, and this increase was only partially inhibited by narigin and resveratrol. The expression of PPARg was several times higher in ethanol. Resveratrol, not naringin, was able to stop this alteration (Oliva et al., 2008). This model's high BALs (505 46 mg percent) caused liver necrosis and fibrosis in some of the rats. These findings highlight the significance of the BALs in identifying the kind of metabolic liver injury brought on by alcohol consumption.

6.2. Oxidative Stress

CYP2E1 induction, which produces free radicals by oxidizing ethanol, is arguably the most significant source of oxidative stress, which damages the liver through multiple pathways. This subject has already been examined and is outlined in French (2013a, b, c). Through several processes, including oxidative stress, lipid peroxidation, fatty acid hydroxylation, hydroxyethyl radical formation, autoimmunity, proteasomal inhibition, epigenetic modifications, and metabolic changes, CYP2E1 plays a significant role in the pathophysiology of ALD. The use of CYP2E1 inhibitors, such as DAS, PIC, CMZ, and CYP2E1 knockout (KO) mice, to stop the injuries is evidence that CYP2E1 is the cause of all of these distinct liver injuries (Zhou et al., 2014; Morimoto et al, 1995; Gouillon et al, 2000; Albano et al,1996). When given ethanol, mice with CYP2E1 overexpression experienced increased oxidative stress (Kathirvel et al., 2010; Morgan et al., 2002). According to Maher (2001), feeding ethanol to CYP2E1 KO mice resulted in less oxidative stress in the liver. Dr. Seitz at Eisenberg will employ a CYP2E1 inhibitor (CMZ) in a clinical trial to treat alcoholic hepatitis (AH) because CYP2E1 is crucial in ALD liver injury. When CYP2E1 oxidizes alcohol, it produces products that result in the formation of protein adducts.

Acetaldehyde, hydroxyethyl free radical, and lipid peroxidation products like 4-hydroxynoneal (4HNE) and malondialdehyde (MDA) are some of these products. These products break down proteins and create adducts that lead to the production of autoantibodies, which cause an autoimmune reaction that damages the liver. Among the cytochromes are P450 3A4 and CYP2E1 are proteins that these produced reactive products target in rats and humans who are fed ethanol (Lytton et al., 1999).

The formation of hydroxyethyl radical-derived protein adducts and the levels of circulating anti-hydroxyethyl radical immunoglobulin G (IgG) in rats fed ethanol and DAS or PIC were significantly impacted by the inhibition of CYP2E1 (Albano et al., 1996). The formation of hydroxyethyl free radicals, liver MDA and plasma lipid hydrogen peroxide levels, and the titers of antibodies against MDA adducts to proteins were all significantly inhibited by the DAS and PIC inhibitors. This suggests a connection between ethanol's induction of CYP2E1, the production of hydroxyethyl radicals, and the stimulation of lipid peroxidation. The levels of hydroxyethyl radical-derived adducts were also correlated with the liver microscopic pathologic severity scores and the CYP2E1 inhibitors. Feeding DAS and PIC significantly decreased the antibodies that the rats fed ethanol intragastrically developed, suggesting that the development of antibodies contributes to the liver damage caused by ethanol consumption.

Experimental liver damage in rats and human alcohol abusers is also caused by the proteins that are adducted to 4HNE and MDA, which are byproducts of lipid peroxidation formed by ethanol oxidation by CYP2E1 (French et al., 1993; Rouach et al., 1997). Rats given intragastrically ethanol for 72 days with high blood ethanol levels continuously monitored 24 hours a day experienced lipid peroxidation severity that paralleled the severity of liver pathology, including centrale central bridging fibrosis and necrosis, upon the addition of isonicotinylhydrazide (INH) to the diet. According to French et al., (1993), MDA and 4HNE were produced in proportion to the severity of liver damage, which included blood AST levels, mega mitochondria (EM) activation of stellate cells (HSC), and lipid peroxidation. To measure additional aspects of oxidative stress, the intragastric feeding experiment was conducted again later. Glutathione and vitamin E levels dropped with ethanol feeding. Additionally, there was less glutathione peroxidation. Protein thiols, carbonyl groups, and glutamine synthetase (GS) activity were measured in addition to protein oxidation. Protein thiol levels and GS activity—an enzyme especially vulnerable to free radical damage—were both decreased by ethanol feeding. Protein carbonyl concentrations rose. The liver pathology score and GS exhibited a strong correlation. This proved that lipid peroxidation brought on by ethanol was the cause of liver damage. It revealed that the antioxidant capacity of the liver is compromised by ethanol. Ethanol-induced oxidative protein functional damage has been demonstrated.

In liver biopsies obtained for AH, 4HNE aggresome formation was demonstrated (Amidi et al., 2007). Fifty-five percent of the macrophages and five percent of the hepatocytes had 4HNE aggresomes. In the hepatocyte cytoplasm, MDBs had no effect on the 4HNE aggresomes. M-30, a piece of cytokeratin 18 (CK-18) that remains after being proteolyzed by caspase during apoptosis, was discovered in the cytoplasm of 45% of AH cases and in MDBs (100%). In 18% of the cases, macrophages contained M-30. Strong electrophile 4HNE reacts with protein Cys, Lys, and His residues as well as nucleophilic functional groups in DNA. Heat shock protein 90 (HSP90), AKTZ, phosphatase and tensin homolog (PTEN), and protein disulfide isomerase are among the proteins that 4HNE modifications target (Shearn et al., 2013). The 4HNE modification of PTEN shows impaired function. Because PTEN can control AKT, it acts as a tumor suppressor. When these proteins are lost, patients experience aberrant growth and proliferation. Because it is a phosphatase, PTEN inhibits AKT. PTEN was carbonylated in a mouse model of ethanol feeding, which resulted in PTEN being carbamylated and losing its function, while AKT activity increased as a result. A plausible mechanism explaining how 4HNE mediated the inhibition of activity resulting in fatty liver from ethanol consumption was discovered (Shearn et al., 2013).

In rats fed ethanol intragastrically, 4HNE also targets the 26s proteasome (Fataccioli et al., 2003). By giving the mice the CYP2E1 inhibitor PIC, the mice's response to ethanol was prevented from inhibiting the function of the 20S proteasome chymotrypsin. This suggested that in rats fed ethanol, ethanol and 4HNE were responsible for the 20s proteasome's loss of control over protein quality. Using the overexpressing CYP2E1 cell line, HepG2 were used in in-vitro experiments. They were cultured for 24 hours with ethanol (100 mM), arachidonic acid, and Fe-NTA of Cederbaum (E47 cells as opposed to control HepG2 cells, C34 cells). Ethanol dramatically reduced the proteasome's chymotrypsin and trypsin activity in the E47 cells. On a Western blot of E47 cells, CYP2E1 was significantly overexpressed. DAS prevented ethanol from inhibiting chymotrypsin. Alongside the appearance of a high band of cytokeratin 8–18 (CK8–18) from the E47 homogenates, polyubiquitin was seen on the E47 Western blot. This high band resembled an MDB-like cytokeratin aggresome. Following a 24-hour exposure to ethanol, immunofluorescent double stains for ubiquitin and CK8–18 stain revealed colocalization in what appeared to be MDBs that had formed in the E47 cells. In the CYP2E1 overexpressing ethanol intragastric mouse model, this correlates with a marked overexpression of CK8 and 18, which correlated with the pathology score severity (Butura et al., 2008). After 24 hours in ethanol, the E47 cells had produced a large amount of carbonyls, as demonstrated by Western blots. In the E47 cells treated with ethanol, the indicator 8-oxyguanine demonstrated that DNA damage was caused by oxygen free radicals. Strongly positive results from a fluorescence stain indicated that the E47 cells had high levels of reactive oxygen species (ROS) caused by ethanol. The E47 ethanol-treated cells were the only ones to exhibit both high- and low-molecular-weight bands on Western blots stained with the 4HNE antibody. Lastly, immunoprecipitated 4HNE-modified proteins stained positively with antibodies to 20s proteasome subunits when subjected to Western blot analysis, i.e., Rpt 4 (19s ATPase subunit), and the a6 subunit (Bardag-Gorce et al., 2006).

We investigated the impact of CYP2E1 induction on the suppression of the 26S proteasome's activity in rats given ethanol intragastrically. After 15 days of ethanol feeding, the CYP2E1 (3.5x) was maximally induced; however, proteasomal chymotrypsin and trypsin activity were only inhibited after 1 month of ethanol feeding. However, following a month of ethanol feeding, the 4HNE adduct formation appeared. Western blots of the livers of the rats and controls fed ethanol at one month of feeding revealed one 4HNE positive band at 44KOa, indicating the isolation of the proteasome fraction. The ATPase RTP4 antibody stained the band positively. The link between the 19s and 20s proteasomes would be harmed by the loss of RTP4 (BardagGorce et al., 2005).

6.3. Inflammasomes

Angiogenesis and MDB production in balloon cells characterize the shift in ALD from reversible to advanced phases. Immunohistochemistry (IHC) staining of human liver biopsies from patients with AH allowed for the protein-level assaying of gene expressions through the use of new technology to measure changes in the expression of inflammasome proteins (Peng et al., 2014) with the creation of MDB. The expression of NIAP was found to be significantly elevated in hepatocytes that were MDB negative as well as MDB forming. MAV5 colocalizes in the mitochondria of liver cells and was markedly upregulated in MDB-negative liver cells in contrast to control liver cells. The amount of Caspase-1 in both MDB-forming and MDB-negative hepatocytes was markedly elevated. Only in liver cells that were forming MDB did interleukin-18 (IL-18) and tumor necrosis factor-a (TNF-a) exhibit significant increases. The abundance of MDBs present was correlated with NLRP3, ASC, caspase-1, IL-18, TL-10, and p65, suggesting a positive correlation between inflammasome formation and MDB formation at the AH stage of ALD. There was no discernible difference in the NLRP3 levels between the liver cells from the AH liver biopsies and the control group.

This is the first concrete evidence linking the pathophysiology of AH in humans to the inflammasome. The NAIP/NLRC4 type of inflammasome would be involved in processes such as phagosomal maturation, T cell activation, regulation of autophagy, secretion of inflammatory mediators, and inducible nitric oxide synthase activation (Lage et al., 2014). DeSantis et al, (2013) concluded that NLRP3 protects the liver from damage in ALD.

The NLRP3 pathway of the inflammasome has received more attention in in-vitro and animal studies than the NIAP pathway, which was seen in liver biopsies from individuals with AH. NLRP3-deficient mice were given a LieberDeCarli ethanol diet to demonstrate this relationship (Petrasek et al., 2015). In mice given alcohol, the development of alcohol-induced liver inflammation was prevented, and liver damage and steatosis were significantly ameliorated. This was due to the lack of NLRP3, a ligand-sensing component of the inflammasome that recognizes uric acid and ATP, mediates paracrine inflammatory cross-talk between damaged hepatocytes and immune cells, and increases the expression of LPS-inducible cytokines, IL-B, and TNF-a from immune cells. The caspase-1-mediated cleavage of IL-1b by the inflammasome, a multiple complex, can detect endogenous danger molecules, indicating that both caspase-1 activation and IL-1b steatosis and inflammation in the liver can occur in ALD (Szabo et al., 2012). Apart from its impact on NLRP3, inflammation has the ability to trigger liver fibrosis through stellate cells in mice lacking NLRP3 (Wree et al., 2014). Inflammasomes can be induced by oxidative stress, and NLRP3 is the primary immune sensor for cellular signals i.e., ROS, which throw off the redox balance within cells (Salminen et al., 2013).

6.4. Macrophages

In the livers of AH patients, macrophages located in the sinusoids and liver scars change from M1 to M2 phenotypes (Lee et al., 2013). The phenotypes of macrophages into M1 and M2abc were identified by immunofluorescence microscopy in a recent survey of liver biopsies from patients with AH. Strong staining for M1 and F4/80 macrophages revealed them all over the sinusoids. TLR4 and TLR2, as well as IL-1b, were also positively stained by the M1 macrophages. TLR4 staining of liver cells was also strongly positive. IFNg, TNF-a, and CXCL9, among other markers for the M1 phenotypes, were negative. Among the M2a markers that stained positively were CD206,

CD163, and CCL18. CCL13 and IL-10 did not stain. CD206 and CD163 both showed strong staining. Macrophages stained with CD206 were distributed throughout the sinusoids. Balloon cells formed MDBs with a concentration of CD163-positive macrophages surrounding them. Serum contains the soluble CD163 molecule, a macrophage activation marker linked to liver fibrosis (Kazankov et al., 2014). The phenotype of M2b macrophages was found to be negative for TNF-a and IL-10 and positive for IL-1b, CCL1, and CXCLL. The M2c macrophage phenotype was found to be negative for CXLL9 and positive for TGFb, CCL18, CD163, CD206, CD14, and TLR8. TGFb-positive is significant because it has been linked to the cell cycle arrest and fibrogenesis seen in AH.

In macrophages found in liver scars, interferon regulatory factor 4 (IRF-4) was overexpressed and colocalized with IL-1b. It has been discovered that IRF-4 is a crucial adaptor molecule engaged in downstream processes that TLR4 initiates, including the production of interferon and the stimulation of proinflammatory cytokines (Seki and Brenner, 2008). In scarred macrophages, IL-1b showed a strong positive stain. It is a cytokine that has been extensively researched for its proinflammatory qualities and is elevated in the serum when AH is present (McClain et al., 1986). A crucial mechanism for the ongoing recruitment of inflammatory cells to the liver and the maintenance of inflammation is highlighted by the induction of MIP-1b expression in hepatic cells by IL-1b (Zhang et al., 2003).

6.5. Neutrophilic Infiltration of the Liver

Neutrophil episodes and multifocal neutrophilic infiltrates in the liver lobules, particularly around MDBs (referred to as satellitosis), occur late in the cirrhosis of AH. After the patient has a fever, sepsis is thought to be the cause. The infiltration of polymorphonuclear leukocytes (PMN) is caused by IL-17 activating IL-8 (Wang et al., 2012). Three days of high-fat diet (HFD) feeding significantly worsened acute binge-induced liver neutrophil infiltration in mice. Steatohepatitis was made worse in mice fed a high-fat diet (HFD) for three months, in addition to a single ethanol binge. This resulted in a 20-fold increase in CXCL 1. Hepatocytes, stellate cells, and endothelium all had elevated CXCL 1 levels, with hepatocytes showing the greatest amount of this (Chang et al., 2015). Mice deficient in osteopontin (OPN) and fed a high-fat diet (HFD) with ethanol bingeing developed PMN infiltrates, and the infiltration of PMN was further enhanced by overexpressing CXCL1 and IL-17a. The findings revealed that, at least in mice, OPN deficiency plays a protective rather than a causative role for AH (Lazaro et al., 2015).

According to Bataller at the 2015 RSA annual meeting in San Antonio, Texas, the prognosis of AH patients is significantly better when PMN infiltrates are present in their livers compared to comparable patients with no PMN infiltration. The purpose of PMNs, including autophagocytosis, is to clear the liver of inflammatory and necrotic debris. In AH patients and experimentally fed mice with alcohol, OPN is overexpressed, particularly in cases of more severe disease (Morales-Ibanez et al., 2013).

In mice given ethanol through chronic binge drinking, e-selectin also contributes to PMN infiltration (Bertola et al., 2013). Neutrophil-mediated inflammation and PMN recruitment are inhibited by blocking CXCR2 signaling (Boppana et al., 2014). IL-8 attraction might be the cause of leukocyte recruitment to MDBs that results in "satellitosis.." In order to test this, mice fed DDC to induce MDB formation and liver biopsies from patients with AH had their levels of IL-8 and CXCR2 expressed by RNA sequencing. In AH and the mouse livers, there was a noticeable increase in the expression of

CXCR2 and IL-8. According to Liu et al. (2015), this may be the mechanism causing satellitosis in response to increased expression of FAT10 and NFkB found in the livers of AH and MDB-forming CXCR2 mice..

6.6. Role of Complement in Alcoholic Hepatitis Pathogenesis

Inflammation is significantly influenced by complement system activation. It has been demonstrated that the pathophysiology of ethanol-induced liver injury in mice is connected to the complement system's activation. Furthermore, Shen et al., (2014) verified that patients with AH also had activated complement in their livers. The complement system antigen immunoreactivity was investigated immunohistochemically and measured using morphometric image analysis using antibodies against Clq, C3, and C5. The activation of Clq, C3, and C5 was observed in the liver biopsies of patients with AH. The formalin-fixed paraffin embedded biopsy tissue underwent polymerase chain reaction (PCR) analysis, which revealed an increase in the expression of Clq and C5, but not C3 mRNA in AH. When comparing balloon hepatocytes that had formed MDBs to hepatocytes that appeared normally, there was an increase in C5aR. In the MDBs, C5aR colocalized with ubiquitin, suggesting that a decrease in the 26s proteasome's ability to digest C5aR resulted in a slower turnover of C5aR and the accumulation of an aggregation of C5aR. As a result, the stabilization of the protein components that cause them to accumulate contributed to the increase in complement factors in the liver cells. Chemotactic factors C3a and C5a can stimulate leukocytes to release inflammatory cytokines (Wang et al., 2012). In the liver, ethanol triggers the classical complement pathway, which causes C1q to attach to apoptotic cells. Eliminating Clq stops the liver's production of TNF-a and IL-6 as well as the ethanol-induced activation of complement (Cohen et al., 2010). Additionally, in primary cultures of HSC, C5a overexpression controls HSC migration through both MCP-1-independent and MCP1-dependent mechanisms (Das et al., 2014).

6.7. Role of Hypoxia

When blood levels of catecholamines rise, the metabolic rate at high BALs also rises, leading to an increase in oxygen consumption and, ultimately, hypoxia of the liver in ALD (Li et al., 2010; 2004 a,b; French, 2015). Rats given ethanol intragastrically only experience a drop in liver ATP levels below controls when BAL levels rise above 200 mg% during the BAL cycle (BardagGorce et al., 2002). On the other hand, a tendency toward hypoxia at the lower BALs was revealed by the pimonidazole adduct formation, a marker of periportal liver hypoxia. Comparing the hypoxyprobe results between controls and lower BALs, however, revealed no discernible variation. These findings contrasted with those of an earlier investigation that claimed hypoxia was present at blood alcohol levels both high and low (Arteel et al., 1997).

When rats fed ethanol were exposed to 6% O_2 levels for six hours, the hypoxia brought on by alcohol consumption increased the liver's vulnerability to necrosis (French et al., 1984). Similarly, feeding rats ethanol along with thyroxin (T4) resulted in a hypermetabolic state that led to widespread liver necrosis because of hypoxia (Li et al., 2001). This was also noted when catecholamines were fed to ethanol (Li et al., 2003), as well as rats given ethanol and exposed to CO (Nanji et al., both following acute hypoxia-induced ATP deficiency (Miyamoto and French, 1988) and 1989a,b).

Rats were given ethanol through a tube in their stomach for a month and their liver surface was monitored for lack of oxygen by checking the pO_2 levels. Gene changes related to lack of oxygen were analyzed using RT-PCR.

Adrenomedilin, adrenergic receptors a 1a and 1d, CDK inhibitor 1a, and erythropoietin were significantly increased during peak alcohol levels compared to lower levels and control rats. HIF-1a concentration was higher in the nuclear fraction during peak alcohol levels. Genes related to the regulation of HIF-1a, such as propyl 4-hydroxylase and von Hippel-Lindau syndrome homology LVh1, were more active during lower alcohol levels. pO_2 levels were lower on the liver surface during peak alcohol levels and dropped quickly when blood flow to the liver was temporarily blocked. The pO_2 levels returned to normal in control rats after the blockage was removed, but not during peak alcohol levels. These findings suggest that lack of oxygen occurs at high levels of alcohol in the blood and slows down recovery from decreased blood flow to the liver. (Li et al., 2004a,b).

There are several potential effects of hypoxia brought on by ethanol abuse. For example, hypoxia stress causes macrophages to express more TLR4 due to hypoxia-inducible factor (Kim et al., 2009). It is possible that alcohol-induced hypoxia causes mice given ethanol to express less of the iron regulatory peptide hepcidin (Heritage et al., 2009).

6.8. The Effect of Nutrition on Alcoholic Liver Disease

Numerous studies have demonstrated that giving different nutrients to rats or mice fed alcohol for one to two months prevents steatosis and steatohepatitis; however, there is no benefit observed when these nutrients are given to patients with AH or cirrhosis. According to one study, 1235 patients' complete abstinence from alcohol did not improve until 135 years later when compared to patients who continue to consume alcohol (Xie et al., 2014). Mendenhall et al., showed that patients with severe AH had a higher survival rate when they followed a high-protein diet (3000 calories via Hepatic Aid/day). S-adenosylmethionine (SAMe), a methyl donor added to the diet, was shown to ameliorate liver pathology in rats fed ethanol intragastrically (Bardag-Gorce et al., 2010a, b, and c). However, a clinical trial feeding SAMe for 6 months during abstinence failed to improve the patients' conditions beyond that of the placebo (Medici et al., 2011). Liver biopsies done before and after feeding SAMe were compared and no difference in the pathology score before or after treatment was observed (Le et al., 2013). Like SAMe, betaine prevents the liver pathology in rats fed ethanol for 1 month (Li et al., 2011). Betaine, such as quercetin and catechin from green tea is an effective antioxidant in vitro in preventing oxidative stress caused by ethanol given to a CYP2E1 overexpressing liver cell line (Oliva et al., 2011). Both betaine and SAMe prevent the alcohol-induced liver pathology by preventing the BALs from rising above 200 mg%. The physiological mechanism involved is the conversion of norepinephrine to epinephrine by providing the methyl group required by the converting enzyme phenylethanolamine N-methyltransferase. Epinephrine increases the metabolic rate which regenerates NADþ from NADH by NADH dehydrogenase in mitochondria (French, 2015). The availability of NAD^+ which is required for oxidation of alcohol increases the elimination rate of the BALs. This keeps the BAL lower than 200 mg% which prevents the development of ALD (French, 2015).

Patients with ALD often struggle with vitamin deficiencies. Low folate intake, intestinal malabsorption, decreased liver uptake and storage, and elevated urinary folate are the causes of folate deficiency in alcoholics (Medici and Halsted, 2013). Due to its effects on methionine metabolism, particularly as a result of DNA synthesis, stability, and epigenetic regulation of gene expression involved in the pathways of liver pathology, folate deficiency contributes to the progression of ALD. Together with a folate deficiency, the effects of ethanol on methionine metabolism work to reduce antioxidant defense and control epigenetic modifications to gene expression. Due to altered folate and methionine metabolism during ALD progression, where DNA nucleotide imbalance and stability develop due to the shunting of 5, 10-MTHF to the MTHFR pathway due to the deficiency of SAMe because of the folate deficiency, the frequency of both colon cancer and HCC increases as ALD progresses. DNA hypomethylation is caused by the interaction of folate and alcohol with histone methylation. The likelihood of developing HCC is associated with the induction of DNA hypomethylation. There is evidence connecting the altered expression of the gene implicated in the pathogenesis of Alzheimer's disease (ALD) to ethanol-induced modifications of the liver's homocysteine metabolism, particularly the decrease in the methyltransferase methyl donor source, SAMe, or the increase in the inhibitor, SAH (Medici & Halsted, 2013).

Rats fed ethanol intragastrically exhibit varying degrees of liver pathology depending on the type of fat in their diet. Saturated fat (tallow) and medium-chain triglycerides totally shield the liver from steatosis. Alcohol-induced steatosis is caused by elevating the amount of unsaturated fat (linoleic acid) to that of lard. Fish oil causes the most severe liver damage, and corn oil exacerbates the steatosis brought on by alcohol (Ronis et al., 2004; Nanji & French, 1989; Morimoto et al., 1994).

6.9. Epigenetic Changes in Gene Expression in Alcoholic Liver Disease

DNA methylation, histone modifications through methylation, acetylation, ubiquitination, phosphorylation, and RNA-based mechanisms are examples of epigenetic modifications. The expression of genes that control the rough endoplasmic reticulum, stress response, and alcoholic liver injury is upregulated in the advanced stage of ALD due to a decrease in liver levels of SAMe, DNA, and histone methylation (Esfandiari et al., 2010). At high BALs, there was an increase in histone acetyltransferase p300, which acetylates histone at lysine 9. In rats given ethanol intragastrically on a continuous basis, it alters gene expression at high BALs in an epigenetic fashion (BardagGorce et al., 2007). p300 activates transcription of numerous genes in response to signal transcription factors such as HIF-1a. The nuclear ubiquitin-proteasome protein quality control pathway is significantly inhibited by prolonged ethanol consumption. This slows down the turnover of transcriptional factors and histone-modifying enzymes, which influences epigenetic mechanisms and raises histone acetylation. The upregulation of p300 led to an increase in the acetylation of H3K9 and H3K27 (histone acetyltransferase) (Park et al., 2005; Oliva et al., 2009a,b).

6.10. Histone Acetylation and Methylation in Experimental Alcoholic Liver Disease

When high urinary ethanol levels (UAL) occur at the peaks of the intragastric tube-fed rat model of ALD, histone modification may be the reason why ethanol feeding alters the expression of so many genes (Bardag-Gorce et al., 2006). At the UAL peaks, a large number of genes were overexpressed in each KEGG pathway. Just 230 genes had altered expression during the urine alcohol cycle's low points. UAL averaged 400–500 mg% during peak conditions and 100–200 mg% during trough conditions. The vast majority of genes whose expression was altered were upregulated, suggesting that at the UAL peaks, histone acetylation rather than methylation predominated. Both H3K9ac and H3K18ac were upregulated at 3 hours after the bolus when the BAL was high (34 mg percent), but not at 12 hours when the BAL was low (29 mg%), in a model of binge drinking in which rats were given 6 g/kg body weights of ethanol bolus.

BAL was at 138 mg% three hours after the ethanol bolus when SAMe was given 1 g/kg (40% reduced by SAMe). Only 640 gene expressions were altered when SAMe was added, compared to 1012 genes whose expressions were altered by the ethanol bolus alone. SAMe was found to ablate the urinary alcohol cycle and significantly reduce BALs (454 mg percent with ethanol alone and 153 mg percent with SAMe added to ethanol) following a month of intragastric feeding of ethanol with or without SAMe (Bardag-Gorce et al., 2010a,b,c). Owing to the low BAL, the ethanol-upregulated genes IIIr2, IIIr1, TNFRsf6, CXC14, CCI6, TLR4, CXCI12, CC14, TLR2, Tgfbr3, TNF, Igfbp2, Falp2 Gadd 45b, Hmox1, PPARa, Herpud1, Col4a1, KIf9, HGF, JAk2, H3K27me3 (a histone that silences genes), PPKCb1, F10, Igflr, Shc1, RXRa, MAPK4, K1f3, MAPK7, F8, C3 (BardagGorce et al., 2010a,b,c).

In the chronic intragastric tube-feeding rat model, where peak BALs occurred every 6–8 days, methyl donor betaine, like SAMe, prevented the high BALs (Li et al., 2011). 50% less BALs were found (450 vs. 220 mg%), as a result of the faster rate of ethanol clearance (Li et al., 2011; French, a, b, and c, 2013). The impact of 2 g/kg body weight of betaine.) in the model of binge drinking rats also decreased the BAL three hours after the ethanol bolus (347 vs. 155 mg%) as a result of the rate of ethanol elimination being accelerated by the methyl donor (French, 2013a,b,c). The 3 and 12 hour post-bolus heat maps were different from both the controls and one another. When betaine was introduced during the three-hour ethanol bolus, the functional pathways indicated a reduction in the changes in gene expression. The metabolic pathways were where this difference was most noticeable. Betaine was found to downregulate 50% of 95 genes, including genes involved in the methionine pathway (Cth, Gnmt, and Ahcyl). Following boluses of both ethanol and betaine, a global shift in gene expression was observed that involved nearly every functional pathway. In the intragastric tube feeding model, betaine (SAMe, for example) inhibited the blood ethanol cycle and liver pathology. These findings suggest that methyl donors, like betaine, when added to alcoholic beverages would stop the development of ALD in humans when fed ethanol (French, 2013a,b,c).

6.11. Microarray Analysis

PCR microplate array analysis specific to the TLR signaling pathway was carried out since SAMe feeding in the intragastric tube feeding model of ALD demonstrated that ethanol upregulated TLR4 and 2 in rats fed alcohol for one month (Oliva et al., 2011). Every TLR, CD14, MyD88, Traf6, FOS, IL-10, Jun oncogene Irf-1, Hspala, Ifnal, Ifng, Trk1, and 2; NFkB, Nr2c2, PPAR, and Traf6 were all upregulated at the BAL peaks. SAMe fed with ethanol totally inhibited TLR2 upregulation but not 4; SAMe, whether fed with or without ethanol, downregulated CD14, MyD88, IL-lr1, lrf1, and TNFRsf1a. Ethanol feeding raised TLR4 and TLR8 protein levels, but SAMe inhibited this. MyD88 protein was elevated by ethanol, but SAMe did not stop this. According to Paradere et al. 2010), , SAMe downregulation of TLR4 expression would stop LPS from activating the TLR4 pathway through NFkB activation, which would stop the production of cytokines that promote hepatic fibrogenesis. Histone methylation changes coincided with changes in gene expression following an ethanol bolus (6 g/kg body weight) at 3 and 12 hours later. H3K9me2 was reduced three hours after an ethanol bolus. H3K4me2 and H3K9me2 levels are raised by SAMe fed with or without ethanol (Bardag-Gorce et al., 2010a,b,c). Gene expression is activated by H3K4me2 (Li et al., Pal-Bhadra et al., (2009), which would account for the upregulation of ADH1, CYP2E1, and ALDH1 and 2 by SAMe. 2007). It is determined that SAMe partially protects the liver from harm through histone methylation. The following alterations were observed in studies employing RTPCR on rat livers fed ethanol continuously via intragastric tube: ALDH1 and 4 were upregulated at the BAL peaks and troughs. PGC-1a was only upregulated at the peaks, PPAR was significantly reduced at the peaks, and SIRT1 was upregulated at both the peak and the trough. According to Bardag-Gorce et al (2009), histone H3K18ac was only elevated at the peaks, while H3K4me2 was significantly elevated and H3K27me3 was elevated at both the peaks and the troughs.

Numerous stages of the disease progression, from steatosis and AH to cirrhosis and end-stage cirrhosis, have been documented in microarray studies on human livers (Seth et al., 2006). As the ALD advanced from steatosis to AH to cirrhosis, the differentially expressed genes with most pathways increased, particularly those linked to fibrogenesis and immunological/ inflammatory responses. The exceptions were the channel transport and protein turnover pathways, which mostly took place during the AH and steatosis stages. 98 genes had altered expression in steatosis patients (30 upregulated and 68 downregulated). The main areas of lipid metabolism, biosynthesis, and transport-related gene expression changes were observed. 211 genes with differential expression were found using AH (100 upregulated, 111 downregulated). Cell adhesions, immunological response, oncogenesis, signal transduction, and embryogenesis were among the pathways that were upregulated. Genes involved in protein biosynthesis, cell growth and maintenance, transcription, signal transduction, and transport had their expression downregulated. In the advanced stages of the disease, RT-PCR verified the expression of seven important genes: CD209 and SAMe synthesis (MAT2A) were downregulated, while OPN, IL-8, annex in A2, TNFRSF 14, and claudin were all upregulated. OPN contributes to inflammation. Fibrinolysis is aided by annexin A2. PMN recruitment is aided by IL-8, while TNFRF14 is a costimulatory molecule that promotes inflammation by inducing IL-8 production in macrophages and matrix-degrading enzymes. Liver cell proliferation is influenced by clonin 10, and LPS is bound by CD209. Following prolonged alcohol exposure, the LPS response is downregulated (Greenberg et al., 1998). SAMe is the predominant methyl donor, and it depends on MATIA. Global gene expression is downregulated, which is a significant epigenetic mechanism (Shukla et al., 2008).

The expression of 46 candidate genes was assessed by quantitative PCR in a second study involving 23 patients with AH (Jung et al., 2008). The outcomes were compared to the morphologic alterations in the liver that were found through biopsy. Portal hypertension and advanced fibrosis were signs of an advanced clinical stage of ALD. Unsurprisingly, there was an upregulation of the genes that code for extracellular matrix, collagen, inflammatory cytokines, fibrinogenesis mediators (TGFb), and apoptosis regulators (Bcl2). Positive correlations were observed between the morphologic features of AH and fibrinogenic regulators, including GRO-a, TIMP-1, and NADPH oxidase components. TGFb was the primary fibrinogen. TIMP-1, matrix metalloproteinase-2 (MMP2), and ut-PA were among the genes that were upregulated in relation to collagen degradation. Disease severity and TIMP were correlated. A severe granulocytic infiltrate was correlated with a 30-fold increase in the cytokine Gro-a's expression. Nox 4 and Duox 1 and 2 were also upregulated, as were the essential elements of the phagocytic NADH oxidase (p22, phos, and Rac-1). A systemic inflammatory response was correlated with TNF-a and IL-6. Procollagen 4a, MMP-1, and UPA increased expression were correlated with mortality within 3 months.

Hepatic gene expression profile was evaluated by DNA microarray in patients with AH in comparison to normal livers in a third study. Gene set enrichment analysis was used to evaluate the functional pathway analysis. Additionally, quantitative PCR was performed, and protein expression was evaluated using Western blot and IHC (Affò et al., 2013). When AH was compared to other liver diseases, FN14 was the only TNF superfamily receptor that was exclusively upregulated, and it was correlated with mortality within 90 days. Hepatocyte populations and regions with fibrinogenesis were found to express the FN14 protein. Progenitor cell expansion and TWEAK's specific receptor FN14 are involved in cellular proliferation, migration, differentiation, apoptosis, angiogenesis, and inflammation (Winkles, 2008; Tirnitz-Parker et al., 2010). This study showed a 56-fold upregulation of FAT10. OPN had a 67-fold upregulation.

6.12. Lipopolysaccharides and Toll-Like Receptor 4 and the Blood Alcohol Cycle

The increase in blood levels of LPS at the peaks of the blood alcoholic cycle is one important factor in the mechanism of liver injury that occurs at these points in the intragastric rat feeding model of ALD (French, 2001). Every time blood alcohol levels reach their peak, blood LPS levels rise (serum LPS to 12–25 EU mL at UAL of 300–350) and fall to low levels when BALs reach trough levels (2–5 EU/mL at 50–75 UAL). Stool weight varies from 6 to 7.5 g/day at the trough, and drops to 0 at the peaks. Feeding SAMe or betaine can prevent high BALs, which in turn prevents the worsening of liver pathology during peaks (French, 2015). This is consistent with the observation that SAMe also inhibits TLR4's increased expression and signaling (Oliva et al., 2011).

Previous studies using the intragastric feeding rat model of ALD demonstrated that feeding SAMe alcohol prevented the upregulation of the TLRs and related proteins, including proinflammatory cytokines and chemokines, as measured by PCR microplate array analysis (Oliva et al., 2011). This is in line with the results of a study that used the methyl signature qPCR Array kit to measure the methylation of 24 genes involved in the TLR4 signaling pathway in rats fed ethanol for a month. Combining the DNA methylation data revealed a highly significant increase in methylation, which was totally stopped by giving SAMe ethanol to eat. Khachatoorian et al., (2013) found a strong correlation between the BAL elevation and the degree of methylation (0.0001)). This suggests that the level of blood alcohol attained is closely correlated with TLR signaling, and that liver damage caused by LPS/TLR4 can be avoided by maintaining a low BAL (even if you continue to drink alcohol night and day at a low rate to maintain a low BAL).

Formalin-fixed/paraffin-embedded liver biopsies from AH patients were used to assess the transcription regulation of the TLR 3/4 signaling pathway by RT-PCR (Liu et al., 2014a). Only liver biopsies demonstrating the formation of MDBs were utilized downstream adaptors for TLRs (such as TRIF and MyD88) all showed upregulation. When compared to normal controls, the livers of alcoholics (AH) had significantly higher levels of MyD88, TLR3, and TLR4. In AH livers, chemokine receptor (CXCR7) mRNA was upregulated in hepatocytes that were positive for FAT10. AH has elevated FAT10 (Liu et al., 2014b). It is brought on in vitro by TNF-a and interferon-gamma (IFNg), which activates NFkB and upregulates CXCR7

(Gao et al., 2014). The TLR4/NFkB pathway, which is dependent on MyD88, was found to be a significant mechanism of liver injury in AH.

TLR4 is involved in the transition of hepatic stem cells, also known as tissue-initiating stem cells (TISCs), to HCC, according to research on the role of the TLR signaling pathway in the development of HCC in ALD (Machida et al., 2012; Machida, 2013). It has been demonstrated that TLR4 may be a proto-oncogene for TISCs in liver oncogenesis. Using FACS, CD133+/CD49f+ TISCs were isolated from HCC developed in diethylnitrosamine-treated mice, ethanol-fed HCV core Tg mice, and alcoholic patients with or without HCV infection. Both in vitro and in a xenograft model, the CD133+/CD49f+ cells that were isolated from the patients and animal models were tumorigenic. The tumor-initiating property was attenuated by TLR4 or Nanog silencing with shRNA.

TISCs had higher levels of TR4 expression than CD133 CD49f+ cells. When combined, TLR4 could be a universal proto-oncogene that causes TLR4-Nanog dependent TISCs to develop. The pluripotency marker Nanog was identified as a direct target of TLR4, which is responsible for the tumor-initiating activity of CD133+ TISCs. It was discovered that TISCs had flaws in the TGFb tumor suppressor pathway. Tumor chemoresistance of the TISCs was abolished, pluripotency genes and tumor genesis were suppressed, and TGFb signaling was reinstated by YAPI and IGF2BP3. Mice with impaired TGFb signaling showed increased TLR4 expression in the liver and TLR4-dependent development of HCCs. In conclusion, TLR4, a critical element of a critical cell regulatory pathway whose dysregulation contributes to the development of HCC, may be indirectly impacted by alcohol (French, 2013a,b,c).

6.13. Balloon Cell Change and Mallory-Denk Body Formation

The primary pathologic alteration in hepatocytes with AH is balloon cell change associated with MDB formation. IHC is used to diagnose it with a high concordance rate for keratin 8/18 (Mookerjee et al., 2011). The degree of AH can be graded through the application of keratin 8/18 immunostaining. The formation of MDBs has a highly intricate mechanism. There are multiple interconnected but distinct mechanisms at play. First off, FAT10 is involved in the key switch. In the DDC feeding model of MDB formation, FAT10 KO mice are unable to form MDBs in response to DDC (French et al., 2012a,b). This is because activating the mechanism of MDB formation requires activating the interferon sequence response element on the FAT10 promoter, which reacts to IFNg and activates the expression of multiple important genes (Oliva et al., 2010). These consist of p38, JNK, and NFKb. After 21 days of incubation, Hepa1–6 cells were shown to produce MDB-like aggresomes by IFNg and TNF-a, according to in vitro research (Oliva et al., 2010).

In the mouse model of MDB formation, increased expression of NFkB was linked to DDC-induced MDB formation. MDB formation in primary cultures was inhibited by a strong NFkB expression inhibitor (Nan et al., 2005a,b). According to the findings, MDB formation was linked to the NFkB pathway, which includes Src, JNK1, and ERK 1/2 expression (Wu et al., 2005). Increased expression of cytokeratins, adhesion molecules, and aggresome-forming proteins, including several kinases like p38, was observed in the livers from the DDC mouse model of MDB formation, according to microarray analysis. When p38 hypophosphorylates cytokeratin, MDB formation is inhibited in vitro by a potent p38 phosphorylation inhibitor (Nan et al., 2006). In the DDC-fed mouse model, two methylation donors, SAMe and betaine, inhibit

MDB formation in vivo (Oliva et al., 2009a,b; Li et al., 2008a,b). MDB formation in primary cell culture was inhibited by SAMe. Modifications in oxidative stress or the production of carbonyl proteins were not linked to MDBs that formed in vivo in response to DDC. Significantly higher expression of FAT10, KLF6, and alpha fetal protein was linked to MDB formation. SAMe feeding inhibited the overexpression of Dnmt1, 3 aPHdac9, and FAT10 that was induced by DDC. Additionally, betaine prevented the proliferation of MDB-forming cells induced by FAT10 and Hdac9 upregulation. The primary mechanism by which the methyl donors inhibit MDB formation is probably through inhibiting FAT10 upregulation.

Moreover, FAT10 overexpression during MDB formation increases the activity of each of the individual catalytic enzymes of the immunoproteasome- with phosphorylation of STAT1 and STAT3 in response to the combination of IFNg and TNF-a, LMP2, LMP7, and MECL-1, as well as in response to IFNg alone, FAT10 alone, and other stimuli (Oliva et al., 2010). Due to a shift in catalytic proteasomal subunits to form the immunoproteasome, there is a possibility that this increase in immunoproteasome activity is one of the mechanisms by which ethanol reduces 26s proteasome activity, which results in a decrease in protein turnover and an accumulation of misfolded proteins in the balloon cells that form MDBs in ALD. Research conducted on human liver from AH patients unequivocally demonstrated that FAT10, LMP2 and LMP7, and MECL-1 were colocalized in the MDBs. The liver cells in AH had higher levels of the immunoproteasome's catalytic proteases (French et al., 2011). The DDC model of MDB formation showed the same thing in the livers of the mice (Bardag-Gorce et al., 2010a,b,c). By stopping the rise in IFNg and TNF-a, SAMe feeding with DDC inhibited the immunoproteasome's induction and maintained the 26s proteasome. The only balloon cells that formed MDBs had elevated levels of MECL-1, FAT10, LMP2 and LMP7. These livers had lower levels of chymotrypsin (Bardag-Gorce et al., 2010a,b,c). As previously mentioned, SAMe feeding stopped MDB formation (Li et al., 2008a,b). These findings corroborate the theory that FAT10-overexpressing hepatocytes are the site of MDB formation, where immunoproteasome upregulation occurs at the expense of 26S proteasome.

In the liver biopsies from normal humans, the immunostain showed colocalization of FAT10, LMP2 and LMP7, and MECL-1 next to mitochondria. Liver biopsies of patients with alcoholic steatohepatitis showed colocalization of FAT10, ubiquitin with LMP2, LMP7, and MECL-1 within the MDBs. This indicated that the shift from the 26 proteasomes to the immunosome had occurred in the MDB-positive hepatocytes (French et al., 2011).

Rats given ethanol continuously via an intragastric tube feeding technique were compared to rats treated with the proteasome inhibitor PS-341 in terms of the epigenetics of 26S proteasome inhibition (Oliva et al., 2009a,b). The liver nuclei's 26S proteasome pathway was inhibited by prolonged ethanol consumption, which resulted in the turnover of transcription factors and histone-modifying enzymes. This had an impact on epigenetic mechanisms, particularly histone acetylation. Similar to chronic alcohol feeding, PS-341 inhibition of the proteasome also resulted in an increase in histone acetylation. Both alcohol and, more significantly, PS-341 inhibited the expression of BHMT, which may account for the observed decrease in histone methylation due to proteasome inhibition.

FAT10ylation is a signal for proteasomal degradation independent of the ubiquitination pathway (Schmidtke et al., 2013). Besides the 26 proteasome, FAT10ylation is involved in autophagia, cell cycle regulation, and apoptosis (Aichem et al., 2012). FAT10ylation was investigated in human liver biopsies from patients with AH and compared with the DDC refed mice MDB formation model (Liu et al., 2014a,b,c). RT-PCR analysis showed that Ufmylation molecules (Ufm, Uba5, Ufc1, and UfSP) were downregulated both in DDC refed mice forming MDBs and AH patients' livers where MDBs had formed indicating that both their protein quality control was downregulated. FAT10 and LMP2 and LMP7 were upregulated. FAT10-specific E1 and 2 enzymes Uba6 and USE1 were both downregulated in both patients and mice in proportion to the number of MDBs that had formed. The ubiquitin fold modifier1 (Ufm1) conjugation pathway (Ufmylation) plays an essential role in protein quality control degradation and signal transduction. In both the human and mouse models it was shown that the betaine fed with DDC prevented transcription silencing of Ufm1, Uba5, and UfSP1 and prevented upregulation of FAT10 and LMP7 in the mouse DDC-fed MDB forming model. Similar downregulation of Ufmylation was seen in AH biopsies where MDB had formed. DNMT1 and DNMT3b mRNA levels were markedly upregulated in AH implying that the maintenance of Ufmylation and methylation might be mediated by DNM1 and DNMT3b. Promoter CpG methylation may be a major mechanism silencing Ufmylation expression. When the immunohistochemical quantitation of 5'methylcytosine and hydroxymethylcytosine were performed on the hepatic nuclei in the AH patient biopsies, 5'methylcytosine was found to be elevated compared to controls establishing the fact that in AH the DNA in the nuclei is hypermethylated (Shen et al., 2015).

Alcohol abuse can impact protein quality control pathways in the liver, leading to alcoholic hepatitis (AH). One pathway involves metacaspase 1 and chaperones. When these mechanisms are unable to clear misfolded proteins, hepatocytes may become ballooned due to osmotic swelling and Mallory-Denk bodies (MDBs) may form(Figure 6.1). Proteins are typically cleared through the use of chaperones and E3 ligases for ubiquitination and subsequent breakdown. Metacaspase 1 (Mea l) and Hsp104 work together in one of these pathways, while P62 assists in linking polyubiquitinated protein aggregates to autophagy machinery. The Hsp70/Hsp40 chaperone system also plays a crucial role in the autophagic system. Ydjl interacts with Ssa1 and promotes ERAD. It is necessary for the ubiquitin-dependent degradation of some aberrant proteins. In order to facilitate the degradation of misfolded proteins labeled with ubiquitin by the 26S proteasome or recycling, VCP/97 collaborates with a variety of partners. The misfolded protein is sequestered into two inclusion bodies, Jun q and IPOD, if none of these pathways are accessible.

Fluorescence intensity semiquantitative morphometric measurements were performed on Mca1, Hsp100, Hsp40, Ydj1, and Ssal in order to assess the suitability of these pathways on AH liver biopsies. We quantitated VCP/97 and 62. In AH, there was a significant upregulation of Mca1, Hsp104, Ydj1, and p62. Upregulated tended to be Ssa1, Hsp40, and VCP/97. The increased expression of Mcal, Hsp104, Ydj1, and p62 in AH may be a sign of autophagy; ERAD, JUNO, and IPOD make up for the decreased activity of the 26S proteasome (Mendoza et al., 2015). The formation of MDB was induced and 26S proteasome activity was inhibited in vitro studies on DDC, MDB-forming hepatocytes in which VCP was chemically inhibited (Wan et al., 2006).

The same approach demonstrated that p62 expression was inhibited in vitro. The formation of MDB was significantly inhibited when p62 was overexpressed (Nan et al., 2004). The 1 month DDC withdrawn mouse model, which exposed the mice to heat shock in vivo, was used to test HPP in vivo. Seven days after heat shock, many MDBs were discovered. By day one following heat shock, there was an increase in HSP25, 70, and 90 in the serum. When fluorescent antibodies were used to stain the livers of ALD patients where MDBs had developed, the results revealed the presence of HSP70 and 90 in the MDBs (Riley et al., 2003). MDBs developed in balloon liver cells when mice were taken out of DDC for a month and given ethanol intragastrically for seven days (ZhangGouillon et al, 1998). This is the first report of animals being fed alcohol to induce the formation of MDB.

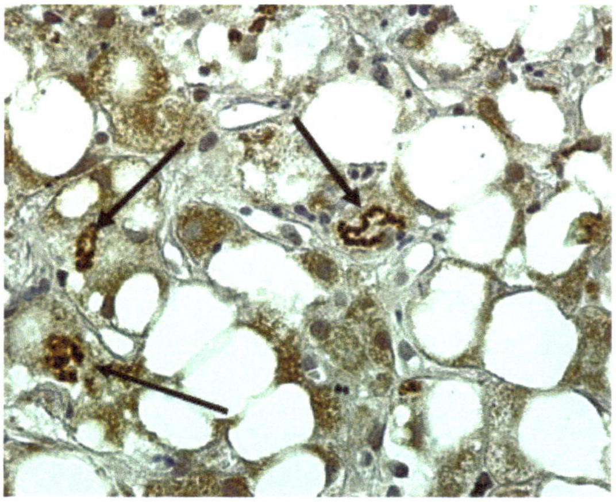

Figure 6.1. *M-30 is localized in Mallory-Denk bodies in ballooned hepatocytes by immunohistochemistry (IHC) stain in a liver from a patient with alcoholic hepatitis 520. Mallory-Denk bodies stained positive with an antibody to CK-18 fragment (arrows).*

Photograph from Amidi, F., et al., Exp. Mol. Pathol. 83, 296–300.

Source: S.W. French, The Pathophysiology of Alcoholic Liver Disease, http://dx.doi.org/10.1016/B978-0-12-804274-8.00010-2.

The significance of measuring CK-18 fragment levels in MDB aggregates for diagnosing AH in clinical settings has been highlighted. Plasma CK-18 fragment levels are a dependable non-invasive marker for severe AH. Bissonnetti et al., (2015) demonstrated that plasma levels of CK-18 fragments align with the diagnosis of AH based on liver biopsy morphology. The CK-18 fragments are derived from MDB aggregates because only MDBs stain positive by IHC antibodies to the CK-18 fragments as shown by Amidi et al., (2007).

6.14. Cell Cycle Arrest in Alcoholic Hepatitis

Patient liver biopsies stained for PCNA, Cyclin D1, p21, p27, and Ki67 revealed a rise in PCNA and Cyclin D1-stained nuclei, but very few Ki67-stained nuclei. There were also lots of P21 and P27 positive nuclei. Seldom do lungs form MDBs stain positively. While the MDBs stained positively for Ki67, the majority of the cells that formed MDBs stained negatively (French et al., 2012a,b). This indicates that the inhibition of the cell cycle between G1 and S and Ki67 is the cause of the cell cycle arrest between Cyclin D and Ki67. Throughout the entire cell cycle, Ki67 is present. The inhibition of regeneration seen in AH can cause a combination of a major loss of liver cells at the same time as an increase in apoptosis occurs (positive TUNEL cell formation) in AH (Medici et al., 2011; Le et al., 2013).

An increase in pEZH2, the MDBs, in both the mouse DDC model of MDB formation and AH is linked to this phenomenon (French et al, 2012a,b), in addition to HCCs where MDBs have developed. In both the mouse model of MDB formation and the MDB-forming cells in AH, H3K27me3 is elevated. DNA is methylated by both EZH2 and H3K27me3, but pEZH2 inhibits this process (Wei et al., 2011). When EZH2 is phosphorylated by CDK1, the 26S proteasome degrades it more quickly (Wu and Zhang, 2011).

Hepatic regeneration and homeostasis are regulated by EZH2 (Bae et al., 2015). In

EZH1 and 2 KO mice, the response of liver regeneration to CCl4-induced necrosis was significantly reduced. The loss of EZH2 can be somewhat offset by EZH1.

There is an increase in p21 expression in the AH nuclei (Crary and Albrecht, 1998; French et al., 2012a,b). When ROS, DNA damage, persistent inflammation, and the development of cirrhosis occur, the levels of p21 rise. Elevated p21 levels promote the cell cycle by inhibiting PCNA replicative function and cyclin-cdk activity. By inhibiting the cyclin/cdk complex activity and PCNA's replicative function, which is necessary for DNA polymerase D activity, p21 stops the cell cycle (Lunz et al., 2005). During the different phases of the cell cycle, either in the steady state or in response to stimuli, ubiquitination and proteasome-mediated degradation tightly and differentially regulate the stability of p21 (Lu and Hunter, 2010). Because ethanol also caused the upregulation of p38 and MAPK, it inhibits regeneration following partial hepatectomy in rats by upregulating p21 expression (Koteish et al., 2002).

A large body of research has been published on the inhibition of the cell cycle and regeneration in human AH. A review of the variables related to regeneration was released in 1994 (Fang et al., PCNA, histones, TGF2, TGF3, and HGF, among others, 1994). In 76% of cases, proliferation markers were found. TGF-a in the bile duct and hepatocytes was linked to a better prognosis ($p < .02$). With Hillan and co. (1996) examined the HGF and Ki67 serum levels in liver biopsies from patients with AH. In all 23 patients, there was an increase in HGF, which was positively correlated with more Ki67-positive liver cell nuclei in the hepatocytes during the biopsies.

Aravinthan et al (2013), conducted a study on the cell cycle in two groups of patients with ALD. One group included ALD patients with cirrhosis, while the other group consisted of ALD patients without cirrhosis. In the first group, there was limited progression in the cell cycle beyond the G1/S phase, along with an increase in p21 expression that was associated with the fibrotic stage of ALD and a negative clinical outcome. In the second group, both an increase in p21 expression and an elevated MELD score were linked to a poor prognosis. Additionally, the increase in p21 expression was connected to the extent of liver fibrosis. Moreover, Dubuquoy et al (2015), discovered that liver explants from patients with AH showed a decrease in the number of Ki67-positive liver cell nuclei, whereas those with alcoholic cirrhosis had a significant increase in Ki67-positive nuclei. The researchers suggested that the reduced Ki67 in AH may be due to lower levels of TNF-a and IL-6 compared to alcoholic cirrhosis, as these cytokines are crucial for liver cell proliferation. Ki67 serves as a mitotic marker expressed from the mid-G1 phase to the end of mitosis, playing a key role in the regulation of mitotic progression. Consequently, impaired hepatocyte mitosis and hindered liver regeneration are possible outcomes (Xia et al., 2013).

6.15. Liver Fibrosis in Alcoholic Liver Disease

The activation of the HSC and its subsequent reversion to the quiescent state have been the main topics of interest in the study of the liver scarring mechanisms in ALD. The issue is that the liver cannot regenerate normally in the presence of persistent and progressive liver injury and inflammation; instead, fibrosis develops (Seki & Brenner, 2015). TGFb and PDGF are the main factors that activate HSCs, causing them to develop into myofibroblasts and cause scarring. The process of scarring involves numerous additional cytokines, intracellular signaling, and transcription factors (Seki & Schwabe, 2015). Ding et al (2014) revealed that the regulation of the transition between regeneration and fibrogenesis is mediated by the chemokine receptors CXCR4 and CXCR7. In the liver biopsies of AH patients activated with TLR-3/4, CXCR7 was markedly upregulated.

Regarding the MyD88 signaling cascade, HSCs are the key cells in TLR4-mediated liver fibrosis (Liu et al., 2014a,b,c) because they upregulate TGFb signaling (Seki et al., 2007). TLR4 activation results in BAMBI repression, which amplifies TGFb-dependent HSC activation (Wallace et al., 2015).

One interesting new type of fibrosis which is markedly increased in the AH stage of ALD is the increase in pericellular laminin and the lumen/fibronectin ratio in areas of bile duct metaplasia (Ray et al., 1993; French et al., 1993) [now called hepatocyte progenitor cell (HPC)] (Dubuquoy et al., 2015). When liver cells switch to a bile duct phenotype (express CK7 and 19 in addition to CK8 and 18), their HSC neighbors produce laminin and fibronectin (basement membrane) type of stroma rather than collagen. This switch was supported by an increase in TWEAK and FN14 expression. The more traditional type of HSC scarring pattern seen in AH is pericellular "chicken wire" deposition of collagen (Bataller & Gao, 2011).

The changes in the HSC environment that cause them to become activated—where vitamin A stores are depleted and smooth muscle actin expression is elevated—are better understood thanks to in vitro research. Alcohol and acetaldehyde cause oxidative stress, which triggers signaling pathways that cause HSC activation, as demonstrated by combined HSC and Kupffer cells (French, 2011). The collagen 1 gene is promoted by Smad 3/4 activation and binding, which is the result of TGFb and its receptors being activated. Acetaldehyde activates PKC and/or PI-3K kinases, which in turn activates ERK 1/2 and JNK, which in turn activates AP-1. Stellate cells' TGFb type II receptor gene expression is regulated by BTEB, which is activated by AP-1. Stellate cell transcription of the collagen 1 gene is increased by the activation of CIEBP and N-1 transcription factors.

Because leptin stimulates HSCs to produce more collagen type I, it has fibrinogenic activity. JAK signaling transducers, STAT, and P13K/AKT signaling pathways are all activated in order to mediate this. By reducing LMP1, which is brought on by the Janus kinase/signal transducers and activators of transcription (JAK/STAT) pathway as well as JAK-mediated H_2O_2-dependent extracellular signal kinase 1/2 and p38 pathways, leptin-induced HSC collagen production is enhanced. In HSCs, leptin promotes the expression of TIMP-1 and causes the generation of H_2O_2. HSCs express adiponectin-like leptin, which induces activated cells to become quiescent. It also prevents HSCs from proliferating and causes them to undergo apoptosis. Alcohol-induced adiponectin reduction facilitates the generation of fibrosis by HSC. When alcohol releases adenosine into the bloodstream, it too mediates HSC function.

A Closer Look

AMP-activated Kinase (AMPK)

AMP-activated kinase (AMPK) is a critical energy sensor and regulator in eukaryotic cells, playing a pivotal role in maintaining cellular energy homeostasis. Structurally, AMPK is a heterotrimeric enzyme composed of three subunits: α (catalytic), β, and γ (regulatory). The α subunit contains the kinase domain responsible for its enzymatic activity, while the β subunit acts as a scaffold facilitating the interaction between α and γ subunits. The γ subunit contains CBS (cystathionine beta-synthase) domains that bind AMP or ATP, which is crucial for AMPK activation. AMPK activation occurs in response to an increase in the AMP/ATP ratio, signifying a low energy state within the cell. AMP binding to the γ subunit induces a conformational change that protects AMPK from dephosphorylation and increases its activity. Additionally, phosphorylation at the threonine-172 residue on the α subunit by upstream kinases such as liver kinase B1 (LKB1), Ca2+/calmodulin-dependent protein kinase β (CaMKKβ), and transforming growth factor-beta-activated kinase 1 (TAK1) further activates AMPK.

Once activated, AMPK initiates responses to restore energy balance by inhibiting anabolic processes that consume ATP, such as fatty acid synthesis, cholesterol synthesis, and protein synthesis. It phosphorylates and inactivates key enzymes like acetyl-CoA carboxylase (ACC) and HMG-CoA reductase, and downregulates mammalian target of rapamycin (mTOR) signaling, which is crucial for protein synthesis. Concurrently, AMPK activates catabolic processes that generate ATP, including glucose uptake by enhancing the translocation of glucose transporter 4 (GLUT4) to the plasma membrane and promoting glycolysis. It also stimulates fatty acid oxidation by phosphorylating and inhibiting ACC, reducing malonyl-CoA levels, and relieving the inhibition of carnitine palmitoyltransferase 1 (CPT1), the rate-limiting enzyme in fatty acid oxidation.

AMPK's influence extends beyond cellular energy regulation to whole-body energy homeostasis, including the hypothalamic control of appetite where it enhances the expression of orexigenic neuropeptides to increase food intake during energy deficiency. Dysfunctions in AMPK signaling are associated with various metabolic disorders such as type 2 diabetes, obesity, and non-alcoholic fatty liver disease (NAFLD). For example, AMPK activation improves insulin sensitivity and reduces hepatic glucose production, presenting a therapeutic target for diabetes management. In the cardiovascular system, AMPK enhances endothelial function, reduces inflammation, promotes angiogenesis, and protects against ischemia-reperfusion injury by regulating mitochondrial function and autophagy. Additionally, AMPK acts as a tumor suppressor by inhibiting cell growth and proliferation through mTOR inhibition, though cancer cells can exploit AMPK pathways to survive in low-energy conditions, making its role in cancer complex and context-dependent.

Given its central role in metabolism, AMPK represents a promising target for therapeutic intervention. Pharmacological agents like metformin and AICAR activate AMPK and are used in the treatment of metabolic diseases. Researchers continue to explore new AMPK modulators with improved specificity and efficacy for various conditions. AMPK is a master regulator of cellular energy homeostasis with significant implications for numerous physiological processes and disease states, making it a vital focus of ongoing biomedical research.

Summary

- The pathophysiology of alcoholic liver disease (ALD) is very complex because the disease progresses slowly over many years where overlapping mechanisms of liver injury come into play, culminating in liver failure.
- Fatty liver disease occurs after acute alcohol ingestion and is generally reversible with abstinence. Fatty liver is not believed to predispose a patient to any chronic form of liver disease if abstinence or moderation is maintained. Alcoholic hepatitis is an acute form of alcohol-induced liver injury that occurs with the consumption of a large quantity of alcohol over a prolonged period.
- CYP2E1 plays an important role in the pathogenesis of ALD through several mechanisms which include oxidative stress, lipid peroxidation, fatty acid hydroxylation, hydroxyethyl radical formation, autoimmunity, proteasomal inhibition, epigenetic changes, and metabolic changes.
- Epigenetic modifications include DNA methylation, histone modifications by methylation, acetylation, ubiquitination, phosphorylation, and RNA-based mechanisms.
- Histone modification could explain how ethanol feeding changes the expression of so many genes when high urinary ethanol levels (UAL) occur at the peaks of the intragastric tube-fed rat model of ALD.
- Liver biopsies from patients with AH stained for PCNA, cycling D1, p21, p27, and Ki67 showed an increase in PCNA and Cyclin D1 stained nuclei, but very few nuclei stained for Ki67. P21 and p27 positive nuclei were also numerous.
- Fatty liver can happen to anyone who drinks a lot. Alcoholic hepatitis and alcoholic cirrhosis are linked to the long-term alcohol abuse seen in alcoholics.
- People with alcohol-induced liver disease are at increased risk of also having hepatitis C virus. Others have hepatitis B virus. Your provider will test you for both and treat you if needed.
- Alcohol-induced liver disease is caused by heavy use of alcohol. The liver breaks down alcohol. If you drink more than it can process, it can become seriously damaged.
- Genetic factors predispose both to alcoholism and to alcoholic liver disease. Both monozygotic twins are more likely to be alcoholics and to develop liver cirrhosis than both dizygotic twins. Polymorphisms in the enzymes involved in the metabolism of alcohol, such as ADH, ALDH, CYP4502E1, mitochondrial dysfunction, and cytokine polymorphism may partly explain this genetic component.
- Cirrhosis is a late stage of serious liver disease marked by inflammation (swelling), fibrosis (cellular hardening) and damaged membranes preventing detoxification of chemicals in the body, ending in scarring and necrosis (cell death).

References

1. Affò, S., Dominguez, M., Lozano, J. J., Sancho-Bru, P., Rodrigo-Torres, D., Morales-Ibanez, O., et al. (2013). Transcriptome analysis identifies TNF superfamily receptors as potential therapeutic targets in alcoholic hepatitis. *Gut, 62*(3), 452–460.
2. Aichem, A., Kalveram, B., Spinnenhirn, V., Kluge, K., Catone, N., Johansen, T., et al. (2012). The proteomic analysis of endogenous FAT10 substrates identifies p62/SQSTM1 as a substrate of FAT10ylation. *Journal of Cell Science, 125*(18), 4576–4585.
3. Albano, E., Clot, P., Morimoto, M., Tamasi, A., Ingelman-Sundberg, M., & French, S. W. (1996). Role of cytochrome P4502E1-dependent formation of hydroxyethyl free radical in the development of liver damage in rats intragastrically fed with ethanol. *Hepatology, 23*(1), 155–163.
4. Amidi, F., French, B. A., Chung, D., Halsted, C., & Medici, V., & French, S. W. (2007). M-30 and 4HNE are sequestered in different aggresomes in the same hepatocytes. *Experimental and Molecular Pathology, 83*(3), 296–300.
5. Aravinthan, A., Pietrosi, G., Hoare, M., Jupp, J., Marshall, A., Verill, C., et al. (2013). Hepatocyte expression of the senescence marker p21 is linked to fibrosis and adverse liver-related outcome in alcohol-related liver disease. *PLoS One, 8*(6), e729003.
6. Arteel, G. E., Limuro, Y., Yin, M., Raleigh, J. A., & Thurman, R. G. (1997). Chronic enteral ethanol treatment causes hypoxia in rat liver tissue in vivo. *Hepatology, 25*(4), 920–926.
7. Bae, W. K., Kang, K., Yu, J. H., Yoo, K. H., Factor, V. M., Kaji, K., et al. (2015). The methyltransferases enhancer of zeste homolog (EZH) 1 and EZH2 control hepatocyte homeostasis and regeneration. *FASEB Journal, 29*(4), 1653–1662.
8. Bardag-Gorce, F., French, B. A., Joyce, M., Baires, M., Montgomery, R. O., Jun, L., et al. (2007). Histone acetyltransferase p300 modulates gene expression in an epigenetic manner at high blood alcoholic levels. *Experimental and Molecular Pathology, 82*(2), 197–202.
9. Bardag-Gorce, F., French, B. A., Li, J., Riley, N. E., Yuan, Q. X., Valinluck, V., et al. (2002). The importance of cycling of blood alcohol levels in the pathogenesis of experimental alcoholic liver disease in rats. *Gastroenterology, 123*(2), 325–335.
10. Bardag-Gorce, F., French, B. A., Nan, L., Song, H., Nguyen, S. K., Yong, H., et al. (2006). CYP2E1 induced by ethanol causes oxidative stress, proteasome inhibition and cytokine aggresome (Mallory body-like) formation. *Experimental and Molecular Pathology, 81*(3), 191–201.
11. Bardag-Gorce, F., Li, J., French, B. A., & French, S. W. (2005). The effect of ethanol-induced CYP2E1 on proteasome activity: The role of hydroxynonenal. *Experimental and Molecular Pathology, 78*(2), 109–115.
12. Bardag-Gorce, F., Li, J., Oliva, J., Lu, S. C., French, B. A., & French, S. W. (2010a). The cyclic pattern of blood alcohol levels during continuous ethanol feeding in rats. The effect of feeding S-adenosylmethionine. *Experimental and Molecular Pathology, 88*(3), 380–387.
13. Bardag-Gorce, F., Oliva, J., Dedes, J., Li, J., French, B. A., & French, S. W. (2009). Chronic ethanol feeding alters hepatocyte memory which is not altered by acute feeding. *Alcoholism: Clinical and Experimental Research, 33*(4), 684–692.

14. Bardag-Gorce, F., Oliva, J., Li, J., French, B. A., & French, S. W. (2010c). SAMe prevents the induction of the immunoproteasome and preserves the 26S proteasome in the DDC-induced MDB mouse model. *Experimental and Molecular Pathology, 88*(3), 353–362.

15. Bardag-Gorce, F., Oliva, J., Lin, A., Wong, W., Fong, S., Li, J., et al. (2010b). S-adenosylmethionine decreases the peak blood alcohol levels 3 h after an acute bolus of ethanol by inducing alcohol metabolizing enzymes in the liver. *Experimental and Molecular Pathology, 89*(3), 217–221.

16. Bataller, R., & Gao, B. (2011). Liver fibrosis in alcoholic liver disease. *Seminars in Liver Disease, 31*(2), 145–156.

17. Bertola, A., Park, O., & Gao, B. (2013). Chronic plus binge ethanol feeding synergistically induces neutrophil infiltration and liver injury in mice: A critical role for E-selectin. *Hepatology, 58*(5), 1814–1823.

18. Bissonnette, J., Altamirana, J. T., Devuc, C., Roux, O., Payance, A., Lebrec, D., et al. (2015). Plasma cytokeratin-18 fragments are an accurate non-invasive tool for the diagnosis of severe alcoholic hepatitis. *Hepatology, 52*(1 Suppl.), 1253A–1254A.

19. Boppana, N. B., Devarajan, A., Gopal, K., Barathan, M., Bakar, S. A., Shankar, E. M., et al. (2014). Blockade of CXCR2 signaling: A potential therapeutic target for preventing neutrophil-mediated inflammatory diseases. *Experimental Biology and Medicine, 239*(4), 509–518.

20. Butura, A., Nilsson, K., Morgan, K., Morgan, T. R., French, S. W., Johansson, I., et al. (2008). The impact of CYP2E1 on the development of alcoholic liver disease as studied in a transgenic mouse model. *Journal of Hepatology, 50*(3), 572–583.

21. Chang, B., Xu, M. J., Zhou, Z., Cai, Y., Li, M., Wang, M., et al. (2015). Short- or long-term high-fat diet feeding plus acute ethanol binge synergistically induce acute liver injury in mice: An important role for CXCL1. *Hepatology, 62*(4), 1070–1085.

22. Cohen, J. I., Roychowdhury, S., McMullen, M. R., Stavitsky, A. B., & Nagy, L. E. (2010). Complement and alcoholic liver disease: Role of C1q in the pathogenesis of ethanol-induced liver injury in mice. *Gastroenterology, 139*(2), 664–674.

23. Crarcy, G. S., & Albrecht, J. H. (1998). Expression of cyclin-dependent kinase inhibitor p21 in human liver. *Hepatology, 28*(3), 738–743.

24. Das, D., Barnes, M. A., & Nagy, L. E. (2014). Anaphylatoxin C5a modulates hepatic stellate cell migration. *Fibrogenesis & Tissue Repair, 7*(1), 1–9.

25. DeSantis, D. A., Ko, C. W., Liu, Y., Liu, X., Hise, A. G., Nunez, G., et al. (2013). Alcohol-induced liver injury is modulated by Nlrp3 and LCRC4 inflammasomes in mice. *Mediators of Inflammation, 2013*, Article ID 751374.

26. Ding, B. S., Cao, Z., Lis, R., Nolan, D. J., Guo, P., Simons, M., et al. (2014). Divergent angiocrine signals from vascular niche balance liver regeneration and fibrosis. *Nature, 505*(7482), 97–102.

27. Dubuquoy, L., Louvet, A., Lassailly, G., Truant, S., Boleslawski, E., Artru, F., et al. (2015). Progenitor cell expansion and impaired hepatocyte regeneration in explanted livers from alcoholic hepatitis. *Gut*. http://dx.doi.org/10.1136/gutjnl-2014-308410.

28. Esfandari, F., Medici, V., Wong, D. H., Jose, S., Dolatshahi, M., Quinlivan, E., et al. (2010). Epigenetic regulation of hepatic endoplasmic reticulum stress pathways in the ethanol fed

cystathionine beta synthase-deficient mouse. *Hepatology, 51*(3), 932–941.

29. Fang, J. W., Bird, G. L., Nakamura, T., Davis, G. L., & Lau, J. Y. (1994). Hepatocyte proliferation as an indicator of outcome in acute alcoholic hepatitis. *Lancet, 343*(8905), 820–823.
30. Fataccioli, V., Andraud, E., Gentil, M., French, S. W., Rouach, H., et al. (2003). Effects of chronic ethanol administration on rat liver proteasome activities: Relationship with oxidative stress. *Hepatology, 29*(1), 14–20.
31. French, B. A., Oliva, J., Bardag-Gorce, F., & French, S. W. (2011). The immunoproteasome in steatohepatitis: Its role in Mallory-Denk body formation. *Experimental and Molecular Pathology, 90*(3), 252–256.
32. French, B. A., Oliva, J., Bardag-Gorce, F., Li, J., Zhong, J., Buslon, V., et al. (2012a). Mallory-Denk bodies form when EZH2/H3k27me3 fails to methylate DNA in the nuclei of human and liver cells. *Experimental and Molecular Pathology, 92*(3), 318–326.
33. French, S. W. (2001). Intragastric ethanol infusion model for cellular and molecular studies of alcoholic liver disease. *Journal of Biomedical Science, 8*(1), 20–27.
34. French, S. W. (2011). Alcoholic liver disease. In S. P. S. Mong (Ed.), *Molecular Pathology of Liver Diseases* (pp. 511–526). Springer Science + Business Media.
35. French, S. W. (2013a). Epigenetic events in liver cancer resulting from alcoholic liver disease. *Alcohol Research, 35*(1), 57–67.
36. French, S. W. (2013b). The importance of CYP2E1 in the pathogenesis of alcoholic liver disease and drug toxicity and the role of the proteasome. In A. Dey (Ed.), *Cytochrome P4502E1: Its Role in Disease and Drug Metabolism* (Subcellular Biochemistry, Vol. 67, pp. 73–100). Springer Science.
37. French, S. W. (2013c). A nutritional approach to prevent alcohol liver disease. In R. Watson et al. (Eds.), *Alcohol and Liver Disease: Alcohol Nutrition Health Consequences* (pp. 473–482). Humana Press.
38. French, S. W. (2015). How to prevent alcoholic liver disease. *Experimental and Molecular Pathology, 98*(3), 304–307.
39. French, S. W., Benson, N. C., & Sun, P. S. (1984). Centrilobular liver necrosis induced by hypoxia in chronic ethanol-fed rats. *Hepatology, 4*(6), 912–917.
40. French, S. W., French, B. A., Oliva, J., Li, J., Bardag-Gorce, F., Tillman, B., et al. (2012b). Fat10 knockout mice fail to develop Mallory-Denk bodies in the DDC mouse model. *Experimental and Molecular Pathology, 93*(3), 309–314.
41. French, S. W., Nash, J., Shitabata, P., Kachi, K., Hara, C., Chedid, A., et al. (1993). Pathology of alcoholic liver disease. *Seminars in Liver Disease, 13*(2), 154–169.
42. Gao, Y., Theng, S. S., Zhuo, J., Teo, W. B., Ren, J., & Lee, C. G. (2014). FAT10, a ubiquitin-like protein, confers malignant properties in nontumorigenic and tumorigenic cells. *Carcinogenesis, 35*(4), 923–934.
43. Gouillon, Z., Lucas, D., Li, J., Hagbjork, A. L., French, B. A., Fu, P., et al. (2000). Inhibition of ethanol-induced liver disease in the intragastric feeding rat model by chlormethiazole. *Proceedings of the Society for Experimental Biology and Medicine, 224*(4), 302–308.
44. Greenberg, S. S., Jie, O., Zhao, X., & Wang, J. F. (1998). Role of PKC and tyrosine kinase in ethanol-mediated inhibition of LPS-inducible nitric oxide synthase. *Alcohol, 16*(3), 167–175.

45. Heritage, M. L., Murphy, T. L., Bridle, K. R., Anderson, G. J., Crawford, D. H., & Fletcher, L. M. (2009). Hepcidin regulation in wild type and Hfe knockout mice in response to alcohol consumption: Evidence for an alcohol-induced hypoxic response. *Alcoholism: Clinical and Experimental Research, 33*(8), 1391–1400.

46. Hillan, K. J., Logan, M. C., Ferrier, R. K., Bird, G. L., Bennett, G. L., McKay, I. C., et al. (1996). Hepatocyte proliferation and serum hepatocyte growth factor levels in patients with alcoholic hepatitis. *Journal of Hepatology, 24*(3), 385–390.

47. Jung, Y., Brown, K. D., Witek, R. P., Omenetti, A., Yang, L., Vandongen, M., et al. (2008). Accumulation of hedgehog-responsive progenitors parallels alcoholic liver disease severity in mice and humans. *Gastroenterology, 134*(6), 1532–1543.

48. Kathirvel, E., Chen, P., Morgan, K., French, S. W., & Morgan, T. R. (2010). Oxidative stress and regulation of anti-oxidant enzymes in cytochrome P4502E1 transgenic mouse model of non-alcoholic fatty liver. *Journal of Gastroenterology and Hepatology, 25*(7), 1136–1143.

49. Kazankov, K., Barrera, F., Moller, H. J., Bibby, B. M., Vilstrup, H., George, J., et al. (2014). Soluble CD163, a macrophage activation marker, is independently associated with fibrosis in patients with chronic viral hepatitis B and C. *Hepatology, 60*(2), 521–530.

50. Khachatoorian, R., Dawson, D., Maloney, E. M., Wang, J., French, B. A., French, S. W., et al. (2013). SAMe treatment prevents the ethanol-induced epigenetic alterations of genes in the Toll-like receptor pathway. *Experimental and Molecular Pathology, 94*(3), 243–246.

51. Kim, S. Y., Choi, Y. J., Joung, S. M., Lee, B. H., Jung, Y. S., & Lee, J. Y. (2009). Hypoxic stress up-regulates the expression of Toll-like receptor 4 in macrophages via hypoxia-inducible factor. *Immunology, 129*(4), 516–524.

52. Koteish, A., Yang, S., Lin, H., Huang, J., & Diehl, A. M. (2002). Ethanol induces redox-sensitive cell-cycle inhibitors and inhibits liver regeneration after partial hepatectomy. *Alcoholism: Clinical and Experimental Research, 26*(11), 1710–1718.

53. Lage, S. L., Longo, C., Branco, L. M., da Costa, T. B., Buzzo, C. D. L., & Bortoluci, K. R. (2014). Emerging concepts about NAIP/NLRC4 inflammasomes. *Frontiers in Immunology, 5*, 309.

54. Lazaro, R., Wu, R., Lee, S., Zhu, N. L., Chen, C. L., French, S. W., et al. (2015). Osteopontin deficiency does not prevent but promotes alcoholic neutrophilic hepatitis in mice. *Hepatology, 61*(1), 129–140.

55. Le, M., Enbom, E., Traum, P. K., Medici, V., Halsted, C. H., & French, S. W. (2013). Alcoholic liver disease patients treated with S-adenosyl-L-methionine: An in-depth look at liver morphologic data comparing pre and post treatment liver biopsies. *Experimental and Molecular Pathology, 95*(2), 187–191.

56. Lee, J., French, B., Morgan, T., French, S. W., et al. (2013). The liver is populated by a broad spectrum of macrophages. In alcoholic hepatitis, the macrophages are M1 and M2. *Experimental and Molecular Pathology, 96*(2), 118–125.

57. Li, J., Bardag-Gorce, F., Dedes, J., French, B. A., Oliva, J., Amidi, F., et al. (2008b). S-adenosylmethionine prevents Mallory-Denk body formation in drug-primed mice by inhibiting the epigenetic memory. *Hepatology, 47*(2), 613–624.

58. Li, J., Bardag-Gorce, F., Oliva, J., Dedes, J., French, B. A., French, S. W., et al. (2010). Gene expression modifications in the liver caused by binge drinking and S-adenosylmethionine feeding: The role of epigenetic changes. *Genes & Nutrition, 5*(3), 169–179.

59. Li, J., French, B. A., Fu, P., & French, S. W. (2001). Liver necrosis induced by thyroid hormone administration in rats fed ethanol. *Experimental and Molecular Pathology, 71*(2), 79–88.

60. Li, J., French, B. A., Fu, P., Bardag-Gorce, F., French, S. W., et al. (2003). Mechanisms of alcoholic cyclic pattern: Role of catecholamines. *American Journal of Physiology–Gastrointestinal and Liver Physiology, 285*(3), G442–G448.

61. Li, J., French, B. A., Fu, P., Bardag-Gorce, F., French, S. W., et al. (2004a). Catecholamines are involved in the mechanism of the urinary alcohol level cycle in rats fed ethanol intragastrically at a constant rate. *Life Sciences, 75*(23), 3043–3051.

62. Li, J., French, B., Wu, Y., Vankatesh, R., Montgomery, R., Bardag-Gorce, F., et al. (2004b). Liver hypoxia and lack of recovery after reperfusion at high blood alcohol levels in the intragastric feeding model of alcohol liver disease. *Experimental and Molecular Pathology, 77*(2), 184–192.

63. Li, J., Li, X. M., Caudill, M., Malysheva, O., Bardag-Gorce, F., Oliva, J., et al. (2011). Betaine feeding prevents the blood alcohol cycle in rats fed alcohol continuously for 1 month using the rat intragastric tube feeding model. *Experimental and Molecular Pathology, 91*(3), 540–547.

64. Li, J., Nguyen, V., French, B. A., Parlow, A. F., Su, G. L., Fu, P., et al. (2008a). Mechanisms of the alcohol cyclic pattern: Role of the hypothalamic-pituitary-thyroid axis. *American Journal of Physiology–Gastrointestinal and Liver Physiology, 279*(1), G118–G125.

65. Li, Y., Cui, Y., Hart, S. N., Klaasen, C. D., & Zhong, X. (2009). Dynamic patterns of histone methylation are associated with ontogenic expression of the Cyp3a genes during mouse liver maturation. *Molecular Pharmacology, 75*(5), 1171–1179.

66. Liu, H., French, B. A., Nelson, T., Li, J., Tillman, B., & French, S. W. (2015). IL-8 signaling is up-regulated in alcoholic hepatitis and DDC fed mice with Mallory-Denk bodies (MDBs) present. *Experimental and Molecular Pathology, 99*(4), 320–325.

67. Liu, H., Gong, M., French, B. A., Li, J., Tillman, B., & French, S. W. (2014c). Mallory-Denk body (MDB) formation modulates ufmylation expression epigenetically in alcoholic hepatitis (AH) and non-alcoholic steatohepatitis (NASH). *Experimental and Molecular Pathology, 97*(3), 477–483.

68. Liu, H., Li, J., Tillman, B., French, B. A., & French, S. W. (2014b). Ufmylation and FATylation pathways are down regulated in human alcoholic and non-alcoholic steatohepatitis and mice fed DDC where Mallory-Denk bodies (MDBs) form. *Experimental and Molecular Pathology, 97*(1), 81–88.

69. Liu, H., Tillman, B., Morgan, T., French, B. A., & French, S. W. (2014a). TLR3/4 signaling is mediated via the NFkB-CXCR4/7 pathway in human alcoholic hepatitis and non-alcoholic steatohepatitis which formed MDB-Denk bodies. *Experimental and Molecular Pathology, 97*(2), 234–240.

70. Lu, Z., & Hunter, T. (2010). Ubiquitylation and proteasomal degradation of the p27Cip1 and p57Kip2 CDK inhibitors. *Cell Cycle, 9*(12), 2342–2352.

71. Lunz III, J. G., Tsuji, H., Nozaki, I., Murase, N., & Demetris, A J. (2005). An inhibitor of cyclin-dependent kinase, stress-induced p21Waf-1/Cip-1, mediates hepatocyte mito-inhibition during the evolution of cirrhosis. *Hepatology, 41*(6), 1262–1271.

72. Lytton, S. D., Helander, A., Zhang-Gouillon, Z. Q., Stokklan, K., Bordone, R., Arico, S., et al. (1999). Autoantibodies against cytochromes P-4502E1 and P-4503A in alcoholics. *American Society of Pharmacology and Experimental Therapeutics, 55*(2), 223–233.

73. Machida, K. (2013). Tumor-initiating stem-like cells and drug resistance: Carcinogenesis through Toll-like receptors, environmental factors, and virus. *Drug Delivery and Translational Research, 3*(2), 152–164.

74. Machida, K., Chen, C. L., Liu, J. C., Kashiwabara, C., Feldman, D., French, S. W., et al. (2012). Cancer stem cells generated by alcohol, diabetes, and hepatitis C virus. *Journal of Gastroenterology and Hepatology, 27*(Suppl. 2), 19–22.

75. Maher, J. (2001). The CYP2E1 knockout delivers another punch: First ASH, now NASH. *Hepatology, 33*(2), 311–312.

76. McClain, C. J., Cohen, D. A., Dinarello, C. A., Cannon, J. G., Shedlofsky, S. I., & Kaplan, A. M. (1986). Serum interleukin-1 (IL-1) activity in alcoholic hepatitis. *Life Sciences, 39*(12), 1479–1485.

77. Medici, V., & Halsted, C. H. (2013). Folate, alcoholic, and liver disease. *Molecular Nutrition & Food Research, 57*(4), 596–606.

78. Medici, V., Virata, M. C., Peerson, J. M., Stabler, S. P., French, S. W., Gregory III, S. F., et al. (2011). S-adenosylmethione treatment for alcoholic liver disease: A double-blinded, randomized, placebo-controlled trial. *Alcoholism: Clinical and Experimental Research, 35*(11), 1960–1965.

79. Mendenhall, C. L., Moritz, T. E., Roselle, G. A., Morgan, T. R., Nemchansky, B. A., Tamburro, C. H., et al. (1995). Protein energy malnutrition in severe alcoholic hepatitis: Diagnosis and response to treatment. *Journal of Parenteral and Enteral Nutrition, 19*(4), 258–265.

80. Mendoza, A. S., Dorce, J., Peng, Y., French, B. A., Tillman, B., Li, J., et al. (2015). Levels of metacaspase 1 and chaperones related to protein quality control in alcoholic and non-alcoholic steatohepatitis. *Experimental and Molecular Pathology, 99*(2), 123–131.

81. Miyamoto, K., & French, S. W. (1988). Hepatic adenine nucleotide metabolism measured in vivo in rats fed ethanol and a high fat-low protein diet: Relation to pathogenesis of alcohol-induced liver injury in the rat. *Hepatology, 8*(1), 53–60.

82. Mookerjee, R. F., Lackner, C., Stauber, R., Stadlbauer, V., Deheragoda, M., et al. (2011). The role of liver biopsy in the diagnosis and prognosis of patients with acute deterioration of alcoholic cirrhosis. *Journal of Hepatology, 55*(5), 1103–1111.

83. Morales-Ibanez, O., Domínguez, M., Ki, S. H., Marcos, M., Chaves, J. F., Nguyen-Khac, E., et al. (2013). Human and experimental evidence supporting a role for osteopontin in alcoholic hepatitis. *Hepatology, 58*(5), 1742–1756.

84. Morgan, K., French, S. W., & Morgan, T. R. (2002). Production of a cytochrome P450 2E1 transgenic mouse and initial evaluation of alcohol liver damage. *Hepatology, 36*(1), 122–134.

85. Morimoto, M., Hagbjörk, A. L., Wan, Y. J., Fu, P. C., Clot, P., Albano, E., et al. (1995). Modulation of experimental alcoholic-induced liver disease by cytochrome P450 2E1 inhibitors. *Hepatology, 21*(6), 1610–1617.

86. Morimoto, M., Zern, M. A., Hagbjörk, A. L., Ingelman-Sundberg, M., & French, S. W. (1994). Fish oil, alcohol, and liver pathology: Role of cytochrome P450/2E1. *Proceedings of the Society for Experimental Biology and Medicine, 207*(2), 197–205.

87. Nan, L., Dedes, J., French, B. A., Bardag-Gorce, F., Li, J., Wu, Y., et al. (2006). Mallory body (cytokeratin aggresomes) formation is prevented in vitro by p38 inhibitor. *Experimental and Molecular Pathology, 80*(3), 228–240.

88. Nan, L., Wu, Y., Bardag-Gorce, F., Li, J., French, B. A., & Wilson, L. T. (2005b). The p150/50 NF-kappaB pathway is essential for Mallory body formation. *Experimental and Molecular Pathology, 78*(3), 198–206.

89. Nan, L., Wu, Y., Bardag-Gorce, F., Li, J., French, B. A., Fun, A. N., et al. (2004). p62 is involved in the mechanism of Mallory body formation. *Experimental and Molecular Pathology, 77*(3), 168–175.

90. Nan, L., Wu, Y., Bardag-Gorce, F., Li, J., French, B. A., Wilson, L. T., Khahn-Nguyen, S., et al. (2005a). RNA interference of VCP/p97 increases Mallory body formation. *Experimental and Molecular Pathology, 78*(1), 1–9.

91. Nanji, A. A., & French, S. W. (1989b). Dietary linoleic acid is required for development of experimentally induced alcoholic liver injury. *Life Sciences, 44*(4), 223–227.

92. Nanji, A. A., Jui, L. T., & French, S. W. (1989c). Effect of chronic carbon monoxide exposure on experimental alcoholic liver injury in rats. *Life Sciences, 45*(7), 885–890.

93. Nanji, A. A., Mendenhall, C. L., & French, S. W. (1989a). Beef fat prevents alcoholic liver disease in the rat. *Alcoholism: Clinical and Experimental Research, 13*(1), 15–19.

94. Oliva, J., Bardag-Gorce, F., Li, J., French, B. A., & French, S. W. (2011). S-adenosylmethionine prevents the up regulation of Toll-like receptor (TLR) signaling caused by chronic ethanol feeding in rats. *Experimental and Molecular Pathology, 90*(3) 329–343.

95. Oliva, J., Bardag-Gorce, F., Li, J., French, B. A., Nguyen, S. K., & Lu, S. C. (2009a). Betaine prevents Mallory-Denk body formation in drug-primed mice by epigenetic mechanisms. *Experimental and Molecular Pathology, 86*(1), 77–86.

96. Oliva, J., Bardag-Gorce, F., Lin, A., French, B. A., & French, S. W. (2010). The role of cytokines in UbD promoter regulation and Mallory-Denk body-like aggresomes. *Experimental and Molecular Pathology, 89*(1), 1–8.

97. Oliva, J., Dedes, J., Li, J., French, S. W., & Bardag-Gorce, F. (2009b). Epigenetics of proteasome exhibition in the liver of rats fed ethanol chronically. *World Journal of Gastroenterology, 15*(6), 705–712.

98. Oliva, J., French, B. A., Li, J., Bardag-Gorce, F., Fu, P., & French, S. W. (2008). Sirt1 is involved in energy metabolism: The role of chronic ethanol feeding and resveratrol. *Experimental and Molecular Pathology, 85*(2), 155–159.

99. Pal-Bhadra, M., Bhadra, U., Jackson, D. E., Mamatha, L., Park, P. H., & Shukla, S. D. (2007). Distinct methylation patterns in histone H3 at Lys-4 and Lys-9 correlate with up- & down-regulation of genes by ethanol in hepatocytes. *Life Sciences, 81*(12), 979–987.

100. Park, P. H., Lim, R. W., & Shukla, S. D. (2005). Involvement of histone acetyltransferase (HAT) in ethanol-induced acetylation of histone H3 in hepatocytes: Potential mechanism for gene expression. *American Journal of Physiology - Gastrointestinal and Liver Physiology, 289*(6), G1124–G1136.

101. Peng, Y., French, B. A., Tillman, B., Morgan, T. R., & French S. W. (2014). The inflammasome in alcoholic hepatitis: Its relationship with Mallory-Denk body formation. *Experimental and Molecular Pathology, 97*(3), 305–313.

102. Petrasek, J., Iracheta-Vallve, A., Saha, B., Satischandran, A, Kodys, K., Fitzgerald, K. A., et al. (2015). Metabolic danger signals, uric acid and ATP, mediate inflammatory cross-talk between

hepatocytes and immune cells in alcoholic liver disease. *Journal of Leukocyte Biology, 98*(2), 249–256.

103. Pradere, J. P., Troeger, J. S., Dapito, D. H., Mencin, A. A., & Schwabe, R. F. (2010). Toll-like receptor 4 and hepatic fibrogenesis. *Seminars in Liver Disease, 30*(3), 232–244.
104. Ray, M. B., Mendenhall, C. L., French, S. W., & Gartside, P. S. (1993). Bile duct changes in alcoholic liver disease: The Veterans Administration Cooperative Study Group. *Liver, 13*(1), 36–45.
105. Resineci, K., & Casey, C. A. (2012). Molecular mechanisms of alcoholic fatty liver. *Indian Journal of Pharmacology, 44*(3), 299–303.
106. Riley, N. E., Li, J., McPhaul, L. W., Bardag-Gorce, F., Lue, Y. H., & French, S. W. (2003). Heat shock proteins are present in Mallory bodies (cytokeratin aggresomes) in human liver biopsy specimens. *Experimental and Molecular Pathology, 74*(3), 168–172.
107. Ronis, M. J., Korourian, S., Zipperman, M., Hakkak, R., Badger, T. M., et al. (2004). Dietary saturated fat reduces alcoholic hepatotoxicity in rats by altering fatty acid metabolism and membrane composition. *Journal of Nutrition, 134*(5), 904–912.
108. Rouach, H., Fataccioli, V., Gentil, M., French, S. W., Morimoto, M., & Nordmann, R. (1997). Effect of chronic ethanol feeding on lipid peroxidation and protein oxidation in relation to liver pathology. *Hepatology, 25*(2), 351–355.
109. Salminen, A., Ojala, J., & Kaarniranta, K. (2013). Mitochondrial dysfunction and oxidative stress activate inflammasomes: Impact on the aging process and age-related diseases. *Cellular and Molecular Life Sciences, 69*(17), 2999–3013.
110. Schmidtke, G., Aichem, A., Groettrup, M., et al. (2013). FAT10ylation as a signal for proteasomal degradation. *Biochimica et Biophysica Acta (BBA)-Molecular Cell Research, 1843*(1), 97–102.
111. Seki, E., & Brenner, D. A. (2008). Toll-like receptors and adaptor molecules in liver disease update. *Hepatology, 48*(1), 322–325.
112. Seki, E., & Brenner, D. A. (2015). Recent advancement of molecular mechanisms of liver fibrosis. *Journal of Hepatobiliary Pancreatic Sciences, 22*(8), 512–518.
113. Seki, E., & Schwabe, R. F. (2015). Hepatic inflammation and fibrosis: Functional links and key pathways. *Hepatology, 61*(3), 1066–1079.
114. Seki, E., De Minicis, S., Osterreicher, C. H., Kluwe, J., Osawa, Y., Brenner, D. A., et al. (2007). TLR4 enhances TGF-β signaling and hepatic fibrosis. *Nature Medicine, 13*(11), 1324–1332.
115. Seth, D., Gorrell, M. D., Cordoba, S., McCaughan, G. W., & Haber, P. S. (2006). Intrahepatic gene expression in human alcoholic hepatitis. *Journal of Hepatology, 45*(3), 306–320.
116. Shearn, C. T., Smathers, R. L., Backos, D. S., Reigan, P., Orlicky, D. J., & Petersen, D. R. (2013). Increased carbonylation of the lipid phosphatase PTEN contributes to Akt2 activation in a murine model of early alcohol-induced steatosis. *Free Radical Biology and Medicine, 65*, 680–692.
117. Shen, H., French, B. A., Liu, H., Tillman, B. C., & French, S. W. (2014). Increased activity of the complement system in the liver of patients with alcoholic hepatitis. *Experimental and Molecular Pathology, 97*(3), 338–344.

118. Shen, H., French, B. A., Tillman, B. C., Li, J., & French, S. W. (2015). Increased DNA methylation in the livers of patients with alcoholic hepatitis. *Experimental and Molecular Pathology, 99*(3), 326–329.

119. Shukla, S., Velasquez, F., French, S. W., Lu, S., Ticku, M. K., & Zahkari, S. (2008). The emerging role of epigenetics in the actions of alcohol. *Alcoholism: Clinical and Experimental Research, 32*(9), 1526–1532.

120. Szabo, G., Petrasek, J., & Bala, S. (2012). Innate immunity and alcoholic liver disease. *Digestive Diseases, 30*(Suppl. 1), 55–60.

121. Tirnitz-Parker, J. E., Viebahn, C. S., Jakubowski, A., Klopcic, B. R., Olynyk, J. K., Yeoh, G. C., et al. (2010). Tumor necrosis factor-like inducer of apoptosis is a mitogen for liver progenitor cells. *Hepatology, 52*(1), 291–302.

122. Wallace, M. C., Friedman, S. L., & Mann, D. A. (2015). Emerging and disease-specific mechanisms of hepatic stellate cell activation. *Seminars in Liver Disease, 35*(2), 107–118.

123. Wan, J. M., Sit, W. H., Lee, C. L., Fu, K. H., & Chan, D. K. (2006) Protection of lethal toxicity of endotoxin by *Salvia miltiorrhiza* BUNGE is via reduction in tumor necrosis factor alpha release and liver injury. *International Immunopharmacology, 6*(5), 750–758.

124. Wan, J. M., Sit, W. H., Wang, H. J., Gao, B., Zakhari, S., & Nagy, L. E. (2012). Inflammation in alcoholic liver disease. *Annual Review of Nutrition, 32*, 343–368.

125. Wei, Y., Chen, Y. H., Li, L. Y., Lang, J., Yeh, S. P., Shi, B., et al. (2011). CDK1-dependent phosphorylation of EZH2 suppresses methylation of H3K27 and promotes osteogenic differentiation of human mesenchymal stem cells. *Nature Cell Biology, 13*(1), 87–94.

126. Winkles, J. A. (2008). The TWEAK-FN14 cytokine-receptor axis: Discovery, biology, and therapeutic targeting. *Nature Reviews Drug Discovery, 7*(5), 411–425.

127. Wree, A., Eguchi, A., McGeough, M. D., Pena, C. A., Johnson, C. D., Canbay, A., et al. (2014). NLRP3 inflammasome activation results in hepatocyte pyroptosis, liver inflammation, and fibrosis in mice. *Hepatology, 59*(3), 898–910.

128. Wu, S. C., & Zhang, Y. (2011). Cyclin-dependent kinase 1. CDK1-mediated phosphorylation of enhancer of Zeste 2 (Ezh2) regulates its stability. *Journal of Biological Chemistry, 286*(32), 28511–28519.

129. Wu, Y., Nan, L., Bardag-Gorce, F., Li, J., French, B. A., Wilson, L T., et al. (2005). The role of laminin-integrin signaling in triggering Mallory-Denk body formation: An in vivo and in vitro study. *Experimental and Molecular Pathology, 79*(1), 1–8.

130. Xia, J., Zhou, Y., Li, H., Wang, Y., Wu, Q., Bao, J., et al. (2013). Loss of histone deacetylases 1 and 2 in hepatocytes impairs murine liver regeneration through Ki67 depletion. *Hepatology, 58*(6), 2089–2098.

131. Xie, Y. D., Feng, B., Gao, Y., & Wei, L. (2014). Effect of abstinence from alcohol on survival of patients with alcoholic cirrhosis: A systematic review and meta-analysis. *Hepatology Research, 44*(4), 436–449.

132. You, M., Fischer, M., Deeg, M. A., & Crabb, D. W. (2002). Ethanol induces fatty acid synthesis pathways by activation of sterol regulatory element-binding protein (SREBP). *Journal of Biological Chemistry, 277*(36), 29342–29347.

133. You, M., Jogasuria, A., Taylor, C., & Wu, J. (2015). Sirtuin 1 signaling and alcoholic fatty liver disease. *Hepatobiliary Surgery and Nutrition, 4*(2), 88–100.

134. Zhang-Gouillon, Z. Q., Yuan, Q. X., Hu, B., Marceau, N., French, B. A., & Gaal, K. (1998). Mallory body formation by ethanol feeding in drug-primed mice. *Hepatology, 27*(1), 116–122.

135. Zhang, T., Guo, C. J., Li, Y., Douglas, S. D., Qi, X. X., Song, L., et al. (2003). Interleukin-1β induces macrophage inflammatory protein 1β expression in human hepatocytes. *Cellular Immunology, 226*(1), 45–53.

136. Zhou, D., Lin, Z., Huang, C., Xie, D., Zhan, S., Kong, L., et al. (2014). Cytochrome P4502E1 inhibitor: A potential oxidative stress regulator in liver disease. *Hepatology Research, 44*(5), 591–592.

Chapter 7

COMPLICATIONS OF CIRRHOSIS AND ASCITES

Contents

Introduction

Fibrosis is a reparative response to chronic liver damage that is usually reversible. The main source of the scar tissue found in fibrosis is hepatic stellate cells. As a result fibrosis often occurs before cirrhosis, and it is the cause of the latter disease's side effects, such as hepatic encephalopathy (HE), ascites (A), portal hypertension (PHT), gastroesophageal varices (GEPV), hepatorenal syndrome (HRS), hepatopulmonary syndrome (HPS), and hepatocellular carcinoma (HCC). Furthermore, cirrhosis can also be diagnosed as uniform micronodular cirrhosis, with nodules measuring less than 3 mm in diameter; larger nodules, on the other hand, are classified as macronodular cirrhosis and typically indicate an advanced stage of the disease. In the end, bacterial infections, large volume paracentesis, and gastrointestinal hemorrhage may be found to be one or more of the precipitating factors in about half of the patients. For this reason, it's critical to discuss the most significant and common cirrhosis complications.

Orientation and Directional Terms

<table>
<tr><th>Term</th><th>Definition</th><th>Illustration</th></tr>
<tr><td>Renin-angiotensin-aldosterone system (RAAS)</td><td>The renin-angiotensin-aldosterone system (RAAS) is the system of hormones, proteins, enzymes and reactions that regulate your blood pressure and blood volume on a long-term basis.</td><td>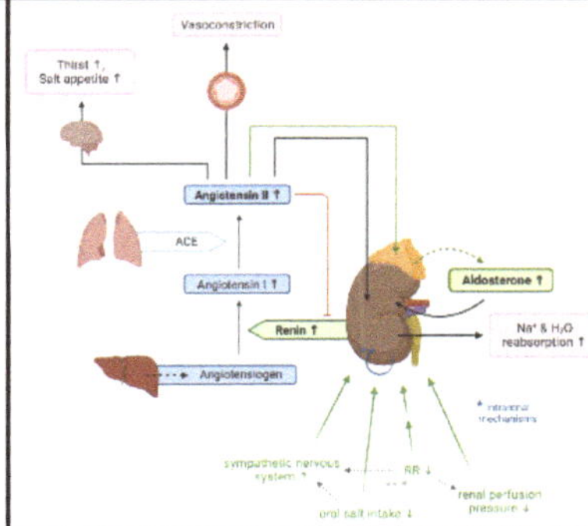
</td></tr>
<tr><td>Hepatorenal syndrome (HRS)</td><td>HRS is characterized by acute onset and rapidly progressing kidney failure with a doubling of serum creatinine to > 2.5 mg/dL (corresponding to a 50% reduction in the creatinine clearance rate) in less than 2 wk, usually associated with multiorgan damage.</td><td>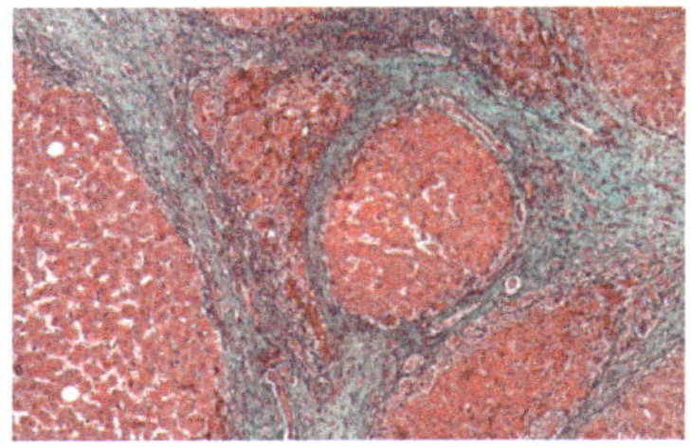</td></tr>
<tr><td>Large-volume paracentesis</td><td>Large-volume paracentesis is the removal of ascitic fluid as much as possible to relieve the symptoms of a tense abdomen and dyspnea.</td><td>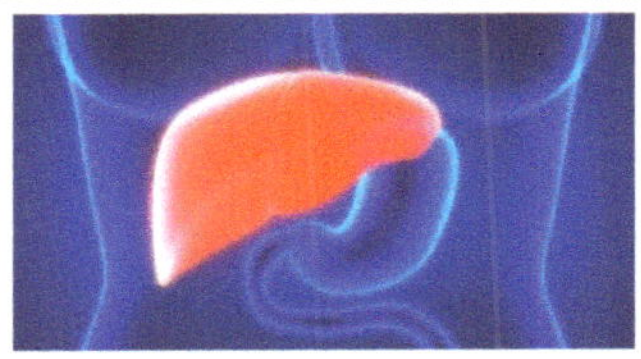</td></tr>
<tr><td>Portal hypertension (PHT)</td><td>Portal hypertension (PHT) indicates increased pressure in portal venous system. Normal portal venous pressure is 10 mmHg (14 cm of H_2O). Patients usually present with splenomegaly, life threatening gastrointestinal bleeding and ascites.</td><td>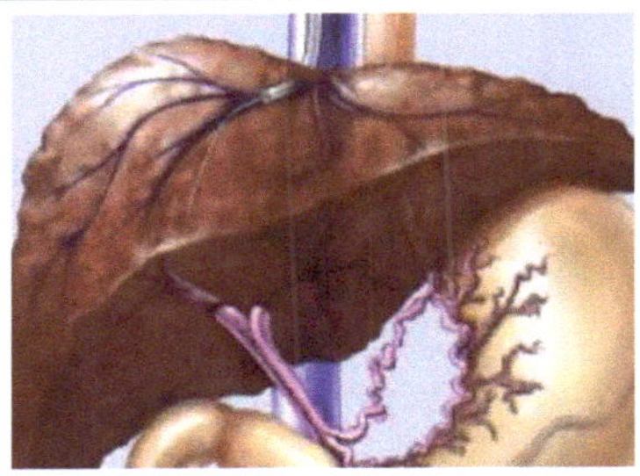</td></tr>
<tr><td>Orthotopic liver transplantation (OLT)</td><td>Orthotopic liver transplantation (OLT) involves the substitution of a diseased native liver with a normal liver (or part of one) taken from a deceased or living donor.</td><td>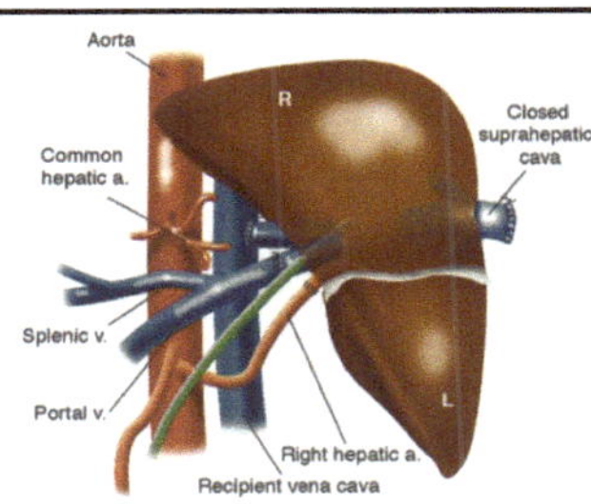
</td></tr>
</table>

7.1. Complications of Cirrhosis

7.1.1. Portal Hypertension

Significant morbidity and mortality in patients with cirrhosis are caused by complications associated with pulmonary hypertension (PH) (Ginès and Cárdenas, 2009; Bloom et al, 2015). Understanding the pathophysiology and etiopathogenesis of the PHT mechanism has advanced significantly in recent years (Figure 7.1).

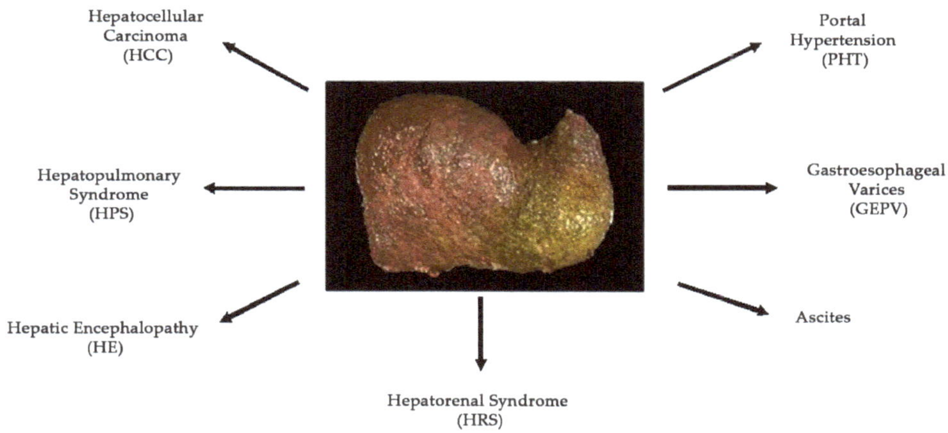

Figure 7.1. *Schematic representation of the main complications of cirrhosis. At the center, a photograph of a human cirrhotic liver is shown, and its relation with portal hypertension (PHT), gastroesophageal varices (GEPV), ascites, hepatorenal syndrome (HRS), hepatic encephalopathy (HE), hepatopulmonary syndrome (HPS), and hepatocellular carcinoma (HCC).*

Source: P. Muriel, et al., Complications of Cirrhosis, http://dx.doi.org/10.1016/B978-0-12-804274-8.00033-3.

A special circulatory system known as the hepatic portal system links the two capillary bed systems in the small intestine and spleen wall and the liver's sinusoidal region. Since the liver receives both oxygenated and deoxygenated blood, its blood flow is distinct. Because of this, the portal vein's pressure and partial pressure of oxygen are lower than those of the body's other organs. Blood from portal vein branches enters the liver through the sinusoids. Blood from the hepatic artery branches also enters the sinusoids and mixes with it to provide oxygen to the liver. This concoction seeps through the sinusoids and gathers in a central vein that empties into the hepatic vein. The inferior vena cava receives the hepatic vein's next drainage. The hepatic artery provides the remaining 20% of blood, with the portal vein providing the other 80%.

According to Cárdenas and Ginès (2005) and de Franchis (2005), PHT is a clinical syndrome that results in hemodynamic changes as a result of difficult blood outflow from the liver. 5 to 10 mmHg is the typical portal pressure. PHT is defined as portal pressure greater than 12 mmHg and an increased wedged hepatic vein pressure (WHVP) gradient larger than 2–6 mmHg between the portal vein and inferior jejunal vein pressure. (Cichoz-Lach et al., 2008). The difference between the WHVP and the free hepatic venous pressure (FHVP) is known as the hepatic vein pressure gradient (HVPG), and it is determined by angiography. PHT is applied if the differential is greater than

5–12 mmHg. From a physical perspective, blood pressure can be expressed as follows: pressure ¼ vascular resistance blood flow. Consequently, elevated blood flow and/or vascular resistance in the portal vascular bed cause PHT. The main cause of resistance increases is mechanical occlusion, which makes it difficult for blood to flow from the portal tract to the inferior vena cava and liver veins (Henderson, 2000).

Another important factor that affects portal pressure is increased blood flow in the portal vein. Hyperkinetic circulation, defined as the cardiac output volume and vasodilation of the vascular bed, including visceral, is related to portal circulation. Consequently, elevated portal flow intensifies additional alterations in blood vessels, amplifying vascular resistance. PHT alters the intrahepatic, systemic, and portosystemic collateral circulations. Vasodilation and vasoconstriction changes contribute significantly to the pathophysiology of PHT by raising intrahepatic resistance and promoting hyperdynamic and collateral circulation expansion. Modifications in the vascular structure, known as vascular remodeling, which is the vessel's adaptive response to persistent alterations caused by shear stress, are another feature of PHT. Vascular remodeling and vasoreactivity are key targets in the treatment of PHT because they cause intrahepatic resistance (Shah, 2007).

Vasodilators play a critical role in increasing portal flow. They are prostaglandins, glucagon, nitric oxide (NO), bile acids, carbon monoxide (CO), tumor necrosis factor-a (TNF-a), and glucagon. Vasoconstrictions or vasodilation result from the malfunction of these physiologically active vasodilators (Gatta et al., 2008). Thus, the primary mechanisms causing the increased vascular tone in the sinusoidal area are the imbalance between the hyperresponsiveness and overproduction of vasoconstrictors (primarily endothelin 1 and cyclooxygenase-derived prostaglandins) and the hyporesponsiveness and impaired production of vasodilators (principally NO). Although the increased intrahepatic vascular resistance associated with cirrhosis is not permanent, various vasoactive molecules that are regulated at different molecular levels can reverse both the structural elements brought about by fibrosis and the active elements brought about by hepatic sinusoidal constriction (Fernandez, 2015). The syndrome is complex and requires more research despite significant advancements in the understanding of its pathophysiology; an intriguing and up-to-date review of liver surgery in cirrhosis and PHT is suggested (Hackl et al., 2016).

7.1.2. Gastroesophageal Varices

Cirrhosis initially leads to portal pressure increases as a consequence of increased resistance to flow because of an architectural distortion of the liver secondary to fibrous tissue (Chen and Ghali, 2012). The pressure within the portal vein is determined by the product of blood flow and resistance, as defined by Ohm's law:

P (Pressure) = Q (Blood Flow) ×R (Resistance)

The hallmark of PHT is a pathologic increase in the pressure gradient between the portal vein and inferior vena cava: the HVPG. The HVPG is the difference between the WHVP, a marker of sinusoidal pressure, and the FHVP (Groszmann et al., 1979), then:

HVPG = WHVP - FHVP

To account for intra-abdominal pressure and obtain a precise portal vein pressure measurement, the FHVP is deducted from the WHVP. At an HVPG of less than 12 mmHg, variations do not form (Viallet & colleagues. 1975; Garcia-Tsao et al, 1985).

According to Triantos and Burroughs (2007), patients with cirrhosis who do not have varices should have repeat endoscopies every two years if their liver function is stable or once a year if they exhibit any symptoms of liver dysfunction. For patients who can handle them, nonselective beta-blockers should be the first line of treatment for medium- or large-sized varices. According to Triantos and Burroughs (2007), this can lower portal vein pressure by about 15–20% and reduce total upper gastrointestinal bleeding by 40%. Beta-blockers are not advised in compensated cirrhotic patients because there is evidence of a decrease in bleeding risk but not in mortality (Triantos & Burroughs, 2007). The beta-blocker dose should be titrated to produce a 25% reduction in the baseline heart rate of the patients or until a resting heart rate of 55–60 beats/min is reached (Poynard et al., 1991). Patients who are unable to tolerate antihypertensive medications may benefit from a prophylactic endoscopy band ligature, which has been shown to have effects comparable to beta-blockers in terms of survival and the initial bleeding episode (Schepke et al., 2004). Patients with medium- to large-sized varices should have band ligation and take beta-blockers. Acute variceal hemorrhage patients may pass away in a matter of weeks from infection, renal failure, early rebleeding, or uncontrollable bleeding. Resuscitation, vasoactive medications (such as 48 hours to 5 days of octreotide), antibiotic therapy, and ligation for esophageal varices or cyanoacrylate infusion for gastric varices must all be started immediately (Thabut & Bernard-Chabert, 2007; Lee et al., 2014). According to Henderson (2006), about 20% of patients will continue to bleed after starting first-line treatment; in this group, portal decompression is advised. Less invasive transjugular intrahepatic portal systemic shunts (TIPS) are often the preferred option. A radiologist places a stent from the portal to the hepatic veins across the hepatic parenchyma as part of the TIPS procedure. A thirty percent chance of encephalopathy is linked to TIPS and surgical shunts (Henderson, 2006). A 75% stenosis was linked to early TIPS experience (LaBerge et al., 1995). The most reliable technique for portal decompression is liver transplantation; additionally, readers may find some recent developments regarding the classification, endoscopic, and ultrasonographic management of gastric varices interesting (Wani et al., 2015).

7.1.3. Ascites

Splanchnic vasodilation, which lowers the effective arterial blood volume, is the primary cause of ascites formation (Schrier et al., 1988; Bloom et al., 2015). Cirrhosis-related increased liver resistance to portal flow results in progressive elevations of PHT and collateral vein formation, which transfers blood to the systemic circulation. Endothelial stretching and possibly bacterial translocation lead to increased local production of various vasodilators, such as substance P, CO, NO, and endogenous cannabinoids, which causes PHT and splanchnic arterial vasodilatation (Iwakiri & Groszmann, 2006; Enomoto et al., 2014). According to recent research, the primary causes of the pathogenesis of the vasodilatation of the hepatic arteries and the related circulatory abnormalities that occur in cirrhosis are thought to be bacterial translocation to mesenteric lymph nodes with increased bacterial products and the subsequent stimulation of cytokine synthesis (Wiest & Garcia-Tsao, 2005; Riordan & Williams, 2006). Because of an increase in plasma volume and cardiac output, arterial blood volume is kept within normal limits during the early stages of cirrhosis despite moderate splanchnic arterial vasodilatation (Ruiz-del-Arbol et al., 2005). Splanchnic arterial vasodilatation is so severe in advanced cirrhosis that it significantly lowers the effective arterial blood volume and arterial pressure. A decrease in cardiac output (perhaps brought on by the existence of cirrhotic cardiomyopathy) may also be a factor in the impairments in the effective arterial blood volume in the later stages of cirrhosis (Ginès et al., 2004; Lee & Liu, 2007); as a consequence, there is a homeostatic activation of vasoconstrictor and antinatriuretic factors to control arterial pressure, leading to renal sodium and fluid retention. The combination of splanchnic arterial vasodilation and PHT alters the intestinal capillary permeability and pressure that facilitates the accumulation of the retained fluid in the abdominal cavity. As the disease progresses, there is a marked dysfunction in renal solute-free water excretion and renal vasoconstriction, leading to dilutional hyponatremia and HRS.

Three groups are created by the International Ascites Club for patients (Ginès et al., 2004). Individuals with grade 1 ascites, in which the condition is only identified by ultrasonography, do not need special care, although they should limit their intake of salty foods. Patients with grade 2 ascites have moderate abdominal distension brought on by the condition, which is accompanied by mild to moderate discomfort. Patients with grade 3 ascites have elevated levels of ascitic fluid, which results in noticeable distension of the abdomen and severe discomfort. Individuals with refractory ascites are those who become unresponsive to high dosages of diuretics or experience adverse effects that prevent them from being used. As a result, the topic of ascites management can be split into three sections: refractory ascites, large-volume ascites (grade 3), and moderate-volume ascites (grade 2).

A low-sodium diet (90 mmol/day) and spironolactone (50–100 mg/day) should be the first steps in the management and treatment of patients with grade 2 ascites in order to achieve the target weight loss of 300–500 g/day. Every seven days, dosages of spironolactone up to 400 mg/day can be increased if necessary.

If necessary, furosemide can be added at a dose of up to 160 mg per day after starting at 20–40 mg per day. Total paracentesis combined with intravenous albumin (g/L of ascites removed) is advised for patients with cirrhosis and grade three ascites. If the patient was able to tolerate them beforehand, a low-sodium diet (90 mmol/day) and diuretics are also advised. In addition to paracentesis, intravenous albumin can be administered as needed to patients with refractory ascites. If the patient is younger than 70 years old and does not have hepatic impairment, transjugular intrahepatic portosystemic shunts may be used in patients with very frequent recurrent ascites without severely impaired hepatic function. Short-term studies and one long-term study have evaluated the clinical utility of these agents in cirrhosis; however, more controlled studies are required to assess the safety, efficacy, and applicability of these agents in patients with ascites and cirrhosis (Ginès et al., 2004). Indeed, the management of cirrhotic ascites has been reviewed by Pedersen et al., (2015).

7.1.4. Hepatorenal Syndrome

Renal tubular function is preserved, renal vasoconstriction is marked, resulting in a decrease in glomerular filtration rate and renal plasma flow, and there are no pathological changes in the renal tissue. These three characteristics define hypertrophic renal syndrome (HRS). The "arterial vasodilation hypothesis" states that cirrhosis is often associated with a marked circulatory dysfunction accompanied by low values of arterial pressure, even though the sympathetic nervous and renin-angiotensin systems are overactive. This marked vasodilation of the splanchnic circulation's artery is the cause of the arterial vasodilation hypothesis (Schrier et al., 1988; Pipili & Cholongitas, 2014).

Orthotopic liver transplantation (OLT) is the best treatment option for cirrhotic patients with HRS because it can eliminate the primary causes of this complication (liver failure and PHT). Regrettably, the transplant outcome as determined by survival, cost, and quality of life is adversely affected by the existence of HRS at the time of transplant (Gonwa et al., 1995). The survival rate at three years is only 60% on average, compared to the expected 70–80% in patients without HRS, so this effect is not very noticeable. OLT patients with HRS have a higher overall in-hospital mortality rate, a higher risk of complications, and longer hospital and intensive care unit stays. Regarding renal function, shortly after OLT, glomerular filtration decreases because of surgical stress, infections, immunosuppressive medication use, and other factors. As a result, a large number of patients (35% vs. 5% of patients without HRS at the time of OLT) require hemodialysis (Gonwa et al., 1995). Despite the prompt correction of the hemodynamic and neurohumoral abnormalities that is clearly apparent within 1 month after OLT (Navasa et al., 1993), the glomerular filtration rate only partially recovers. This partial renal insufficiency persists during follow-up and may progress to an end-stage renal failure if the immunosuppressive strategy is not adequate (Schlitt et al., 2001).

Due to the quick progression of HRS, the majority of patients with cirrhosis and HRS passed away before undergoing OLT until the late 1990s. This issue has been partially resolved by the development of a model of end-stage liver disease (MELD) and a strategy for stratifying OLT priority based on MELD. Specifically, patients with elevated serum creatinine values now have a higher priority for OLT. Furthermore, since the late 1990s, new approaches to treating HRS have been put forth. Using vasoconstrictors and albumin has been shown to be a successful "treatment bridge" toward OLT, increasing the proportion of HRS patients who receive OLT (Gonwa et al., 1995; Restuccia et al., 2004); in fact, a comprehensive update on diagnosis and treatment of HRS is herein suggested (Baraldi et al., 2015).

7.1.5. Hepatic Encephalopathy

One of the primary causes of HE is the buildup of ammonia (Holecek, 2015). Blood-brain barrier-crossing increases in ammonia concentration are caused by liver dysfunction and portosystemic collaterals in cirrhosis. Ammonia causes structural changes in neurons in the brain, which causes astrocyte swelling (Häussinger & Schliess, 2008). The condition known as Alzheimer type II astrocytosis is caused by swollen astrocytes with enlarged nuclei and displaced chromatin, which is displaced to the perimeter of the cell, in autopsy studies of brain tissue from patients with cirrhosis (Pilbeam et al., 1983).

The "Trojan horse" hypothesis (Albrecht & Norenberg, 2006) links glutamine buildup to one of the processes causing neuronal edema. The excitatory neurotransmitter glutamate interacts with ammonia when it enters astrocytes, and glutamine is synthesized by the enzyme glutamine synthetase (Corbalán et al., 2002). After glutamine enters the mitochondria, glutaminase cleaves it into glutamate and ammonia, raising the intracellular ammonia levels (Schliess et al., 2002; Montes et al., 2003). This causes a feed-forward loop, as the elevation of ammonia in the mitochondria in turn produces reactive oxygen and nitrogen species, leading to further edema (Albrecht & Norenberg, 2006; Corbalán et al., 2002; Schliess et al., 2004; Rama Rao & Norenberg, 2007). Research has also demonstrated the function of aquaporin-4, a water channel expressed in astrocytes, which is potentiated by ammonia (Chepkova et al., 2006). Taurine, an antioxidant that mitigates ammonia-induced toxicity, is also depleted as a result of astrocyte edema (Jalan et al., 2003). The non-digestible disaccharides consist of lactitol and lactulose. Their role in treating HE is to decrease intestinal ammonia production and absorption. They accomplish this by acting as a laxative, transferring ammonia from the portal circulation into the colon, and interfering with the intestinal mucosa's absorption of glutamine and its subsequent metabolism to ammonia (Córdoba et al., 2005). When treating acute HE, nonabsorbable disaccharides are thought to be the best option; 67–87% of patients report improved symptoms. Lactulose dramatically enhances cognitive function and health-related quality of life in patients with HE, according to a placebo-controlled trial (Prasad et al., 2007). The overall treatment effect was modest but statistically significant, with a relative risk of no improvement ranging from 0.62 to 0.92 in a recent review of the effectiveness of nonabsorbable disaccharides compared with either no intervention or placebo (Als-Nielsen et al., 2004). A significantly increased risk of no improvement was observed in patients taking nonabsorbable disaccharides, with a relative risk of 1.24. The authors also evaluated the relative efficacy of antibiotics and nonabsorbable disaccharides. 2004). Both the review by Liu et al., (2015) and the excellent reference by Sundaram and Shaikh (Sundaram & Shaikh, 2009) address antibiotics and other therapies. regarding HE management is advised.

7.1.6. Hepatopulmonary Syndrome

The majority of HPS treatment is based on research on lung hypertension patients from other causes, however prostacyclin appears to be helpful (Nacif et al., 2014). Studies conducted recently have shown that sildenafil can reduce pulmonary hypertension (Bruix & Sherman, 2005; Reichenberger et al., 2006). Because of the risk of bleeding, anticoagulation treatments should not be used in cases of severe liver disease. Since these patients do not respond to NO, beta-blockers are contraindicated because they reduce stroke volume and exacerbate effective hypovolemia, and calcium channel blockers are not advised (Herve et al., 2007). Oxygen therapy is an option, even though severe hypoxemia in portopulmonary hypertension is uncommon. TIPS plays no part in this situation, and liver transplantation produces inconsistent results. Because of the over 50% perioperative mortality associated with liver transplantation, it is not recommended when the pulmonary arterial pressure is higher than 35–45 mmHg (Herve et al., 2007).

A defect in arterial oxygenation brought on by intrapulmonary vascular dilatations is known as HPS. Eight to seventeen percent of cirrhosis patients have this entity, and their median survival is eleven months (Reichenberger et al., 2006). Usually, patients arrive with cyanosis, platypnea (increased dyspnea from the supine to the upright position), and progressive dyspnea. Even in the presence of established chronic cardiopulmonary disease, there is a high suspicion of HPS when there is a combination of arterial intrapulmonary vascular dilatation, arterial deoxygenation, and liver disease or PHT. It has not been demonstrated that TIPS is helpful. Most of the time, liver transplantation is helpful in treating HPS (Herve et al., 2007); additionally, an updated review (Lv & Fan, 2015) may provide more details.

7.1.7. Hepatocellular Carcinoma

Throughout the world, HCC is among the most prevalent malignant tumors (BRUIX & Sherman, 2005; Spangenberg et al., 2009; Nault, 2014), and it has a significant correlation with morbidity and death. In certain regions of Africa and Asia, where HCC accounts for a sizable share of cancer-related deaths, the incidence of HCC varies from less than 10 cases per 100,000 people annually in North America and Western Europe to more than 50–150 cases per

100,000 people annually (Forner et al., 2008, Nault 2014). The context of HCC is distinct, as it arises in the presence of established and potentially avoidable environmental risk factors. Monitoring enhances the identification and management of cancers.

The target population is easily identifiable, and the test that has been used in the US—abdominal ultrasonography—is both widely accepted by the public and has a high diagnostic accuracy, making the detection of HCC feasible. The suitability of potentially curative treatments for early detection of HCC is enhanced if the test and recall procedures are standardized. The term "very early tumor," which denotes a nodule of less than 2 cm with an indistinct nodular pattern and a hypoattenuated vascular pattern on contrast imaging, has long been incorporated into the definition of early cancer (Forner et al., 2008). Proteomic and gene expression profiling are two examples of new technologies that should make it possible to better understand the molecular processes underlying the development of HCC and may also help identify new therapeutic targets and diagnostic markers. Additionally, this platform ought to facilitate increasingly individualized patient-centered care concerning diagnosis, prognosis, treatment, and recurrence prevention. Consistent with this idea, research results indicate that the liver tissue's gene expression signature next to an HCC lesion could potentially indicate a patient's prognosis (Spangenberg et al., 2009). These advancements suggest that tailored, targeted treatment might actually take the lead as the preferred course of treatment for HCC patients (Mazzanti et al., 2016).

7.2. Ascites

The "end-stage" of any chronic liver disease, cirrhosis can present with a wide range of clinical symptoms that stem from liver insufficiency, portal hypertension, and/or the hyperdynamic circulatory state. Nowadays, most people understand that cirrhosis is a dynamic, heterogeneous illness that progresses through several prognostic stages, the two most important of which are compensated and decompensated (D'Amico et al., 2006; Ripoll et al., 2015). Patients with compensated cirrhosis have a median survival of more than 12 years (D'Amico et al, 2006), although the median survival for patients in the decompensated stage is only 1–1½ years (D'Amico et al., 1986; Gines et al., 1987b).

Ascites is the most common clinically evident complication that characterizes the decompensated stage of cirrhosis (Gines et al., 1987b; Planas et al., 2004), the pathological accumulation of fluid in the peritoneal cavity. Ascites is characterized as clinically overt ascites requiring specific therapy with diuretics as a decompensating event in cirrhosis (Figure 7.2). The patient is deemed decompensated even if the ascites subsides when diuretics are used. However, studies have shown that patients with subclinical ascites—ascites that is only detected by ultrasound or other imaging studies—have an intermediate mortality between those who do not have ascites and those who do. As a result, subclinical ascites is not clearly a decompensating event (Zipprich et al., 2012).

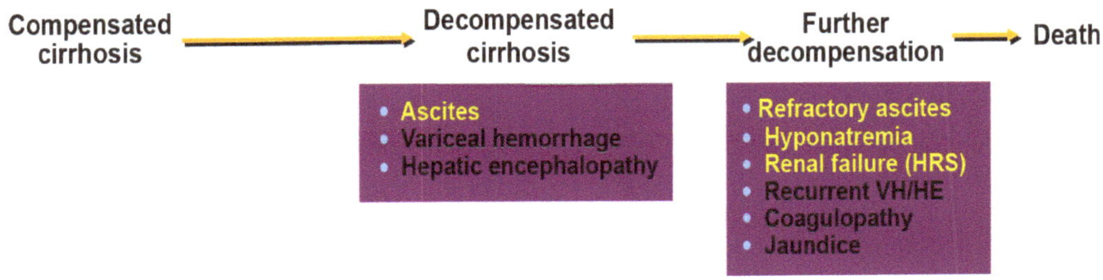

Figure 7.2. *Progression of cirrhosis through different prognostic stages. Ascites is one of the most important complications defining decompensated cirrhosis. The most important mechanism leading to decompensation is portal hypertension. The stage of "further decompensation" is mostly characterized by the development of refractory ascites, hyponatremia, and acute kidney injury (hepatorenal syndrome). The most important mechanism leading to further decompensation is worsening vasodilatation. HE, hepatic encephalopathy; HRS, hepatorenal syndrome; VH, variceal hemorrhage.*

Source: G. Garcia-Tsao, Ascites, http://dx.doi.org/10.1016/B978-0-12-804274-8.00036-9.

This condition is comparable to the increased death rate seen in patients with varices and compensated cirrhosis as opposed to those without varices (Bruno et al., 2009). Ascites is associated with the highest mortality rate when compared to the other complications that define decompensation, which include variceal hemorrhage (VH) and overt hepatic encephalopathy (HE) (Bruno et al., 2013). According to D'Amico et al., the 5-year mortality rate is approximately 30% when it happens as the sole decompensating event and increases to approximately 88% when it is linked to VH. 2014). As the pathophysiological mechanisms leading to ascites worsen, patients with cirrhosis are more likely to experience complications such as hyponatremia and the hepatorenal syndrome (HRS), which are linked to a higher mortality rate (Llach et al., 1988; Kim et al., 2008). Ascitic fluid infection known as spontaneous bacterial peritonitis (SBP) is one of the most common complications that cause the pathophysiology to worsen and result in a high death rate.

7.3. Pathogenesis

Fluid extravasates from the hepatic sinusoids in cirrhosis as opposed to the splanchnic capillaries. Thus, fluid leakage into the peritoneal space is caused by sinusoidal hypertension, which is a consequence of a blockage in the hepatic venous outflow caused by fibrosis and regenerative nodules. But sinusoidal hypertension on its own is insufficient to cause ascites to continuously form. The other crucial element in the pathophysiology of cirrhotic ascites is plasma volume expansion, which is achieved by sodium and water retention and permits the replenishment of intravascular volume.

7.3.1. Sinusoidal Hypertension

The hepatic venous pressure gradient (HVPG), a measurement of sinusoidal pressure, has been demonstrated to be the most reliable indicator of the onset of decompensation in patients with compensated cirrhosis (Ripoll et al., 2007; Rincon et al., 2013). Normal HVPG is between 3 and 5 mmHg and an HVPG greater or equal to 10 mmHg is the cutoff with the best predictive accuracy (this HVPG has now been called "clinically significant portal hypertension") (Ripoll et al., 2007).

These studies have confirmed that ascites is the most frequent decompensating event accounting for 69% (Rincon et al., 2013) and 74% (Ripoll et al., 2007) of all decompensating events. These studies have also shown that serum albumin is the second strongest predictor of decompensation, indicating that, in addition to portal hypertension, liver insufficiency plays a role in the development of cirrhosis decompensation. In the same way that most patients with gastroesophageal varices have an HVPG of at least 12 mmHg (Garcia-Tsao et al., 1985), patients with ascites also have an HVPG of at least 12 mmHg (Morali et al., 1992, Casado et al., 1998). Importantly, ascites development is significantly delayed in patients in whom the portosystemic gradient is reduced to levels below 12 mmHg (Casado et al., 1998).

7.3.2. Increased Intravascular Volume

If there was not a simultaneous rise in intravascular volume, ascites formation would be a self-limiting process. As a consequence of portal hypertension, there is concurrent arterial splanchnic and systemic vasodilatation during the formation of portosystemic collaterals, which lowers the effective arterial blood volume (Sikuler et al., 1985). The renin-angiotensin-aldosterone system (RAAS) and the sympathetic nervous system are two examples of the neurohumoral systems that are activated as a result of this underfilling. These systems cause renal sodium and water retention as well as an increase in intravascular volume that sustains the formation of ascites. Additionally, these systems are activated through baroreceptor stimulation (Schrier et al., 1988). Sodium retention has in fact been shown to precede the development of ascites (Wong et al., 2001).

The hyperdynamic circulatory state characteristic of patients with decompensated cirrhosis is characterized by vasodilatation (low peripheral resistance), increased plasma volume, and consequently elevated cardiac output. The primary cause of vasodilatation in cirrhosis is increased production of the vasodilator nitric oxide (NO). An upregulation in vascular endothelial growth factor, which happens with even slight increases in portal pressure, seems to be the initial stimulus for increased NO (Abraldes et al., 2006). Shear stress will then cause vasodilatation and an increase in blood flow, which will cause endothelial NO expression. Vasodilatation plays a role in the formation of ascites and is demonstrated in experimental cirrhosis, wherein NO blockade lowers the volume of ascites while upregulating the activation of the RAAS, raising systemic blood pressure and sodium excretion (Martin et al., 1998; Lee et al., 1993). The RAAS is further activated in cirrhotic patients receiving vasodilators such as phosphodiesterase inhibitors, angiotensin receptor blockers, and prazosin (Albillos et al., 1995; Thiesson et al., 2005) with associated sodium retention (Albillos et al., 1995; Thiesson et al., 2005), and ascites (Albillos et al., 1995).

7.3.3. Progression of Pathogenic Mechanisms

Vasodilatation causes avid sodium retention (ascites that is now resistant to diuretics) and the nonosmotic release of arginine vasopressin (AVP), an antidiuretic hormone, in a stage of more advanced cirrhosis decompensation. Water permeability is increased when AVP activates V2 receptors in the kidney tubule, allowing the translocation of aquaporins—selective water channels—from the cytosol to the collecting ducts' luminal plasma membrane. Dilutional hyponatremia results from this increase in water reabsorption exceeding that of sodium retention (Gines & Guevara, 2008).

Renal vasoconstriction and reduced renal blood flow are the results of progressive vasodilatation's additional stimulation of the vasoconstrictive systems, primarily renin and angiotensin. Furthermore, in this high-output cardiac state, or "cirrhotic cardiomyopathy," a relative decrease in cardiac output adds to the reduction in renal blood flow (Ruizdel-Arbol et al., 2005). Due to this reduction in renal blood flow, patients with decompensated cirrhosis only experience the prerenal form of kidney injury known as the HRS (Garcia-Tsao et al., 2008).

A further increase in NO production, which most likely stems from bacterial translocation and the ensuing systemic inflammation, is the mechanism that worsens vasodilatation. The process by which live bacteria from the intestinal lumen move to the mesenteric lymph nodes and other extraintestinal locations is known as "bacterial translocation." In a study involving ascites-ridden rats, rats with bacterial translocation had even higher NO levels than ascites-ridden rats without bacterial translocation; as a result, both their systemic and splanchnic circulations experienced greater vasodilatation (Wiest et al., 1999). Increased endothelial NO synthase, the primary enzymatic source of NO overproduction, was linked to increased production of tumor necrosis factor-alpha following bacterial translocation. Bacterial translocation has been suggested as one of the primary mechanisms in the pathophysiology of SBP, one of the main complications of ascites, in addition to exacerbating the vasodilatory state of cirrhosis.

7.4. Pathophysiological Bases for the Treatment of Ascites

Figure 7.3 illustrates the pathophysiology of ascites and refractory ascites as well as the sites of action of the currently advised therapies. Since large-volume paracentesis (LVP) and salt restriction are first-line therapies for ascites and refractory ascites, respectively, they act downstream of the pathophysiological cascade and are primarily symptomatic, so it is not surprising that they have not improved survival. However, managing ascites is crucial to enhancing patient satisfaction and lowering the risk of developing SBP, the most serious ascites complication.

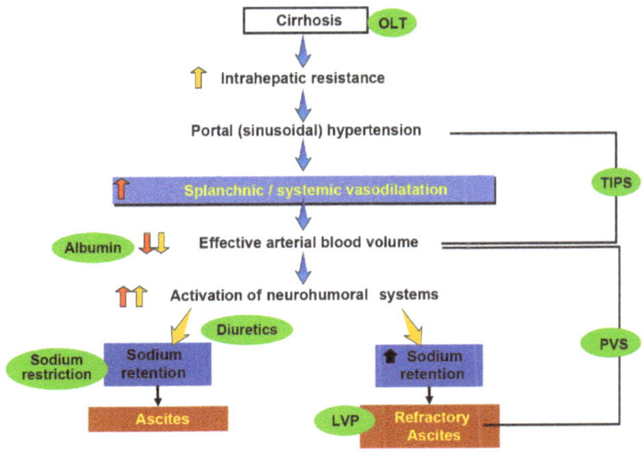

Figure 7.3. *Pathophysiology of ascites and site of action of different therapies.*

Source: G. Garcia-Tsao, Ascites, http://dx.doi.org/10.1016/B978-0-12-804274-8.00036-9.

In the following section, therapies that are currently used in the treatment of ascites are placed in the context of the pathophysiological cascade.

7.4.1. Therapies That Remove Ascites

LVP is a local therapy in which a needle is used to remove ascites. Recurrence of ascites is the norm because it has no effect on the pathophysiological mechanisms of the condition. Furthermore, this procedure is not completely benign because some patients, especially those who have had more than five liters of ascites removed, may develop a condition called "paracentesis circulatory dysfunction" (PCD), which deteriorates vasodilatation (Ruiz del Arbol et al., as a result of which there was a higher risk of hyponatremia, renal failure, and mortality (Gines et al., 1996). The rate of PCD has been reduced by concurrent intravenous albumin use. Although albumin works by increasing intravascular volume, it may also have a positive vasoconstrictive effect because it binds vasodilators like NO. An automated low-flow plump, a comparable form of therapy, is an indwelling device implanted surgically that transfers ascites from the peritoneum to the bladder more carefully (approximately 1 L of ascites removed during the day) (Bellot et al., 2013). As for LVP, on the other hand, it is linked to complications like a progressive drop in serum albumin and a higher risk of bacterial peritonitis and does not address the pathophysiological mechanisms of ascites.

7.4.2. Therapies That Act on Sodium Retention

Diuretics and salt restriction work by creating an unfavorable sodium balance. Spironolactone and other diuretics that block the action of aldosterone are referred to as "core" diuretics because hyperaldosteronism is the primary cause of sodium retention in cirrhosis. Although loop diuretics, like furosemide, are more powerful natriuretics, their efficacy will be reduced because of the hyperaldosteronism that results from taking up sodium that is not reabsorbed in the loop of Henle through the action of furosemide at the distal and collecting tubules (Perez-Ayuso et al., 1983). Additionally, furosemide used alone has been demonstrated in randomized controlled trials to be significantly less effective than spironolactone used alone (Fogel et al., 1981; Perez-Ayuso et al., 1983), or to the combination spironolactone/furosemide (Fogel et al., 1981).

7.4.3. Therapies That Act on Decreased Intravascular Volume

To avoid post-PCD, intravenous albumin is advised as an intravascular volume expander following LVP. Various plasma volume expanders, such as dextran, gelatin, hydroxyethyl starch, and hypertonic saline, have been compared with albumin in this context. In a meta-analysis, the question of whether patient morbidity and death varied between studies comparing albumin vs. Compared to other volume expanders, albumin was demonstrated to lower the incidence of hyponatremia and PCD with a potential decrease in mortality (Bernardi et al., 2012). Albumin is therefore the recommended plasma volume expander in cirrhosis.

The LeVeen shunt, also known as the Denver shunt, is a technique for performing continuous abdominal paracentesis that involves recirculating the protein-rich ascitic fluid back into the central circulation via a subcutaneous plastic cannula that is surgically inserted and has a one-way pressure valve. Following the insertion of the peritoneovenous shunt (PVS), there was a marked increase in plasma volume as well as natriuresis and diuresis. PVS has been demonstrated to be as effective as LVP in randomized controlled trials (RCTs), with a comparable survival rate and complication rate (Gines et al., 1991, 1995). But because PVS obstructs shunts frequently and can cause other complications (like infection or heart failure), its use has decreased as a result of these high rates of obstruction.

7.4.4. Therapies That Act on Vasodilatation

The primary pathogenic mechanism of vasodilatation is not specifically addressed by any of the available treatments. Vasoconstrictors may be useful in certain situations. In order to ascertain whether patient morbidity and death varied between studies that compared albumin vs. Vasoconstrictors have been demonstrated to be just as successful in preventing PCD as albumin (Bernardi et al., 2012). Terlipressin, a vasoconstrictor that is unavailable in the US, was primarily used in these trials. An investigation comparing the efficacy of octreotide/midodrine, a combination of weak vasoconstrictor drugs, vs. There was a tendency for albumin to be more effective than PCD in preventing recurrent ascites (Bari et al., 2012). Albumin may have beneficial effects that go beyond plasma expansion, as it will bind vasodilators (such as NO) and act as a vasoconstrictor and can also act against systemic inflammation (Garcia-Martinez et al., 2013), the main driver of vasodilatation.

7.4.5. Therapies That Act on Increased Intrahepatic Resistance and Sinusoidal Hypertension

The only treatment for ascites that acts upstream in the pathophysiological cascade is the transjugular intrahepatic portosystemic shunt or TIPS. An intrahepatic stent is inserted via jugular vein catheterization between a normotensive hepatic vein and a hypertensive portal vein. This procedure is typically carried out by an interventional radiologist. It also acts by increasing effective arterial blood volume as blood sequestered in the splanchnic circulation is transferred to the systemic circulation, relieving sinusoidal pressure, the primary mechanical mechanism in the formation of ascites. Meta-analyses of five prospective RCTs comparing TIPS vs. LVP (Lebrec et al., 1996; Salerno et al., 2004) showed, as expected, that TIPS was more effective in preventing the recurrence of ascites (Albillos et al., 2005; D'Amico et al., 2005). However, TIPS was associated with a higher risk for severe encephalopathy without differences in survival (Albillos et al., 2005; D'Amico et al., 2005). A meta-analysis of patient data from individual RCTs, as well as a subgroup of those previously mentioned, revealed that TIPS is linked to significantly lower mortality when compared to LVP, most likely because of lower rates of GI bleeding, SBP, and HRS (Salerno et al., 2007).

With MELD scores <15, a median survival of more than 12 months was noted in this study. TIPS stents that were exposed, or bare, were used in these trials. Polytetrafluoroethylene-covered stents have largely replaced uncovered stents, which obstruct frequently (18–78%) and are linked to a significantly lower obstruction rate and a decreased risk of encephalopathy (Bureau et al., Retrospective studies (Maleux et al., 2004) have demonstrated improved survival, especially in patients with a baseline MELD of <16. 2010). A recent RCT comparing TIPS using covered stents versus LVP showed a higher resolution of ascites and a significantly higher probability of survival in the group randomized to TIPS, with no differences in encephalopathy. Notably, the average MELD score in the TIPS group was 12 (Bureau et al., 2017).

7.4.6. Therapies That Act on the Diseased Liver

A patient with cirrhosis who develops ascites has a poor prognosis and should be evaluated for a liver transplant. Therefore, transplantation constitutes the ultimate treatment for ascites and its complications.

7.5. Management of Cirrhotic Ascites

Diuretics and salt restriction are the mainstays of treatment for most cirrhosis patients who first develop ascites. Later, the patient is said to have developed refractory ascites when the pathophysiological mechanisms leading to the formation of ascites worsen and the ascites becomes resistant to diuretics. The following section outlines particular suggestions for the treatment of these two distinct stages of cirrhosis ascites.

7.5.1. New Onset Ascites

While preliminary research indicates that LVP treatment expedites the removal of ascites and may be linked to a reduced rate of complications compared to diuretics (Gines et al., 1987a), therapy based on sodium restriction and diuretics continues to be the cornerstone of care due to its wide applicability, affordability, and simplicity of use (EASL, 2010; Runyon, 2013). However, it makes sense to start therapy with an LVP before or concurrently with sodium restriction/ diuretics in patients with tense ascites in order to relieve patient discomfort. Patients with concomitant cirrhosis complications, such as VH and SBP, that are known to be associated with a decreased effective arterial blood volume, should not start diuretics.

Sodium should be restricted to approximately 2 g of sodium per day (equivalent to 90 mEq/ day or 5.2 g of dietary salt per day) (Moore et al., 2003). There are virtually no complications associated with sodium restriction. However, the nonpalatability of a sodium-restricted diet may lead to inadequate food intake with further alteration of the already compromised nutritional status of patients with ascites. In these cases, it is preferable to allow a higher sodium intake while increasing the dose of diuretics.

Dietary sodium should be limited to amounts less than sodium excretion in the urine in order to create a negative sodium balance. Diuretics should be used to raise sodium excretion because it is typically low in patients with cirrhosis and ascites. As was previously mentioned, the preferred course of treatment is spironolactone-based diuretics. You can start diuretic therapy with either spironolactone or spironolactone plus furosemide. Eliminating ascites with spironolactone alone takes longer and may be linked to hyperkalemia (Angeli et al., 2009). On the other hand, while ascites is eliminated faster when spironolactone and furosemide are combined, this combination may require more frequent monitoring and dose adjustments (Fogel et al., 1981; Santos et al., 2003). Therefore, starting spironolactone alone may be preferred in an outpatient setting, while starting spironolactone and furosemide together may be preferred in an inpatient setting (or in settings where patients can be monitored every week). Starting at an oral dosage of 50–100 mg per day, spironolactone is gradually increased to a maximum of 400 mg per day. If and when weight loss is not ideal or hyperkalemia appears, furosemide should be added. Furosemide should be taken in conjunction with spironolactone. The recommended starting dose for furosemide is 20–40 mg once daily, which can be gradually increased to a maximum of 160 mg per day. We define an inadequate diuretic response as weight loss of less than 1 kg in the first week and less than 2 kg/week in the following weeks, requiring an increase in the dose of diuretics (Moore et al., 2003). It is important to find out if the patient has followed the recommended sodium-restricted diet and has abstained from using nonsteroidal anti-inflammatory drugs before concluding that they are not responding to diuretic therapy. Nonadherence to dietary sodium restriction should be suspected if patients fail to lose weight despite a 24-h urine excretion >78 mEq/L or a spot urine sodium concentration greater than its potassium concentration (this correlates with a 24-h sodium excretion >78 mmol/L).

The more common complications of diuretic therapy are prerenal azotemia due to intravascular volume depletion (25%), hyponatremia (28%), and HE (26%) (Gines et.al., 1987a; Salerno et al., 1987; Sola et al., 1994). Encephalopathy occurs mostly as a result of prerenal azotemia with increases in urea nitrogen that lead to increased ammonia levels. In patients who develop any of these complications, the dose of diuretics should be reduced or diuretics should be temporarily discontinued and restarted at a lower dose once they resolve. To minimize the rate of complications, weight loss in patients without edema should be maintained at a maximum of 1 lb/day (0.5 kg/day), whereas patients with edema can safely lose up to 2 lb/day (1 kg/day). Due to its antiandrogenic properties, spironolactone is frequently linked to side effects, the most common of which is painful gynecomastia. Another aldosterone antagonist with less antiandrogenic activity, eplerenone, has been approved for the treatment of congestive heart failure and essential hypertension. It appears to be effective in reducing painful gynecomastia without compromising its therapeutic effects (Mimidis et al., 2007). About 25 mg of spironolactone is equal to 50 mg of eplerenone in terms of the mineralocorticoid effect. Although it has a much weaker natriuretic effect than spironolactone, amiloride, another potassium-sparing diuretic, does not cause gynecomastia and may be used in patients with excruciatingly painful gynecomastia (Angeli et al., 1994).

7.5.2. Refractory Ascites

Ascites that is no longer responding to diuretics is known as refractory ascites. This can be due to two reasons: either the maximum dose (400 mg/day of spironolactone and 180 mg/day of furosemide) has been reached without causing natriuresis or weight loss, or the development of ascites complications has made it impossible to reach this maximum dose. LVP is currently the accepted treatment for ascites that is refractory. The preferred LVP modality is total paracentesis, which involves removing all ascites in a single procedure and concurrently infusing 6–8 g of albumin per liter of ascites removed. This method is just as safe as repeated partial paracentesis (Moore et al., 2003; EASL, 2010; Runyon, 2013). The rate of ascites reaccumulation and, ultimately, the need to ease the patient's discomfort dictate how frequently LVP is performed. As a result, the patient decides whether or not LVP is necessary. Diuretics at the highest dose that can be tolerated and sodium restriction should be used in addition to serial LVP to extend the interval between doses. However, diuretics should be discontinued if associated with complications or if urinary sodium is less than 30 mEq/L (indicating lack of any effect of diuretics). The development of post-PCD, which is characterized as a marked increase in plasma renin activity six days after LVP and a decrease in effective arterial blood volume, is one of the main side effects of LVP. A higher death rate, the onset of renal dysfunction, and a quicker recurrence of ascites are all linked to PCD development (Gines et al., 1996; Ruiz del Arbol et al., 1997). Two factors are independent predictors of the development of PCD: the amount of ascites extracted and the type of volume expander used in association with LVP (Gines et al., 1996), with the lowest rates observed when less than 5 L is removed and/or when albumin is used as a plasma volume expander (rate approximately 16%; Gines et al., 1988; Sola-Vera et al., 2003). Albumin administration has been recommended at a dose of 6–8 g of albumin IV per liter of ascites removed; however, a randomized trial has shown that albumin at a dose of 4 g/L of ascites removed is as effective as 8 g/L in preventing PCD (Alessandria et al., 2011). Patients with renal dysfunction or hyponatremia (who are more vasodilated and therefore more prone to develop PCD) should always receive albumin irrespective of the volume of ascites removed.

Procedure-related complications of LVP consist mainly of bleeding and ascites leakage (De Gottardi et al., 2009). Major bleeding occurs rarely but may be lethal (Arnold et al., 1997; De Gottardi et al., 2009), and although it is mostly related to the puncture of mesenteric vessels, it has been recently suggested that a platelet count less than 50,000/ mm^3 may be a predictor of severe complications and platelet transfusion before LVP may be recommended in these cases (De Gottardi et al., 2009). Leakage of ascitic fluid is rare and occurs with incomplete ascites removal. This complication can be solved by completing the LVP preferably in a site remote from the leaking puncture site. Patients who require more than two or three LVP per month or whose ascites is loculated and cannot be completely removed with a single LVP should have a TIPS placed (Moore et al., 2003). Evidence for better survival with TIPS in patients with refractory ascites and an MELD of 15 or lower (Salerno et al., 2007; Maleux et al., 2010) suggests that earlier placement of TIPS, as soon as ascites becomes refractory, may be the preferred strategy. In general, TIPS should not be performed in patients with serum bilirubin >3 mg/dL, a Child score >11, age >70 or evidence of heart failure (ejection fraction < 60%), and/or severe pulmonary hypertension. Patients who receive TIPS for refractory ascites are typically more hyperdynamic than those who receive TIPS for VH, which raises the possibility of heart failure following TIPS. Given that covered stents are associated with a better survival rate than LVP and have a significantly lower incidence of shunt occlusion (Bureau et al., 2017), they are favored over stents with just the TIPS. The primary long-term consequence of TIPS is the development of new HE or a worsening of preexisting HE. About 9% of procedure-related complications occur, with intraperitoneal hemorrhage being the most frequent (Boyer and Haskal, 2005). Although PVS is an alternative to LVP, its application has essentially been abandoned because LVP is an easier process that can be carried out in an outpatient setting. Additionally, because PVS can cause peritoneal adhesions, placing one could make it more difficult to place TIPS in the future and complicate liver transplant surgery. PVS is therefore primarily recommended for patients who frequently need LVP and who are not suitable candidates for TIPS or transplant. In uncontrolled studies conducted in centers outside of the United States, a peritoneo-vesical automated pump system that shunts ascites from the peritoneal cavity into the urinary bladder has been tested more recently. The pump removes about 1000 cc of fluid per day and needs to be surgically implanted under general anesthesia. Although it greatly lowers the need for LVP, which enhances the quality of life, it is linked to serious side effects such as surgical site infections (even in the presence of antibiotic prophylaxis), surgical complications, fluid loss that results in prerenal azotemia, and a drop in serum albumin levels (Bellot et al., 2013; Thomas et al., 2015). Results of prospective randomized trials vs. LVP are awaited.

7.5.3. Prevention of Further Decompensation

Preventing further decompensation (hyponatremia, acute kidney injury) by preventing the pathophysiological mechanisms that cause ascites formation from getting worse is one of the main objectives in the treatment of ascites patients. Therefore, it is best to avoid or prevent factors that worsen vasodilatation or further decrease the intravascular effective volume in patients with ascites, especially in those who are refractory to the condition. Vasodilators, such as carvedilol, angiotensin-converting enzyme inhibitors, and angiotensin receptor blockers, shouldn't be administered to these patients, especially if there has been even a slight drop in arterial blood pressure. The use of nonselective beta-blockers (NSBB) in this situation carries a risk of further decompensation, acute kidney injury, and death because it may further reduce cardiac output and destabilize patients already in this precarious hemodynamic state. This has been a contentious topic because some studies have indicated that patients with refractory ascites have a higher risk of acute kidney injury and/or mortality (Serste et al., 2010) or SBP (Mandorfer et al., 2014). Nevertheless, contradicting results have been found in larger, more recent studies. In a particular study, a propensity score-matched analysis conducted on a cohort of patients with cirrhosis waiting for a transplant revealed that patients with refractory ascites who were on NSBB had a higher chance of survival than those who were not. Interestingly, the use of carvedilol, an NSBB with vasodilatory properties that has been demonstrated to cause a larger drop in blood pressure, compared to propranolol produced an intermediate survival between patients who were prescribed propranolol (lowest mortality) and those who were not on NSBB (highest mortality) (Leithead et al., 2015). A second study, a post hoc analysis of data on three placebo-controlled randomized trials of V2-receptor antagonists in the treatment of ascites, showed no differences in mortality between those on and off NSBB, even when adjusted by MELD, mean arterial pressure, and dose of beta-blockers or study group (satavaptan vs. placebo) (Bossen et al., 2016). Furthermore, a third trial performed in patients with cirrhosis and multiorgan failure showed a benefit in survival in patients admitted with NSBB probably as a result of a decrease in inflammation (Mookerjee et al., 2016).

The mean arterial pressure is significantly lower in patients in the NSBB group in studies demonstrating a deleterious effect of NSBB, suggesting that this could be the clinical indicator that would prompt NSBB dose reduction or discontinuation (Garcia-Tsao, 2016). The Baveno VI consensus conference recommended that, until additional evidence is available, NSBB should be used cautiously in patients with refractory ascites and that the dose be reduced or discontinued in the event of acute kidney injury development, a systolic blood pressure of less than 90 mmHg, or serum sodium of less than 130 mEq/L. This recommendation was made due to the benefits of NSBB, particularly in the prevention of recurrent VH (de Franchis, 2015).

Preventing VH, using albumin in the presence of SBP, using diuretics with caution, and preventing further decrease in the intravascular effective volume are all ways to stop further decompensation.

Ascites is the most common decompensating event in cirrhosis and is associated with a poor prognosis. Patients with ascites should initiate evaluation to determine liver transplant candidacy. Mainstay of therapy is sodium restriction and diuretics. Patients in whom ascites is refractory to diuretic therapy, should be treated with LVP accompanied by intravenous infusion of albumin. TIPS should be reserved for patients who require frequent LVP and should be particularly considered in those with a MELD score < 15. Knowledge of the pathophysiological mechanisms of ascites and its complications should lead to more effective therapies and procedures/drugs that should be avoided.

A Closer Look

Cirrhosis of the Liver

Liver cirrhosis is a chronic, progressive disease that causes scar tissue to progressively replace healthy liver tissue, impairing liver function. The liver's capacity to produce necessary proteins, detoxify the blood, and control metabolism is compromised by this scarring. Chronic liver diseases like hepatitis B or C, excessive alcohol use, or non-alcoholic fatty liver disease (NAFLD) can cause long-term damage that can lead to cirrhosis. Portal hypertension is a condition where the portal vein experiences elevated pressure due to restricted blood flow caused by the liver's increasing scarring. Ascites, or an accumulation of fluid in the abdomen, variceal hemorrhage, and hepatic encephalopathy—a condition in which toxins build up in the brain and impair cognition and confusion—can all result from this. Cirrhosis may not cause any symptoms in the early stages, but as the condition worsens, signs and symptoms like weakness, jaundice (yellowing of the skin and eyes), and unexplained weight loss may appear. Usually, a combination of blood tests, imaging studies, and occasionally a liver biopsy are used to make the diagnosis. Even though cirrhosis cannot be reversed, it can be slowed down in course with the right care and alterations in lifestyle. This can entail giving up alcohol, taking care of underlying illnesses like hepatitis, and changing to a nutritious diet. Liver transplantation might be the only effective course of treatment in severe cases. The severity of the disease and the existence of complications affect a person's prognosis for cirrhosis, but improving results requires early detection and treatment. Cirrhosis is a serious and potentially fatal condition that emphasizes the significance of liver health and the necessity of routine medical monitoring for individuals who are at risk.

Summary

- Chronic liver damage frequently leads to fibrosis, which is a reversible scarring response. Hepatic stellate cells are the primary source of the scar tissue present in fibrosis.
- PHT is defined as a clinical syndrome that produces hemodynamic changes due to difficult blood outflow from the liver.
- Portal circulation is connected with hyperkinetic circulation, which is observed as the cardiac output volume and vasodilation of the vascular bed, including visceral.
- Liver dysfunction and portosystemic collaterals in cirrhosis produce rise in the ammonia concentration in the bloodstream that crosses the blood-brain barrier. In the brain, ammonia results in structural alterations in neurons, producing astrocyte swelling.
- Cirrhosis is the "end-stage" of any chronic liver disease with a broad spectrum of clinical manifestations that are due to portal hypertension, the hyperdynamic circulatory state, and/or liver insufficiency.
- Salt restriction and diuretics act by inducing a negative sodium balance. Because hyperaldosteronism is the main cause of sodium retention in cirrhosis, diuretics that block the action of aldosterone, such as spironolactone, are considered the "core" diuretics.
- Refractory ascites is defined as ascites that is no longer responding to diuretics, either because the highest dose (spironolactone 400 mg/day, furosemide 180 mg/day) has been reached and no natriuresis/weight loss is obtained or because this maximum dose cannot be reached because of the development of complications of ascites.

References

1. Abraldes, J. G., Iwakiri, Y., Loureiro-Silva, M., Haq, O., Sessa, W. C., & Groszmann, R. J. (2006). Mild increases in portal pressure upregulate vascular endothelial growth factor and endothelial nitric oxide synthase in the intestinal microcirculatory bed, leading to a hyperdynamic state. *American Journal of Physiology–Gastrointestinal and Liver Physiology, 290*(5), G980–G987.
2. Albillos, A., Banares, R., Gonzalez, M., Catalina, M. V., & Molinero, L. M. (2005). A meta-analysis of transjugular intrahepatic portosystemic shunt versus paracentesis for refractory ascites. *Journal of Hepatology, 43*(6), 990–996.
3. Albillos, A., Lledo, J. L., Rossi, I., Perez-Paramo, M., Tabueca, M. J., Banares, R., Iborra, J., Garrido, A., Escartin, P., & Bosch, J. (1995). Continuous prazosin administration in cirrhotic patients: Effects on portal hemodynamics and on liver and renal function. *Gastroenterology, 109*(4), 1257–1265.
4. Albrecht, J., & Norenberg, M. D. (2006). Glutamine: A Trojan horse in ammonia neurotoxicity. *Hepatology, 44*(4), 788–794.
5. Alessandria, C., Elia, C., Mezzabotta, L., Risso, A., Andrealli, A., Spandre, M., Morgando, A., Marzano, A., & Rizzetto, M. (2011). Prevention of paracentesis-induced circulatory dysfunction in cirrhosis: Standard vs half albumin doses. A prospective, randomized, unblinded pilot study. *Digestive and Liver Disease, 43*(11), 881–886.

6. Als-Nielsen, B., Gluud, L. L., & Gluud, C. (2004). Non-absorbable disaccharides for hepatic encephalopathy: Systematic review of randomised trials. *BMJ, 328*(7449), 1046.
7. Angeli, P., Dalla Pria, M., DeBei, E., Albino, G., Caregaro, L., Merkel, C., Ceolotto, G., & Gatta, A. (1994). Randomized clinical study of the efficacy of amiloride and potassium canrenoate in nonazotemic cirrhotic patients with ascites. *Hepatology, 19*(1), 72–79.
8. Angeli, P., Fasolato, S., Mazza, E., Okolicsanyi, L., Maresio, G., Velo, E., Galioto, A., Salinas, F., D'Aquino, M., Sticca, A., & Gatta, A. (2009). Combined versus sequential diuretic treatment of ascites in nonazotemic patients with cirrhosis: Results of an open randomized clinical trial. *Gut, 59*(1), 98–104.
9. Arnold, C., Haag, K., Blum, H. E., & Rossle, M. (1997). Acute hemoperitoneum after large-volume paracentesis. *Gastroenterology, 113*(3), 978–982.
10. Baraldi, O., Valentini, C., Donati, G., Comai, G., Cuna, V., Capelli, I., et al. (2015). Hepatorenal syndrome: Update on diagnosis and treatment. *World Journal of Nephrology, 6*(6), 511–520.
11. Bari, K., Minano, C., Shea, M., Inayat, I. B., Hashem, H. J., Gilles, H., Heuman, D., & Garcia-Tsao, G. (2012). The combination of octreotide and midodrine is not superior to albumin in preventing recurrence of ascites after large-volume paracentesis. *Clinical Gastroenterology and Hepatology, 10*(10), 1169–1175.
12. Bellot, P., Welker, M. W., Soriano, G., von, S. M., Appenrodt, B., Wiest, R., Whittaker, S., Tzonev, R., Handshiev, S., Verslype, C., Moench, C., Zeuzem, S., Sauerbruch, T., Guarner, C., Schott, E., Johnson, N., Petrov, A., Katzarov, K., Nevens, F., Zapater, P., & Such, J. (2013). Automated low flow pump system for the treatment of refractory ascites: A multi-center safety and efficacy study. *Journal of Hepatology, 58*(5), 922–927.
13. Bernardi, M., Caraceni, P., Navickis, R. J., & Wilkes, M. M. (2012). Albumin infusion in patients undergoing large-volume paracentesis: A meta-analysis of randomized trials. *Hepatology, 55*(4), 1172–1181.
14. Bloom, S., Kemp, W., & Lubel, J. (2015). Portal hypertension: Pathophysiology, diagnosis and management. *Internal Medicine Journal, 45*(1), 16–26.
15. Bossen, L., Krag, A., Vilstrup, H., Watson, H., & Jepsen, P. (2016). Non-selective beta-blockers do not affect mortality in cirrhosis patients with ascites: Post hoc analysis of three RCTs with 1198 patients. *Hepatology, 63*(6), 1968–1976.
16. Boyer, T. D., & Haskal, Z. J. (2005). The role of transjugular intrahepatic portosystemic shunt in the management of portal hypertension. *Hepatology, 41*(2), 386–400.
17. Bruix, J., & Sherman, M. (2005). Management of hepatocellular carcinoma. *Hepatology, 42*(5), 1208–1236.
18. Bruno, S., Saibeni, S., Bagnardi, V., Vandelli, C., De Luca, M., Felder, M., Fracanzani, A. L., Prisco, C., Vitaliani, G., Simone, L., Gaeta, G. B., Stanzione, M., Persico, M , Furlan, C., Stroffolini, T., Salerno, F., & Maisonneuve, P. (2013). Mortality risk according to different clinical characteristics of first episode of liver decompensation in cirrhotic patients: A nationwide, prospective, 3-year follow-up study in Italy. *American Journal of Gastroenterology, 108*(7), 1112–1122.
19. Bruno, S., Zuin, M., Crosignani, A., Rossi, S., Zadra, F., Roffi, L., Borzio, M., Redaelli, A., Chiesa, A., Silini, E. M., Almasio, P. L., & Maisonneuve, P. (2009). Predicting mortality risk in patients with compensated HCV-induced cirrhosis: A long-term prospective study. *American Journal of Gastroenterology, 104*(5), 1147–1158.

20. Bureau, C., Garcia-Pagan, J. C., Otal, P., Pomier-Layrargues, G., Chabbert, V., Cortez, C., Perreault, P., Peron, J. M., Abraldes, J. G., Bouchard, L., Bilbao, J. I., Bosch, J., Rousseau, H., & Vinel, J. P. (2004). Improved clinical outcome using polytetrafluoroethylene-coated stents for TIPS: Results of a randomized study. *Gastroenterology, 126*(2), 469–475.

21. Bureau, C., Thabut, D., Oberti, F., Dharancy, S., Carbonell, N., Bouvier, A., Mathurin, P., Otal, P., Cabarrou, P., Peron, J. M., & Vinel, J. P. (2017). Transjugular intrahepatic portosystemic shunts with covered stents increase transplant-free survival of patients with cirrhosis and recurrent ascites. *Gastroenterology, 152*(1), 157–163.

22. Cárdenas, A., & Ginès, P. (2005). Management of complications of cirrhosis in patients awaiting liver transplantation. *Journal of Hepatology, 42*(S1), S124–S133.

23. Cárdenas, A., & Ginès, P. (2009). Portal hypertension. *Current Opinion in Gastroenterology, 25*(3), 195–201.

24. Casado, M., Bosch, J., Garcia-Pagan, J. C., Bru, C., Banares, R., Bandi, J. C., Escorsell, A., Rodriguez-Laiz, J. M., Gilabert, R., Feu, F., Schorlemer, C., & Echenagusia, A. (1998). Clinical events after transjugular intrahepatic portosystemic shunt: Correlation with hemodynamic findings. *Gastroenterology, 114*(6), 1296–1303.

25. Chen, Y. I., & Ghali, P. (2012). Prevention and management of gastroesophageal varices in cirrhosis. *International Journal of Hepatology, 2012*, 750150.

26. Chepkova, A. N., Sergeeva, O. A., & Haas, H. L. (2006). Taurine rescues hippocampal long-term potentiation from ammonia-induced impairment. *Neurobiology of Disease, 23*(3), 512–521.

27. Cichoz-Lach, H., Celiński, K., Słomka, M., & Kasztelan-Szczerbińska, B. (2008). Pathophysiology of portal hypertension. *Journal of Physiology and Pharmacology, 59*(S2), 231–238.

28. Corbalán, R., Hernández-Viadel, M., Llansola, M., Montoliu, C., & Felipo, V. (2002). Chronic hyperammonemia alters protein phosphorylation and glutamate receptor-associated signal transduction in brain. *Neurochemistry International, 41*(2–3), 103–108.

29. Córdoba, J., Mínguez, B., & Vergara, M. (2005). Treatment of hepatic encephalopathy. *Lancet, 365*(9464), 1384–1385.

30. D'Amico, G., Garcia-Tsao, G., & Pagliaro, L. (2006). Natural history and prognostic indicators of survival in cirrhosis. A systematic review of 118 studies. *Journal of Hepatology, 44*(1), 217–231.

31. D'Amico, G., Luca, A., Morabito, A., Miraglia, R., & D'Amico, M. (2005). Uncovered transjugular intrahepatic portosystemic shunt for refractory ascites: A meta-analysis. *Gastroenterology, 129*(4), 1282–1293.

32. D'Amico, G., Morabito, A., Pagliaro, L., & Marubini, E. (1986). Survival and prognostic indicators in compensated and decompensated cirrhosis. *Digestive Diseases and Sciences, 31*(5), 468–475.

33. D'Amico, G., Pasta, L., Morabito, A., D'Amico, M., Caltagirone, M., Malizia, G., Tine, F., Giannuoli, G., Traina, M., Vizzini, G., Politi, F., Luca, A., Virdone, R., Licata, A., & Pagliaro, L. (2014). Competing risks and prognostic stages of cirrhosis: A 25-year inception cohort study of 494 patients. *Alimentary Pharmacology & Therapeutics, 39*(10), 1180–1193.

34. de Franchis, R. (2005). Evolving consensus in portal hypertension. Report of the Baveno IV consensus Workshops on methodology of diagnosis and therapy in portal hypertension. *Journal of Hepatology, 43*(1), 167–176.

35. de Franchis, R. (2015). Expanding consensus in portal hypertension. Report of the Baveno VI Consensus Workshop: Stratifying risk and individualizing care for portal hypertension. *Journal of Hepatology, 63*(3), 743–752.

36. De Gottardi, A., Thevenot, T., Spahr, L., Morard, I., Bresson-Hadni, S., Torres, F., Giostra, E., & Hadengue, A. (2009). Risk of complications after abdominal paracentesis in cirrhotic patients: A prospective study. *Clinical Gastroenterology and Hepatology, 7*(8), 906–909.

37. European Association for the Study of the Liver (EASL). (2010). EASL clinical practice guidelines on the management of ascites, spontaneous bacterial peritonitis, and hepatorenal syndrome in cirrhosis. *Journal of Hepatology, 53*(3), 397–417.

38. Enomoto, H., Inoue, S., Matsuhisa, A., & Nishiguchi, S. (2014). Diagnosis of spontaneous bacterial peritonitis and an in-situ hybridization approach to detect an "unidentified" pathogen. *International Journal of Hepatology, 2014*, 634617.

39. Fernandez, M. (2015). Molecular pathophysiology of portal hypertension. *Hepatology, 61*(4), 1406–1415.

40. Fogel, M. R., Sawhney, V. K., Neal, A., Miller, R. G., Knauer, C. M., & Gregory, P. B. (1981). Diuresis in the ascitic patient: A randomized controlled trial of three regimens. *Journal of Clinical Gastroenterology, 3*(S1), 73–80.

41. Forner, A., Vilana, R., Ayuso, C., Bianchi, L., Solé, M., Ayuso, J. R., et al. (2008). Diagnosis of hepatic nodules 20 mm or smaller in cirrhosis: Prospective validation of the noninvasive diagnostic criteria for hepatocellular carcinoma. *Hepatology, 47*(1), 97–104.

42. Garcia-Martinez, R., Caraceni, P., Bernardi, M., Gines, P., Arroyo V., & Jalan, R. (2013). Albumin: Pathophysiologic basis of its role in the treatment of cirrhosis and its complications. *Hepatology*. http://dx.doi.org/10.1002/hep.26338.

43. Garcia-Tsao, G., Groszmann, R. J., Fisher, R. L., Conn, H. O., Atterbury, C. E., & Glickman, M. (1985). Portal pressure, presence of gastroesophageal varices and variceal bleeding. *Hepatology, 5*(3), 419–424.

44. Garcia-Tsao, G. (2016). Beta blockers in cirrhosis: The window re-opens. *Journal of Hepatology, 64*(3), 532–534.

45. Garcia-Tsao, G., Parikh, C. R., & Viola, A. (2008). Acute kidney injury in cirrhosis. *Hepatology, 48*(6), 2064–2077.

46. Gatta, A., Bolognesi, M., & Merkel, C. (2008). Vasoactive factors and hemodynamic mechanisms in the pathophysiology of portal hypertension in cirrhosis. *Molecular Aspects of Medicine, 29*(1–2), 119–129.

47. Ginès, A., Fernandez-Esparrach, G., Monescillo, A., Vila, C., Domenech, E., Abecasis, R., Angeli, P., Ruiz-del-Arbol, L., Planas, R., Sola, R., Ginès, P., Terg, R., Inglada, L., Vaque, P., Salerno, F., Vargas, V., Clemente, G., Quer, J. C., Jimenez, W., Arroyo, V., & Rodes, J. (1996). Randomized trial comparing albumin, dextran-70 and polygeline in cirrhotic patients with ascites treated by paracentesis. *Gastroenterology, 111*(4), 1002–1010.

48. Ginès, A., Planas, R., Angeli, P., Guarner, C., Salerno, F., Ginès, P., Salo, J., Rodriguez, N., Domenech, E., Soriano, G., Anibarro, Gassull, M. A., Gatta, A., Arroyo, V., & Rodes, J. (1995). Treatment of patients with cirrhosis and refractory ascites by LeVeen shunt with titanium tip: Comparison with therapeutic paracentesis. *Hepatology, 22*(1), 124–131.

49. Ginès, P., Arroyo, V., Quintero, E., Planas, R., Bory, F., Cabrera, J., Rimola, A., Viver, J., Camps, J., Jimenez, W., Mastai, R., Gaya, J., & Rodes, J. (1987a). Comparison of paracentesis and diuretics in the treatment of cirrhotics with tense ascites: Results of a randomized study. *Gastroenterology, 93*(2), 234–241.

50. Ginès, P., Arroyo, V., Vargas, V., Planas, R., Casafont, F., Panes, J., Hoyos, M., Viladomiu, L., Rimola, A., Morillas, R., Salmeron, J. M., Ginès, A., Esteban, R., & Rodes, J. (1991). Paracentesis with intravenous infusion of albumin as compared with peritoneovenous shunting in cirrhosis with refractory ascites. *New England Journal of Medicine, 325*(12), 829–835.

51. Ginès, P., Cárdenas, A., Arroyo, V., & Rodés, J. (2004). Management of cirrhosis and ascites. *New England Journal of Medicine, 350*(16), 1646–1654.

52. Ginès, P., & Guevara, M. (2008). Hyponatremia in cirrhosis: Pathogenesis, clinical significance, and management. *Hepatology, 48*(3), 1002–1010.

53. Ginès, P., Quintero, E., & Arroyo, V. (1987b). Compensated cirrhosis: Natural history and prognosis. *Hepatology, 7*(1), 122–128.

54. Ginès, P., Tito, L., Arroyo, V., Planas, R., Panes, J., Viver, J., Torres, M., Humbert, P., Rimola, A., Llach, J., Badalamenti, S., Jimenez, W., Gaya, J., & Rodes, J. (1988). Randomized comparative study of therapeutic paracentesis with and without intravenous albumin in cirrhosis. *Gastroenterology, 94*(6), 1493–1501.

55. Gonwa, T. A., Klintmalm, G. B., Levy, M., Jennings, L. S., Goldstein, R. M., & Husberg, B. S. (1995). Impact of pretransplant renal function on survival after liver transplantation. *Transplantation, 59*(3), 361–365.

56. Groszmann, R. J., Glickman, M., Blei, A. T., Storer, E., & Conn, H. O. (1979). Wedged and free hepatic venous pressure measured with a balloon catheter. *Gastroenterology, 76*(2), 253–258.

57. Hackl, C., Schlitt, H. J., Renner, P., & Lang, S. A. (2016). Liver surgery in cirrhosis and portal hypertension. *World Journal of Gastroenterology, 22*(11), 2725–2735.

58. Häussinger, D., & Schliess, F. (2008). Pathogenetic mechanism of hepatic encephalopathy. *Gut, 57*(8), 1156–1165.

59. Henderson, J. M. (2000). Surgical treatment of portal hypertension. *Best Practice & Research Clinical Gastroenterology, 14*(6), 911–925.

60. Henderson, J. M. (2006). Surgery versus transjugular intrahepatic portal systemic shunt in the treatment of severe variceal bleeding. *Clinical Liver Disease, 10*(3), 599–612.

61. Herve, P., Le Pavec, J., Sztrymf, B., Decante, B., Savale, L., & Sitbon, O. (2007). Pulmonary vascular abnormalities in cirrhosis. *Best Practice & Research Clinical Gastroenterology, 21*(1), 141–150.

62. Holecek, M. (2015). Ammonia and amino acid profiles in liver cirrhosis: Effects of variables leading to hepatic encephalopathy. *Nutrition, 31*(1), 14–20.

63. Iwakiri, Y., & Groszmann, R. (2006). The hyperdynamic circulation of chronic liver diseases: From the patient to the molecule. *Hepatology, 43*(S1), S121–S131.

64. Jalan, R., Olde Damink, S. W., Lui, H. F., Glabus, M., Deutz, N. E., Hayes, P. C., et al. (2003). Oral amino acid load mimicking hemoglobin results in reduced regional cerebral perfusion and deterioration in memory tests in patients with cirrhosis of the liver. *Metabolic Brain Disease, 18*(1), 37–49.

65. Kim, W. R., Biggins, S. W., Kremers, W. K., Wiesner, R. H., Kamath, P. S., Benson, J. T., Edwards, E., & Therneau, T. M. (2008). Hyponatremia and mortality among patients on the liver-transplant waiting list. *New England Journal of Medicine, 359*(10), 1018–1026.

66. LaBerge, J. M., Somberg, K. A., Lake, J. R., Gordon, R. L., Kerlan Jr., R. K., Ascher, N. L., et al. (1995). Two-year outcome following transjugular intrahepatic portosystemic shunt for variceal bleeding: Results in 90 patients. *Gastroenterology, 108*(4), 1143–1151.

67. Lebrec, D., Giuily, N., Hadengue, A., Vilgrain, V., Moreau, R., Poynard, T., Gadano, A., Lassen, C., Benhamou, J. P., & Erlinger, S. (1996). Transjugular intrahepatic portosystemic shunts: Comparison with paracentesis in patients with cirrhosis and refractory ascites: A randomized trial. *Journal of Hepatology, 25*(2), 135–144.

68. Lee, F. Y., Colombato, L. A., Albillos, A., & Groszmann, R. J. (1993). Nw-nitro-L-arginine administration corrects peripheral vasodilation and systemic capillary hypotension, and ameliorates plasma volume expansion and sodium retention in portal hypertensive rats. *Hepatology, 17*(1), 84–90.

69. Lee, S. S., & Liu, H. (2007). Cardiovascular determinants of survival in cirrhosis. *Gut, 56*(6), 746–748.

70. Lee, Y. Y., Tee, H. P., & Mahadeva, S. (2014). Role of prophylactic antibiotics in cirrhotic patients with variceal bleeding. *World Journal of Gastroenterology, 20*(7), 1790–1796.

71. Leithead, J. A., Rajoriya, N., Tehami, N., Hodson, J., Gunson, B. K., Tripathi, D., & Ferguson, J. W. (2015). Non-selective beta-blockers are associated with improved survival in patients with ascites listed for liver transplantation. *Gut, 64*(7), 1111–1119.

72. Liu, A., Perumpail, R. B., Kumari, R., Younossi, Z. M., Wong, R. J., & Ahmed, A. (2015). Advances in cirrhosis: Optimizing the management of hepatic encephalopathy. *World Journal of Hepatology, 18*(34), 2871–2879.

73. Llach, J., Gines, P., Arroyo, V., Rimola, A., Tito, L., Badalamenti, S., Jimenez, W., Gaya, J., Rivera, F., & Rodes, J. (1988). Prognostic value of arterial pressure, endogenous vasoactive systems, and renal function in cirrhotic patients admitted to the hospital for the treatment of ascites. *Gastroenterology, 94*(2), 482–487.

74. Lv, Y., & Fan, D. (2015). Hepatopulmonary syndrome. *Digestive Diseases and Sciences, 60*(7), 1914–1923.

75. Maleux, G., Perez-Gutierrez, N. A., Evrard, S., Mroue, A., Le, M. O., Laleman, W., & Nevens, F. (2010). Covered stents are better than uncovered stents for trans jugular intrahepatic portosystemic shunts in cirrhotic patients with refractory ascites: A retrospective cohort study. *Acta Gastroenterologica Belgica, 73*(3), 336–341.

76. Mandorfer, M., Bota, S., Schwabl, P., Bucsics, T., Pfisterer, N., Kruzik, M., Hagmann, M., Blacky, A., Ferlitsch, A., Sieghart, W., Trauner, M., Peck-Radosavljevic, M., & Reiberger, T. (2014). Nonselective beta blockers increase risk for hepatorenal syndrome and death in patients with cirrhosis and spontaneous bacterial peritonitis. *Gastroenterology, 146*(7), 1680–1690.

77. Martin, P. Y., Ohara, M., Gines, P., Xu, D. L., St John, J., Niederberger, M., & Schrier, R. W. (1998). Nitric oxide synthase (NOS) inhibition for one week improves renal sodium and water excretion in cirrhotic rats with ascites. *Journal of Clinical Investigation, 101*(1), 235–242.

78. Mazzanti, R., Arena, U., & Tassi, R. (2016). Hepatocellular carcinoma: Where are we? *World Journal of Experimental Medicine, 20*(1), 21–36.

79. Mimidis, K., Papadopoulos, V., & Kartalis, G. (2007). Eplerenone relieves spironolactone-induced painful gynecomastia in patients with decompensated hepatitis B-related cirrhosis. *Scandinavian Journal of Gastroenterology, 42*(12), 1516–517.

80. Montes, S., Alcaraz-Zubeldia, M., Muriel, P., & Ríos, C. (2003). Role of manganese accumulation in increased brain glutamine of the cirrhotic rat. *Neurochemical Research, 28*(6), 911–917.

81. Mookerjee, R. P., Pavesi, M., Thomsen, K. L., Mehta, G., MacNaughtan, J., Bendtsen, F., Coenraad, M., Sperl, J., Gines, P., Moreau, R., Arroyo, V., & Jalan, R. (2016). Treatment with non-selective beta-blockers is associated with reduced severity of systemic inflammation and improved survival of patients with acute-on-chronic liver failure. *Journal of Hepatology, 64*(3), 574–582.

82. Moore, K. P., Wong, F., Gines, P., Bernardi, M., Ochs, A., Salerno, F., Angeli, P., Porayko, M., Moreau, R., Garcia-Tsao, G., Jimenez, W., Planas, R., & Arroyo, V. (2003). The management of ascites in cirrhosis: Report on the consensus conference of the International Ascites Club. *Hepatology, 38*(1), 258–266.

83. Morali, G. A., Sniderman, K. W., Deitel, K. M., Tobe, S., Witt-Sullivan, H., Simon, M., Heathcote, J., & Blendis, L. M. (1992). Is sinusoidal portal hypertension a necessary factor for the development of hepatic ascites? *Journal of Hepatology, 16*(3), 249–250.

84. Nacif, L. S., Andraus, W., Pinheiro, R. S., Ducatti, L., Haddad, L. B., & D'Albuquerque, L. C. (2014). The hepatopulmonary syndrome. *Arquivos Brasileiros de Cirurgia Digestiva, 27*(2), 145–147.

85. Nault, J. C. (2014). Pathogenesis of hepatocellular carcinoma according to aetiology. *Best Practice & Research Clinical Gastroenterology, 28*(5), 927–947.

86. Navasa, M., Feu, F., García-Pagán, J. C., Jiménez, W., Llach, J., Rimola, A., et al. (1993). Hemodynamic and humoral changes after liver transplantation in patients with cirrhosis. *Hepatology, 17*(3), 355–360.

87. Pedersen, J. S., Bendtsen, F., & Møller, S. (2015). Management of cirrhotic ascites. *Therapeutic Advances in Chronic Disease, 6*(3), 124–137.

88. Perez-Ayuso, R. M., Arroyo, V., Planas, R., Gaya, J., Bory, F., Rimola, A., Rivera, F., & Rodes, J. (1983). Randomized comparative study of efficacy of furosemide versus spironolactone in nonazotemic cirrhosis with ascites. Relationship between the diuretic response and the activity of the renin-aldosterone system. *Gastroenterology, 84*(5), 961–968.

89. Pilbeam, C. M., Anderson, R. M., & Bhathal, P. S. (1983). The brain in experimental portal systemic encephalopathy. I. Morphological changes in three animal models. *Journal of Pathology, 140*(4), 331–345.

90. Pipili, C., & Cholongitas, E. (2014). Renal dysfunction in patients with cirrhosis: Where do we stand? *World Journal of Gastrointestinal Pharmacology and Therapeutics, 5*(3), 156–168.

91. Planas, R., Balleste, B., Alvarez, M. A., Rivera, M., Montoliu, S., Galeras, J. A., Santos, J., Coll, S., Morillas, R. M., & Sola, R. (2004). Natural history of decompensated hepatitis C virus-related cirrhosis. A study of 200 patients. *Journal of Hepatology, 40*(5), 823–830.

92. Poynard, T., Calès, P., Pasta, L., Ideo, G., Pascal, J. P., Pagliaro, L., et al. (1991). Beta-adrenergic-antagonist drugs in the prevention of gastrointestinal bleeding in patients with cirrhosis

and esophageal varices. An analysis of data and prognostic factors in 589 patients from four randomized clinical trials. Franco-Italian Multicenter Study Group. *New England Journal of Medicine, 324*(22), 1532–1538.

93. Prasad, S., Dhiman, R. K., Duseja, A., Chawla, Y. K., Sharma, A., & Agarwal, R. (2007). Lactulose improves cognitive functions and health-related quality of life in patients with cirrhosis who have minimal hepatic encephalopathy. *Hepatology, 45*(3), 549–559.
94. Rama Rao, K. V., & Norenberg, M. D. (2007). Aquaporin-4 in hepatic encephalopathy. *Metabolic Brain Disease, 22*(3–4), 265–275.
95. Reichenberger, F., Voswinckel, R., Steveling, E., Enke, B., Kreckel, A., Olschewski, H., et al. (2006). Sildenafil treatment for Porto pulmonary hypertension. *European Respiratory Journal, 28*(3), 563–567.
96. Restuccia, T., Ortega, R., Guevara, M., Ginès, P., Alessandria, C., Ozdogan, O., et al. (2004). Effects of treatment of hepatorenal syndrome before transplantation on post transplantation outcome. A case control study. *Journal of Hepatology, 40*(1), 140–146.
97. Rincon, D., Lo, I. O., Tejedor, M., Hernando, A., Ripoll, C., Catalina, M. V., Salcedo, M., Matilla, A., Senosiain, M., Clemente, G., Molinero, L. M., Albillos, A., & Banares, R. (2013). Prognostic value of hepatic venous pressure gradient in patients with compensated chronic hepatitis C-related cirrhosis. *Scandinavian Journal of Gastroenterology, 48*(4), 487–495.
98. Riordan, S. M., & Williams, R. (2006). The intestinal flora and bacterial infection in cirrhosis. *Journal of Hepatology, 45*(5), 744–757.
99. Ripoll, C., Bari, K., & Garcia-Tsao, G. (2015). Serum albumin can identify patients with compensated cirrhosis with a good prognosis. *Journal of Clinical Gastroenterology, 49*(7), 613–619.
100. Ripoll, C., Groszmann, R., Garcia-Tsao, G., Grace, N., Burroughs, A., Planas, R., Escorsell, A., Garcia-Pagan, J. C., Makuch, R., Patch, D., Matloff, D. S., & Bosch, J. (2007). Hepatic venous pressure gradient predicts clinical decompensation in patients with compensated cirrhosis. *Gastroenterology, 133*(2), 481–488.
101. Ruiz del Arbol, L., Monescillo, A., Jimenez, W., Garcia-Plaza, A., Arroyo, V., & Rodes, J. (1997). Paracentesis-induced circulatory dysfunction: Mechanism and effect on hepatic hemodynamics in cirrhosis. *Gastroenterology, 113*(2), 579–586.
102. Ruiz-del-Arbol, L., Monescillo, A., Arocena, C., Valer, P., Ginès, P., Moreira, V., Milicua, J. M., Jimenez, W., & Arroyo, V. (2005). Circulatory function and hepatorenal syndrome in cirrhosis. *Hepatology, 42*(2), 439–447.
103. Runyon, B. A. (2013). Introduction to the revised American Association for the Study of Liver Diseases Practice Guideline management of adult patients with ascites due to cirrhosis 2012. *Hepatology, 57*(4), 1651–1653. Available from: PM: 23463403.
104. Salerno, F., Badalamenti, S., Incerti, P., Tempini, S., Restelli, B., Bruno, S., Bellati, G., & Roffi, L. (1987). Repeated paracentesis and i.v. albumin infusion to treat "tense" ascites in cirrhotic patients: A safe alternative therapy. *Journal of Hepatology, 5*(1), 102–108.
105. Salerno, F., Camma, C., Enea, M., Rossle, M., & Wong, F. (2007). Transjugular intrahepatic portosystemic shunt for refractory ascites: A meta-analysis of individual patient data. *Gastroenterology, 133*(3), 825–834.

106. Salerno, F., Merli, M., Riggio, O., Cazzaniga, M., Valeriano, V., Pozzi, M., Nicolini, A., & Salvatori, F. (2004). Randomized controlled study of TIPS versus paracentesis plus albumin in cirrhosis with severe ascites. *Hepatology, 40*(3), 629–635.

107. Santos, J., Planas, R., Pardo, A., Durandez, R., Cabre, E., Morillas, R. M., Granada, M. L., Jimenez, J. A., Quintero, E., & Gassull, M. A. (2003). Spironolactone alone or in combination with furosemide in the treatment of moderate ascites in nonazotemic cirrhosis: A randomized comparative study of efficacy and safety. *Journal of Hepatology, 39*(2), 187–192.

108. Schepke, M., Kleber, G., Nürnberg, D., Willert, J., Koch, L., Veltzke-Schlieker, W., et al. (2004). Ligation versus propranolol for the primary prophylaxis of variceal bleeding in cirrhosis. *Hepatology, 40*(1), 65–72.

109. Schliess, F., Foster, N., Görg, B., Reinehr, R., & Häussinger, D. (2004). Hypoosmotic swelling increases protein tyrosine nitration in cultured rat astrocytes. *Glia, 47*(1), 21–29.

110. Schliess, F., Görg, B., Fischer, R., Desjardins, P., Bidmon, H. J., Herrmann, A., et al. (2002). Ammonia induces MK-801-sensitive nitration and phosphorylation of protein tyrosine residues in rat astrocytes. *FASEB Journal, 16*(7), 739–741.

111. Schlitt, H. J., Barkmann, A., Böker, K. H., Schmidt, H. H., Emmanouilidis, N., Rosenau, J., et al. (2001). Replacement of calcineurin inhibitors with mycophenolate mofetil in liver-transplant patients with renal dysfunction: A randomized controlled study. *Lancet, 357*(9256), 587–591.

112. Schrier, R. W., Arroyo, V., Bernardi, M., Epstein, M., Henriksen, J. H., & Rodés, J. (1988). Peripheral arterial vasodilation hypothesis: A proposal for the initiation of renal sodium water retention in cirrhosis. *Hepatology, 8*(5), 1151–1157.

113. Schrier, R. W., Arroyo, V., Bernardi, M., Epstein, M., Henriksen, J. H., & Rodés, J. (1988). Peripheral arterial vasodilation hypothesis: A proposal for the initiation of renal sodium and water retention in cirrhosis. *Hepatology, 8*(5), 1151–1157.

114. Serste, T., Melot, C., Francoz, C., Durand, F., Rautou, P. E., Valla, D., Moreau, R., & Lebrec, D. (2010). Deleterious effects of beta-blockers on survival in patients with cirrhosis and refractory ascites. *Hepatology, 52*(3), 1017–1022.

115. Shah, V. (2007). Molecular mechanisms of increased intrahepatic resistance in portal hypertension. *Journal of Clinical Gastroenterology, 41*(Supplement 3), S259–S261.

116. Sikuler, E., Kravetz, D., & Groszmann, R. J. (1985). Evolution of portal hypertension and mechanisms involved in its maintenance in a rat model. *American Journal of Physiology, 248*(5), G618–G625.

117. Sola, R., Vila, M. C., Andreu, M., Oliver, M. I., Coll, S., Gana, J., Ledesma, S., Ginès, P., Jimenez, W., & Arroyo, V. (1994). Total paracentesis with dextran 40 vs. diuretics in the treatment of ascites in cirrhosis: A randomized controlled study. *Journal of Hepatology, 20*(2), 282–288.

118. Sola-Vera, J., Minana, J., Ricart, E., Planella, M., Gonzalez, B., Torras, X., Rodriguez, J., Such, J., Pascual, S., Soriano, G., Perez-Mateo, M., & Guarner, C. (2003). Randomized trial comparing albumin and saline in the prevention of paracentesis-induced circulatory dysfunction in cirrhotic patients with ascites. *Hepatology, 37*(5), 1147–1153.

119. Spangenberg, H. C., Thimme, R., & Blum, H. E. (2009). Targeted therapy for hepatocellular carcinoma. *Nature Reviews Gastroenterology & Hepatology, 6*(7), 423–432.

120. Sundaram, V., & Shaikh, O. S. (2009). Hepatic encephalopathy: Pathophysiology and emerging therapies. *Medical Clinics of North America, 93*(4), 819–836.

121. Thabut, D., & Bernard-Chabert, B. (2007). Management of acute bleeding from portal hypertension. *Best Practice & Research Clinical Gastroenterology, 21*(1), 19–29.

122. Thiesson, H. C., Jensen, B. L., Jespersen, B., Schaffalitzky de Muckadell, O. B., Bistrup, C., Walter, S., Ottosen, P. D., Veje, A., & Skott, O. (2005). Inhibition of cGMP-specific phosphodiesterase type 5 reduces sodium excretion and arterial blood pressure in patients with NaCl retention and ascites. *American Journal of Physiology-Renal Physiology, 288*(5), F1044–F1052.

123. Thomas, M. N., Sauter, G. H., Gerbes, A. L., Stangl, M., Schiergens, T. S., Angele, M., Werner, J., & Guba, M. (2015). Automated low flow pump system for the treatment of refractory ascites: A single-center experience. *Langenbeck's Archives of Surgery, 400*(8), 979–983. Available from: PM: 26566989.

124. Triantos, C. K., & Burroughs, A. K. (2007). Prevention of the development of varices and first portal hypertensive bleeding episode. *Best Practice & Research Clinical Gastroenterology, 21*(1), 31–42.

125. Viallet, A., Marleau, D., Huet, M., Martin, F., Farley, A., Villeneuve, J. P., et al. (1975). Hemodynamic evaluation of patients with intrahepatic portal hypertension: Relationship between bleeding varices and the porto hepatic gradient. *Gastroenterology, 69*(6), 1297–1300.

126. Wani, Z. A., Bhat, R. A., Bhadoria, A. S., Maiwall, R., & Choudhury, A. (2015). Gastric varices: Classification, endoscopic and ultrasonographic management. *Journal of Research in Medical Sciences, 20*(12), 1200–1207.

127. Wiest, R., Das, S., Cadelina, G., Garcia-Tsao, G., Milstien, S., & Groszmann, R. J. (1999). Bacterial translocation to lymph nodes of cirrhotic rats stimulates eNOS-derived NO production and impairs mesenteric vascular contractility. *Journal of Clinical Investigation, 104*(9), 1223–1233.

128. Wiest, R., & Garcia-Tsao, G. (2005). Bacterial translocation (BT) in cirrhosis. *Hepatology, 41*(3), 422–433.

129. Wong, F., Liu, P., & Blendis, L. (2001). Sodium homeostasis with chronic sodium loading in preascitic cirrhosis. *Gut, 49*(6), 847–851.

130. Zipprich, A., Garcia-Tsao, G., Rogowski, S., Fleig, W. E., Seufferlein, T., & Dollinger, M. M. (2012). Prognostic indicators of survival in patients with compensated and decompensated cirrhosis. *Liver International, 32*(9), 1407–1414.

Chapter

8

HEPATORENAL SYNDROME, HEPATOPULMONARY SYNDROME, AND PORTOPULMONARY HYPERTENSION

Contents

Introduction

Acute kidney injury is a common complication among patients with liver cirrhosis and is often fatal. Hepatorenal syndrome, a type of acute kidney injury first described in the mid-20th century, is characterized by intense narrowing of the renal arteries due to circulatory issues in cirrhotic patients. This type of kidney injury does not improve with volume expansion or renal vasodilators. However, kidney function usually returns to normal after a liver transplant. Studies have shown that kidney function can also be restored in many patients with pharmacological treatment using terlipressin or norepinephrine in combination with albumin (Alessandria et al., 2007; Neri et al., 2008;Rodriguez et al., 2014; Cavallin et al., 2015). Thus, there are compelling reasons to support the idea that HRS is a distinct type of kidney failure that only affects patients who have cirrhosis and has a functional cause. Significant side effects of chronic liver disease include portopulmonary hypertension (PoPH) and hepatopulmonary syndrome (HPS), which affect the pulmonary vasculature and have different pathophysiological mechanisms and clinical implications.

Liver disease, intrapulmonary vascular dilatation, and arterial hypoxemia are the hallmarks of hepatopulmonary syndrome. It is brought on by the lungs' dilated blood vessels, which cause an irregular oxygen exchange and hypoxemia. Breathlessness, cyanosis, and digital clubbing are among the symptoms. HPS is linked to a higher death rate in patients with liver disease and can have a serious negative influence on quality of life. Conversely, portopulmonary hypertension is the emergence of pulmonary arterial hypertension within the framework of portal hypertension. Because of vascular remodeling and vasoconstriction, it is characterized by elevated pulmonary vascular resistance. Dyspnea, exhaustion, and symptoms of right heart failure are examples of clinical manifestations. PoPH makes liver transplantation more difficult and dangerous during surgery because of elevated pulmonary pressures. Both conditions need to be diagnosed and treated with caution. While PoPH may be treated with vasodilators and careful consideration of liver transplantation eligibility, HPS primarily depends on supportive measures and liver transplantation as the final form of treatment. Comprehending these syndromes is essential to enhancing treatment and enhancing results for individuals suffering from chronic liver disease.

Orientation and Directional Terms

<table>
<tr><th>Term</th><th>Definition</th><th>Illustration</th></tr>
<tr><td>Bacterial translocation (BT)</td><td>Bacterial translocation is defined as the passage of viable bacteria from the gastrointestinal (GI) tract to extraintestinal sites, such as the mesenteric lymph node complex (MLN), liver, spleen, kidney, and bloodstream.</td><td>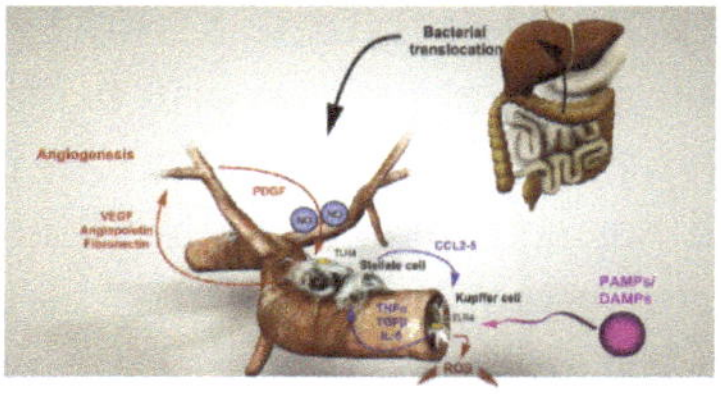
</td></tr>
<tr><td>Gastrointestinal (GI)</td><td>The gastrointestinal tract is the tract or passageway of the digestive system that leads from the mouth to the anus. The GI tract contains all the major organs of the digestive system, in humans and other animals, including the esophagus, stomach, and intestines.</td><td>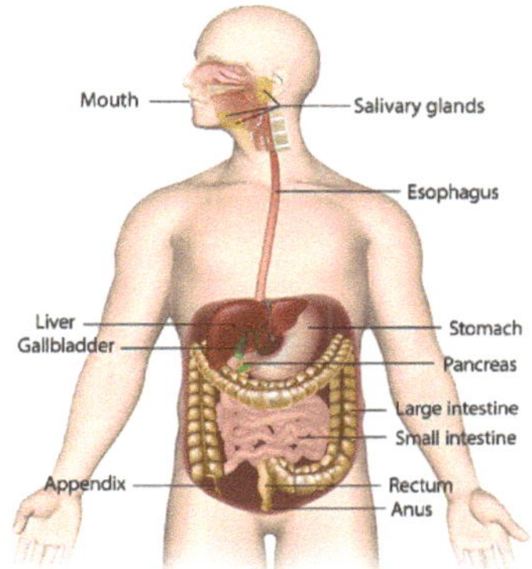
</td></tr>
<tr><td>Dyspnea</td><td>Dyspnea is a sensation of running out of the air and of not being able to breathe fast enough or deeply enough. It results from multiple interactions of signals and receptors in the CNS, peripheral receptors chemoreceptors, and mechanoreceptors in the upper airway, lungs, and chest wall.</td><td>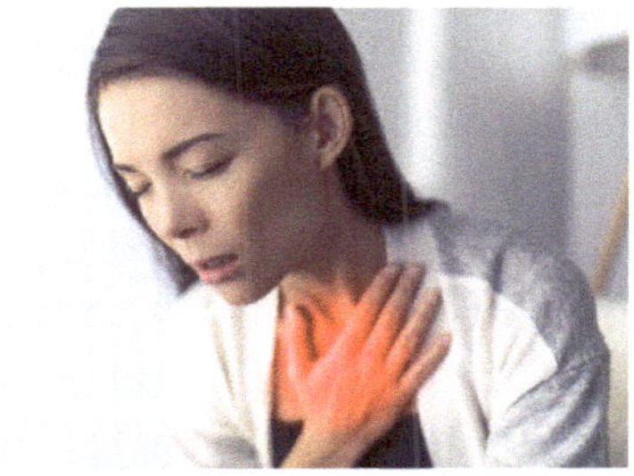</td></tr>
<tr><td>Angiogenesis</td><td>Angiogenesis is the formation of new blood vessels. This process involves the migration, growth, and differentiation of endothelial cells, which line the inside wall of blood vessels. The process of angiogenesis is controlled by chemical signals in the body.</td><td>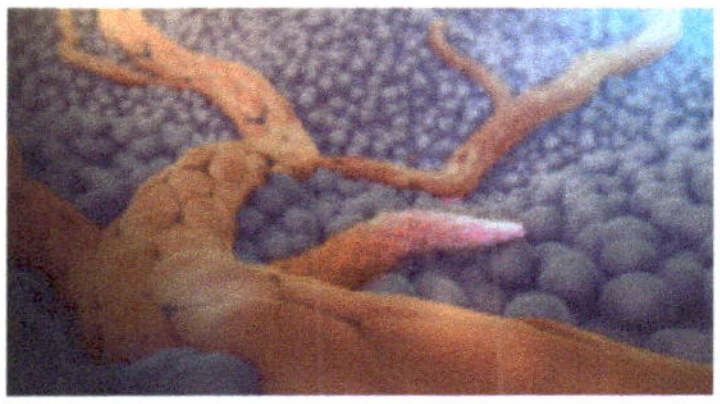</td></tr>
<tr><td>Right heart catheterization (RHC)</td><td>Right heart catheterization is an invasive test that can show how well your heart is pumping. It measures blood pressure and oxygen in your lungs and the right side of your heart. It's also called pulmonary artery catheterization.</td><td>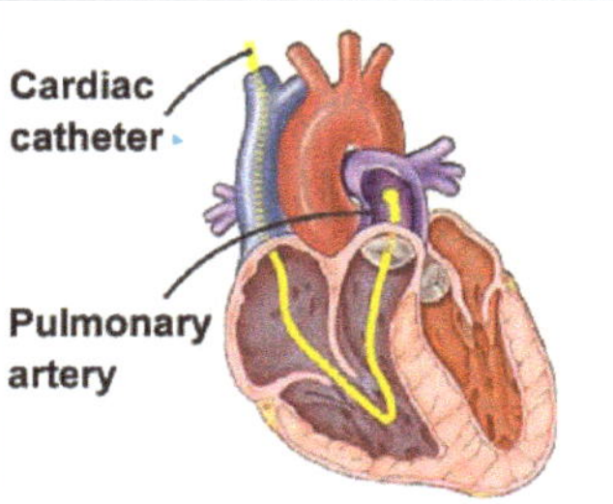
</td></tr>
</table>

8.1. Pathophysiology of HRS

The final stage of all chronic liver diseases is liver cirrhosis, which is characterized by a long-term buildup of fibrosis and inflammation of the liver that disrupts the normal architecture of the liver. According to Lee and Friedman (2011), these structural alterations are linked to significant anomalies in the hepatic microcirculation that result in elevated vascular resistance. Additionally, a synthesis of local splanchnic vasodilator molecules occurs, which increases portal venous flow and causes arterial splanchnic vasodilation. Increased hepatic vascular resistance and increased portal venous inflow are the two factors that contribute to portal hypertension. For many years, the pathophysiological hallmark of the progression of cirrhosis and the development of HRS has been recognized as the peripheral arterial vasodilation theory in the context of systemic circulatory dysfunction due to portal hypertension (Schrier et al., 1988). But new research suggests that other mechanisms, such as inflammation and gut-liver interaction, may also be important in explaining HRS, and that the conditions of portal hypertension and circulatory dysfunction alone cannot fully account for the condition.

8.1.1. The Arterial Vasodilation Theory

In a nutshell, the arterial vasodilation theory describes a dysfunction in the systemic arterial circulation that is primarily caused by portal hypertension-induced primary arterial vasodilation of the splanchnic circulation, which results in a decrease in systemic vascular resistance (SVR) (Schrier et al., 1988; Gines and Schrier, 2009).

Patients with compensated cirrhosis in the early stages of the disease have moderate portal hypertension. Here, splanchnic arterial vasodilation results in a small drop in SVR, which in turn lowers arterial pressure and, eventually, the effective systemic arterial blood volume. This drop is initially made up for by an increase in cardiac output. The splanchnic circulation vasodilates intensely in patients with decompensated cirrhosis in the advanced stages of the disease because of increased synthesis of vasodilator factors, nitric oxide (NO), carbon monoxide, and/or endogenous cannabinoids (Schrier et al., 1988; Arroyo et al., 1996), among others. Other factors, such as neoangiogenesis in mesenteric arteries and impaired response to vasoconstrictors may also contribute to the reduced vascular resistance in the splanchnic circulation. The splanchnic circulation has a strong vasodilation that causes a progressive decrease in SVR that is unbalanced by the heart's increased output. As a result of the difference between the intravascular blood volume and the significantly increased intravascular arterial circulation brought on by the vasodilator factors, there is an arterial underfilling at this point, which is referred to as effective arterial hypovolemia. Additionally, evidence points to a decrease in cardiac output that is likely related to cirrhotic cardiomyopathy and contributes to arterial underfilling (Ruiz-del-Arbol et al., 2005; Wiese et al., 2014).

Systemic vasoconstrictor systems, such as the renine angiotensin system (RAAS), the sympathetic nervous system (SNS), and arginine vasopressin (AVP), are activated in response to the severe arterial underfilling. Vasoconstrictor systems that are activated cause water and sodium retention as well as increased plasma volume and vasoconstriction, which help to keep arterial pressure within normal bounds (Henriksen et al., 1984; Macgilchrist et al., 1991). As the disease progresses, deleterious effects secondary to an intense activation of the vasoconstrictor systems arise with ascites formation, hypervolemic hyponatremia, and hypoperfusion (Henriksen et al., 1984; Claria et al., 1991; Oliver and Verna, 2010) of kidney circulation favoring the onset of HRS.

Furthermore, the altered relationship between blood flow and pressure in the kidney is probably a result of the SNS's increased activity. Research indicates that patients with significantly advanced cirrhosis exhibit a shift in the renal blood flow autoregulation curve. This indicates that their renal blood flow is lower than that of patients with compensated cirrhosis for a given level of renal perfusion pressure (Stadlbauer et al., 2008).

- ***Other Vasoactive Factors:*** Extravasoactive substances such as endothelin, prostaglandins (PGs), and natriuretic hormones may also contribute to hemodynamic abnormalities in cirrhosis patients. Although there is an increase in endothelin and natriuretic hormone plasma levels in cirrhosis, it is unclear how these hormones contribute to the pathophysiology of kidney and circulatory dysfunction in cirrhosis patients (Gines et al., 1988; La Villa et al., 1992; Moore et al., 1992; Wong et al., 2008). There has also been evidence of an increase in PGs, the metabolites of arachidonic acid generated through the cyclooxygenase pathway, in cirrhosis. PGI2 and PGE2, which are elevated in patients with cirrhosis and ascites, have renal vasodilator effects and are crucial in balancing the vasoconstrictor effects of RAAS, SNS, and AVP. In fact, AKI development is often linked to the use of nonsteroidal anti-inflammatory drugs (NSAIDs), which inhibit the synthesis of prostaglandins (PGs) (Elia et al., 2015).

8.1.2. Systemic Inflammation Theory

The most widely recognized theory to explain the systemic circulatory dysfunction associated with cirrhosis is arterial vasodilation. Nevertheless, a growing body of research from both human and experimental studies suggests that advanced cirrhosis is associated with a systemic inflammatory state that worsens as the disease progresses and probably plays a part in the physiopathology of HRS by causing systemic circulatory dysfunction on various levels (Arroyo et al., 2015; Bernardi et al., 2015).

A persistent systemic inflammatory state in cirrhosis may result from three distinct mechanisms that trigger the immune system: (1) bacterial translocation (BT) from the gut accompanied by the release of pathogenassociated molecular patterns (PAMPs); (2) release of danger-associated molecular patterns (DAMPs) from hepatocytes that have been injured; and (3) bacterial infections. A systemic inflammatory response is triggered by any of these mechanisms, which activate the pattern recognition receptors (PPRs) found in innate immune cells (Bernardi et al., 2015). Dysbiosis and bacterial overgrowth in the gut are made easier by advanced cirrhosis, which is linked to decreased bile flow, impaired gastric secretion, and impaired intestinal motility. In addition to the increased intestinal permeability associated with cirrhosis, these quantitative and qualitative changes in the microbiota result in BT to the mesenteric lymph nodes. BT is linked to higher rates of systemic inflammation and bacterial infections (Wiest et al., 2014).

Actually, proinflammatory cytokines (primarily tumor necrosis factor-a [TNF-a] and interleukin-6 [IL-6]) and vasoactive factors (i.e., NO) in the splanchnic region as well as elevated cytokine levels in the serum, which may result in a decrease in SVR and an increase in cardiac output in contrast to individuals without BT (Albillos et al., 2003). BT and TNF-a increase NO production and endothelial nitric oxide synthase activity in mesenteric arterioles in experimental models of cirrhosis (Tazi et al., 2005). The idea that systemic inflammation contributes to splanchnic arterial vasodilation, thereby exacerbating systemic circulatory dysfunction, is bolstered by the connection observed among BT, inflammatory pathways, and NO production. Interventional studies that lower BT provide more evidence for the significance of both BT and inflammation in the pathophysiology of HRS. This is because, in patients with advanced cirrhosis, norfloxacin treatment for primary prophylaxis of spontaneous bacterial peritonitis (SBP) lowers the risk of HRS without preventing SBP (Fernandez et al., 2007), supporting the hypothesis that the prevention of BT may reduce systemic inflammation and subsequently decreases the risk of HRS (Figure 8.1).

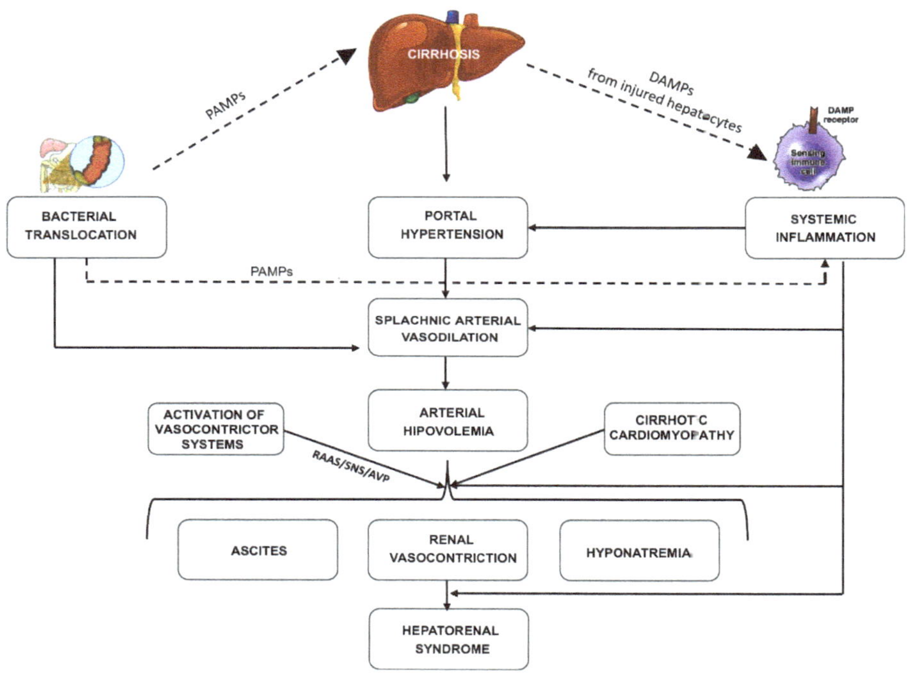

Figure 8.1. *Proposed pathophysiology of heptorenal syndrome. PAMPS, pathogen-associated molecular patterns; DAMPS, damage-associated molecular patterns; RAAS, renin-angiotensin aldosterone system; SNS, sympathetic nervous system; AVP, vasopressin.*

Source: I. Graupera, et al., Hepatorenal Syndrome, http://dx.doi.org/10.1016/B978-0-12-804274-8.00038-2.

Studies conducted in the 1990s provided clinical evidence that patients with SBP and HRS had significantly higher levels of IL-6 and TNF-a in their plasma and ascitic fluid than did patients with SBP but not HRS (Navasa et al., 1998). Furthermore, elevated levels of vasodilator substances, such as carbon monoxide and NO, were linked to this rise in circulating cytokines (De las Heras et al., 2003). All kinds of infections may be linked to HRS, despite the fact that the condition was initially identified in SBP patients (Terra et al., 2005; Fasolato et al., 2007; Pereira et al.,2012).

According to a prospective study, about one-third of patients with cirrhosis and bacterial infections experience HRS, and nearly half of those patients experience rapidly progressive HRS (type-1) (Barreto et al., 2014).

A prospective study comprising 100 patients with cirrhosis and AKI evaluated the association between systemic inflammation and the type of kidney failure (Thabut et al., 2007). While only 14% of patients with kidney failure due to hypovolemia had associated infections and/or systemic inflammatory response syndrome (SIRS), the majority of patients with HRS (78%) did. Surprisingly, SIRS was present in nearly one-third of patients with HRS even though no bacterial infection was reported. These data indicate that systemic inflammation, with or without infection, is common in HRS and seems to be characteristic of this condition and not related to impaired kidney function per se as it does not occur in kidney failure due to hypovolemia. These results imply that systemic and local proinflammatory responses are induced by BT, the release of PAMPs and DAMPs, and bacterial infections. This could result in a highly inflammatory state that exacerbates impaired circulatory function and progressive renal hypoperfusion, which could be a trigger for the development of HRS.

8.2. Diagnosis

The International Club of Ascites (ICA) first proposed the current definition of HRS in 1996, and it was revised in 2007 (Arroyo et al., 1996; Salerno et al., 2007). The following factors were used to determine the diagnosis: (1) the existence of advanced liver disease; (2) an increase in serum creatinine to a level greater than 2.5 mg/dL over a 2-week period for HRS-type 1; and (3) clinical and analytical standards to exclude other possible causes of renal failure. A limitation of this definition was that serum creatinine levels had to double from baseline to a value greater than 2.5 mg/dL in order to diagnose type 1 HRS (HRS-1).

There are two distinct types of HRS, each with a distinct clinical evolution and prognosis, based on the severity of kidney failure. Serum creatinine levels rise extremely quickly to levels greater than 2.5 mg/dL in HRS-1, which is characterized as an AKI. With a median survival of just two weeks without treatment, it is linked to an extremely poor prognosis. However, type 2 HRS (HRS-2) is characterized by a moderate impairment of kidney function with serum creatinine levels typically ranging from 1 to 2 mg/dL. It can progress less quickly over a variable period of time or remain stable. With a median survival of six months, these patients have a better prognosis than those with HRS-1, despite the fact that they are also linked to a poor prognosis (Table 8.1).

A revised definition of HRS has been proposed recently, though, and it incorporates the criteria of the Acute Kidney Injury Network (AKIN). AKI has been defined differently for the general population over the last ten years, with relative changes in serum creatinine being suggested as the definition rather than a specific cut-off value. AKI is defined by the AKIN criteria as a rise in serum creatinine of more than 0.3 mg/dL from baseline (Mehta et al., 2007). Additionally, based on the progression and serum creatinine value, it divides AKI into several stages. It has been demonstrated that even slight increases in serum creatinine levels have an effect on prognosis, and these criteria have also been validated in the cirrhotic population.

Table 8.1. *Classical Diagnostic Criteria of HRS (Barreto et al., 2014)*

Classical Diagnostic Criteria of HRS
• Cirrhosis with ascites. • Serum creatinine >133 mmol/L (1.5 mg/dL). • No improvement of serum creatinine (decrease to a level of ≤133 mmol/L) after at least 2 days with diuretic withdrawal and volume expansion with albumin. The recommended dose of albumin is 1 g/kg of body weight per day up to a maximum of 100 g/day. • Absence of shock. • No current or recent treatment with nephrotoxic drugs. • Absence of parenchymal kidney disease as indicated by proteinuria >500 mg/day, microhematuria (>50 red blood cells per high-power field), and/or abnormal renal ultrasonography.
HRS, hepatorenal syndrome.

Source: I. Graupera, et al., Hepatorenal Syndrome, http://dx.doi.org/10.1016/B978-0-12-804274-8.00038-2.

Additionally, it has been noted that in patients with HRS, the likelihood of responding to vasoconstrictors is inversely correlated with the serum creatinine levels at diagnosis (Rodriguez et al., 2014). In light of this, the most recent ICA consensus has proposed a revised definition of HRS based on the classification of AKI and the removal of the serum creatinine threshold value for the diagnosis of HRS (ICA-AKI criteria; Angeli et al.) as well as a new definition for the diagnosis of AKI in cirrhosis. , 2015), making it possible to diagnose and treat these patients earlier.

8.3. Differential Diagnosis

AKI can occur in patients with cirrhosis for a variety of reasons, the most frequent being hypovolemia, acute tubular necrosis (ATN), and HRS. Given that these causes have entirely different prognoses and courses of treatment, the differential diagnosis between them is crucial (Martin-Llahi et al., 2011). Particularly difficult is the differential diagnosis between ATN and HRS (Table 8.2 & 8.3). Both disorders can occur in very sick cirrhosis patients, and while ATN is a structural kidney failure that, in extreme circumstances, should be treated with dialysis, HRS is a functional kidney failure that can be treated with certain pharmaceuticals (Schrier, 2010; Gill et al., 2005; Gines & Fagundes 2012). Currently, clinical diagnostic criteria that involve some subjectivity are used to differentiate between the various causes of AKI in cirrhosis.

The biomarker most frequently used in routine clinical practice to diagnose AKI is serum creatinine. However, serum creatinine is unable to differentiate between the various kidney failure causes. Thus, objective techniques that reliably aid in the differential diagnosis of AKI in cirrhosis patients—particularly between functional kidney failure (HRS) and ATN—are desperately needed. Nephrology research over the past few years has revealed many urine biomarkers of kidney injury that seem to be helpful in the differential diagnosis of AKI causes, early detection of AKI, and prediction of AKI progression. The most promising of these biomarkers are liver-type fatty acid-binding protein (L-FABP), kidney injury molecule-1 (KIM-1), IL-18, and neutrophil gelatinase-associated lipocalin (NGAL).

Table 8.2. *ICA-AKI New Definitions for the Diagnosis of AKI in Patients With Cirrhosis (Piano et al., 2013)*

Subject	Definition
Baseline sCr	A value of sCr obtained in the previous 3 months, when available, can be used as baseline sCr. In patients with more than one value within the previous 3 months, the value closest to the admission time to the hospital should be used. In patients without a previous sCr value, the sCr on admission should be used as baseline.
Definition of AKI	• Increase in sCr ≥0.3 mg/dL (≥26.5 μmol/L) within 48 h. • A percentage increase sCr ≥50% from baseline which is known, or presumed, to have occurred within the prior 7 days.
Staging of AKI	**Stage 1:** Increase in sCr ≥0.3 mg/dL (26.5 μmol/L) or an increase in sCr ≥1.5-fold −2-fold from baseline. **Stage 2:** Increase in sCr greater than twofold to threefold from baseline. **Stage 3:** Increase of sCr greater than threefold from baseline or sCr ≥4.0 mg/dL (353.6 μmol/L) with an acute increase ≥0.3 mg/dL (26.5 μmol/L) or initiation of renal replacement therapy.

ICA-AKI, International Club of Ascites—Acute Kidney Injury; *sCr,* serum creatinine.
Adapted from Angeli, P., Gines, P., Wong, F., et al., 2015. Diagnosis and management of acute kidney injury in patients with cirrhosis: revised consensus recommendations of the International Club of Ascites. J. Hepatol. 62 968–974.

Source. I. Graupera, et al., Hepatorenal Syndrome, http://dx.doi.org/10.1016/B978-0-12-804274-8.00038-2.

Table 8.3. *New Proposed Diagnostic Criteria of HRS According to the ICA-AKI Criteria (Piano et al., 2013)*

HRS AKI Diagnosis

- Diagnosis of cirrhosis and ascites.
- Diagnosis of AKI according to ICA-AKI criteria.
- No response after 2 consecutive days of diuretic withdrawal and plasma volume expansion with albumin 1 g/kg of body weight.
- Absence of shock.
- No current or recent use of nephrotoxic drugs (NSAIDs, aminoglycosides, iodinated contrast media, etc.).
- No macroscopic signs of structural kidney injury, defined as:
  - Absence of proteinuria (>500 mg/day)
  - Absence of microhematuria (>50 RBCs per high-power field)
  - Normal findings on renal ultrasonography

HRS, hepatorenal syndrome; *ICE-AKI,* International Club of Ascites—Acute Kidney Injury; *NSAIDs,* nonsteroidal anti-inflammatory drugs; *RBCs,* red blood cells.

Source. I. Graupera, et al., Hepatorenal Syndrome, http://dx.doi.org/10.1016/B978-0-12-804274-8.00038-2

Damaged kidney tubular epithelia cause the overexpression of the 24 kDa glycoprotein known as NGAL. Before serum creatinine elevates during AKI, urinary NGAL (uNGAL) levels increase exponentially (Koyner et al., 2010). The possible contribution of uNGAL to the differential diagnosis of AKI causes in cirrhosis has been examined in four different studies (Fagundes et al., 2012; Verna et al., 2012; Belcher et al., 2014; Ariza et al., 2015). uNGAL levels were higher in AKI patients than in non-AKI patients. The primary discovery of these investigations, however, is that uNGAL levels aid in the differential diagnosis of AKI in cirrhosis. When comparing uNGAL levels between patients with prerenal azotemia and HRS, patients with ATN have the highest levels. The lowest uNGAL levels are seen in patients with prerenal azotemia, which is comparable to those in patients without AKI. It's interesting to note that patients with HRS have intermediate uNGAL levels, which are considerably higher than those of hypovolemia patients and significantly lower than those of ATN patients. (Fagundes et al., 2012; Verna et al., 2012; Belcher et al., 2014; Ariza et al., 2015). These studies' data demonstrate that uNGAL, with areas under the receiver-operating characteristic curves of 0.8, has a good predictive accuracy for differentiating ATN from other causes of AKI (Fagundes et al., 2012; Belcher et al., 2014). In addition to NGAL, two other studies assessed the significance of other urine biomarkers in the differential diagnosis of AKI in cirrhosis patients (Belcher et al., 2014; Ariza et al., 2015) (Figure 8.2).

The consistent findings from both studies demonstrate that patients with ATN have significantly higher levels of IL-18 and albumin than patients with a non-ATN cause of AKI, with good predictive accuracy. In patients with ATN, L-FABP and KIM-1 likewise exhibit a similar pattern at higher levels. KIM-1, a 105 kDa transmembrane glycoprotein, has been demonstrated to rise in the kidney's proximal tubule in response to injury (i.e., ischemia, nephrotoxicity) (Han et al., 2002). L-FABP belongs to FABP family, which are cytoplasmic proteins of 13–14 kDa that bind long-chain fatty acids. They are expressed in different cell types; particularly, L-FABP is expressed in liver, kidney, and intestine, among others (Nakamura et al., 2006).

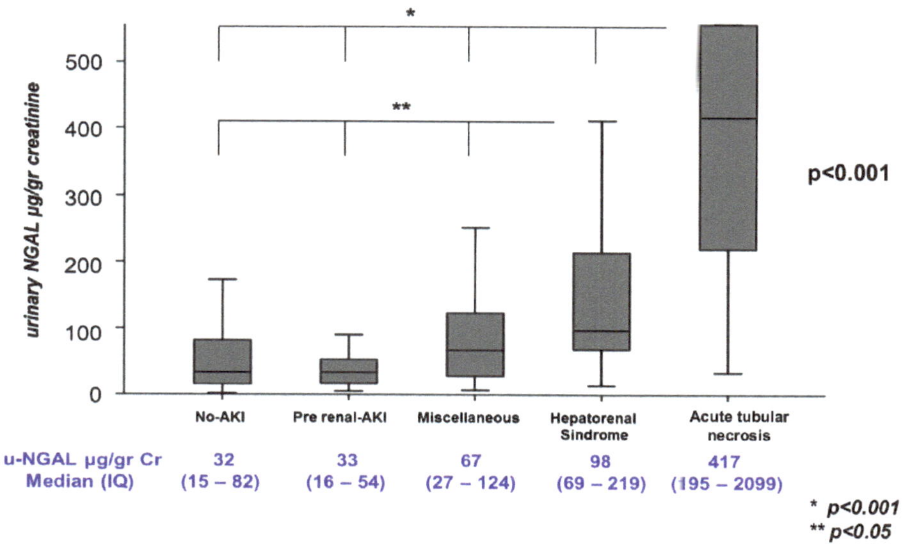

Figure 8.2. *Urine neutrophil gelatinase-associated lipocalin (NGAL) levels in patients with cirrhosis without acute kidney injury (AKI) and AKI due to different causes.*

Source: Adapted from Fagundes, C., Pepin, M.N., Guevara, M., et al., 2012. Urinary neutrophil gelatinase-associated lipocalin as biomarker in the differential diagnosis of impairment of kidney function in cirrhosis. J. Hepatol. 57, 267–273.

Urinary biomarkers, particularly NGAL, appear to be a useful and promising tool for the differential diagnosis of AKI in cirrhosis. The usefulness of these biomarkers in clinical practice will be made clear by prospective studies assessing them in the differential diagnosis algorithm.

8.4. Precipitating Factors

When HRS develops on its own without any apparent trigger, it is most likely the result of the disease's advancement and can further impair circulatory function. On the other hand, a precipitating factor that exacerbates pre-existing circulatory dysfunction may also cause HRS. Though all other types of infections can also cause HRS to develop, their frequency is usually lower. Bacterial infections, especially SBP, are the most common precipitating factors (Fagundes and Gines, 2012). Therefore, patients with cirrhosis and bacterial infections need a close monitoring to enable early diagnosis of the potential development of AKI.

Another circumstance that can potentially result in the development of HRS in about 15% of patients is large-volume paracentesis without concurrent intravenous (IV) albumin administration (Fagundes & Gines, 2012). In fact, the primary indication for IV albumin administration following large-volume paracentesis is the prevention of HRS-1.

Finally, gastrointestinal (GI) bleeding is another complication of cirrhosis that can act as a precipitating factor of HRS. However, kidney failure in the setting of GI bleeding is uncommon (<10%) and is usually associated with prerenal AKI rather than HRS (Cardenas et al., 2001).

8.5. Treatment of HRS

8.5.1. General Management

General management is dependent on the kind of HRS and any related issues (EASL, 2010; Fagundes & Gines, 2012). Hospitalization is necessary for the management of patients with HRS-1, ideally in an intensive care unit or an intermediate care unit. These patients require close monitoring to detect treatment-related adverse events and associated cirrhosis complications, especially bacterial infections, early in the course of treatment. The management of patients with HRS-1 who are not candidates for liver transplantation should be decided individually due to the poor prognosis of HRS1 (EASL, 2010; Fagundes & Gines, 2012).

For patients undergoing treatment with vasoconstrictors and albumin, central venous catheterization is advised to track central venous pressure. However, because there is a significant risk of urinary tract infections, using a bladder catheter is not always necessary and should even be avoided. It is only advised for patients with severe oliguria to use a bladder catheter. Lastly, because these patients have severe kidney failure and pronounced sodium and solute-free water retention, it is important to administer IV fluid with caution. Thus, the administration of excessive IV fluids may raise the risk of developing pulmonary edema as well as increase ascites and edema (EASL, 2010; Durand et al., 2016). In contrast to patients with HRS-1, patients with HRS-2 without associated complications can be managed in the outpatient clinic.

8.5.2. Vasoconstrictor Drugs

Currently, the therapy of choice for managing HRS-1 as a stopgap to liver transplantation is treatment with vasoconstrictor medications combined with IV albumin (EASL, 2010; Fagundes and Gines, 2012;). Vasoconstrictor medications include alpha-adrenergic agonists like noradrenaline and midodrine as well as vasopressin analogs like terlipressin that are used to treat HRS. The majority of available data and published evidence relates to the use of albumin and terlipressin.

- ***Terlipressin:*** About 40–50% of patients with HRS-1 who receive treatment with terlipressin and albumin see a significant improvement in their kidney function, according to data from randomized, controlled trials and systematic reviews (Sanyal et al., 2008; Martin-Llahi et al., 2008; Gluud et al., 2010). Additionally, a systematic review revealed that this treatment increased patients' survival rates who had type 1 HRS (Gluud et al., 2010). Classically the scheme of treatment with terlipressin is based on repeated IV boluses (EASL, 2010; Fagundes and Gines, 2012). It is recommended to start terlipressin treatment at a dose of 1 mg/4–6 h. If after 3 days of treatment, there is no improvement of kidney function, defined as a reduction of serum creatinine of more than 25% from pretreatment value, the dose should be increased up to 2 mg/4–6 h. The course of treatment is continued for a maximum of 14 days or until there is a complete response, which is indicated by a drop in serum creatinine to less than 10.5 mg/dL (EASL, 2010). Terlipressin treatment recipients need to be closely watched in order to identify any possible side effects as soon as possible. Terlipressin is a potent vasoconstrictor that can cause heart palpitations or ischemia. About 10% of patients experience ischemic side effects that force them to stop their medication (EASL, 2010; Sanyal et al., 2008; Martin-Llahi et al., 2008). Patients taking terlipressin must also receive concurrent IV albumin treatment, starting on the first day at 1 g/kg body weight and increasing to 20–40 g/day (Fagundes & Gines, 2012; EASL, 2010). It is advised to keep an eye on central venous pressure while receiving treatment, as was previously mentioned. IV albumin should be temporarily stopped if patients experience elevated central venous pressure levels during treatment, with values greater than 12–15 mmHg.

Nonrandomized research has indicated that administering terlipressin by continuous IV infusion rather than IV boluses may increase its effectiveness and reduce side effects (Piano et al., 2011). Recently, the first randomized, controlled trial comparing the safety and efficacy of terlipressin given by continuous IV infusion versus IV boluses has been published. This study shows that the percentage of response to treatment was not significantly different between patients treated with continuous IV infusion versus patients treated with IV boluses (76% vs. 65%, respectively; P ¼ NS) (Cavallin et al., 2016).

Nonetheless, the group receiving continuous infusion therapy had a noticeably lower mean daily effective dose of terlipressin. Additionally, compared to the group of patients treated with IV boluses, the rate of adverse events was significantly lower in the continuous IV infusion group (35% vs. $P < .025$) 62%, respectively. Consequently, the study's findings imply that terlipressin administered via continuous IV infusion is more effective and well-tolerated at lower dosages than terlipressin administered via IV boluses (Cavallin et al., 2016).

Lastly, it is important to note that while patients with ongoing bacterial infections were not included in the original definition of HRS, this has changed with the publication of a revised definition in 2007 (Salerno et al., 2007). Patients with active bacterial infections were excluded from all trials evaluating the safety and effectiveness of terlipressin and albumin for HRS-1 in this particular context. As a result, data on the effectiveness and security of albumin and vasoconstrictors in patients with persistent infections were unavailable. A recent prospective proof-of-concept study examined the safety and effectiveness of terlipressin and albumin treatment in patients with type-1 HRS who were still experiencing sepsis. According to another study, treating HRS-1 linked to sepsis with terlipressin and albumin is both safe and effective. As a result, this treatment may be suggested in this particular clinical setting (Rodriguez et al., 2014).

- ***Alpha-Adrenergic Agonists:*** When terlipressin is unavailable in a given country, other vasoconstrictors serve as an alternate pharmaceutical intervention. These consist of subcutaneous octreotide plus oral midodrine plus IV noradrenaline; both are connected to IV albumin at the same dosage as suggested for terlipressin treatment. Noradrenaline seems to be useful for managing HRS-1, despite the paucity of available data (Alessandria et al., 2007; Sharma et al., 2008; Singh et al., 2012; Junior Nassar et al., 2014). In a recent randomized-controlled study, the effectiveness and safety of treating patients with HRS with terlipressin versus noradrenaline were compared. In both groups, about 40% of patients responded to treatment, and the adverse event profile was likewise comparable (Singh et al., 2012). Therefore, noradrenaline seems to be as effective and safe as terlipressin for the management of HRS-1.

It has also been proposed that patients with HRS-1 may benefit from a combination of subcutaneous octreotide linked to albumin and oral midodrine to enhance kidney function. However, there have only been a few studies conducted thus far, and no randomized comparison trials with other vasoconstrictors have been conducted (Esrailian et al., 2007; Skagen et al., 2009). A recent randomized controlled trial examined the efficacy of treating patients with HRS with terlipressin plus albumin versus midodrine and octreotide plus albumin. According to this study, the combination of midodrine and octreotide plus albumin is not as effective as terlipressin plus albumin therapy (response rate 70% vs. 29%, respectively; P ¼ .01) (Cavallin et al., 2016).

8.5.3. Liver Transplantation

Liver transplantation is the preferred treatment for patients with HRS as it provides a definitive solution for the underlying liver disease (EASL, 2010; Fagundes & Gines, 2012; Durand et al., 2016). Given the extremely short survival times of all patients with HRS, these patients ought to be referred to hospitals that have established liver transplant programs and ought to be regarded as candidates for liver transplantation. These patients should be evaluated for a liver transplant alone rather than a combined liver and kidney transplant because HRS is reversible following liver transplantation. Only patients with HRS who have not responded to treatment and who have needed renal replacement therapy (RRT) for longer than 6–8 weeks—and who therefore have a low chance of recovering kidney function—should be evaluated for a combined liver and kidney transplant (Charlton et al., 2009). The fact that patients with HRS-1 have a high waiting list mortality rate is an important consideration. As a result, these patients ought to receive transplant consideration with top priority. Giving these patients high priority in the organ allocation process is made possible by the utilization of the model for end-stage liver disease (MELD) score, which incorporates serum creatinine. It is advised to keep the MELD score determined using the serum creatinine value prior to treatment while these patients are on the waiting list in order to prevent a decrease in the MELD score in those patients who respond to medical treatment with vasoconstrictors and albumin. (Fagundes & Gines, 2012; Boyer et al., 2011; Angeli & Gines, 2012).

Finally, although there are no prospective studies, it is recommended that patients with HRS-1 should be treated with vasoconstrictors and albumin before transplantation because this strategy may improve outcomes after transplantation (EASL, 2010; Fagundes and Gines, 2012).

8.5.4. Transjugular Intrahepatic Portosystemic Shunt

As an alternative therapy for the management of HRS, TIPS has been proposed because it lowers portal pressure, improves circulatory dysfunction, and may therefore improve kidney function. The use of TIPS in patients with HRS-1, who have a very advanced form of liver disease, is, however, extremely limited because many of them are not suitable candidates for TIPS insertion. TIPS improves kidney function in about 60% of patients with HRS by reducing the activity of endogenous vasoconstrictor systems, according to two small studies. These studies did not include patients with prior hepatic encephalopathy or those with advanced liver disease, which is defined as a Child-Pugh score of 12 or serum bilirubin levels greater than 5 mg/dL (Brensing et al., 2000; Mitzner et al., 2000). Therefore, existing data are very limited and the applicability of TIPS in patients with HRS-1 is very low because TIPS is considered contraindicated in patients with severe liver failure, which is very common in the setting.

8.5.5. Renal Replacement Therapy

Studies evaluating the function of RRT in HRS-1 patients are nonexistent. When vasoconstrictors fail to treat patients with HRS-1 and they meet the requirements for emergent RRT (hypervolemia, hyperkalemia, and metabolic acidosis), RRT may be used. Clinical experience, however, suggests that, at least initially, the development of criteria leading to the indication of RRT is uncommon in patients with HRS-1. Novel dialysis techniques for the treatment of HRS-1 have been proposed, including the use of the fractionated plasma separation and adsorption (Prometheus) system and the molecular readsorbent recirculating system. These techniques are predicated on the removal of various chemicals, including endogenous vasodilators, from the bloodstream. They seem promising, but more research is required to fully understand their potential as therapeutic alternatives for HRS because the available data are still sparse and the results ambiguous (Mitzner et al., 2000; Kribben et al., 2012).

8.6. Hepatopulmonary Syndrome

8.6.1. Definition and Prevalence

Hepatopulmonary syndrome (HPS) is identified by a combination of gas exchange problems resulting from the growth of vascular dilations within the lungs and shunting between arteries and veins in individuals with liver disease and/or portal hypertension. It appears to affect between 4–47% of patients with chronic liver disease (Hopkins et al., 1992; Stoller et al., 1995). The diverse study populations and applied diagnostic criteria are to blame for the wide range of prevalence. Although its presence has also been reported in patients with acute or chronic inflammatory liver disease, Budde-Chiari syndrome, and portal hypertension without chronic liver disease, HPS is most frequently linked to liver cirrhosis (De et al., 2000; Gupta et al., 2001; Regev et al., 2001; Teuber et al., 2002).

8.6.2. Clinical Features

Since HPS cases can be asymptomatic, patients on the waiting list for liver transplantation (LT) should be actively screened for the disease. Dyspnea is the most common symptom of HPS. Digital clubbing, cyanosis, and spider angiomas are related clinical symptoms that are not particular to the diagnosis of HPS (Teuber et al., 2002). Platypnea and orthodeoxia, dyspnea, and hypoxemia that worsens when standing are characteristics specific to HPS. These result from the pulmonary blood being redistributed to the basal regions of the lungs during the transition from a supine to an upright position, along with the predominance of vasodilation in these areas, which raises the ventilation-perfusion mismatch (Teuber et al., 2002). These clinical indications, however, do not necessarily indicate HPS.

Research findings regarding the relationship between the severity of liver disease, as indicated by the Child-Pugh or MELD score, and HPS are inconsistent. While many studies show a weak correlation between liver disease severity and oxygenation levels, some conflicting data exists (Teuber et al., 2002; Regev et al., 2001; Abrams et al., 1995; Krowka et al., 2000b; Mandell, 2004; Hoeper et al., 2004; Singh and Sager, 2009), other studies indeed show an association between them (Vachiery et al., 1997; Schenk et al., 2002; Younis et al., 2015). Generally, one can agree that HPS may occur in each Child-Pugh class, although it most often occurs in Child-Pugh C patients (Grace and Angus, 2013).

8.6.3. Diagnosis

The combination of impaired gas exchange and IPVDs in patients with cirrhosis and/or portal hypertension is one of the diagnostic criteria for HPS. It is important to look into concurrent cardiopulmonary disease because HPS can coexist with other intrinsic heart or lung conditions, which can make clinical symptoms worse. The European Respiratory Society Task Force recommends diagnosing gas exchange disturbances by calculating the P(A-a) O_2 gradient (arterial blood gas in an upright position, breathing room air): $[(\text{Patm}-\text{PH}_2\text{O}) \times 0.21-\text{PaCO}_2/0.8]-\text{PaO}_2$. The severity of HPS is classified based on PaO_2 measurements (Rodriguez-Roisin et al., 2004). Orthodeoxia can be diagnosed as a PaO_2 decrease of ≥ 4 mmHg or $\geq 5\%$ from a supine to the upright position. However, one should keep in mind that hypoxemia may also occur due to hepatic hydrothorax, ascites, chronic obstructive pulmonary disease, and interstitial lung disease (Table 8.4).

Table 8.4. *Diagnostic Criteria for Hepatopulmonary Syndrome and Portopulmonary Hypertension*

HPS	1. Presence of liver disease 2. Intrapulmonary shunting 3. P(A–a) O_2 gradient $\geq$ 15 mmHg (or >20 mmHg when >65 years of age)
PPHT	1. Presence of portal hypertension 2. mPAP > 25 mmHg 3. PCWP > 15 mmHg 4. PVR > 240 dyne s/cm^5

HPS, hepatopulmonary syndrome; *mPAP*, mean pulmonary artery pressure; *PCWP*, pulmonary capillary wedge pressure; *PPHT*, portopulmonary hypertension; *PVR*, pulmonary vascular resistance.

Source: S. Raevens and I. Colle, Hepatopulmonary Syndrome and Portopulmonary Hypertension, http://dx.doi.org/10.1016/B978-0-12-804274-8.00039-4.

Table 8.5. *Staging of Severity of Hepatopulmonary Syndrome and Portopulmonary Syndrome*

Stage	HPS, PaO_2	PPHT, mPAP
Mild	$\geq$80 mmHg	>25–<35 mmHg
Moderate	60–79 mmHg	$\geq$35–<45 mmHg
Severe	50–59 mmHg	$\geq$45 mmHg
Very severe	<50 mmHg	–

HPS, hepatopulmonary syndrome; *mPAP*, mean pulmonary artery pressure, *PPHT*, portopulmonary hypertension.

Source: S. Raevens and I. Colle, Hepatopulmonary Syndrome and Portopulmonary Hypertension, http://dx.doi.org/10.1016/B978-0-12-804274-8.00039-4.

Microbubble transthoracic echocardiography (MTTE) or a 99m-Technetium-labeled macroaggregated albumin (MAA) scan are used to document IPVDs. The accepted gold standard is MTTE. In this procedure, an intravenous injection of hand-shaken saline is used to create microbubbles larger than 10 mm in diameter. When the body is healthy, these bubbles get stuck in the <8–15 mm lung capillaries and are then taken up by the alveoli. Intrapulmonary shunting and IPVDs (15–100 mm) are present in cases of HPS when the left atrium opacifies three to six cardiac cycles after the appearance of microbubbles in the right atrium (Table 8.5).

Differentiating intrapulmonary shunting from intracardiac right-to-left shunts, which cause microbubbles to form in the left atrium as soon as three cardiac cycles, is critically important. When compared to transthoracic echocardiography, transesophageal contrast echocardiography offers superior imaging quality, which increases the sensitivity of HPS detection (Aller et al., 1999).

However, because it requires sedation, has a higher cost, and has a theoretical but low risk of esophageal variceal bleeding, this technique is not frequently used in practice (Rodriguez-Roisin et al., 2004) (Figure 8.3).

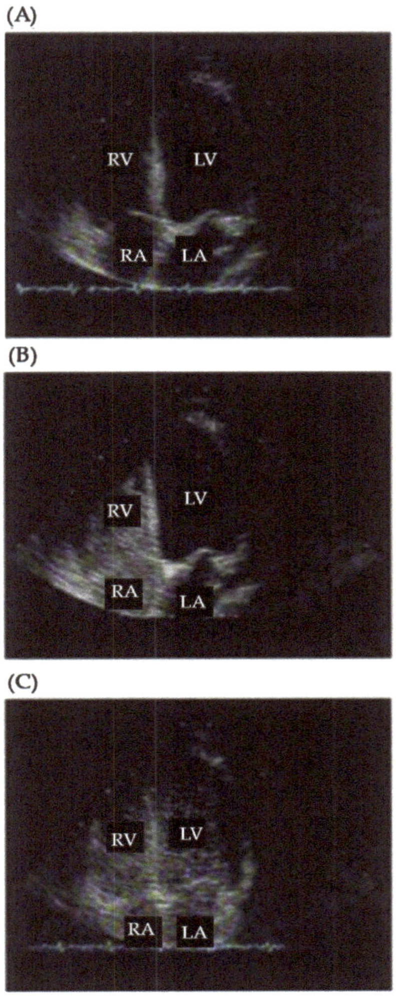

Figure 8.3. *Contrast echocardiogram for detecting intrapulmonary vasodilatation. (A) Parasternal four-chamber view of the heart (LA, left atrium; LV, left ventricle; RA, right atrium; RV, right ventricle) prior to the administration of agitated saline contrast. (B) Four-chamber view immediately after the administration of contrast, demonstrating the presence of echogenic microbubbles in the right atrium and ventricle immediately after injection of agitated saline into the antecubital vein. (C) Visualization of echogenic microbubbles in the left atrium and ventricle three cardiac cycles after visualization on the right due to intrapulmonary vasodilatation in a patient with hepatopulmonary syndrome. Intracardiac shunting results in the immediate passage of microbubbles from the right-to-left chambers without a three cycle delay and can be excluded using this technique.*

Source: Reproduced from Fallon, M.B., Arguedas, M.R., 2006. Pulmonary complications of liver disease. In: Boyer, T.D., Wright, T.L., Manns, M.P., Zakim and Boyer's Hepatology, fifth ed. Elsevier, pp. 477–488, with permission.

During MAA scanning, 99m-Technetium-labeled albumin is injected intravenously and radionuclide uptake in the brain and kidneys is studied. Normally, the particles (>20 mm in diameter) are trapped in the pulmonary capillaries (<8–15 mm diameter). In the case of intracardiac or intrapulmonary shunts, these aggregates can pass through the pulmonary vasculature and are subsequently retained in the brain and kidneys (Wolfe et al., 1977). The pulmonary and systemic radionuclide uptake can be quantified using an MAA scan, which has the benefit of helping to identify patients who are more likely to die from LT-associated causes. The inability of the MAA scan to distinguish between intracardiac and intrapulmonary shunting is its main drawback (Krowka et al., 2000b; Arguedas et al., 2003; Rodriguez-Roisin et al., 2004).

Since MTTE can distinguish between intracardiac and intrapulmonary shunting, it is more sensitive (Abrams et al., 1995), MTTE is regarded as the most effective screening method for HPS detection. Furthermore, one benefit of MTTE is its ability to identify pulmonary hypertension. Investigating concurrent cardiopulmonary disease requires additional testing. Chest radiographs can be normal or reveal evidence of IPVDs, such as high-resolution computed tomography (HRDT) (Herve et al., 2007; Singh & Sager, 2009). When large arteriovenous malformations that are amenable to embolization are suspected, pulmonary angiography is indicated in cases of severe hypoxemia (PaO2 < 60 mmHg) (Singh and Sager, 2009 July). Pulmonary angiography allows for the distinction between two types of HPS patterns. Normal angiography or diffuse vascular dilatation characterize type I, while focal arteriovenous malformations characterize type II. Coil embolization should be taken into consideration because these type II arteriovenous communications may continue after LT and because they pose a risk for paradoxal embolism and cerebral abscesses (Krowka et al., 2000b, 1993; Poterucha et al., 1995; Molleston et al., 1999; Anel & Sheagren, 2001; Porres-Aguilar et al., 2012). Patients with HPS may have abnormal results from lung function tests, particularly from the diffusing capacity for carbon monoxide (CO), which can range from mild to more severe forms (Martinez et al., 2001).

While arterial blood gas analysis and MTTE are considered the gold standard tests for diagnosis, simpler and more widely available noninvasive techniques are commonly used to screen for the presence of HPS. Research indicates that pulse oximetry, which measures the difference in oxygen saturation between when a person is supine and standing, is a highly sensitive screening method for HPS (Arguedas et al., 2007; Abrams et al., 2002; Krowka, 2011). An oxygen saturation threshold value of < 60 mmHg (Arguedas et al., 2007). Because of the shape of the oxyhemoglobin dissociation curve, minor fluctuations in oxygen saturation can result in significant changes in PaO_2 levels. Therefore, it is necessary to perform additional arterial blood gas analysis if oxygen saturation drops below 96%. Pulse oximetry is a noninvasive and cost-effective method that can be utilized for screening and continuous monitoring of gas exchange issues in patients with liver disease. It may also be possible to detect HPS by measuring left atrial and ventricular enlargement or the serum concentration of biomarkers (vascular cell adhesion molecule 1, intercellular cell adhesion molecule 3, and von Willebrand Factor). However, these methods still need to be validated in larger patient populations (Zamirian et al., 2007; Pouriki et al., 2011; Raevens et al., 2014; Horvatits et al., 2014) (Figure 8.4).

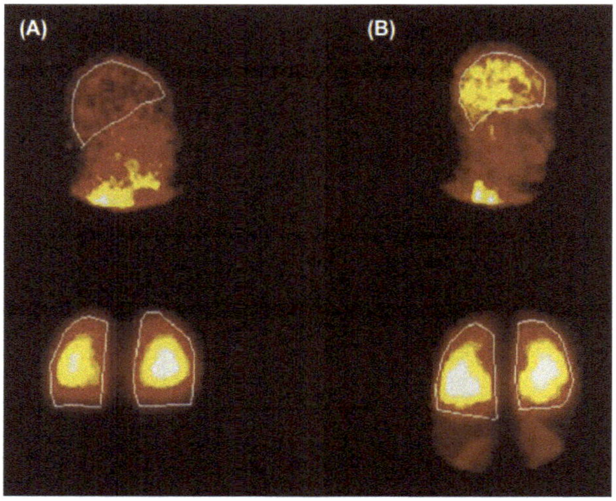

Figure 8.4. *Technetium-labeled macroaggregated albumin (MAA) scanning to detect and quantify intrapulmonary shunting in hepatopulmonary syndrome (HPS).*

Source: Reproduced from Abrams, G.A., et al., 1998. Use of macroaggregated albumin lung perfusion scan to diagnose hepatopulmonary syndrome: a new approach. Gastroenterology 114, 308, with permission.

8.6.4. Pathophysiology and Pathogenesis

Intrapulmonary vasodilation and angiogenesis, which result in arterial deoxygenation through three mechanisms (intrapulmonary right-to-left shunting, diffusion restriction, and ventilation-perfusion (V/Q) mismatch) are characteristics of HPS (Rodriguez-Roisin et al., 2004). V/Q mismatch is the primary mechanism causing impaired oxygenation; increased blood flow is produced by vasodilation at the alveolar capillary level while ventilation stays constant. Limitations on oxygen diffusion are a second mechanism that causes disruptions in gas exchange. Oxygen exchange is restricted because vasodilation lengthens the distance that oxygen molecules must travel to reach the capillary's center. In patients with liver disease, this diffusional barrier is made worse by a fast blood flow brought on by hyperdynamic circulation, which reduces the transit time of erythrocytes. Third, HPS is associated with direct intrapulmonary arteriovenous communications, which results in blood avoiding the alveoli. The mixed venous blood that enters the central circulation is the outcome of these three mechanisms (Berthelot et al., 1966; Schraufnagel et al., 1997). Although the pathogenesis of HPS is not completely understood, several mechanisms contributing to its development have been revealed in experimental studies.

- ***Vasodilation:*** An imbalance favoring vasodilation between vasoconstrictors and vasodilators is linked to abnormal intrapulmonary vasodilation in HPS. This imbalance is primarily caused by an increase in nitric monoxide (NO), which is produced by endothelial and inducible nitric oxide synthase (eNOS and iNOS) (Ling et al., 2004). Patients with HPS have been reported to have elevated exhaled NO levels; following LT, these levels returned to normal (Rolla et al., 1997) and elevated endothelin-1 (ET-1) blood levels have been linked to HPS in both humans and animals. Depending on the kind of receptor it binds to, ET-1 can cause either vasodilation or constriction of the blood vessels. Prior research has shown that experimental portal hypertension is associated with selective intrapulmonary ET-1B receptor upregulation (Zhang et al., 1999; Luo et al., 2003). The binding of ET-1 to the ET1B receptor leads to eNOS activation and NO-mediated vasodilation. The main source of this increase in circulating ET-1 is cholangiocyte production (Yang et al., 2014b). Experimental studies have shown that selective ET-1B receptor blocking was able to decrease pulmonary eNOS expression and prevent the onset of HPS (Ling et al., 2004; Zhang et al., 2009).

Second, HPS has been linked to a proinflammatory state that is typified by increased intrapulmonary recruitment and macrophage activation. This results in intestinal endotoxemia and is caused by intestinal bacterial translocation with dysfunctional liver endotoxin clearance. Tumor necrosis factor-alpha (TNF-a) and other proinflammatory cytokines stimulate iNOS, which causes a second pathway leading to NO-mediated vasodilation (Nunes et al., 2001). Treatment with either monoclonal anti-TNF-a antibodies or pentoxifyllin has been shown to improve HPS in rats by inhibiting TNF-a, iNOS, and angiogenesis (Liu et al., 2012; Sztrymf et al., 2004). Administration of the antibiotic norfloxacin was able to reduce the severity of experimental HPS by its intestinal decontaminating properties (Rabiller et al., 2002). Another mechanism leading to vasodilation is through CO. CO is primarily produced from the degradation of heme by heme oxygenase (HO) (Zhang et al., 2003). Arterial carboxyhemoglobin levels are raised in patients with HPS (Arguedas et al., 2005) and HO inhibition with tin protoporphyrin IX has been shown to be able to improve arterial blood gases and intrapulmonary vasodilation in experimental HPS (Zhang et al., 2003).

- ***Angiogenesis:*** Pathological pulmonary angiogenesis contributes to the development of pulmonary capillary proliferation and arteriovenous shunts. Angiogenesis, the process of forming new blood vessels, is controlled by various angiogenic factors, with vascular endothelial growth factor A (VEGF-A) being extensively studied in multiple liver diseases and complications (Fernandez et al., 2009; Coulon et al., 2011). Accumulation of activated macrophages, which stimulate VEGF signaling pathways, leads to pulmonary angiogenesis. Depletion of these macrophages prevented and reversed the hemodynamic and histological features of HPS, according to experimental studies (Thenappan et al., 2011). Chemokines that are specific to the pulmonary vasculature control the homing of monocytes. Endothelial chemokine ligand 1 (fractalkine, CX3CL1) binds to its chemokine receptor 1 (fractalkine receptor, CX3CR1) to sequester monocytes, and this activates VEGF-A-mediated angiogenesis (Zhang et al., 2012).

Interestingly, administration of physiological doses of ET-1 triggers an increase in CX3CL1/CX3CR1 expression, which suggests a link between ET-1 and CX3CL1 in mediating intrapulmonary monocyte accumulation and induction of angiogenesis (Zhang et al., 2014). VEGF-A is involved in both normal and pathological angiogenesis. By binding to its receptor, VEGF-A stimulates (Stoller et al., 1995) the phosphoinositide 3-kinase/protein kinase B (PI3K/Akt) and PI3K/eNOS pathway, leading to endothelial cell survival and increased NO levels, and (Hopkins et al., 1992) the phospholipase C gamma (PLCg)/mitogen-activated protein kinase/extracellular-signal-regulated kinase and the PLCg/ prostaglandin pathway, leading to endothelial cell proliferation and vascular cell permeability (Coulon et al., 2011; Dimmeler & Zeiher, 2000). It has been demonstrated in experimental studies that reducing angiogenesis with sorafenib, a small molecule with tyrosine kinase and Raf kinase inhibition properties, reduces the severity of HPS (Chang et al., 2013; Yang et al., 2014b). Treatment with rosuvastatin has been shown to improve HPS in experimental cirrhosis by acting as an antiangiogenic and anti-inflammatory agent via VEGF-A/VEGFR1,2/Rho-A kinase inhibition and TNF-a/nuclear factor kappa B (NF-kB)/iNOS inhibition (Chang et al., 2015).

- ***Respiratory Epithelial Compartment:*** The majority of research to date has concentrated on the roles that inflammation, angiogenesis, and vasodilation play in HPS. Recent data, however, also suggests that surfactant and type II epithelial cells in the alveoli play a part. In experimental HPS, a few studies showed decreased surfactant production and pneumocyte II apoptosis (Yang et al., 2014a). Further research in this area is necessary, but these changes in alveolar structure and function might offer fresh targets for upcoming therapeutic interventions.

8.6.5. Prognosis and Clinical Course

Death rates rise and life quality significantly declines as a result of HPS. In patients with HPS without LT, the 5-year survival rate is 23% and the median survival is about 24 months, while in patients without HPS, the 5-year survival rate is 63% and the median survival is 87 months (Swanson et al., 2005). The primary cause of death is not pulmonary deterioration, but rather complications from an underlying liver disease.

8.6.6. Treatment Options

Numerous pharmacological interventions have been investigated for the treatment of HPS. In the past, the majority of clinical research aimed at elucidating the pathogenic basis of NO and CO-mediated vasodilation and angiogenesis was unsatisfactory. Case studies and brief observational research using guanylate cyclase inhibitors, such as methylene blue (Rolla et al., 1994; Schenk et al., 2000; Jounieaux et al., 2001; Roma et al., 2010), nebulized NG-nitro-L-arginine methyl ester (L-NAME, NO inhibition) (Brussino et al., 2003; Gomez et al., 2006), pentoxifylline (Gupta et al., 2008; Tanikella et al., 2008; Kianifar et al., 2012), norfloxacin (Anel & Sheagren, 2001; Gupta et al., 2010a), aspirin (Song et al., 1996), somatostatin (Krowka et al., 1993), indomethacin (Machicao and Fallon, 2012), garlic (Abrams & Fallon, 1998; Najafi et al., 2006; De et al., 2010), or mycophenolate mofetil (angiogenesis and NO production inhibitor) (Moreira et al., 2013) were administered or a transjugular intrahepatic portosystemic shunt was placed had contradictory results and failed to show a clear beneficial effect as therapy for HPS in humans. As a result, no effective medical therapies for HPS are available up till now (Figure 8.5).

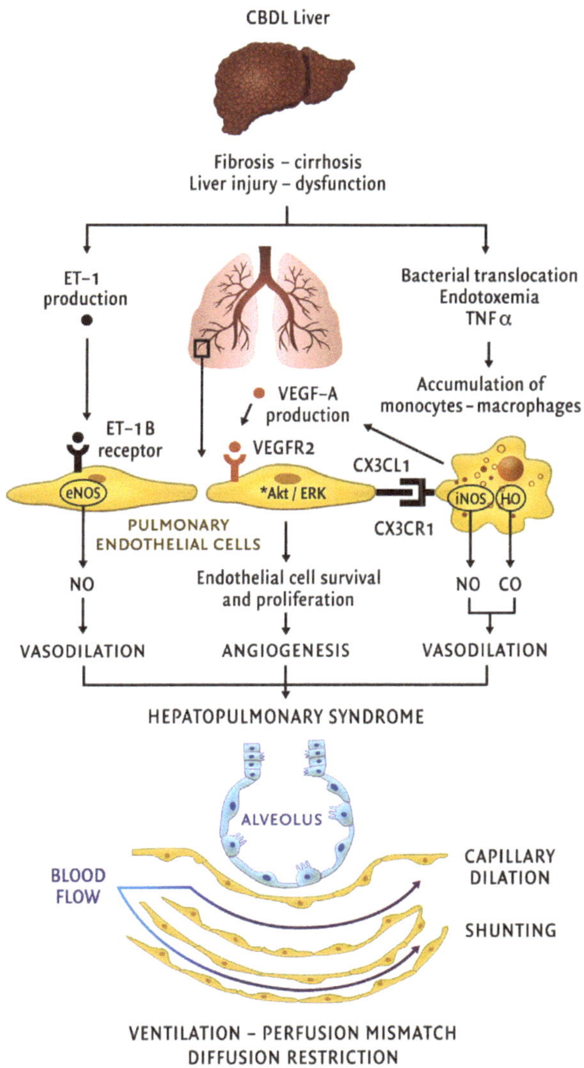

Figure 8.5. *Pathogenesis and pathophysiology of hepatopulmonary syndrome (HPS).*

Source: Reproduced from Raevens, et al., June 2015. Hepatopulmonary syndrome and portopulmonary hypertension: recent knowledge in pathogenesis and overview of clinical assessment. Liver Int. 35 (6), 1646–1660, with permission.

In cases of severe hypoxemia (PaO_2 < 60 mmHg) at rest, the only effective supportive therapy is low-flow oxygen provided continuously over an extended period of time. Arteriovenous malformations embolotherapy is a potential palliative treatment for HPS patients who are not candidates for LT (Herve et al., 2007).

HPS was once thought to be a contraindication for LT because of the high mortality rate linked to LT in HPS patients. However, after subsequent studies reported improvements in IPVDs, arterial oxygenation, and survival, HPS was deemed a sign of lung transplantation. The posttransplantation oxygenation improvement can occur months or years after the transplant. In more than 80% of cases, HPS resolves completely after LT (Rodriguez-Roisin et al., 2004; Pascasio et al., 2014), mostly within 6–12 months (Arguedas et al., 2003; Pascasio et al., 2014; Gupta et al., 2010b; Schiffer et al., 2006). A 5-year survival of 76% post-LT is reported in HPS patients, a rate which not significantly differs from that of patients without HPS (Swanson et al., 2005). However, very severe HPS (PaO2 < 50 mmHg) is associated with significantly increased posttransplantation mortality, up to 50%e100% (Taille et al., 2003). The strongest predictors of death posttransplantation are a preoperative hypoxemia ≤50 mmHg and brain uptake of ≤ 20% on MAA scan (Arguedas et al., 2003). MELD exception points are allocated to patients with advanced HPS (PaO_2 < 60 mmHg) to increase priority for LT. This policy is based on the fact that hypoxemia in HPS is progressive and that post-LT mortality is highest in patients with very severe forms of HPS. Several studies observed a trend for better survival since the implementation of the MELD exception policy for HPS compared to earlier HPS transplantation (Iyer et al., 2013). Nevertheless, it has also been reported that HPS recurs after LT (Casey et al., 2013). A recent study examined the overall pre- and post-transplantation results of patients who met the standard exception for HPS (Goldberg et al., 2014). These results indicate that the present HPS-MELD standard exception policy provides a survival advantage to wait-listed patients with HPS compared to patients without HPS exceptions. As a result, the discussion arose about whether the time has come to recalibrate the HPS-MELD standard exception policy (Sulieman et al., 2008; Ghabril and Lucey, 2014 Goldberg et al., 2014).

HPS results from abnormal intrapulmonary capillary dilation and development of arteriovenous shunts. Patients with liver disease should be screened by pulse oximetry, after which a definitive diagnosis can be made based on hypoxemia on arterial blood gas analysis and positive MTTE. As hypoxemia is generally progressive and HPS may resolve after LT, patients with severe forms of HPS can apply for MELD exception.

8.7. Portopulmonary Hypertension

8.7.1. Definition and Epidemiology

A raised mean pulmonary artery pressure (mPAP) of more than 25 mmHg is referred to as pulmonary arterial hypertension. Measurements of hemodynamic status are carried out during right heart catheterization (RHC). Portopulmonary hypertension (PPHT) is the term for pulmonary artery hypertension that occurs in conjunction with portal hypertension, either with or without liver disease, and is defined by an increased resistance to pulmonary arterial blood flow. Diagnostic hemodynamic criteria include mPAP > 25 mmHg, pulmonary vascular resistance (PVR) > 240 dyne s/cm^5, and a normal pulmonary capillary wedge pressure (PCWP) < 15 mmHg (Rodriguez-Roisin et al., 2004).

Patients with noncirrhotic portal hypertension as well as those with liver cirrhosis have PPHT. It is estimated that approximately 5% of patients with advanced liver disease and those undergoing LT evaluation have PPHT (Colle et al., 2003; Krowka et al., 2006). According to Rodriguez-Roisin et al. (2004) mPAP measurements are used to classify the severity of PPHT. There is no correlation between the degree of portal hypertension and the presence of PPHT or the severity of liver disease.

8.7.2. Clinical Signs, Screening, and Diagnosis

PPHT can present in a variety of clinical ways. Long periods of time may pass before patients show any symptoms at all, and the first ones are usually mild and nonspecific, such as weariness and dyspnea with effort. In the case of LT candidates, screening should proceed even in the absence of symptoms. Clinical signs associated with PPHT include cardiomegaly or enlarged pulmonary arteries on chest radiography, right atrial enlargement, right ventricular hypertrophy, right axis deviation, and right bundle branch block on electrocardiography (Pilatis et al., 2000). These symptoms, however, are primarily seen in PPHT cases that are more advanced. Transthoracic echocardiography (TTE) regularly screens for the presence of PPHT, even though RHC is still the gold standard for diagnosing the condition (Herve et al., 2007; Pilatis et al. (2000). To facilitate the early detection of elevated right ventricular systolic pressures (RVSP), dilatation, hypertrophy, and dysfunction in the right ventricle, routine TTE screening of LT candidates is advised (Pilatis et al., 2000; Carithers and Murray, 2005; Herve et al., 2007). Tricuspid regurgitant velocity is used to calculate the RVSP as an estimation of the systolic pulmonary artery pressure (sPAP) using the Bernoulli equation: $\text{sPAP} = 4 \times (\text{TR}^2) + \text{mRAP}$, where TR is the tricuspid regurgitant peak velocity and mRAP is the mean right atrial pressure, depending on the degree of vascular filling of the inferior cava vein. RHC is mandatory to confirm PPHT in case of elevated sPAP on TTE (Figure 8.6).

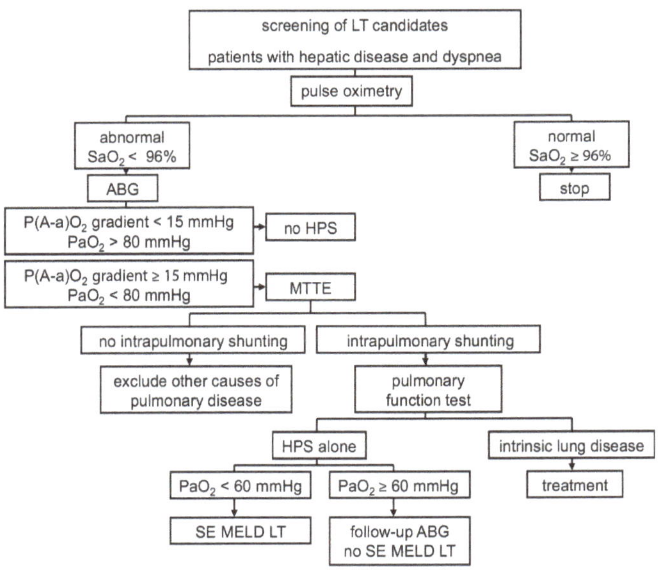

Figure 8.6. *Algorithm for screening and treatment of hepatopulmonary syndrome (HPS) in symptomatic patients and liver transplantation (LT) candidates.*

Source: Adapted from Raevens, et al., June 2015. Hepatopulmonary syndrome and portopulmonary hypertension: recent knowledge in pathogenesis and overview of clinical assessment. Liver Int. 35 (6), 1646–1660.

There is still disagreement over the sPAP cutoff point that determines when an RHC investigation is required. In various transplantation centers, cutoff values ranging from 30 to 50 mmHg are employed. Moderate to severe PPHT can be reliably detected with a cutoff of 50 mmHg (Krowka et al., 2006), but a lower cutoff of 30 mmHg can identify all PPHT types, including the mildest ones (Colle et al., 2003). The most recently published study evaluating different cutoffs for RHC referral determined a new cutoff of 38 mmHg, which is associated with high specificity (82%) maintaining a 100% negative predictive value (Raevens et al., 2013). This approach guarantees no patients with PPHT will be missed in the screening phase. The accuracy of TTE to detect PPHT can further be increased by also incorporating signs of right ventricular dysfunction, e.g., right ventricle dilation (Raevens et al., 2013). Although the optimal cutoff for estimated sPAP is not universally decided, everyone agrees that screening for PPHT with TTE is mandatory before LT. The main goal of this screening policy is to identify those patients who are at high risk of adverse cardiovascular events during LT. As PPHT may develop within time periods as short as 2–3 months (Colle et al., 2003), hemodynamic measurements should be repeated regularly (e.g., every 3 months) on the LT waiting list.

RHC is still the gold standard for diagnosing PPHT because TTE is unable to differentiate between volume overload or real PPHT, which is a hyperdynamic state with normal to low PVR (Colle et al., 2003). Up to 50% of cirrhosis patients have documented elevated mean arterial pressure (mPAP) as a result of high cardiac output, but normal or low PVR. Furthermore, the transpulmonary gradient (TPG) can be computed, and an elevated PVR is correlated with a TPG > 12 mmHg (Krowka, 2006; Golbin & Krowka, 2007; Feltracco et al., 2009), and reflects the severity of obstruction to pulmonary blood flow (Krowka, 2006). Through a Swan Ganz catheter in the right or left jugular vein, sPAP, diastolic pulmonary artery pressure, mPAP, PCWP, and mRAP can be measured. PVR and TPG can be calculated using the following formulas: PVR = (mPAP × PCWP) 80/cardiac output and TPG = mPAP × mPCWP.

8.7.3. Pathophysiology and Pathogenesis

Histologically, PPHT and other types of pulmonary arterial hypertension (PAH) are identical. The pulmonary arterial blood flow is obstructed in both conditions due to media hypertrophy, smooth muscle cell proliferation, and intima proliferation. In situ thrombosis and platelet aggregates may develop later (Krowka & Edwards, 2000; Pietra et al., 2004). An elevated PVR results from thicker arterial walls and blood vessel blockage. There are currently no experimental models that can replicate PPHT. The majority of our understanding of the development of PPHT comes from research on PAH, and its pathogenesis is unknown.

Similar to HPS, PPHT results from an imbalance between vasoconstrictors and vasodilators, with pulmonary vasoconstriction being the cause in this instance. The development of PPHT is partly due to the hyperdynamic circulation: elevated pulmonary blood flow results in shear stress, which can cause endothelial dysfunction and injury, which can then cause vasoconstriction and progressive vascular remodeling. The most widely accepted theory is that of neurohumoral activation, in which the pulmonary circulation is reached through portosystemic shunts by vasoconstrictive and proliferative substances that are either produced by the diseased liver or would normally be metabolized by a healthy liver. ET-1, tromboxane A2, interleukin-1, interleukin-6, angiotensin-1, glucagon, and serotonin are the compounds that have been identified (Giaid & Saleh, 1995; Egermayer et al., 1999; Rubens et al., 2001; Maruyama et al., 2005; Budhiraja & Hassoun, 2003). Patients with PPHT showed elevated levels of ET-1 (Pellicelli et al., 2010). Patients with PPHT are characterized by an upregulation of ET-1A receptors, which causes vasoconstriction in the event of ET-1 binding, in contrast to patients with HPS, who exhibit an upregulation of the ET-1B receptor. Since PPHT develops in only a small proportion of patients with portal hypertension, factors other than portal hypertension must play a role in its development. This gave rise to the theory that PPHT is hereditarily predisposed to develop. After examining various single nucleotide polymorphisms, it was discovered that PPHT, aromatase, phosphodiesterase 5, angiopoietin 1, calcium-binding protein A4, and estrogen receptor 1 were associated (Roberts et al., 2009).

8.7.4. Prognosis and Clinical Course

PPHT is linked to a poor prognosis since it can cause death and right heart failure. A mean survival of roughly 15 months and 1- and 5-year survival rates of 46% and 14%, respectively, can be anticipated in the absence of treatment or LT (Krowka et al., 2000a; Pilatis et al., 2000; Budhiraja & Hassoun, 2003; Neuhofer et al., 2006; Colle et al., 2007; Swanson et al., 2008).

LT might treat PPHT (Bozbas et al., 2009), however PPHT alone may make LT more difficult due to the significant hemodynamic changes and high perioperative and postoperative risks involved. It is possible to rule out transplantation in patients with PPHT based on mPAP measurements. A study conducted by Krowka et al. (2000a) showed that a right heart failure or persistent pulmonary hypertension-related death risk is 50% for an mPAP between 35 and 50 mmHg and 100% for an mPAP > 50 mmHg. These results suggest that a minimum arterial pressure of 35–50 mmHg is regarded as a relative contraindication to transplantation, while a minimum arterial pressure of 50 mmHg is known as an absolute contraindication. To ensure a successful outcome after transplantation, it is therefore necessary to lower pulmonary pressure with vasodilator therapy, aiming for mPAP < 35 mmHg, before LT. An investigation by Krowka et al., (2000a) showed that a right heart failure or persistent pulmonary hypertension-related death risk is 50% associated with an mPAP between 35 and 50 mmHg and 100% associated with an mPAP > 50 mmHg. These results indicate that a mPAP of 35–50 mmHg is regarded as a relative contraindication for transplantation, while a mPAP of 50 mmHg or higher is regarded as an absolute contraindication. Therefore, in order to ensure a successful outcome after transplantation, pulmonary pressure must be reduced by vasodilator treatment, with a target mPAP of less than 35 mmHg, before lung transplantation.

Patients with an mPAP of 35 to 45 mmHg are advised by the European Respiratory Society Task Force to receive vasodilator therapy before LT, and patients with an mPAP of 45 or higher should only receive vasodilator therapy (Rodriguez-Roisin et al., 2004). Furthermore, according to Ramsay (2010), right ventricular function must be adequate to manage the reperfusion phase of transplantation. Patients with PPHT are eligible for MELD exception points since 2006, which prioritizes them for transplantation. This is because PPHT is linked to poor outcomes, and vasodilator therapy enables successful bridging to LT, which may be curative. As long as RHC is conducted again, the MELD score may be modified every three months. However, PPHT may worsen after LT and PPHT may develop in patients with pretransplantation HPS as well. Previous case reports described possible transition between

HPS and PPHT (Martinez-Palli et al., 1999; Ioachimescu et al., 2007; Zopey et al., 2013) or coexistence of HPS and PPHT in the same patient (Pham et al., 2010).

8.7.5. Treatment Options

Advanced therapy for PPHT-related pulmonary arterial hypertension involves the administration of endothelin receptor (ETR) antagonists, phosphodiesterase type 5 (PDE-5) inhibitors, prostacyclin analogs, and soluble guanylate cyclase (sGC) stimulators. This therapy targets three pathways: the ET pathway, the NO pathway, and the prostacyclin pathway. Regretfully, there is currently insufficient information available to direct the medical management of PPHT (Figure 8.7). The majority of knowledge comes from research done on PAH patients because patients with PPHT are frequently left out of clinical trials. The role of novel medications (macitentan, oral treprostinil, and riociguat) remains to be determined. Several reports describe the effective use of oral ETR antagonists, PDE-5 inhibitors, and intravenous prostacyclin therapy to lower pulmonary pressure, even as a bridge to transplantation.

- ***Endothelin Pathway:*** There are various therapeutic options for blocking ETRs. Vasodilation is the outcome of bosentan, ambrisentan, and macitentan's antagonistic action on the ET-1 receptor. Bosentan is a nonspecific antagonist of the ET-1A and ET-1B receptors with a 20:1 selectivity for ET-1A and ET-1B receptors. It also lowers portal hypertension (Reichen et al., 1998), but disadvantage of hepatotoxicity (Reichen et al., 1998; Eriksson et al., 2011).

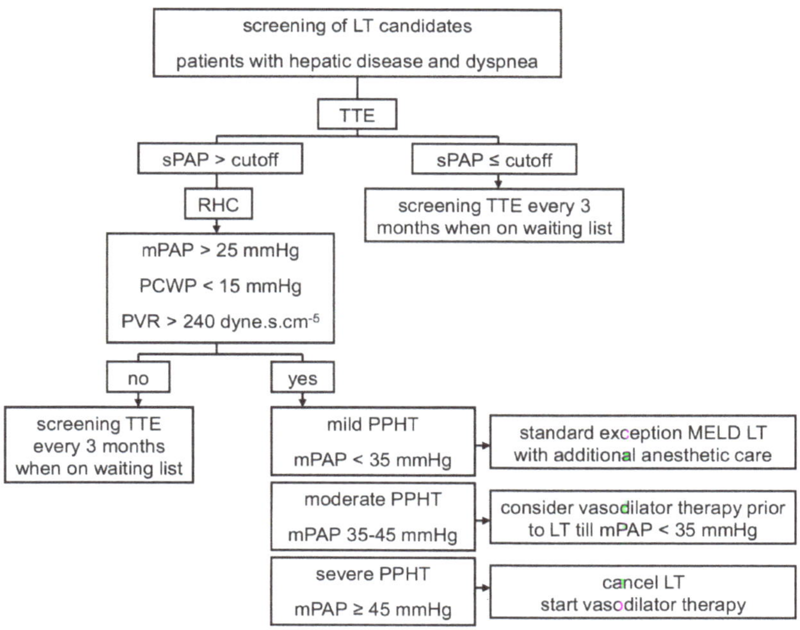

Figure 8.7. *Algorithm for screening and treatment of portopulmonary hypertension (PPHT) in symptomatic patients and liver transplantation (LT) candidates.*

Source: Adapted from Raevens, et al., June 2015. Hepatopulmonary syndrome and portopulmonary hypertension: recent knowledge in pathogenesis and overview of clinical assessment. Liver Int. 35 (6), 1646–1660.

Ambrisentan is a selective ET1A receptor antagonist (100:1 ET-1A/ET-1B selectivity) with minimal effect on liver function (Cartin-Ceba et al., 2011; Halank et al., 2011). A new dual receptor antagonist is macitentan (50:1 ET-1A/ET-1B selectivity), which is approved for the treatment of PAH and which is currently being studied in a randomized controlled trial for treatment of PPHT (ClinicalTrial.gov number NCT02382016). Sitaxentan was withdrawn from the market because of two cases of fatal liver injury (Lee et al., 2011).

- ***Nitric Oxide Pathway:*** PDE-5 inhibitors, such as sildenafil and the longer-acting drugs vardenafil and tadalafil, are currently prescribed to treat PAH. By blocking the metabolism of cyclic guanosine monophosphate (cGMP), they mediate their vasodilator effect (Ramsay, 2010 April; Swanson and Krowka, 2008; Park, 2008; Austin et al., 2008; Tam and He, 2007). They should be used with caution as they may increase portal hypertension by splanchnic vasodilation (Table 8.6).

Riociguat is a recently developed sGC stimulator drug that boosts cGMP production. Unlike the oral medications macitentan and trepostinil, Riociguat's efficacy has been demonstrated in PPHT patients (Ghofrani et al., 2013). One common side effect is hypotension, experienced by 10% of patients in clinical studies (Ghofrani et al., 2013).

Table 8.6. *Therapies for Treatment of Pulmonary Arterial Hypertension*

Class	Drug	Route
Prostacyclin analogs	Epoprostenol	IV
	Treprostinil	IV and SC, INH, PO
	Iloprost	INH
Endothelin receptor antagonists	Bosentan	PO
	Ambrisentan	PO
	Macitentan	PO
Phosphodiesterase 5 inhibitors	Sildenafil	PO
	Vardenafil	PO
	Tadalafil	PO
Soluble guanylate cyclase stimulators	Riociguat	PO

INH, inhalation; *IV*, intravenous; *PO*, oral; *SC*, subcutaneous.

Source. S. Raevens and I. Colle, Hepatopulmonary Syndrome and Portopulmonary Hypertension, http://dx.doi.org/10.1016/B978-0-12-804274-8.00039-4.

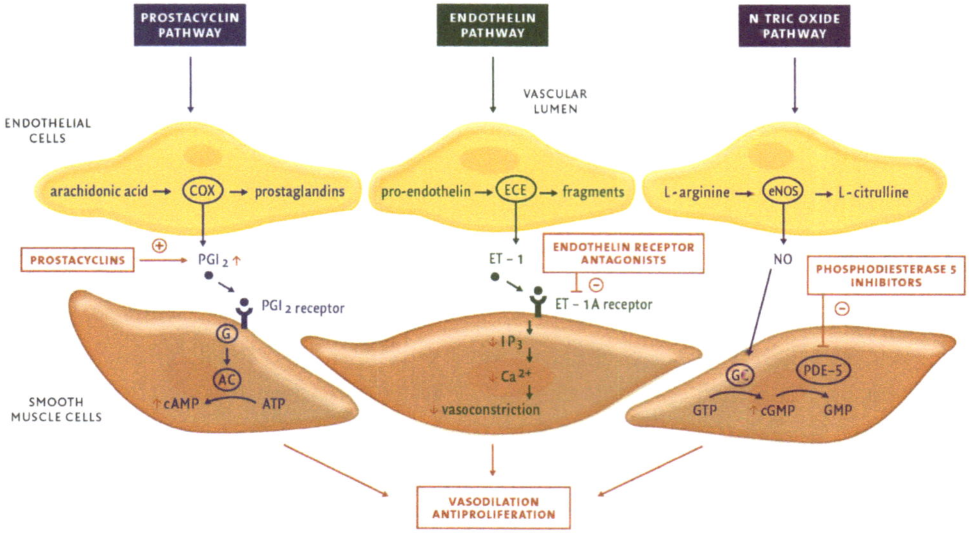

Figure 8.8. *Mechanism of action of current vasodilator therapies as treatment of portopulmonary hypertension (PPHT).*

Source. Reproduced from Raevens, et al., June 2015. Hepatopulmonary syndrome and portopulmonary hypertension: recent knowledge in pathogenesis and overview of clinical assessment. Liver Int. 35 (6), 1646–1660, with permission.

In mild cases of post-prostata hypoxic hemorrhage (PPHT), nitric oxide by inhalation may be administered perioperatively. Inhaled oxygen may also provide an extra short-term benefit (Findlay et al., 1999; Roberts et al., 2001).

- ***Prostacyclin Pathway:*** Epoprostenol, iloprost, treprostinil, and other prostacyclin analogs have antiplatelet-aggregating, antiproliferative, and vasodilatory properties. Despite the effectiveness of intravenous epoprostenol therapy, there are unfavorable effects related to safety, tolerability, and administration method (Benza et al., 2007; Park, 2008). Rebound pulmonary hypertension, headaches, gastrointestinal side effects, worsening hepatic function, and portal hypertension are among the side effects (Park, 2008; Tam & He, 2007; Le Pavec et al., 2008). Recently, treprostinil has been approved as the first oral prostacyclin analog for the treatment of pulmonary hypertension (Jing et al., 2013) (Figure 8.8).
- ***Other Therapies:*** Patients with PPHT should not have transjugular intrahepatic portosystemic shunts inserted because this procedure can cause an acute rise in preload, which can lead to acute heart failure. β-Blockade is associated with decreased exercise capacity and worse hemodynamics so it should be stopped and replaced by endoscopic ligature in case of medium to large varices (Provencher et al., 2006).

Increased PVR is a hallmark of PPHT, a portal hypertension complication. If ignored and untreated, it is linked to a lower chance of survival. TTE is used as part of routine screening for the presence of PPHT, while RHC is the preferred method for diagnosing PPHT. If the patient's mPAP is less than 35 mmHg while on vasodilator therapy or if their PPHT is mild, LT may be given priority.

A Closer Look

Hepatopulmonary Syndrome in Adults

When a person has chronic liver disease, they may experience hepatopulmonary syndrome (HPS), a complicated and dangerous condition marked by liver dysfunction, intrapulmonary vascular dilatations, and arterial hypoxemia (low blood oxygen levels). Affected people experience severe breathing difficulties as a result of the poor oxygen exchange caused by these aberrant blood vessel alterations in the lungs. Although hepatitis and non-cirrhotic portal hypertension are two other chronic liver diseases that can cause HPS, cirrhosis is the most common cause of it. Although the precise causes of HPS remain unclear, it is thought that liver dysfunction triggers the release of vasoactive chemicals like nitric oxide, which results in the atypical dilatation of pulmonary blood vessels. This dilation causes an imbalance between the lungs' perfusion (blood flow) and ventilation (airflow), which ultimately prevents oxygen from reaching the alveoli, where gas exchange usually takes place. The result is hypoxemia.

Individuals diagnosed with HPS frequently exhibit symptoms like orthodeoxia, or shortness of breath, and cyanosis, or bluish discoloration of the skin and mucous membranes caused by low oxygenation. The quality of life may be greatly impacted by these symptoms, which may get worse as the liver disease worsens. A combination of clinical evaluation, imaging tests such as contrast-enhanced echocardiography, and arterial blood gas analysis to verify hypoxemia are usually used in the diagnosis of HPS. Even though HPS is a severe condition, its management is difficult because there are currently no specific medical treatments that can reverse it. While oxygen therapy can alleviate symptoms, it doesn't deal with the underlying vascular abnormalities. Liver transplantation is the most effective treatment for HPS and has been demonstrated to alleviate pulmonary symptoms by treating underlying liver dysfunction in many cases. On the other hand, patients with severe hypoxemia may have increased perioperative risks, so timing of the transplant is crucial. The severity of the hypoxemia and the underlying liver disease determine the prognosis, but in the absence of a transplant, HPS can worsen respiratory failure and increase mortality. Because HPS affects liver and respiratory function, hepatologists, pulmonologists, and transplant specialists must collaborate to provide the best possible care for patients. For adults with this difficult syndrome, early diagnosis and evaluation for possible liver transplantation are essential to improving prognosis.

Summary

- Hepatorenal Syndrome (HRS) is a life-threatening condition that affects kidney function in people with advanced liver disease. HRS is most common in people with advanced cirrhosis (or scarring of the liver) and ascites, an abnormal buildup of fluid in the abdomen that is often related to liver disease.
- Hepatopulmonary syndrome is characterized by the presence of liver disease, arterial hypoxemia, and intrapulmonary vascular dilations. It results from the dilation of blood vessels in the lungs, leading to abnormal oxygen exchange and hypoxemia.
- Pulmonary hypertension is a type of high blood pressure that affects the arteries in the lungs and the right side of the heart.
- PPH is associated with high morbidity and mortality in patients undergoing liver transplantation, necessitating the screening for PPH during the evaluation of potential liver transplant recipients.
- Portopulmonary hypertension, on the other hand, involves the development of pulmonary arterial hypertension in the context of portal hypertension. It is marked by increased pulmonary vascular resistance due to vasoconstriction and vascular remodeling.
- Liver cirrhosis is the end-stage of all forms of chronic liver disease and is characterized by disruption of the normal architecture of the liver secondary to liver inflammation and deposition of fibrosis over a long period of time.
- Patients with cirrhosis may develop AKI due to several different causes, the most common being hypovolemia, acute tubular necrosis (ATN), and HRS. The differential diagnosis between these causes is essential as they have completely different prognosis and treatment
- HRS may develop spontaneously without any identifiable precipitating factor, probably due only to the progression of the disease, leading to a further impairment in circulatory function. However, HRS may also be triggered by a precipitating factor that impairs the already existing circulatory dysfunction.
- The use of TIPS has been suggested as an alternative therapy for the management of HRS because it reduces portal pressure and, as a consequence, improves circulatory dysfunction leading to potential improvement of kidney function.
- Hepatopulmonary syndrome (HPS) is characterized as a triad of disturbed gas exchange caused by the development of intrapulmonary vascular dilations (IPVDs) and arteriovenous shunting in patients with liver disease and/or portal hypertension.
- Abnormal intrapulmonary vasodilation in HPS is related to an imbalance between vasodilators and vasoconstrictors in favor of vasodilation, mainly by an increase in nitric monoxide (NO), caused by endothelial and inducible nitric oxide synthase (eNOS and iNOS).
- Pulmonary artery hypertension is defined as an elevated mean pulmonary artery pressure (mPAP) > 25 mmHg. Hemodynamic measurements are performed during right heart catheterization (RHC).

References

1. Abrams, G. A., & Fallon, M. B. (1998). Treatment of hepatopulmonary syndrome with *Allium sativum* L. (garlic): A pilot trial. *Journal of Clinical Gastroenterology, 27*(3), 232–235.

2. Abrams, G. A., Jaffe, C. C., Hoffer, P. B., Binder, H. J., & Fallon, M. B. (1995). Diagnostic utility of contrast echocardiography and lung perfusion scan in patients with hepatopulmonary syndrome. *Gastroenterology, 109*(4), 1283–1288.

3. Abrams, G. A., Sanders, M. K., & Fallon, M. B. (2002). Utility of pulse oximetry in the detection of arterial hypoxemia in liver transplant candidates. *Liver Transplantation, 8*(4), 391–396.

4. Albillos, A., de la Hera, A., Gonzalez, M., et al. (2003). Increased lipopolysaccharide binding protein in cirrhotic patients with marked immune and hemodynamic derangement. *Hepatology, 37*(1), 208–217.

5. Alessandria, C., Ottobrelli, A., Debernardi-Venon, W., et al. (2007). Noradrenalin vs terlipressin in patients with hepatorenal syndrome: A prospective, randomized, unblinded, pilot study. *Journal of Hepatology, 47*(4), 499–505.

6. Aller, R., Moya, J. L., Moreira, V., Boixeda, D., Cano, A., Picher, J., et al. (1999). Diagnosis of hepatopulmonary syndrome with contrast transesophageal echocardiography: Advantages over contrast transthoracic echocardiography. *Digestive Diseases and Sciences, 44*(6), 1243–1248.

7. Anel, R. M., & Sheagren, J. N. (2001). Novel presentation and approach to management of hepatopulmonary syndrome with use of antimicrobial agents. *Clinical Infectious Diseases, 32*(10), E131–E136.

8. Angeli, P., & Gines, P. (2012). Hepatorenal syndrome, MELD score and liver transplantation: An evolving issue with relevant implications for clinical practice. *Journal of Hepatology, 57*(5), 1135–1140.

9. Angeli, P., Gines, P., Wong, F., et al. (2015). Diagnosis and management of acute kidney injury in patients with cirrhosis: Revised consensus recommendations of the International Club of Ascites. *Journal of Hepatology, 62*(4), 968–974.

10. Arguedas, M. R., Abrams, G. A., Krowka, M. J., & Fallon, M. B. (2003). Prospective evaluation of outcomes and predictors of mortality in patients with hepatopulmonary syndrome undergoing liver transplantation. *Hepatology, 37*(1), 192–197.

11. Arguedas, M. R., Drake, B. B., Kapoor, A., & Fallon, M. B. (2005). Carboxyhemoglobin levels in cirrhotic patients with and without hepatopulmonary syndrome. *Gastroenterology, 128*(2), 328–333.

12. Arguedas, M. R., Singh, H., Faulk, D. K., & Fallon, M. B. (2007). Utility of pulse oximetry screening for hepatopulmonary syndrome. *Clinical Gastroenterology and Hepatology, 5*(6), 749–754.

13. Ariza, X., Sola, E., Elia, C., et al. (2015). Analysis of a urinary biomarker panel for clinical outcomes assessment in cirrhosis. *PLoS One, 10*(6), e0128145.

14. Arroyo, V., Gines, P., Gerbes, A. L., et al. (1996). Definition and diagnostic criteria of refractory ascites and hepatorenal syndrome in cirrhosis. International Ascites Club. *Hepatology, 23*(1), 164–176.

15. Arroyo, V., Moreau, R., Jalan, R., et al. (2015). Acute-on-chronic liver failure: A new syndrome that will re-classify cirrhosis. *Journal of Hepatology, 62*(1 Suppl), S131–S143.

16. Austin, M. J., McDougall, N. I., Wendon, J. A., Sizer, E., Knisely, A. S., Rela, M., et al. (2008). Safety and efficacy of combined use of sildenafil, bosentan, and iloprost before and after liver transplantation in severe port pulmonary hypertension. *Liver Transplantation, 14*(3), 287–291.

17. Barreto, R., Fagundes, C., Guevara, M., et al. (2014). Type-1 hepatorenal syndrome associated with infections in cirrhosis: Natural history, outcome of kidney function, and survival. *Hepatology, 59*(4), 1505–1513.

18. Belcher, J. M., Sanyal, A. J., Peixoto, A. J., et al. (2014). Kidney biomarkers and differential diagnosis of patients with cirrhosis and acute kidney injury. *Hepatology, 60*(2), 622–632.

19. Benza, R. L., Park, M. H., Keogh, A., & Girgis, R. E. (2007). Management of pulmonary arterial hypertension with a focus on combination therapies. *Journal of Heart and Lung Transplantation, 26*(5), 437–446.

20. Bernardi, M., Moreau, R., Angeli, P., et al. (2015). Mechanisms of decompensation and organ failure in cirrhosis: From peripheral arterial vasodilation to systemic inflammation hypothesis. *Journal of Hepatology, 63*(5), 1272–1284.

21. Berthelot, P., Walker, J. G., Sherlock, S., & Reid, L. (1966). Arterial changes in the lungs in cirrhosis of the liver and lung spider nevi. *The New England Journal of Medicine, 274*(6), 291–298.

22. Boyer, T. D., Sanyal, A. J., Garcia-Tsao, G., et al. (2011). Impact of liver transplantation on the survival of patients treated for hepatorenal syndrome type 1. *Liver Transplantation, 17*(11), 1328–1332.

23. Bozbas, S. S., Eyuboglu, F. O., Arslan, N. G., Ergur, F. O., Karakayali, H., & Haberal, M. (2009). The prevalence and the impact of portopulmonary hypertension on postoperative course in patients undergoing liver transplantation. *Transplantation Proceedings, 41*(7), 2860–2863.

24. Brensing, K. A., Textor, J., Perz, J., et al. (2000). Long term outcome after transjugular intrahepatic portosystemic stent-shunt in non-transplant cirrhotics with hepatorenal syndrome: A phase II study. *Gut, 47*(2), 288–295.

25. Brussino, L., Bucca, C., Morello, M., Scappaticci, E., Mauro, M., & Rolla, G. (2003). Effect on dyspnoea and hypoxaemia of inhaled N(G)-nitro-L-arginine methyl ester in hepatopulmonary syndrome. *The Lancet, 362*(9377), 43–44.

26. Budhiraja, R., & Hassoun, P. M. (2003). Porto pulmonary hypertension: A tale of two circulations. *Chest, 123*(2), 562–576.

27. Cardenas, A., Gines, P., Uriz, J., et al. (2001). Renal failure after upper gastrointestinal bleeding in cirrhosis: Incidence, clinical course, predictive factors, and short-term prognosis. *Hepatology, 34*(4), 671–676.

28. Cartin-Ceba, R., Swanson, K., Iyer, V., Wiesner, R. H., & Krowka, M. J. (2011). Safety and efficacy of ambrisentan for the treatment of Porto pulmonary hypertension. *Chest, 139*(1), 109–114.

29. Casey, S., Schelleman, A., & Angus, P. (2013). Recurrence of hepatopulmonary syndrome post-orthotopic liver transplantation in a patient with noncirrhotic portal hypertension. *Hepatology, 58*(6), 2205–2206.

30. Cavallin, M., Kamath, P. S., Merli, M., et al. (2015). Terlipressin plus albumin versus midodrine and octreotide plus albumin in the treatment of hepatorenal syndrome: A randomized trial. *Hepatology, 62*(2), 567–574.

31. Cavallin, M., Piano, S., Romano, A., et al. (2016). Terlipressin given by continuous intravenous infusion versus intravenous boluses in the treatment of hepatorenal syndrome: A randomized controlled study. *Hepatology, 63*(3), 983–992.

32. Chang, C. C., Chuang, C. L., Lee, F. Y., Wang, S. S., Lin, H. C., Huang, H. C., et al. (2013). Sorafenib treatment improves hepatopulmonary syndrome in rats with biliary cirrhosis. *Clinical Science (London), 124*(7), 457–466.

33. Chang, C. C., Wang, S. S., Hsieh, H. G., Lee, W. S., Chuang, C. L., Lin, H. C., et al. (2015). Rosuvastatin improves hepatopulmonary syndrome through inhibition of inflammatory angiogenesis of lung. *Clinical Science (London), 129*(6), 449–460.

34. Charlton, M. R., Wall, W. J., Ojo, A. O., et al. (2009). Report of the first international liver transplantation society expert panel consensus conference on renal insufficiency in liver transplantation. *Liver Transplantation, 15*(1 Suppl), S1–S34.

35. Claria, J., Jimenez, W., Arroyo, V., et al. (1991). Effect of V1-vasopressin receptor blockade on arterial pressure in conscious rats with cirrhosis and ascites. *Gastroenterology, 100*(2), 494–501.

36. Colle, I. O., Moreau, R., Godinho, E., Belghiti, J., Ettori, F., Cohen-Solal, A., et al. (2003). Diagnosis of Porto pulmonary hypertension in candidates for liver transplantation: A prospective study. *Hepatology, 37*(2), 401–409.

37. Colle, I., Van Steenkiste, C., Geerts, A., & Van Vlierberghe, H. (2007). Hepatopulmonary syndrome and Porto pulmonary hypertension: What's new? *Acta Gastroenterologica Belgica, 70*(2), 203–209.

38. Coulon, S., Heindryckx, F., Geerts, A., Van Steenkiste, C., Colle, I., & Van Vlierberghe, H. (2011). Angiogenesis in chronic liver disease and its complications. *Liver International, 31*(2), 146–162.

39. De las Heras, D., Fernandez, J., Gines, P., et al. (2003). Increased carbon monoxide production in patients with cirrhosis with and without spontaneous bacterial peritonitis. *Hepatology, 38*(2), 452–459.

40. De, B. K., Dutta, D., Pal, S. K., Gangopadhyay, S., Das, B. S., & Pani, A. (2010). The role of garlic in hepatopulmonary syndrome: A randomized controlled trial. *Canadian Journal of Gastroenterology, 24*(3), 183–188.

41. De, B. K., Sen, S., Biswas, P. K., Sanyal, R., Majumdar, D., & Biswas, J. (2000). Hepatopulmonary syndrome in inferior vena cava obstruction responding to cavoplasty. *Gastroenterology, 118*(1), 192–196.

42. Dimmeler, S., & Zeiher, A. M. (2000). Akt takes center stage in angiogenesis signaling. *Circulation Research, 86*(1), 4–5.

43. Durand, F., Graupera, I., Gines, P., et al. (2016). Pathogenesis of hepatorenal syndrome: Implications for therapy. *American Journal of Kidney Diseases, 67*(2), 318–328.

44. EASL (European Association for the Study of the Liver). (2010). Clinical practice guidelines on the management of ascites, spontaneous bacterial peritonitis, and hepatorenal syndrome in cirrhosis. *Journal of Hepatology, 53*(3), 397–417.

45. Egermayer, P., Town, G. I., & Peacock, A. J. (1999). Role of serotonin in the pathogenesis of acute and chronic pulmonary hypertension. *Thorax, 54*(2), 161–168.

46. Elia, C., Graupera, I., Barreto, R., et al. (2015). Severe acute kidney injury associated with non-steroidal anti-inflammatory drugs in cirrhosis: A case-control study. *Journal of Hepatology, 63*(3), 593–600.

47. Eriksson, C., Gustavsson, A., Kronvall, T., & Tysk, C. (2011). Hepatotoxicity by bosentan in a patient with Porto pulmonary hypertension: A case-report and review of the literature. *Journal of Gastrointestinal and Liver Diseases, 20*(1), 77–80.

48. Esrailian, E., Pantangco, E. R., Kyulo, N. L., et al. (2007). Octreotide/Midodrine therapy significantly improves renal function and 30-day survival in patients with type 1 hepatorenal syndrome. *Digestive Diseases and Sciences, 52*(3), 742–748.

49. Fagundes, C., & Gines, P. (2012). Hepatorenal syndrome: A severe, but treatable, cause of kidney failure in cirrhosis. *American Journal of Kidney Diseases, 59*(6), 874–885.

50. Fagundes, C., Barreto, R., Guevara, M., et al. (2013). A modified acute kidney injury classification for diagnosis and risk stratification of impairment of kidney function in cirrhosis. *Journal of Hepatology, 59*(3), 474–481.

51. Fagundes, C., Pepin, M. N., Guevara, M., et al. (2012). Urinary neutrophil gelatinase-associated lipocalin as biomarker in the differential diagnosis of impairment of kidney function in cirrhosis. *Journal of Hepatology, 57*(2), 267–273.

52. Fasolato, S., Angeli, P., Dallagnese, L., et al. (2007). Renal failure and bacterial infections in patients with cirrhosis: Epidemiology and clinical features. *Hepatology, 45*(1), 223–229.

53. Feltracco, P., Serra, E., Brezzi, M. L., Milevoj, M., Rizzi, S., & Furnari, M., et al. (2009). Hemodynamic profile of Porto pulmonary hypertension. *Transplantation Proceedings, 41*(4), 1235–1239.

54. Fernandez, J., Navasa, M., Planas, R., et al. (2007). Primary prophylaxis of spontaneous bacterial peritonitis delays hepatorenal syndrome and improves survival in cirrhosis. *Gastroenterology, 133*(3), 818–824.

55. Fernandez, M., Semela, D., Bruix, J., Colle, I., Pinzani, M., & Bosch, J. (2009). Angiogenesis in liver disease. *Journal of Hepatology, 50*(3), 604–620.

56. Findlay, J. Y., Harrison, B. A., Plevak, D. J., & Krowka, M. J. (1999). Inhaled nitric oxide reduces pulmonary artery pressures in Porto pulmonary hypertension. *Liver Transplantation and Surgery, 5*(5), 381–387.

57. Ghabril, M., & Lucey, M. (2014). Is it time to recalibrate the MELD exception points attributed for hepatopulmonary syndrome? *Gastroenterology, 146*(5), 1158–1160.

58. Ghofrani, H. A., Galie, N., Grimminger, F., Grunig, E., Humbert, M., Jing, Z. C., et al. (2013). Riociguat for the treatment of pulmonary arterial hypertension. *The New England Journal of Medicine, 369*(4), 330–340.

59. Giaid, A., & Saleh, D. (1995). Reduced expression of endothelial nitric oxide synthase in the lungs of patients with pulmonary hypertension. *The New England Journal of Medicine, 333*(4), 214–221.

60. Gill, N., Nally Jr., J. V., & Fatica, R. A. (2005). Renal failure secondary to acute tubular necrosis: Epidemiology, diagnosis, and management. *Chest, 128*(4), 2847–2863.

61. Gines, P., & Schrier, R. W. (2009). Renal failure in cirrhosis. *New England Journal of Medicine, 361*, 1279–1290.

62. Gines, P., Jimenez, W., Arroyo, V., et al. (1988). Atrial natriuretic factor in cirrhosis with ascites: Plasma levels, cardiac release and splanchnic extraction. *Hepatology, 8*, 636–642.

63. Gluud, L. L., Christensen, K., Christensen, E., et al. (2010). Systematic review of randomized trials on vasoconstrictor drugs for hepatorenal syndrome. *Hepatology, 51*, 576–584.

64. Golbin, J. M., & Krowka, M. J. (2007). Porto pulmonary hypertension. *Clinics in Chest Medicine, 28*(1), 203–218.

65. Goldberg, D. S., Krok, K., Batra, S., Trotter, J. F., Kawut, S. M., & Fallon, M. B. (2014). Impact of the hepatopulmonary syndrome MELD exception policy on outcomes of patients after liver transplantation: An analysis of the UNOS database. *Gastroenterology, 146*(5), 1256–1265.

66. Gomez, F. P., Barbera, J. A., Roca, J., Burgos, F., Gistau, C., & Rodriguez-Roisin, R. (2006). Effects of nebulized N(G)-nitro-L-arginine methyl ester in patients with hepatopulmonary syndrome. *Hepatology, 43*(5), 1084–1091.

67. Grace, J. A., & Angus, P. W. (2013). Hepatopulmonary syndrome: Update on recent advances in pathophysiology, investigation, and treatment. *Journal of Gastroenterology and Hepatology, 28*(2), 213–219.

68. Gupta, D., Vijaya, D. R., Gupta, R., Dhiman, R. K., Bhargava, M., & Verma, J., et al. (2001). Prevalence of hepatopulmonary syndrome in cirrhosis and extrahepatic portal venous obstruction. *American Journal of Gastroenterology, 96*(12), 3395–3399.

69. Gupta, L. B., Kumar, A., Jaiswal, A. K., Yusuf, J., Mehta, V., & Tyagi, S., et al. (2008). Pentoxifylline therapy for hepatopulmonary syndrome: A pilot study. *Archives of Internal Medicine, 168*(16), 1820–1823.

70. Gupta, S., Castel, H., Rao, R. V., Picard, M., Lilly, L., & Faughnan, M. E., et al. (2010b). Improved survival after liver transplantation in patients with hepatopulmonary syndrome. *American Journal of Transplantation, 10*(2), 354–363.

71. Gupta, S., Faughnan, M. E., Lilly, L., Hutchison, S., Fowler, R., & Bayoumi, A. M. (2010a). Norfloxacin therapy for hepatopulmonary syndrome: A pilot randomized controlled trial. *Clinical Gastroenterology and Hepatology, 8*(12), 1095–1098.

72. Halank, M., Knudsen, L., Seyfarth, H. J., Ewert, R., Wiedemann, B., & Kolditz, M., et al. (2011). Ambrisentan improves exercise capacity and symptoms in patients with Porto pulmonary hypertension. *Zeitschrift für Gastroenterologie, 49*(9), 1258–1262.

73. Han, W. K., Bailly, V., Abichandani, R., Thadhani, R., & Bonventre, J. V. (2002). Kidney injury molecule-1 (KIM-1): A novel biomarker for human renal proximal tubule injury. *Kidney International, 62*, 237–244.

74. Henriksen, J. H., Ring-Larsen, H., Kanstrup, I. L., et al. (1984). Splanchnic and renal elimination and release of catecholamines in cirrhosis. Evidence of enhanced sympathetic nervous activity in patients with decompensated cirrhosis. *Gut, 25*, 1034–1043.

75. Herve, P., Le, P. J., Sztrymf, B., Decante, B., Savale, L., & Sitbon, O. (2007). Pulmonary vascular abnormalities in cirrhosis. *Best Practice & Research Clinical Gastroenterology, 21*(1), 141–159.

76. Hoeper, M. M., Krowka, M. J., & Strassburg, C. P. (2004). Porto pulmonary hypertension and hepatopulmonary syndrome. *The Lancet, 363*(9419), 1461–1468.

77. Hopkins, W. E., Waggoner, A. D., & Barzilai, B. (1992). Frequency and significance of intrapulmonary right-to-left shunting in end-stage hepatic disease. *American Journal of Cardiology, 70*(4), 516–519.

78. Horvatits, T., Drolz, A., Roedl, K., Herkner, H., Ferlitsch, A., & Perkmann, T., et al. (2014). Von Willebrand factor antigen for detection of hepatopulmonary syndrome in patients with cirrhosis. *Journal of Hepatology, 61*(3), 544–549.

79. Ioachimescu, O. C., Mehta, A. C., & Stoller, J. K. (2007). Hepatopulmonary syndrome following Porto pulmonary hypertension. *European Respiratory Journal, 29*(6), 1277–1280.

80. Iyer, V. N., Swanson, K. L., Cartin-Ceba, R., Dierkhising, R. A., Rosen, C. B., & Heimbach, J. K., et al. (2013). Hepatopulmonary syndrome: Favorable outcomes in the MELD exception era. *Hepatology, 57*(6), 2427–2435.

81. Jing, Z. C., Parikh, K., Pulido, T., Jerjes-Sanchez, C., White, R. J., Allen, R., et al. (2013). Efficacy and safety of oral treprostinil monotherapy for the treatment of pulmonary arterial hypertension: A randomized, controlled trial. *Circulation, 127*(5), 624–633.

82. Jounieaux, V., Leleu, O., & Mayeux, I. (2001). Cardiopulmonary effects of nitric oxide inhalation and methylene blue injection in hepatopulmonary syndrome. *Intensive Care Medicine, 27*(6), 1103–1104.

83. Kianifar, H. R., Khalesi, M., Mahmoodi, E., & Afzal, A. M. (2012). Pentoxifylline in hepatopulmonary syndrome. *World Journal of Gastroenterology, 18*(35), 4912–4916.

84. Koyner, J. L., Vaidya, V. S., Bennett, M. R., et al. (2010). Urinary biomarkers in the clinical prognosis and early detection of acute kidney injury. *Clinical Journal of the American Society of Nephrology, 5*, 2154–2165.

85. Kribben, A., Gerken, G., Haag, S., et al. (2012). Effects of fractionated plasma separation and adsorption on survival in patients with acute-on-chronic liver failure. *Gastroenterology, 142*, 782–789.

86. Krowka, M. J. (2006). Evolving dilemmas and management of Porto pulmonary hypertension. *Seminars in Liver Disease, 26*(3), 265–272.

87. Krowka, M. J. (2011). Hepatopulmonary syndrome: Monitoring at your fingertip. *Digestive Diseases and Sciences, 56*(6), 1599–1600.

88. Krowka, M. J., & Edwards, W. D. (2000). A spectrum of pulmonary vascular pathology in Porto pulmonary hypertension. *Liver Transplantation, 6*(2), 241–242.

89. Krowka, M. J., Dickson, E. R., & Cortese, D. A. (1993). Hepatopulmonary syndrome: Clinical observations and lack of therapeutic response to somatostatin analogue. *Chest, 104*(2), 515–521.

90. Krowka, M. J., Plevak, D. J., Findlay, J. Y., Rosen, C. B., Wiesner, R. H., & Krom, R. A. (2000a). Pulmonary hemodynamics and perioperative cardiopulmonary-related mortality in patients with Porto pulmonary hypertension undergoing liver transplantation. *Liver Transplantation, 6*(4), 443–450.

91. Krowka, M. J., Swanson, K. L., Frantz, R. P., McGoon, M. D., & Wiesner, R. H. (2006). Porto pulmonary hypertension: Results from a 10-year screening algorithm. *Hepatology, 44*(6), 1502–1510.

92. Krowka, M. J., Wiseman, G. A., Burnett, O. L., Spivey, J. R., Therneau, T., & Porayko, M. K.,

et al. (2000b). Hepatopulmonary syndrome: A prospective study of relationships between severity of liver disease, PaO_2 response to 100% oxygen, and brain uptake after (99m) Tc MAA lung scanning. *Chest, 118*(3), 615–624.

93. La Villa, G., Romanelli, R. G., Casini Raggi, V., et al. (1992). Plasma levels of brain natriuretic peptide in patients with cirrhosis. *Hepatology, 16*, 156–161.
94. Lee, U. E., & Friedman, S. L. (2011). Mechanisms of hepatic fibrogenesis. *Best Practice & Research Clinical Gastroenterology, 25*, 195–206.
95. Lee, W. T., Kirkham, N., Johnson, M. K., Lordan, J. L., Fisher, A. J., & Peacock, A. J. (2011). Sitaxentan-related acute liver failure in a patient with pulmonary arterial hypertension. *European Respiratory Journal, 37*(2), 472–474.
96. Ling, Y., Zhang, J., Luo, B., Song, D., Liu, L., & Tang, L., et al. (2004). The role of endothelin-1 and the endothelin B receptor in the pathogenesis of hepatopulmonary syndrome in the rat. *Hepatology, 39*(6), 1593–1602.
97. Liu, L., Liu, N., Zhao, Z., Liu, J., Feng, Y., & Jiang, H., et al. (2012). TNF-alpha neutralization improves experimental hepatopulmonary syndrome in rats. *Liver International, 32*(6), 1018–1026.
98. Luo, B., Liu, L., Tang, L., Zhang, J., Stockard, C. R., Grizzle, W. E., et al. (2003). Increased pulmonary vascular endothelin B receptor expression and responsiveness to endothelin-1 in cirrhotic and portal hypertensive rats: A potential mechanism in experimental hepatopulmonary syndrome. *Journal of Hepatology, 38*(5), 556–563.
99. Macgilchrist, A. J., Howes, L. G., Hawksby, C., et al. (1991). Plasma noradrenaline in cirrhosis: A study of kinetics and temporal relationship to ascites formation. *European Journal of Clinical Investigation, 21*, 238–243.
100. Machicao, V. I., & Fallon, M. B. (2012). Hepatopulmonary syndrome. *Seminars in Respiratory and Critical Care Medicine, 33*(1), 11–16.
101. Mandell, M. S. (2004). Hepatopulmonary syndrome and Porto pulmonary hypertension in the model for end-stage liver disease (MELD) era. *Liver Transplantation, 10*(10 Suppl. 2), S54–S58.
102. Martin-Llahi, M., Guevara, M., & Torre, A., et al. (2011). Prognostic importance of the cause of renal failure in patients with cirrhosis. *Gastroenterology, 140*, 488–496.
103. Martin-Llahi, M., Pepin, M. N., Guevara, M., et al. (2008). Terlipressin and albumin vs albumin in patients with cirrhosis and hepatorenal syndrome: A randomized study. *Gastroenterology, 134*, 1352–1359.
104. Martinez-Palli, G., Barbera, J. A., Taura, P., Cirera, I., Visa, J., & Rodriguez-Roisin, R. (1999). Severe Porto pulmonary hypertension after liver transplantation in a patient with preexisting hepatopulmonary syndrome. *Journal of Hepatology, 31*(6), 1075–1079.
105. Martinez, G. P., Barbera, J. A., Visa, J., Rimola, A., Pare, J. C., Roca, J., et al. (2001). Hepatopulmonary syndrome in candidates for liver transplantation. *Journal of Hepatology, 34*(5), 651–657.
106. Maruyama, T., Ohsaki, K., Shimoda, S., Kaji, Y., & Harada, M. (2005). Thromboxane-dependent Porto pulmonary hypertension. *American Journal of Medicine, 118*(1), 93–94.

107. Mehta, R. L., Kellum, J. A., Shah, S. V., et al. (2007). Acute Kidney Injury Network: Report of an initiative to improve outcomes in acute kidney injury. *Critical Care, 11*, R31.

108. Mitzner, S. R., Stange, J., Klammt, S., et al. (2000). Improvement of hepatorenal syndrome with extracorporeal albumin dialysis MARS: Results of a prospective, randomized, controlled clinical trial. *Liver Transplantation, 6*, 277–286.

109. Molleston, J. P., Kaufman, B. A., Cohen, A., Shackelford, P. G., Keating, J. P., Lowell, J. A., et al. (1999). Brain abscess in hepatopulmonary syndrome. *Journal of Pediatric Gastroenterology and Nutrition, 29*(2), 225–226.

110. Moore, K., Wendon, J., Frazer, M., et al. (1992). Plasma endothelin immunoreactivity in liver disease and the hepatorenal syndrome. *New England Journal of Medicine, 327*, 1774–1778.

111. Moreira, S. H., Reis, G., Guedes, M., Cleto, E., Vizcaino, J. R., Kelly, D., et al. (2013). A case of hepatopulmonary syndrome solved by mycophenolate mofetil (an inhibitor of angiogenesis and nitric oxide production). *Journal of Hepatology, 58*(3), 630–633.

112. Murray, K. F., & Carithers Jr., R. L. (2005). AASLD practice guidelines: Evaluation of the patient for liver transplantation. *Hepatology, 41*(6), 1407–1432.

113. Najafi, S. M., Kianifar, H. R., Kianee, A., & Khatami, G. (2006). Effect of oral garlic on arterial oxygen pressure in children with hepatopulmonary syndrome. *World Journal of Gastroenterology, 12*(15), 2427–2431.

114. Nakamura, T., Sugaya, T., Node, K., et al. (2006). Urinary excretion of liver-type fatty acid-binding protein in contrast medium-induced nephropathy. *American Journal of Kidney Diseases, 47*, 439–444.

115. Nassar Junior, A. P., Farias, A. Q., LA DA, et al. (2014). Terlipressin versus norepinephrine in the treatment of hepatorenal syndrome: A systematic review and meta-analysis. *PLoS One, 9*, e107466.

116. Navasa, M., Follo, A., Filella, X., et al. (1998). Tumor necrosis factor and interleukin-6 in spontaneous bacterial peritonitis in cirrhosis: Relationship with the development of renal impairment and mortality. *Hepatology, 27*, 1227–1232.

117. Neri, S., Pulvirenti, D., Malaguarnera, M., et al. (2008). Terlipressin and albumin in patients with cirrhosis and type I hepatorenal syndrome. *Digestive Diseases and Sciences, 53*, 830–835.

118. Neuhofer, W., Gulberg, V., & Gerbes, A. L. (2006). Endothelin and endothelin receptor antagonism in Porto pulmonary hypertension. *European Journal of Clinical Investigation, 36*(Suppl. 3), 54–61.

119. Nunes, H., Lebrec, D., Mazmanian, M., Capron, F., Heller, J., Tazi, K. A., et al. (2001). Role of nitric oxide in hepatopulmonary syndrome in cirrhotic rats. *American Journal of Respiratory and Critical Care Medicine, 164*(5), 879–885.

120. Oliver, J. A., & Verna, E. C. (2010). Afferent mechanisms of sodium retention in cirrhosis and hepatorenal syndrome. *Kidney International, 77*, 669–680.

121. Park, M. H. (2008). Advances in diagnosis and treatment in patients with pulmonary arterial hypertension. *Catheterization and Cardiovascular Interventions, 71*(2), 205–213.

122. Pascasio, J. M., Grilo, I., Lopez-Pardo, F. J., Ortega-Ruiz, F., Tirado, J. L., Sousa, J. M., et al. (2014). Prevalence and severity of hepatopulmonary syndrome and its influence on survival

in cirrhotic patients evaluated for liver transplantation. *American Journal of Transplantation, 14*(6), 1391–1399.

123. Pellicelli, A. M., Barbaro, G., Puoti, C., Guarascio, P., Lusi, E. A., Bellis, L., et al. (2010). Plasma cytokines and Porto pulmonary hypertension in patients with cirrhosis waiting for orthotopic liver transplantation. *Angiology, 61*(8), 802–806.
124. Pereira, G., Guevara, M., Fagundes, C., et al. (2012). Renal failure and hyponatremia in patients with cirrhosis and skin and soft tissue infection: A retrospective study. *Journal of Hepatology, 56*, 1040–1046.
125. Pham, D. M., Subramanian, R., & Parekh, S. (2010). Coexisting hepatopulmonary syndrome and portopulmonary hypertension: Implications for liver transplantation. *Journal of Clinical Gastroenterology, 44*(7), e136–e140.
126. Piano, S., Morando, F., Fasolato, S., et al. (2011). Continuous recurrence of type 1 hepatorenal syndrome and long-term treatment with terlipressin and albumin: A new exception to MELD score in the allocation system to liver transplantation? *Journal of Hepatology, 55*, 491–496.
127. Piano, S., Rosi, S., Maresio, G., et al. (2013). Evaluation of the Acute Kidney Injury Network criteria in hospitalized patients with cirrhosis and ascites. *Journal of Hepatology, 59*, 482–489.
128. Pietra, G. G., Capron, F., Stewart, S., Leone, O., Humbert, M., Robbins, I. M., et al. (2004). Pathologic assessment of vasculopathies in pulmonary hypertension. *Journal of the American College of Cardiology, 43*(12 Suppl. S), 25S–32S.
129. Pilatis, N. D., Jacobs, L. E., Rerkpattanapipat, P., Kotler, M. N., Owen, A., Manzarbeitia, C., et al. (2000). Clinical predictors of pulmonary hypertension in patients undergoing liver transplant evaluation. *Liver Transplantation, 6*(1), 85–91.
130. Porres-Aguilar, M., Altamirano, J. T., Torre-Delgadillo, A., Charlton, M. R., & Duarte-Rojo, A. (2012). Porto pulmonary hypertension and hepatopulmonary syndrome: A clinician-oriented overview. *European Respiratory Review, 21*(125), 223–233.
131. Poterucha, J. J., Krowka, M. J., Dickson, E. R., Cortese, D. A., Stanson, A. W., & Krom, R. A. (1995). Failure of hepatopulmonary syndrome to resolve after liver transplantation and successful treatment with embolotherapy. *Hepatology, 21*(1), 96–100.
132. Pouriki, S., Alexopoulou, A., Chrysochoou, C., Raftopoulos, L., Papatheodoridis, G., Stefanadis, C., et al. (2011). Left ventricle enlargement and increased systolic velocity in the mitral valve are indirect markers of the hepatopulmonary syndrome. *Liver International, 31*(9), 1388–1394.
133. Provencher, S., Herve, P., Jais, X., Lebrec, D., Humbert, M., Simonneau, G., et al. (2006). Deleterious effects of beta-blockers on exercise capacity and hemodynamics in patients with portopulmonary hypertension. *Gastroenterology, 130*(1), 120–126.
134. Rabiller, A., Nunes, H., Lebrec, D., Tazi, K. A., Wartski, M., Dulmet, E., et al. (2002). Prevention of gram-negative translocation reduces the severity of hepatopulmonary syndrome. *American Journal of Respiratory and Critical Care Medicine, 166*(4), 514–517.
135. Raevens, S., Colle, I., Reyntjens, K., Geerts, A., Berrevoet, F., Rogiers, X., et al. (2013). Echocardiography for the detection of Porto pulmonary hypertension in liver transplant candidates: An analysis of cutoff values. *Liver Transplantation, 19*(6), 602–610.

136. Raevens, S., Coulon, S., Van Steenkiste, C., Colman, R., Verhelst, X., Van Vlierberghe, H., et al. (2015). Role of angiogenic factors/cell adhesion markers in serum of cirrhotic patients with hepatopulmonary syndrome. *Liver International, 35*(5), 1499–1507.

137. Ramsay, M. (2010). Portopulmonary hypertension and right heart failure in patients with cirrhosis. *Current Opinion in Anesthesiology, 23*(2), 145–150.

138. Regev, A., Yeshurun, M., Rodriguez, M., Sagie, A., Neff, G. W., Molina, E. G., et al. (2001). Transient hepatopulmonary syndrome in a patient with acute hepatitis A. *Journal of Viral Hepatitis, 8*(1), 83–86.

139. Reichen, J., Gerbes, A. L., Steiner, M. J., Sagesser, H., & Clozel, M. (1998). The effect of endothelin and its antagonist Bosentan on hemodynamics and microvascular exchange in cirrhotic rat liver. *Journal of Hepatology, 28*(6), 1020–1030.

140. Roberts, D. H., Lepore, J. J., Maroo, A., Semigran, M. J., & Ginns, L. C. (2001). Oxygen therapy improves cardiac index and pulmonary vascular resistance in patients with pulmonary hypertension. *Chest, 120*(5), 1547–1555.

141. Roberts, K. E., Fallon, M. B., Krowka, M. J., Brown, R. S., Trotter, J. F., Peter, I., et al. (2009). Genetic risk factors for Porto pulmonary hypertension in patients with advanced liver disease. *American Journal of Respiratory and Critical Care Medicine, 179*(9), 835–842.

142. Rodriguez-Roisin, R., Krowka, M. J., Herve, P., & Fallon, M. B. (2004). Pulmonary-hepatic vascular disorders (PHD). *European Respiratory Journal, 24*(5), 861–880.

143. Rodriguez, E., Elia, C., Sola, E., et al. (2014). Terlipressin and albumin for type-1 hepatorenal syndrome associated with sepsis. *Journal of Hepatology, 60*, 955–961.

144. Rolla, G., & Bucca, C. (1994). Methylene blue in the hepatopulmonary syndrome. *New England Journal of Medicine, 331*(16), 1098.

145. Rolla, G., Brussino, L., Colagrande, P., Dutto, L., Polizzi, S., Scappaticci, E., et al. (1997). Exhaled nitric oxide and oxygenation abnormalities in hepatic cirrhosis. *Hepatology, 26*(4), 842–847.

146. Roma, J., Balbi, E., Pacheco-Moreira, L., Gonzalez, A. C., Leal, C. G., Pousa, F., et al. (2010). Methylene blue used as a bridge to liver transplantation postoperative recovery: A case report. *Transplantation Proceedings, 42*(2), 601–604.

147. Rubens, C., Ewert, R., Halank, M., Wensel, R., Orzechowski, H. D., Schultheiss, H. P., et al. (2001). Big endothelin-1 and endothelin-1 plasma levels are correlated with the severity of primary pulmonary hypertension. *Chest, 120*(5), 1562–1569.

148. Ruiz-del-Arbol, L., Monescillo, A., Arocena, C., et al. (2005). Circulatory function and hepatorenal syndrome in cirrhosis. *Hepatology, 42*, 439–447.

149. Salerno, F., Gerbes, A., Gines, P., et al. (2007). Diagnosis, prevention, and treatment of hepatorenal syndrome in cirrhosis. *Gut, 56*, 1310–1318.

150. Sanyal, A. J., Boyer, T., Garcia-Tsao, G., et al. (2008). A randomized, prospective, double-blind, placebo-controlled trial of terlipressin for type 1 hepatorenal syndrome. *Gastroenterology, 134*, 1360–1368.

151. Schenk, P., Fuhrmann, V., Madl, C., Funk, G., Lehr, S., Kandel, O., et al. (2002). Hepatopulmonary syndrome: Prevalence and predictive value of various cutoffs for arterial oxygenation and their clinical consequences. *Gut, 51*(6), 853–859.

152. Schenk, P., Madl, C., Rezaie-Majd, S., Lehr, S., & Muller, C. (2000). Methylene blue improves the hepatopulmonary syndrome. *Annals of Internal Medicine, 133*(9), 701–706.

153. Schiffer, E., Majno, P., Mentha, G., Giostra, E., Burri, H., Klopfenstein, C. E., et al. (2006). Hepatopulmonary syndrome increases the postoperative mortality rate following liver transplantation: A prospective study in 90 patients. *American Journal of Transplantation, 6*(6), 1430–1437.

154. Schraufnagel, D. E., Malik, R., Goel, V., Ohara, N., & Chang, S. W. (1997). Lung capillary changes in hepatic cirrhosis in rats. *American Journal of Physiology, 272*(1 Pt 1), L139–L147.

155. Schrier, R. W. (2010). ARF, AKI, or ATN? *Nature Reviews Nephrology, 6*, 125.

156. Schrier, R. W., Arroyo, V., Bernardi, M., et al. (1988). Peripheral arterial vasodilation hypothesis: A proposal for the initiation of renal sodium and water retention in cirrhosis. *Hepatology, 8*, 1151–1157.

157. Sharma, P., Kumar, A., Shrama, B. C., et al. (2008). An open label, pilot, randomized controlled trial of noradrenaline versus terlipressin in the treatment of type 1 hepatorenal syndrome and predictors of response. *American Journal of Gastroenterology, 103*, 1689–1697.

158. Singh, C., & Sager, J. S. (2009). Pulmonary complications of cirrhosis. *Medical Clinics of North America, 93*(4), 871–883.

159. Singh, V., Ghosh, S., Singh, B., et al. (2012). Noradrenaline vs. terlipressin in the treatment of hepatorenal syndrome: A randomized study. *Journal of Hepatology, 56*, 1293–1298.

160. Skagen, C., Einstein, M., Lucey, M. R., et al. (2009). Combination treatment with octreotide, midodrine, and albumin improves survival in patients with type 1 and type 2 hepatorenal syndrome. *Journal of Clinical Gastroenterology, 43*, 680–685.

161. Song, J. Y., Choi, J. Y., Ko, J. T., Bae, E. J., Kim, H. S., Noh, C. I., et al. (1996). Long-term aspirin therapy for hepatopulmonary syndrome. *Pediatrics, 97*(6 Pt 1), 917–920.

162. Stadlbauer, V., Wright, G. A., Banaji, M., et al. (2008). Relationship between activation of the sympathetic nervous system and renal blood flow autoregulation in cirrhosis. *Gastroenterology, 134*, 111–119.

163. Stoller, J. K., Lange, P. A., Westveer, M. K., Carey, W. D., Vogt, D., & Henderson, J. M. (1995). Prevalence and reversibility of the hepatopulmonary syndrome after liver transplantation: The Cleveland Clinic experience. *West Journal of Medicine, 163*(2), 133–138.

164. Sulieman, B. M., Hunsicker, L. G., Katz, D. A., & Voigt, M. D. (2008). OPTN policy regarding prioritization of patients with hepatopulmonary syndrome: Does it provide equitable organ allocation? *American Journal of Transplantation, 8*(5), 954–964.

165. Swanson, K. L., & Krowka, M. J. (2008). Screen for Porto pulmonary hypertension, especially in liver transplant candidates. *Cleveland Clinic Journal of Medicine, 75*(2), 121–130, 133.

166. Swanson, K. L., Wiesner, R. H., & Krowka, M. J. (2005). Natural history of hepatopulmonary syndrome: Impact of liver transplantation. *Hepatology, 41*(5), 1122–1129.

167. Swanson, K. L., Wiesner, R. H., Nyberg, S. L., Rosen, C. B., & Krowka, M. J. (2008). Survival in portopulmonary hypertension: Mayo Clinic experience categorized by treatment subgroups. *American Journal of Transplantation, 8*(11), 2445–2453.

168. Sztrymf, B., Rabiller, A., Nunes, H., Savale, L., Lebrec, D., Le, P. A., et al. (2004). Prevention of hepatopulmonary syndrome and hyperdynamic state by pentoxifylline in cirrhotic rats. *European Respiratory Journal, 23*(5), 752–758.

169. Taille, C., Cadranel, J., Bellocq, A., Thabut, G., Soubrane, O., Durand, F., et al. (2003). Liver transplantation for hepatopulmonary syndrome: A ten-year experience in Paris, France. *Transplantation, 75*(9), 1482–1489.

170. Tam, N. L., & He, X. S. (2007). Clinical management of Porto pulmonary hypertension. *Hepatobiliary & Pancreatic Diseases International, 6*(5), 464–469.

171. Tanikella, R., Philips, G. M., Faulk, D. K., Kawut, S. M., & Fallon, M. B. (2008). Pilot study of pentoxifylline in hepatopulmonary syndrome. *Liver Transplantation, 14*(8), 1199–1203.

172. Tazi, K. A., Moreau, R., Herve, P., et al. (2005). Norfloxacin reduces aortic NO synthases and proinflammatory cytokine up-regulation in cirrhotic rats: Role of Akt signaling. *Gastroenterology, 129*, 303–314.

173. Terra, C., Guevara, M., Torre, A., et al. (2005). Renal failure in patients with cirrhosis and sepsis unrelated to spontaneous bacterial peritonitis: Value of MELD score. *Gastroenterology, 129*, 1944–1953.

174. Teuber, G., Teupe, C., Dietrich, C. F., Caspary, W. F., Buhl, R., & Zeuzem, S. (2002). Pulmonary dysfunction in non-cirrhotic patients with chronic viral hepatitis. *European Journal of Internal Medicine, 13*(5), 311–318.

175. Thabut, D., Massard, J., Gangloff, A., et al. (2007). Model for end-stage liver disease score and systemic inflammatory response are major prognostic factors in patients with cirrhosis and acute functional renal failure. *Hepatology, 46*, 1872–1882.

176. Thenappan, T., Goel, A., Marsboom, G., Fang, Y. H., Toth, P. T., Zhang, H. J., et al. (2011). A central role for CD68(+) macrophages in hepatopulmonary syndrome. Reversal by macrophage depletion. *American Journal of Respiratory and Critical Care Medicine, 183*(8), 1080–1091.

177. Vachiery, F., Moreau, R., Hadengue, A., Gadano, A., Soupison T., Valla, D., et al. (1997). Hypoxemia in patients with cirrhosis: Relationship with liver failure and hemodynamic alterations. *Journal of Hepatology, 27*(3), 492–495.

178. Verna, E. C., Brown, R. S., Farrand, E., et al. (2012). Urinary neutrophil gelatinase-associated lipocalin predicts mortality and identifies acute kidney injury in cirrhosis. *Digestive Diseases and Sciences, 57*, 2362–2370.

179. Wiese, S., Hove, J. D., Bendtsen, F., et al. (2014). Cirrhotic cardiomyopathy: Pathogenesis and clinical relevance. *Nature Reviews Gastroenterology & Hepatology, 11*, 177–186.

180. Wiest, R., Lawson, M., & Geuking, M. (2014). Pathological bacterial translocation in liver cirrhosis. *Journal of Hepatology, 60*, 197–209.

181. Wolfe, J. D., Tashkin, D. P., Holly, F. E., Brachman, M. B., & Genovesi, M. G. (1977). Hypoxemia of cirrhosis: Detection of abnormal small pulmonary vascular channels by a quantitative radionuclide method. *American Journal of Medicine, 63*(5), 746–754.

182. Wong, F., Moore, K., Dingemanse, J., et al. (2008). Lack of renal improvement with nonselective endothelin antagonism with tezosentan in type 2 hepatorenal syndrome. *Hepatology, 47*, 160–168.

183. Wong, F., Nadim, M. K., Kellum, J. A., et al. (2011). Working Party proposal for a revised classification system of renal dysfunction in patients with cirrhosis. *Gut, 60*, 702–709.

184. Yang, W., Hu, B., Wu, W., Batra, S., Blackburn, M. R., Alcorn, J. L., et al. (2014a). Alveolar type II epithelial cell dysfunction in rat experimental hepatopulmonary syndrome (HPS). *PLoS One, 9*(11), e113451.

185. Yang, W., Zhang, J., Hu, B., Wu, W., Venter, J., Alpini, G., et al. (2014b). The role of receptor tyrosine kinase activation in cholangiocytes and pulmonary vascular endothelium in experimental hepatopulmonary syndrome. *American Journal of Physiology - Gastrointestinal and Liver Physiology, 306*(1), G72–G80.

186. Younis, I., Sarwar, S., Butt, Z., Tanveer, S., Qaadir, A., & Jadoon, N. A. (2015). Clinical characteristics, predictors, and survival among patients with hepatopulmonary syndrome. *Annals of Hepatology, 14*(3), 354–360.

187. Zamirian, M., Aslani, A., & Shahrzad, S. (2007). Left atrial volume: A novel predictor of hepatopulmonary syndrome. *American Journal of Gastroenterology, 102*(7), 1392–1396.

188. Zhang, J., Ling, Y., Luo, B., Tang, L., Ryter, S. W., Stockard, C. R., et al. (2003). Analysis of pulmonary heme oxygenase-1 and nitric oxide synthase alterations in experimental hepatopulmonary syndrome. *Gastroenterology, 125*(5), 1441–1451.

189. Zhang, J., Ling, Y., Tang, L., Luo, B., Pollock, D. M., & Fallon, M. B. (2009). Attenuation of experimental hepatopulmonary syndrome in endothelin B receptor-deficient rats. *American Journal of Physiology - Gastrointestinal and Liver Physiology, 296*(4), G704–G708.

190. Zhang, J., Yang, W., Hu, B., Wu, W., & Fallon, M. B. (2014). Endothelin-1 activation of the endothelin B receptor modulates pulmonary endothelial CX3CL1 and contributes to pulmonary angiogenesis in experimental hepatopulmonary syndrome. *American Journal of Pathology, 184*(6), 1706–1714.

191. Zhang, J., Yang, W., Luo, B., Hu, B., Maheshwari, A., & Fallon, M. B. (2012). The role of CX3CL1/CX3CR1 in pulmonary angiogenesis and intravascular monocyte accumulation in rat experimental hepatopulmonary syndrome. *Journal of Hepatology, 57*(4), 752–758.

192. Zhang, M., Luo, B., Chen, S. J., Abrams, G. A., & Fallon, M. B. (1999). Endothelin-1 stimulation of endothelial nitric oxide synthase in the pathogenesis of hepatopulmonary syndrome. *American Journal of Physiology, 277*(5 Pt 1), G944–G952.

193. Zopey, R., Susanto, I., Barjaktarevic, I., & Wang, T. (2013). Transition from hepatopulmonary syndrome to Porto pulmonary hypertension: A case series of 3 patients. *Case Reports in Pulmonology, 2013*, 561870.

Chapter 9

MONITORING OF LIVER FIBROGENESIS AND BIOCHEMICAL DIAGNOSIS OF FIBROSIS

Contents

Introduction

Biomedical research over the past 20 years has yielded a wealth of new understandings regarding the pathophysiology of liver fibrosis. the nature of the molecular mediators regulating the expression of the fibrotic extracellular matrix (ECM), the composition of the ECM, the cellular sources of the ECM, the resolution of the ECM, the apoptosis of contributing cells [hepatocytes and hepatic stellate cells (HSCs)], and the reversibility of fibrosis. The objectives are to identify novel noninvasive biomarkers that indicate the activity (progression) of development (fibrogenesis) rather than the stage (extent) of fibrotic organ transition and to identify therapeutic options, at least in the experimental stage.

As "surrogate markers," liver biopsies must be complemented by frequent, dependable, impartial, and reasonably priced diagnostic and follow-up procedures for therapeutic trials. In addition to invasiveness (mortality rate $1:10^3$ to $1:10^4$, severe complications in 0–57% of cases) and sampling error (1/50,000th, or about 30 mg, of the liver mass (~1500 g) can hardly be representative for the whole organ), biopsy histological examination is dependent on sample quality, or the length and size of the tissue specimen (coefficient of variation between 45 and 55%, accuracy 65–75%), and subjective evaluation of morphological changes (also known as "observer error"), which includes grading of necroinflammatory activity (the catalyst for fibrogenesis) and staging (the extent) of fibrotic organ transition (Bedossa et al., 2003). Therefore, caution must be exercised when considering the diagnostic value of the biopsy as the "gold standard" in the detection of fibrosis/fibrogenesis. The necessity for safe, complementary, or alternative serum biomarkers is highlighted by this circumstance.

Orientation and Directional Terms

Term	Definition	Illustration
Enhanced Liver Fibrosis (ELF)	Enhanced Liver Fibrosis (ELF) score is an ECM marker set consisting of tissue inhibitor of metalloproteinases 1 (TIMP-1), amino-terminal propeptide of type III procollagen (PIIINP) and hyaluronic acid (HA) showing good correlations with fibrosis stages in chronic liver disease.	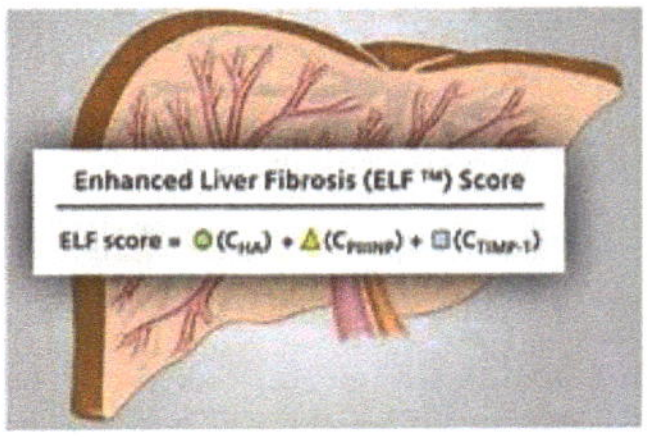
Platelet-derived growth factor (PDGF)	Platelet-derived growth factor (PDGF) is one among numerous growth factors that regulate cell growth and division. In particular, PDGF plays a significant role in blood vessel formation, the growth of blood vessels from already-existing blood vessel tissue, mitogenesis, i.e. proliferation, of mesenchymal cells such as fibroblasts, osteoblasts, tenocytes, vascular smooth muscle cells and mesenchymal stem cells as well as chemotaxis, the directed migration, of mesenchymal cells.	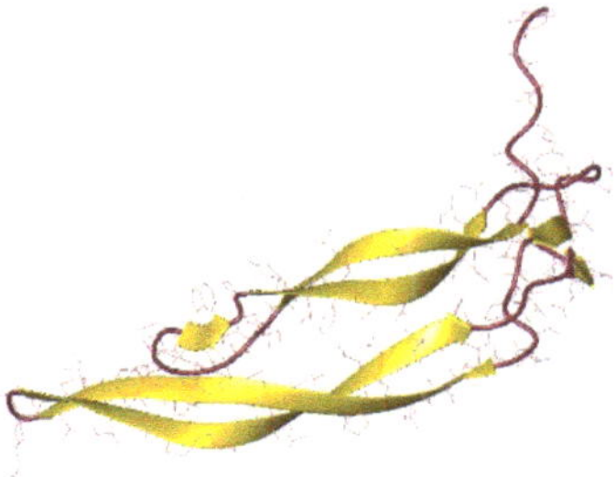
Fibroblast Growth Factors (FGFs)	Fibroblast Growth Factors (FGFs) are potent regulators of cell proliferation and differentiation. They are critically important in normal development, tissue maintenance, wound repair, and angiogenesis in somatic stem cells.	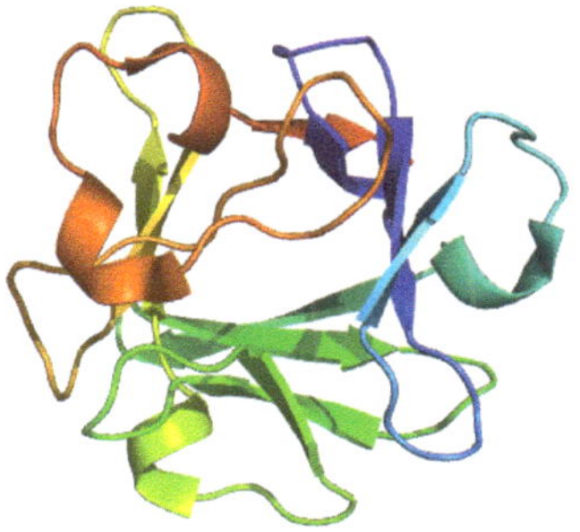
Primary biliary cholangitis (PBC)	Primary biliary cholangitis (PBC), formerly termed primary biliary cirrhosis, is an autoimmune disorder that leads to the gradual destruction of intrahepatic bile ducts, resulting in periportal inflammation and cholestasis. Prolonged hepatic cholestasis subsequently causes cirrhosis and portal hypertension.	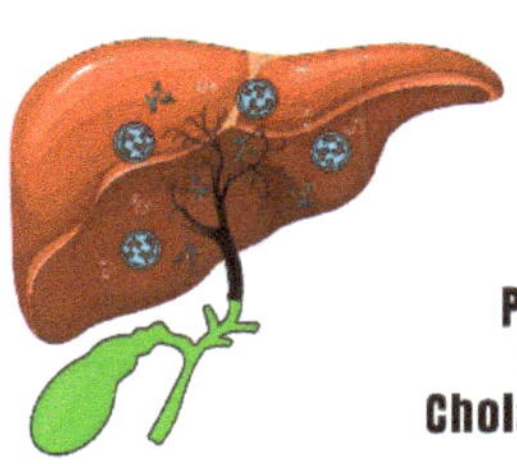

9.1. Current Biomarkers of Hepatic Fibrogenesis

There is presently no serum-based biomarker that can adequately replace liver biopsy in the assessment of liver fibrosis, despite its acknowledged limitations. A plausible explanation could be a vague and imprecise categorization of putative biomarkers. Fibrosis biomarkers are typically categorized into one of two groups. Biomarkers for class I fibrosis are pathophysiologically derived from changes in fibrogenic cell types, specifically induced stem cells (Ito-Cells) and their transdifferentiated counterparts, i.e., degradation of extracellular matrix according to Grressner and Weiskirchen (2006), myofibroblasts (MFB). They have to show the fibrogenic and/or fibrolytic process activity and, consequently, the ECM remodeling. The degree of connective tissue deposition is not indicated by these biomarkers, i.e., the organ's stage of fibrotic transition. They are often expensive laboratory tests that arise from the clinical application of fibrogenic mechanisms. Their selection is therefore based on conjecture.

The majority of class II fibrosis biomarkers gauge the degree of fibrosis (amount of extracellular matrix deposition). They typically consist of standard clinical-chemical tests (e.g., coagulation factors, proteins, enzymes), which may not accurately represent alterations in fibrogenic cells or ECM metabolism. If they have any pathobiochemical relationship at all with fibrogenesis, it is indirect. Their selection is therefore empirical rather than based on theory. The markers are integrated into multiparametric panels and are standard laboratory tests. In general, both types of serum biomarkers follow different pathophysiological concepts. Class I markers inform about "what is going on" (i.e., grade of fibrogenic activity); class II markers indicate "where fibrosis is" (i.e., stage of fibrosis).

9.2. Class I Fibrosis Biomarkers

Due to metabolic dysfunction and/or hemodynamic bypasses, class I biomarkers are matrix components that are increasingly expressed by activated HSC and MFBs, have a delayed clearance by Kupffer cells or sinusoidal endothelial cells in the liver or are increasingly expressed mediators of fibrogenesis like transforming growth factor (TGF)-b. Table 9.1 and Figure 9.2 provide a summary of the class I biomarkers of fibrosis that are currently available.

All things considered, only the N-terminal propeptide of type III-procollagen (PIIINP), which has been proposed as a combination of several procollagen and collagen fragments, has found limited clinical application and is not widely accepted (Collazos and Diaz, 1994). There have been reports of sensitivity levels between 76 and 78% and specificity levels between 71 and 81%. These results can be further raised by combining the results with other collagen fragment markers. It is important to note that PIIINP is not a biomarker unique to the liver.

Similarly, structural glycoproteins (e.g., such as tenascin and undulin), biosynthetic (e.g., prolylhydroxylase), or enzymes that break down. collagen's matrix metalloproteinases) and other extracellular matrix (ECM) constituents have not demonstrated efficacy in identifying, classifying, and advancing fibrosis (Figure 9.1). When cirrhosis in nonalcoholic fatty liver disease (NAFLD) and other etiologies are taken into account, hyaluronan, formerly known as hyaluronic acid, has been shown in multiple studies to be the relatively best class I biomarker of fibrosis, with sensitivities and specificities of 86–100% and 88%, respectively (Lydatakis et al., 2006). Hyaluronan's high negative predictive value (98–100%) at a cut-off concentration of 60 mg/L—significantly higher than its positive predictive value of 61%—underpins its diagnostic efficacy. Because of this, serum hyaluronan's primary use is concentrated on its capacity to rule out advanced fibrosis and cirrhosis. Good hypotheses for a reliable fibrosis biomarker include its stimulated synthesis in activated HSC, secretion into the sinusoidal bloodstream, and short half-life of 2–9 minutes in the circulation.

Laminin was reported to be a predictor of portal hypertension because significantly elevated concentrations were found under these conditions (Kropf et al., 1991). TGF-b concentrations in plasma are elevated and correlate with the severity of liver disease and were suggested as noninvasive biomarker of fibrosis. However, the significant correlation with aspartate-aminotransferase (AST) and alanine-aminotransferase (ALT) activity (Flisiak et al., 2002) and the pathobiochemical finding that substantial amounts of TGF-b are localized in hepatocytes and released into the medium if hepatocytes are permeabilized suggest the elevation of TGF-b as a marker of necrosis instead of fibrogenesis. However, it is functionally and immunologically quite difficult to detect TGF-b in body fluids such as blood due to binding to latent TGF-binding proteins (Breitkopf et al., 2001; Hyytiainen et al., 2004), alpha 2-macroglobulin (Crookston et al., 1993), and other ligands. Thus the measurement of an easier-to-detect mediator of TGF-b activity would generate important analytical advantages over the measurement of TGF-b itself (Grainger et al., 2000).

Table 9.1. *Class I Biomarkers of Liver Fibrogenesis*

	Specimen			
	Serum	Urine	Liver Biopsy	Analytical Method
Extracellular Matrix–Related Enzymes				
Prolyl hydroxylase	+	–	+	Radioenzymatic, RIA
Monoamine oxidase	+	–	(+)	Enzymatic
Lysyl oxidase	+	–	+	RIA
Lysyl hydroxylase	+	–	–	RIA
Galactosyl hydroxylysyl–glucosyl transferase	+	–	+	RIA
Collagen peptidase	+	–	+	Enzymatic
N-Acetyl-β-D-glucosaminidase	+	+	+	Enzymatic
Collagen Fragments and Split Products				
Type I procollagen				
• N-terminal propeptide	+	–	+	ELISA
• C-terminal propeptide	+	–	+	RIA
Type III procollagen				
• Intact procollagen	+	–	–	RIA
• N-terminal propeptide				
• Complete propeptide (Col 1–3)	+	–	–	RIA
• Globular domain of propeptide (Col-1)	+	–	–	RIA
Type IV collagen				
NC1-fragment [C-terminal] cross-linking domain	+	+	–	ELISA, RIA

7S domain ("7S collagen")	+	+	–	RIA
Type VI collagen	+	+	+	RIA
Glycoproteins and Matrix Metalloproteinase (Inhibitors)				
Laminin, P1-fragment	+	–	–	RIA, ELISA
Undulin	+	–	–	ELISA
Vitronectin	+	–	–	ELISA
Tenascin	+	–	–	ELISA
YKL-40	+	–	+	RIA/ELISA
(Pro)matrix metalloproteinase (MMP-2)	+	–	–	ELISA
Tissue inhibitor of metalloproteinases (TIMP-1, TIMP-2)	+	–	–	ELISA
sICAM-1 (soluble intercellular adhesion molecule, sCD54)	+	–	–	ELISA
Glycosaminoglycans				
Hyaluronic acid (hyaluronan)	+	–	–	Radioligand assay
Molecular Mediators				
TGF-β	+	–	+	ELISA
CCN2	+	?	+	ELISA

CCN2, connective tissue growth factor; *ELISA*, enzyme-linked immunosorbent assay; *RIA*, radioimmunoassay; *TGF-β*, transforming growth factor beta.

Source. O.A. Gressner, Monitoring of Liver Fibrogenesis and Biochemical Diagnosis of Fibrosis, http://dx.doi.org/10.1016/B978-0-12-804274-8.00041-2.

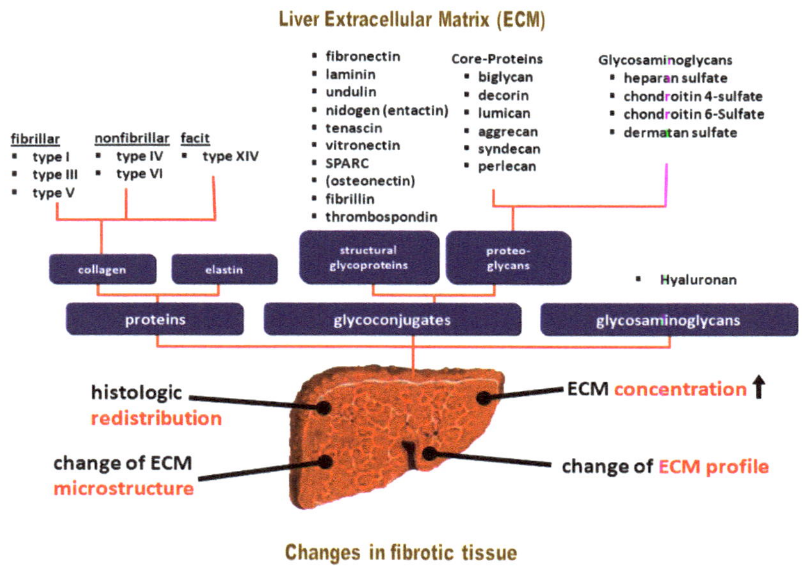

Figure 9.1. *Components of the extracellular matrix (connective tissue) of the fibrotic liver and their major changes. The binding of glycosaminoglycans (GAG) to the respective core proteins (CP) of proteoglycans (PG) is shown. BM, basement membranes; FACIT, fibril-associated collagens with interrupted triple helices.*

Source: O.A. Gressner, Monitoring of Liver Fibrogenesis and Biochemical Diagnosis of Fibrosis, http://dx.doi.org/10.1016/B978-0-12-804274-8.00041-2.

9.3. Class II Fibrosis Biomarkers

This category includes a wide range of biochemical scores that are expanding quickly as well as multiparameter combinations (i.e., biomarker panels), which are chosen using a variety of mathematical algorithms and statistical models (e.g., the analysis of multiple logistic regression). They meet the best diagnostic standards for fibrosis detection and staging and, to a lesser degree, for grading fibrogenic activity. The panels are typically made up of fairly basic (standard) laboratory tests that can be affected by variations in the serum or plasma of patients with cirrhosis and fibrosis. The more than 20 scores that are currently available contain several parameters that have no pathophysiological connection to fibrogenesis or fibrosis. Only a small number of parameters can be thought of as having a direct relationship with the fibrogenic process, and some of them have indirect relationships. Necrosis-related parameters like ALT and AST, coagulation-dependent tests, transport proteins, bilirubin, and certain ECM parameters are among those that need to be measured. The decrease in platelet counts in patients with cirrhosis is often included. The most widely used are the Actitest (Biopredictive, Paris, France) for necroinflammatory activity and the Fibrotest: glutamyl transferase, total bilirubin, haptoglobin, a2-macroglobulin, apolipoprotein A1, and, in the case of Actitest, ALT as well (Poynard et al., 2004). A patented artificial intelligence algorithm is used to calculate the data from Fibrotest and Actitest, yielding the respective measures of fibrosis stage and necroinflammatory grade (activity).

Based on platelet count, alkaline phosphatase, and AST, the WAI score (Wai et al., 2003), the TIMP-1, PIIINP, and hyaluronan-based enhanced liver function (ELF) test (Rosenberg et al, 2004), and the Hepascore determined by factors such as age, gender, gamma-glutamyl transpeptidase, hyaluronan, bilirubin, and a2-macrofulin (Adams et al., 2005) are additional scores that have little bearing on clinical practice. Siemens Healthcare Diagnostics currently offers the ELF test as a ready-made application for the Centaur immunological systems. It is currently the first fibrosis score that is further developed for application in routine medical laboratories (Siemens, 2014). It was suggested that fibrotest would be a more accurate indicator of hepatitis C complications and mortality than biopsy staging (Poynard et al., 2005).

Recently, Fibrotest and Actitest were added to a set of biomarkers that were adjusted for age, gender, and body mass index in order to predict liver steatosis (steatotest), alcoholic steatohepatitis, and nonalcoholic steatohepatitis (NASH-test). These biomarkers were obtained by supplementing serum cholesterol, triglycerides, glucose, and (for the NASH-test) AST. 2005). The NASH-test is a helpful screening tool for advanced fibrosis and NASH in patients with various metabolic syndromes, according to the diagnostic criteria developed in a large number of patients. The steatotest is a straightforward and noninvasive quantitative measure of liver steatosis (Poynard et al., 2005). FibroMax (Biopredictive) is a technique designed to calculate these fibrosis-related tests all at once in a single procedure. However, a comparative analysis of class II serum biomarker panels was unable to demonstrate their superior clinical performance (Parkes et al., 2006) (Table 9.2). Because only roughly 40% of the results were classified as accurate, between 50 and 70% of the results had errors in the staging of the severity of the fibrosis, and a tiny percentage of results were downright wrong (Parkes et al., 2006). Therefore, care must be taken in clinical practice when implementing the currently recommended multiparameter approaches with class II fibrosis biomarker panels. Their stepwise combination may be a successful strategy to increase the panel markers' diagnostic accuracy in chronic hepatitis C (Parkes et al., 2006).

Table 9.2. *Class II Biomarkers of Liver Fibrogenesis*

Index	Parameters	Chronic Liver Disease	Sensitivity (%)	Specificity (%)
Actitest	Fibrotest + ALT	HCV		
Bonacini index	ALT/AST-ratio, INR, platelet count	HCV	46	19
ELF score	PIIINP, hyaluronan, TIMP-1	Mixed	11	41
FIB-4	Platelet count, AST, ALT, age	HCV/HIV	70	74
FibroIndex	Platelet count, AST, γ-globulin	HCV	38	18
Fibrometer test	Platelet count, prothrombin index, AST, α2-macroglobulin, hyaluronan, urea, age	Mixed	81	5
Fibrotest (fibro-score)	Haptoglobin, α2-macroglobulin, apolipoprotein A1, GGT, bilirubin	HCV, HBV	75	6
Forns-index	Age, platelet count, GGT, cholesterol	HCV	15	51
Fortunato-score	Fibronectin, prothrombin time, PCHE, ALT, Mn-SOD, β-NAG	HCV		15
Hepascore	Bilirubin, GGT, hyaluronan, α2-macroglobulin, age, gender	HCV	63	10
Leroy-score	PIIINP, MMP-1	HCV	60	13
NAFLD fibrosis score	Age, BMI, IFG, diabetes, AST/ALT, platelet count, albumin			
Park-index		HCV	47	17
Patel-index (FibroSpect)	Hyaluronan, TIMP-1, α2-macroglobulin	HCV	77	73
PGAA-index	Prothrombin time, GGT, apolipoprotein A1, α2-macroglobulin	Alcohol	79	10
PGA-index	Prothrombin time, GGT, apolipoprotein A1	Mixed	12	81
Pohl-score	AST/ALT-ratio, platelet count	HCV	41	20
Sheth-index	AST/ALT (De Ritis)	HCV	53	21
Sud-index (FPI)	Age, AST, cholesterol, insulin resistance (HOMA), past alcohol intake	HCV	17	44
Testa-index	Platelet count/spleen diameter ratio	HCV	78	79
WAI index (APRI)	AST, platelet count	HCV	10	75

ALT, alanine aminotransferase; *APRI,* AST-to-platelet ratio index; *AST,* aspartate-aminotransferase; *BMI,* body mass index; *ELF,* enhanced liver function test; *FIB,* fibrosis; *FPI,* fibrosis probability index; *GGT,* gamma-glutamyltransferase; *HBV,* hepatitis B virus; *HCV,* hepatic C virus; *HOMA,* homeostasis model assessment; *IFG,* impaired fasting glucose; *INR,* international normalized ratio; *MMP,* matrix metalloproteinases; *Mn-SOD,* manganese superoxide dismutase; *NAFLD,* nonalcoholic fatty liver disease; *β-NAG,* N-acetyl-β-glucosaminidase; *PCHE,* Plasma cholinesterase; pseudocholinesterase; butyrylcholinesterase; *PIIINP,* N-terminal propeptide of type III-procollagen; *TIMP,* tissue inhibitors of metalloproteinases.

Source: O.A. Gressner, Monitoring of Liver Fibrogenesis and Biochemical Diagnosis of Fibrosis, http://dx.doi.org/10.1016/B978-0-12-804274-8.00041-2.

The diagnostic performance could be greatly enhanced by combining the sequential algorithms of AST-to-platelet ratio index (APRI), Forns' index, and Fibrotest; this would reduce the need for liver biopsy by 50–70% (Sebastiani et al., 2006). It should be noted, though, that because of analytical imprecision and widely nonstandardized methods for measuring biochemical routine parameters, the combination of individually assessed parameters inevitably results in relatively high variance (Gressner et al., 2009). For common clinical-chemical analytes, coefficients of variation vary from 3 to 6% for series to 4 to more than 12%for hyaluronan, PIIINP, and other matrix parameters. As a result, there may be significant variation in the comparability and reproducibility of activity grading and staging the degree of fibrotic tissue transition amongst researchers, which restricts their large-scale application and comparison. More significantly, many of these parameters lack standardized assay procedures (methods), which precludes the widespread application of cut-offs and algorithms (Rosenthal-Allieri et al., 2005).

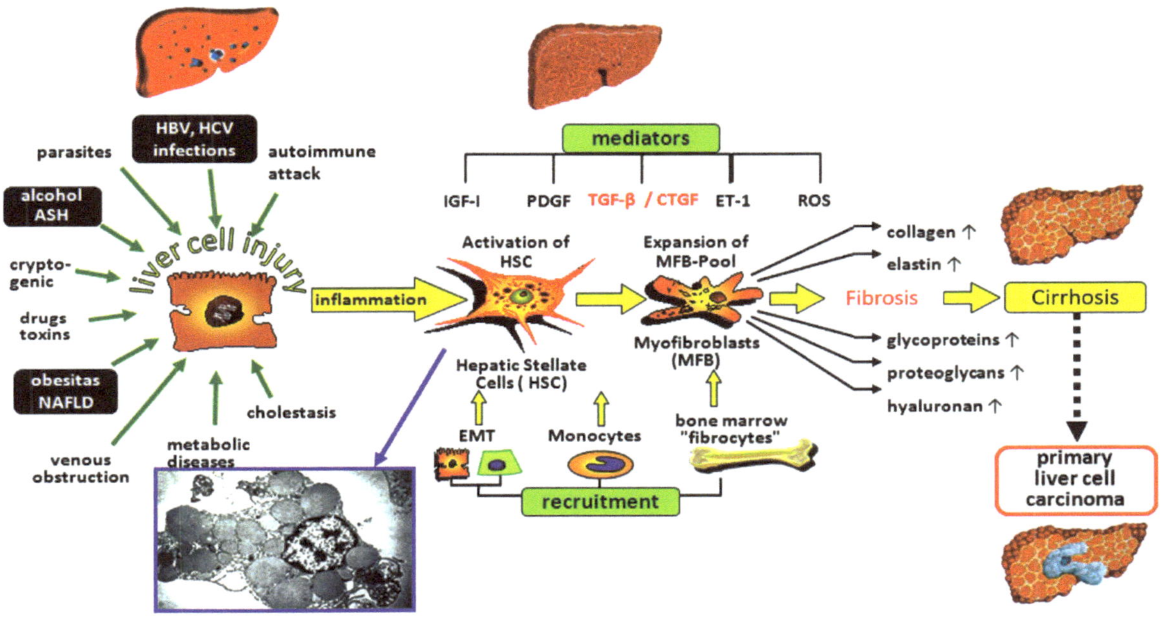

Figure 9.2. *Synopsis of pathogenetic mechanisms of liver fibrosis (fibrogenesis).*

Source: O.A. Gressner, Monitoring of Liver Fibrogenesis and Biochemical Diagnosis of Fibrosis, http://dx.doi.org/10.1016/B978-0-12-804274-8.00041-2.

9.4. Development of Innovative Biomarkers

There may be strong, noninvasive (blood) biomarkers of hepatic fibrogenesis and fibrosis, according to our expanding understanding of the pathophysiology of hepatic fibrosis. Table 9.3 lists a number of recently discovered or suggested biomarkers.

9.4.1. Contribution of Bone Marrow-Derived Cells to HSCs, MFBs, and Fibroblasts in Fibrotic Liver Tissue

Numerous studies have suggested that the bone marrow is a source of multipotent, immature cells that can develop into different organs. If the proper liver microenvironment is present, bone marrow cells can differentiate into hepatocytes, cholangiocytes, sinusoidal endothelial cells, and Kupffer cells (Gao et al., 2001; Fujii et al., 2002). The significance of this phenomenon for regenerative medicine (e.g., therapy using bone marrow stem cells). It was recently expanded to include HSC and MFB in both clinical and experimental settings. It was shown that up to 30% of HSC in the liver originate from the bone marrow and acquire the MFB phenotype under injurious conditions by transplanting male bone marrow (Y chromosome) or genetically tagged bone marrow into female mice (Baba et al., 2004). According to another study, the bone marrow provides up to 68% of HSC and 70% of MFB in the livers of experimental CCl4-cirrhotic mice (Russo et al., 2006). Although it has been demonstrated that bone marrow cells play a significant role in the population of MFBs even in human liver fibrosis, it is currently unknown which particular type of bone marrow cells or mesenchymal stem cells is important for the production of hepatic MFBs (Forbes et al., 2004). According to Kisseleva et al., (2006) the liver contains myelogenic fibrocytes that can be differentiated into collagen-producing MFB by TGF-b. They belong to a subset of circulating leukocytes and have a distinct surface phenotype that includes type I collagen (capability of matrix synthesis), CD34+ (progenitor cell), and CD45+ (hematopoietic origin) (Quan et al., 2006), and demonstrate strong immunostimulatory effects (Abe et al., 2001). In a variety of fibrotic lesions, including lung, keloids, scleroderma, and fibrotic changes of the kidney, fibrocytes are a systemic source of contractile MFB (Quan et al., 2004).

Table 9.3. *Future Candidate Biomarkers of Noninvasive Diagnosis and Follow-Up of Liver Fibrogenesis*

Biomarker	Specimen	Analytical Method	Pathobiochemical Bias
BMP-7	Serum	Immunoassay	Antagonist of TGF-β, inhibitor of EMT
Colony stimulating factors (CSF): G-CSF GM-CSF M-CSF	Whole blood	Immunoassays	Mobilization of bone marrow–derived fibrocytes
CTGF	Serum	Immunoassay	TGF-β induced expression in and secretion by hepatocytes and HSCs
Glycomics	Serum	Adaptation of DNA sequencer/fragment analyzer technology to profiling of desialylated *N*-linked oligosaccharides	Fibrosis-specific profiles of desialylated serum protein linked oligo-saccharides (*N*-glycans)
NX-DCP	Serum	Immunoassay	Increased release as result of fibrosis-induced hypoxia of liver parenchyma
Proteomics	Serum	Mass spectrometry (MS)	Fibrosis-specific serum protein profiles
Xylosyl transferase	Serum	Liquid chromatography tandem MS	Key enzyme of the biosynthesis of glycosaminoglycan chains in proteoglycans, e.g., in HSCs and hepatocytes

BMP, bone morphogenetic protein; *CTGF*, connective tissue growth factor; *EMT*, epithelial–mesenchymal transition; *G-CSF*, granulocyte-colony stimulating factor; *GM-CSF*, Granulocyte macrophage colony-stimulating factor; *HSCs*, hepatic stellate cells; *NX-DCP*, NX-des-γ-carboxyprothrombin; *TGF-β*, transforming growth factor beta.

Source: O.A. Gressner, Monitoring of Liver Fibrogenesis and Biochemical Diagnosis of Fibrosis, http://dx.doi.org/10.1016/B978-0-12-804274-8.00041-2.

One common mechanism of tissue fibrosis and wound healing is the mobilization of bone marrow cells and their recruitment into the damaged tissue (Ishii et al., 2005), which is most likely controlled by CSF (colonial stimulating factors), like granulocyte-CSF (GCSF) (Higashiyama et al., 2007). This mediator controls bone marrow cell migration to tissue damage sites in conjunction with chemokines, as well as bone marrow efflux into the bloodstream (Abe et al., 2001). Because activated HSC secrete a wide range of inflammatory mediators, including chemokines, stem cell factor, platelet activating factor, and macrophage colony-stimulating factor (M-CSF), as well as leukocyte adhesion molecules, such as intercellular adhesion molecule 1, vascular cell adhesion molecule 1, and neural cell adhesion molecule, necessary for the recruitment, activation, and maturation of blood-born cells at the site of injury, these cells are likely important (Marra, 1999). Because myelogenic cells express matrix metalloproteinases, which enhance the breakdown of fibrotic extracellular matrix, it has been suggested that locating these cells in the injured liver will also help resolve liver fibrosis (Higashiyama et al., 2007).

9.4.2. Transformation of Peripheral Blood Cells to MFBs of the Liver

According to recent research, a subset of circulating blood monocytes has highly developed multidifferentiation potential and can be quickly recruited for tissue repair processes (Romagnani et al., 2006). Furthermore, it has been proposed that the quantity of myelogenic stem cells in the bloodstream plays a crucial role in regenerative processes resulting from ischemic and degenerative illnesses (i.e., coronary ischemic stroke).

Investigations over the last years have proven that peripheral blood monocytes can be differentiated in vitro to hepatocyte-like cells if they are exposed to the M-CSF and specific interleukins (monocyte-derived neo-hepatocytes) (Ruhnke et al., 2005a, 2005b). Although liver fibrogenesis is not yet proven, subgroups of monocytes can differentiate into fibroblast-like cells (fibrocytes) after migration into the damaged tissue. There, they participate in fibrotic processes, e.g., of the lung and kidney. The differentiation is positively influenced by granulocyte colony-stimulating factor (G-CSF), M-CSF, monocyte chemotactic peptide 1 (MCP-1), and other chemokines and hematopoietic growth and differentiation factors, which are expressed and secreted by activated HSC (Kisseleva et al., 2006; Pinzani et al., 1992; Marra et al., 1993; Sprenger et al., 1997) and other liver cell types (Marra et al., 1998). It is of interest that very recently an inhibitory effect of the acute-phase protein serum amyloid P (SAP) on the process of differentiation of monocytes to fibrocytes could be established (Pilling et al., 2003) and, consequently, a preventive effect of SAP-injections on the development of bleomycin-induced lung fibrosis was found (Pilling et al., 2007). C-reactive protein failed to show an inhibitory effect on the differentiation of monocytes to fibrocytes. Because SAP is synthesized in hepatocytes, severe liver injury might facilitate the monocyte fibrocyte differentiation process due to the reduction of the inhibitory SAP. Although this mechanism is presently speculative for the liver, circulating monocytes might nonetheless be a pool for immediate repair processes of liver damage. Besides special monocytes as a source of fibroblasts in the fibrotic liver, circulating stem cells have to be considered, which are $CD34^{+}$ and C-X-C chemokine receptor type 4 ($CXCR4^{+}$) (a chemokine receptor) (Romagnani et al., 2006). G-CSF and the stromal derived factor are probably the most important regulators of stem cell mobilization from bone marrow and their integration into the damaged tissue followed by differentiation to fibroblasts and other cells.

9.4.3. Parameters of Epitheliale-Mesenchymal Transition

An increasing body of experimental research suggests a mechanism other than HSC activation and transdifferentiation for the fibrotic response of injured organs, such as the enlargement of the resident (local) pool of fibroblasts in the lung and kidney (Lee et al., 2006). Known as epithelial-mesenchymal transition (EMT), this process is now recognized as a key mechanism in the production of fibroblasts during fibrogenesis in adult tissues, although it was first identified in the context of embryonic development (Kalluri and Neilson, 2003). The ability of tubular epithelial cells to transdifferentiate into fibroblasts that express the fibroblast specific protein 1 (FSP-1), also referred to as the S21A4 calcium-binding protein, and to express collagens has been demonstrated in fibrotic kidney disease (Kalluri and Neilson, 2003). Comparably, cardiac endothelial cells can transform into fibroblasts in situations of damage (mesenchymal-mesenchymal transition) and alveolar epithelial cells of the lung are susceptible to EMT. It has been demonstrated that tubular epithelial cells can transdifferentiate into fibroblasts in fibrotic kidney disease, expressing collagens and the fibroblast specific protein 1 (FSP-1), also referred to as the S21A4 calcium-binding protein (Kalluri & Neilson, 2003). Similar to this, lung alveolar epithelial cells can undergo epithelial-mesenchymal transition (EMT) and cardial endothelial cells can also differentiate into fibroblasts in response to injury.

An estimated 66% of fibroblasts in the kidney and 20% in the heart are thought to be the result of EMT (R. Kalluri, individual correspondence). The idea that endothelial cell transformation to MFB-like cells may account for the rise in matrix proteins and MFB pathognomonic of fibrotic diseases is supported by observations made in blood vessels both in vitro and in vivo after prolonged inflammation (Karasek, 2007). Following the demonstration of a transition from albumin-positive hepatocytes to FSP-1-positive and albumin-negative fibroblasts, very recent studies have also addressed EMT in liver fibrogenesis. About 40% of hepatic fibroblasts are thought to be derived from hepatocytes, according to preliminary research, but more research is required to confirm these findings (R. Kalluri, individual correspondence). Evidence of EMT of mature mouse hepatocytes in vitro and of the mouse hepatocyte cell line alpha mouse liver 12 has been reported recently (Kaimori et al., 2007).

Type I collagen deposition and a significant upregulation of a1(I) collagen mRNA expression were indicators of the EMT state. Hepatocytes can therefore produce type I collagen and undergo EMT changes. Bile duct epithelial cells, or cholangiocytes, are an additional source of EMT. It has been established that bile duct epithelial cells in primary biliary cirrhosis (PBC) express vimentin and FSP-1 (S21A4), which are early indicators of fibroblasts (Robertson et al., 2007). Ductopania, or the narrowing of the bile ducts, and the proliferation of the portal fibroblast pool are the two-way effects of cholangiocyte EMT, and they both play a major role in the development of portal fibrosis. Studies conducted in vitro using human cholangiocytes in culture have validated the reported clinical observations. According to Rygiel et al., (2008), EMT thus demonstrates to be a general pathogenetic principle of chronic cholestatic liver diseases. Furthermore, bile duct epithelial cells stimulate the activation and proliferation of portal/periportal mesenchymal cells to peribiliary MFB in a paracrine manner through TGF-b, platelet-derived growth factor BB, and endothelin-1 (Kinnman et al., 2003), it became apparent that this pathway was crucial for the development of septa and portal fibrosis in cholestatic liver diseases. In fact, Beaussier et al., (2007), found that in obstructive cholestatic injuries, only a small percentage of MFB that produce ECM originates from HSC. (Saile & Ramadori, 2004). This highlights the significance of the underlying fibrogenic liver disease and highlights the heterogeneous origin of MFB in fibrogenesis (Torok et al., 2015).

TGF-b (Kalluri and Neilson, 2003), epidermal growth factor (EGF), insulin-like growth factor (IGF)-II, and fibroblast growth factor (FGF)-2 are the molecular inducers of epithelial-mesenchymal transition (EMT) because they facilitate the genetic and phenotypic programming of epithelial cells into mesenchymal cells (fibroblasts). TGF-b is the prototype for the strongest EMT inducer. The activation of Smad2/3 phosphorylation, the inhibition of Smad4 silencing with small interfering RNA (siRNA), and the induction of the snail transcription factor demonstrated the inducing role of TGF-b for the mesenchymal transition of mouse hepatocytes (described earlier) (Karasek, 2007). Remarkably, TGF-b only causes EMT in hepatocytes that are resistant to this cytokine's proapoptotic effects (Yang et al., 2006; Del Castillo et al., 2006). The subpopulation of surviving hepatocytes exhibits an overexpression of Snail by TGF-b conferring resistance to programmed cell death (Vega et al., 2004). Several additional pathways are involved in the generation of apoptosis resistance, e.g., protein kinase A (Yang et al., 2006) and EGF/TGF-a (Del Castillo et al., 2006). Hepatocyte EMT is therefore reliant on the equilibrium of apoptotic and survival mechanisms. In order to release epithelial cells from cell-to-cell and cell-basement membrane binding, EMT also necessitates the activity of metalloproteinases and a TGF-b-dependent downregulation of E-cadherin. The most significant molecular analog is the TGF-b superfamily member bone morphogenetic protein (BMP)-7. BMP-7 can cause a mesothelial to-epithelial transition (reverse EMT, or MET), in addition to inhibiting EMT (Zeisberg et al., 2003). It has antiapoptotic properties and antiinflammatory and proliferation-stimulating effects (Sugimoto et al., 2007). BMP-7 inhibits TGF-b signaling via Smads (Wang and Hirschberg, 2004), which transduce the effect of the latter cytokine from its receptor; a serine/threonine kinase to the Smad-binding element of respective target genes in the nucleus (ten Dijke and Hill, 2004). In addition, several trapping proteins such as the small proteoglycans decorin and biglycan, latency-associated peptide, BMP and activin membrane-bound inhibitor, kielin-chordinelike protein, gremlin, and a2- macroglobulin change the balance between TGF-b and BMP-7 in favor of an anti-EMT effect due to binding a neutralization of TGF-b (Neilson, 2005).

9.4.4. Connective Tissue Growth Factor

Connective tissue growth factor (CTGF; CCN2) in serum is a novel class I biomarker of fibrogenesis that appears to reflect TGF-b activity, according to preliminary research (Gressner et al., 2006). This 38-kDa protein, which belongs to the secreted, cysteine-rich glycoprotein CCN superfamily, has been linked to the development of hepatic fibrosis and is now thought to play a significant role as a downstream amplifier of the profibrogenic master cytokine TGF-b's effects (Leask and Abraham, 2006). Although the precise molecular mechanism of action of this cytokine is still unknown, it is expressed in cholangiocytes, portal fibroblasts, hepatocytes, and HSC (Abreu et al., 2002; Gressner et al., 2007), and appears to alter the TGF-b/BMP-7 functional ratio (Abreu et al., 2002). CTGF is overexpressed in experimental and human liver cirrhosis (Rachfal and Brigstock, 2003; Abou-Shady et al., 2000; Paradis et al., 1999), which is mediated mainly by TGF-b, but also by endothelin-1, tumor necrosis factor-a, vascular endothelial growth factor (VEGF), nitrogen oxide, prostaglandin E2, thrombin, high glucose, and hypoxia (Blom et al., 2002). CTGF inhibits

BMP, but activates TGF-b signaling by modulation of the receptor-binding of these ligands (Abreu et al., 2002). Additionally, CCN2/CTGF expression is sensitively upregulated by TGF-b. The crucial role in fibrogenesis was documented by recent studies in which knock-down of CCN2/CTGF by siRNA leads to substantial attenuation of experimental liver fibrosis (Li et al., 2006; George and Tsutsumi, 2007). Thus depletion of CTGF greatly attenuates the development of experimental liver fibrosis (Figure 9.3).

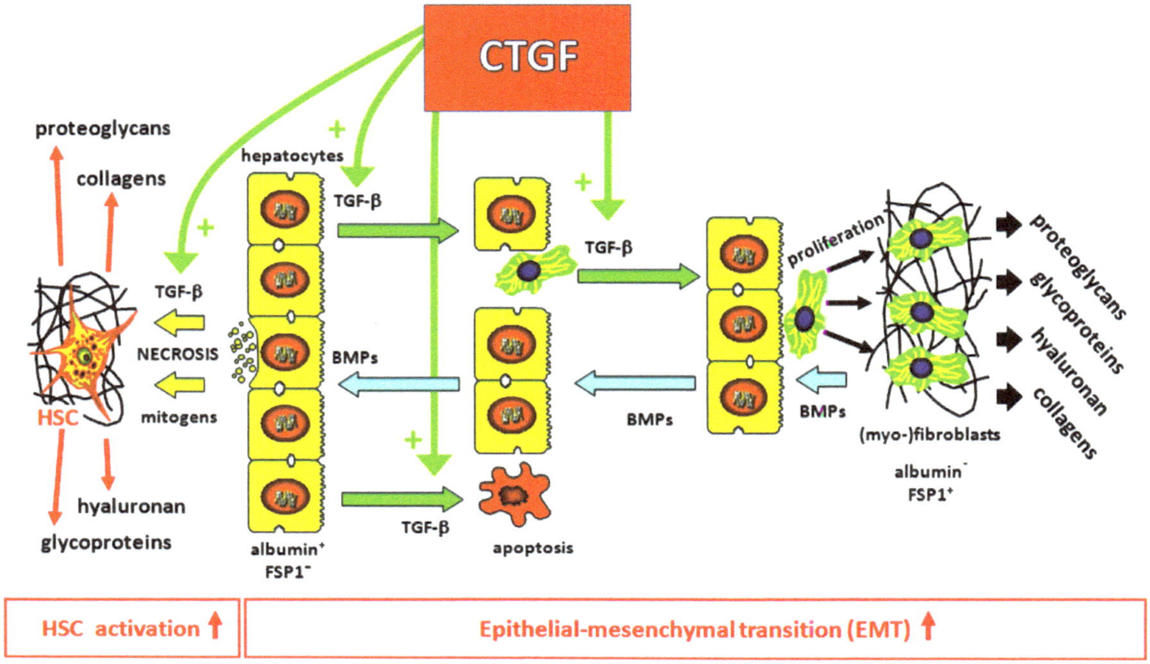

Figure 9.3. *Role of connective tissue growth factor (CTGF) in hepatic fibrogenesis.*

Source: O.A. Gressner, Monitoring of Liver Fibrogenesis and Biochemical Diagnosis of Fibrosis, http://dx.doi.org/10.1016/B978-0-12-804274-8.00041-2.

Significant increases of CTGF in serum/plasma of patients with fibrogenic CLD were previously shown in this study using an in-house immunoassay for CTGF (Kovalenko et al., 2009; Gressner et al., 2013). The area under the curve (AUC) for fibrosis versus control and cirrhosis versus control were calculated to be 0.165 and 0.9, respectively; the sensitivities were 21% and 5%, respectively, and the specificities 10% and 6%, respectively (Gressner et al., 2006). Thus there is good evidence for CTGF as a diagnostic relevant fibrogenic master switch in fibrotic CLD.

The levels of CTGF exhibit a biphasic pattern, wherein patients with fibrotic and cirrhotic conditions have ascending concentrations, whereas patients with HCC have slightly descending levels. Moreover, CTGF concentrations declined with tumor size and progression, showing reduced levels in TNM stage II and stage III compared to TNM stage I in the tumor, nodes, and metastases (TNM) (Gressner et al., 2013). The course of CTGF serum concentrations may therefore be additionally advised as a "negative" tumor marker in patients with established cirrhosis, in addition to its diagnostic utility in reflecting the degree of fibrosis.

When combined, MET and EMT, as well as, in certain cases, MMT (mesothelial to mesenchymal transition, e.g., vascular endothelial cells to fibroblasts), as well as the regulation of the bioactive TGF-b/BMP-7 ratio and the proteins that act as adaptors and trapping agents, provide a variety of regulatory options for impacting fibrogenesis. For the kidney, these mechanisms are fairly well understood (Zeisberg, 2006); however, additional experimental evidence is required for the liver, particularly concerning the liver's quantitative role in fibrogenesis (Figure 9.3).

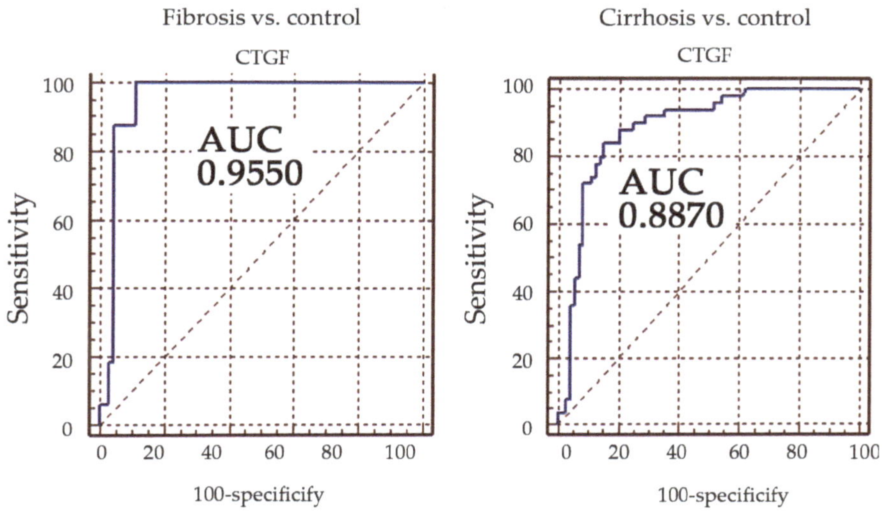

Figure 9.4. *Potential of connective tissue growth factor (CTGF) in serum for monitoring hepatic fibrogenesis.*

Source: O.A. Gressner, Monitoring of Liver Fibrogenesis and Biochemical Diagnosis of Fibrosis, http://dx.doi.org/10.1016/B978-0-12-804274-8.00041-2.

9.4.5. YKL-40

The glycoprotein YKL-40, also known as "chondrex," has been observed to exhibit strong expression in human liver tissue. This protein is thought to function as a growth factor for endothelial and fibroblast cells. Its molecular mass is 40 kDa. YKL-40 mRNA is specifically present in HSCs. YKL-40 concentrations in the sera of patients with liver diseases have been found to be elevated in several studies. For hepatic C virus (HCV) patients, an 80% sensitivity, 77% specificity, and an AUC of 0.81 for fibrosis are reported (Saitou et al., 2005); for those with alcoholic liver disease, a specificity of 88.5%, but a sensitivity of only 50.8%, however, was determined. Only 11.5% of the patients without severe fibrosis displayed a Chondrex plasma level above this threshold (Tran et al., 2000). Serum concentrations of this protein correlate with other ECM products secreted by MFB (e.g., PIIINP, hyaluronan, MMP-2, and TIMP-1) (Tran et al., 2000). It is claimed that YKL-40 concentrations reflect the degree of liver fibrosis, but extensive clinical evaluation is required and other inflammatory and malignant diseases as potential conditions of YKL-40 elevations have to be excluded.

9.4.6. Xylosyl Transferase

Increased activity of Xylosyl transferase (XT), a crucial enzyme that links the glycosaminoglycan side chain to the proteoglycan moiety's core protein, has been observed in the serum of patients suffering from connective tissue diseases. It is possible to measure a large number of liver fibrotic patients using high-performance liquid chromatography-tandem mass spectrometry (Kuhn et al., 2006). Due to the highly stimulated proteoglycan synthesis of MFB in fibrotic livers (Gressner, 1994), XT activity in serum may be a promising class I biomarker of fibrogenesis. However, the test's analytic performance and lack of standardization make it difficult to evaluate this parameter further.

9.4.7. Glycomics

The identification of unique serum proteomic fingerprints in patients with fibrosis has led to advancements in differentiation between stages of fibrosis and prediction of fibrosis and cirrhosis in chronic hepatitis B infection patients. Studies have shown that serum proteome profiling and total serum protein glycomics, specifically N-glycan patterns, have the potential for further successful developments (Callewaert et al., 2004; Poon et al., 2005). Sensitivities, specificities, and accuracy of prediction for cirrhosis have been reported to be around 10%. Additionally, N-glycan profiling has shown the ability to differentiate between compensated cirrhosis and noncirrhotic chronic liver diseases with sensitivities and specificities of 79% and 7% (Callewaert et al., 2004).

The integration of objective and reliable noninvasive biomarkers for the diagnosis and follow-up of fibrogenic (liver) diseases would be greatly aided by the addition of contemporary high-resolution or molecular imaging analyses to all of these laboratory tests.

9.5. NX-DES-g-Carboxyprothrombin

There are various variations of des-g-carboxyprothrombin (DCP) depending on how many glutamic acid (Glu) residues there are, ranging from 0 to 10. The DCP variation known as NX-des-g-carboxyprothrombin (NX-DCP) has fewer Glu residues. Previous research revealed that NX-DCP is released more and more when parenchymal hypoxia caused by fibrosis occurs (Toyoda et al., 2012).

A study from Japan performed a prospective cohort study on a consecutive group of 22 patients who underwent liver biopsy for HCV-related liver disease. Detected serum concentrations of NX-DCP correlated positively with the fibrosis stage ($p = 0.006$). Moreover, NX-DCP was a multivariate factor associated with the presence of significant fibrosis F 3–4 (median 21 of F0–2 group vs. median 22 of F3–4 group with $p = 0.002$). The AUC of NX-DCP showed no significant differences compared with multiparametric type II fibrosis markers such as the APRI, the modified-APRI, and the Pohl score ($p > .05$). Moreover, NX-DCP had a similar predictive ability to the models (mentioned earlier), and thereby should be furthermore evaluated as a potential new noninvasive prediction tool for fibrosis (Saito et al., 2015).

Serum biomarkers of types I and II that are currently on the market should be used cautiously because neither single nor panel markers fully meet the criteria for the perfect noninvasive fibrosis biomarker. These include, in particular: (1) ease of analysis; (2) robust test system standardization; (3) cost-effectiveness; and (4) high specificity and sensitivity in identifying fibrogenic liver diseases. Even the most highly regarded and current type I (i.e., hyaluronan) as well as type II (i.e., Serum biomarkers (Actitest and Fibrotest) do not fit all of these requirements. Therefore, in order to inspire new ideas for the noninvasive assessment of fibrosis using biochemical or physical means, more in-depth insights into the mechanism of liver fibrosis and advancements in analytical techniques are required.

Novel approaches for treating liver fibrogenesis and noninvasive diagnostic techniques are made possible by the recently identified pathogenetic mechanisms of fibrosis that were previously discussed (Mehal and Schuppan, 2015; Torok et al., 2015). Finding the TGF-b/BMP-7 ratio in serum or plasma may be beneficial as it may indicate the EMT process and, consequently, at least some of the fibrosis progression rate. Patients with slow progression (slow fibroser) may have a decreasing ratio; those with rapid progression (rapid fibroser) may have an increasing ratio. However, there are a few things to keep in mind. First, the circulation's cytokine ratio may not accurately reflect the activity of these molecules in close proximity to fibroblasts and epithelial cells, respectively, and a significant portion of these molecules may be in a biologically latent form. As a result, the protein ratio does not always correspond to the crucial activity ratio for the diagnosis of these mediators. Because this modulator protein is highly upregulated in the fibrotic liver and is produced and secreted by both parenchymal and nonparenchymal cells, measuring CTGF in serum or plasma is proposed as an innovative fibrogenesis parameter (Gressner et al., 2007) and the antifibrogenic BMP-7 is inhibited while the profibrogenic TGF-b is stimulated (Abreu et al., 2002). Preliminary studies point to significantly enhanced concentrations of CTGF in the blood of patients with active liver fibrogenesis (Gressner et al., 2006) in contrast to advanced cirrhosis with low concentration of active fibrogenesis, which is reflected by a relative decrease of serum CTGF.

One approach to assess their diagnostic potential could be to use flow cytometric detection of circulating fibrocytes in blood or in buffy coat leukocytes using $CD34^+$, $CD45^+$, and collagen I positivities as identifying markers. As an alternative, these antigens could be found by employing a quantitative PCR technique to amp up their mRNA. Furthermore, a reassessment of the elevated levels of M-CSF, G-CSF, and granulocyte macrophage colony-stimulating factor (GMCSF) in the serum of patients with cirrhosis was previously published (Kubota et al., , 1995) as facilitators of the integration of bone marrow cells and fibrocytes into the injured liver tissue (Yannaki et al., 2005) could be a worthwhile endeavor. It is worth examining if there is a relationship between the activity of liver fibrogenesis and a systemic increase in hematopoietic growth factors.

Numerous publications discuss antifibrotic therapeutic strategies by inhibition of TGF-b (AbouShady et al., 2000; Abe et al., 2001; Liu et al., 2006; Torok et al., 2015), but the systemic application of inhibitors and, consequently, an overall and ubiquitous reduction of TGF-b activity will most likely have severe side effects, e.g., on tumor development and progression, autoimmunopathy, and degenerative diseases (Gressner and Weiskirchen, 2003). Therefore, the therapeutic application of recombinant human BMP-7 or functionally active BMP-7 fragments might be advantageous because BMP-7 inhibits experimental fibrosis in rats (Kinoshita et al., 2007), stimulates liver regeneration (Sugimoto et al., 2007), and inhibits TGF-driven parenchymal cell apoptosis due to its antagonism of TGF-b.

Successful antifibrotic outcomes have been observed in experimental trials utilizing thioacetamide-induced rat liver fibrosis (Kinoshita et al., 2007). Similar to this, a number of studies conducted on kidney diseases in experimental settings demonstrate that BMP-7 can cause MET, which has regenerative and antifibrotic properties (Zeisberg & Shah, 2005). As of right now, it is unclear if the successful

CTGF-inhibitory trials for the prevention of experimental fibrosis (Li et al., 2006; George & Tsutsumi, 2007) can be applied to clinical settings; however, investigations demonstrating a reduction in CTGF activity through systemic administration of a humanized monoclonal blocking antibody (F-3019) that neutralizes and expedites the protein's clearance (Liu, 2007) are ongoing and show encouraging early outcomes.

Pathophysiologically, the TGF-b/BMP-7 ratio is switched in favor of BMP-7, which is why CTGF inhibitors should have fibrosuppressive effects. Recently, CTGF expression was shown to be inhibited (Li et al., 2006; Tsutsumi & George, 2007). To sum up, in-depth research is still needed to convert the promising outcomes of animal and cell culture studies into practical applications. Strong optimism is justified by the new pathogenetic insights, as they greatly expand the range of possible strategies to disrupt the fibrogenic pathway.

Rethinking the exclusive role of HSC in the development of fibrosis is clearly necessary, as evidenced by the evolving understanding of the pathogenetic mechanisms of liver fibrosis (discussed previously). HSC-derived fibrogenic cells are just one of several sources of distinct MFB/fibroblast subpopulations found in fibrosing livers, though some of the recently proposed fibrogenic mechanisms still need further experimental evidence in vitro and in situ. Most importantly, the etiology of fibrosis can affect the composition of MFBs. PBC may cause a distinct pathogenetic pathway from that of alcoholic fibrosis. These data highlight the crucial idea that because distinct classes of MFBs are produced by different pathways, findings from different experimental fibrogenesis models cannot be broadly applied. Furthermore, unlike in the past, HSC activation in culture cannot be considered the nearly universal paradigm of the liver fibrogenic mechanism. We now know that a number of the intracellular fibrogenic signaling molecular cascades are specifically cell type modulated, thanks to the availability of detailed information on these pathways. Therefore, it is conceivable that distinct subpopulations of fibroblasts and their transient precursor cell types respond differently to major fibrogenic cytokines, e.g., TGF-b. If so, there will be a significant future increase in the complexity of the fibrogenic mechanisms.

New methods for the noninvasive evaluation of fibrosis using biochemical or physical methods will be developed as a result of a thorough understanding of the mechanism underlying liver fibrosis and the advancement of analytical techniques. These biochemical serum-based indicators of liver fibrosis/fibrogenesis will supplement quantitative elastography methods, which have been widely used in clinical settings to measure liver stiffness. These methods include magnetic resonance elastography, acoustic radiation force impulse, and monodimensional ultrasound transient elastography (FibroScan) (Patel et al., 2015). Furthermore, the examination of genetic susceptibility markers or the identification of unique single nucleotide polymorphism signatures linked to the degree of fibrosis may serve as additional supplementary diagnostic methods.

A Closer Look

Pulmonary Fibrosis

Pulmonary fibrosis is a chronic, progressive lung disease characterized by the thickening and scarring (fibrosis) of lung tissue, leading to a decline in lung function and difficulty in breathing. The causes of pulmonary fibrosis are diverse and often unknown, with idiopathic pulmonary fibrosis (IPF) being the most common type where no clear cause is identified. Known causes include environmental and occupational exposures to pollutants like silica dust and asbestos, radiation therapy for cancers, certain medications such as chemotherapy drugs, and autoimmune diseases like rheumatoid arthritis and scleroderma. Genetic predisposition also plays a role in some cases. Symptoms of pulmonary fibrosis typically develop gradually and include shortness of breath, especially during physical activity, a persistent dry cough, fatigue, chest discomfort, loss of appetite, weight loss, and clubbing of the fingers and toes. Diagnosis involves a combination of medical history, physical examination, high-resolution CT scans, pulmonary function tests, blood tests, and sometimes bronchoscopy and biopsy. There is no cure for pulmonary fibrosis, but treatment focuses on managing symptoms and slowing disease progression. Medications such as antifibrotic agents (pirfenidone and nintedanib) can help slow progression, while corticosteroids and immunosuppressive drugs may reduce inflammation. Oxygen therapy and pulmonary rehabilitation programs can improve quality of life, and in severe cases, a lung transplant may be considered. Lifestyle changes, including quitting smoking, maintaining a healthy diet, and staying active, are also important. The prognosis for pulmonary fibrosis varies; some patients experience a slow progression, while others face a rapid decline in lung function. Early diagnosis and treatment are crucial for improving quality of life and potentially extending survival. Research continues to focus on understanding the disease's mechanisms and developing more effective treatments, with particular interest in genetic research, biomarkers for predicting disease progression and treatment response, and new therapeutic approaches. Patients can find support and resources through organizations like the Pulmonary Fibrosis Foundation, which offers information, community support, and advocacy. Understanding pulmonary fibrosis involves recognizing its complex and multifactorial nature, emphasizing early detection, and adopting a comprehensive and personalized management approach.

Summary

- The growing understanding of the pathogenesis of hepatic fibrosis indicates potentially powerful, noninvasive (blood) biomarkers of hepatic fibrogenesis and fibrosis.
- Liver fibrosis represents a scarring response to either acute or chronic cellular injury. Following acute liver injury, parenchymal cells regenerate to successfully preserve hepatocellular mass and function. This acute process is associated with an inflammatory and fibrogenic response but limited deposition of extracellular matrix (ECM).
- The field of hepatic fibrosis is flourishing thanks to continued experimental advances complemented by exciting progress in the treatment of chronic liver disease. Control of chronic hepatitis B and C by antiviral therapies has established that advanced fibrosis can regress in association with improved clinical outcomes, there by intensifying enthusiasm to uncover the mechanistic basis for hepatic fibrogenesis and its attenuation.
- The anatomical arrangement of parenchymal and nonparenchymal cells of the liver contributes to its unique role as an immunity-modulating organ and helps explain how the liver responds to an insult. The liver is composed primarily of epithelial cells, hepatocytes and cholangiocytes, and resident nonparenchymal cells that include hepatic macrophages (Kupffer cells), sinusoidal endothelium, and HSCs.
- The liver capsule extends as septa into the liver, delineating hepatic lobules that form the structural units of the liver. The lobule forms a hexagonal structure with portal triads—including branches of the hepatic portal vein, the hepatic artery, and the bile duct—localized in the periphery of the lobule and with a portal vein branch in the center.
- Besides activation and transdifferentiation of HSC, an increasing number of experimental studies point to an additional mechanism for the enlargement of the resident (local) pool of fibroblasts during the fibrotic reaction of the damaged organs, e.g., in the kidney and lung.
- Xylosyltransferase (XylT) initiates the process using UDP-Xyl as donor and PG core protein as acceptor. No defined consensus amino-acid sequence for xylosylation exists, except that a glycine residue consistently lies immediately carboxy-terminal to target serine residues.
- Glycomics is a subset of the field of glycobiology that aims to identify the structure and function of the complete set of glycans (the glycome) produced in a given cell or organism and identify all the genes that encode glycoproteins.

References

1. Abe, R., Donnelly, S. C., Peng, T., Bucala, R., & Metz, C. N. (2001). Peripheral blood fibrocytes: Differentiation pathway and migration to wound sites. *Journal of Immunology, 166*, 7556–7562.
2. Abou-Shady, M., Friess, H., Zimmermann, A., di Mola, F. F., Guo, X. Z., Baer, H. U., et al. (2000). Connective tissue growth factor in human liver cirrhosis. *Liver, 20*, 296–304.
3. Abreu, J. G., Ketpura, N. I., Reversade, B., & De Robertis, E. M. (2002). Connective-tissue growth factor (CTGF) modulates cell signaling by BMP and TGF-beta. *Nature Cell Biology, 4*, 599–604.
4. Adams, L. A., Bulsara, M., Rossi, E., DeBoer, B., Speers, D., & George, J. (2005). Hepascore:

An accurate validated predictor of liver fibrosis in chronic hepatitis C infection. *Clinical Chemistry, 51*, 1867–1873.

5. Baba, S., Fujii, H., Hirose, T., Yasuchika, K., Azuma, H., Hoppo, T., et al. (2004). Commitment of bone marrow cells to hepatic stellate cells in mouse. *Journal of Hepatology, 40*, 255–260.
6. Beaussier, M., Wendum, D., Schiffer, E., Dumont, S., Rey, C., Lienhart, A., et al. (2007). Prominent contribution of portal mesenchymal cells to liver fibrosis in ischemic and obstructive cholestatic injuries. *Laboratory Investigation, 87*, 292–303.
7. Bedossa, P., Dargère, D., & Paradis, V. (2003). Sampling variability of liver fibrosis in chronic hepatitis C. *Hepatology, 38*, 659–667.
8. Blom, I. E., Goldschmeding, R., & Leask, A. (2002). Gene regulation of connective tissue growth factor: New targets for antifibrotic therapy? *Matrix Biology, 21*, 473–482.
9. Breitkopf, K., Lahme, B., Tag, C. G., & Gressner, A. M. (2001). Expression and matrix deposition of latent transforming growth factor beta binding proteins in normal and fibrotic rat liver and transdifferentiating hepatic stellate cells in culture. *Hepatology, 33*, 387–396.
10. Callewaert, N., Van Vlierberghe, H., Van Hecke, A., Laroy, W., Delanghe, J., & Contreras, R. (2004). Noninvasive diagnosis of liver cirrhosis using DNA sequencer-based total serum protein glycomics. *Nature Medicine, 10*, 429–434.
11. Collazos, J., & Diaz, F. (1994). Role of the measurement of serum procollagen type III N-terminal peptide in the evaluation of liver diseases. *Clinical Chimica Acta, 227*, 37–43.
12. Crookston, K. P., Webb, D. J., Lamarre, J., & Gonias, S. L. (1993). Binding of platelet-derived growth factor-BB and transforming growth factor-beta 1 to alpha 2-macroglobulin in vitro and in vivo: Comparison of receptor-recognized and non-recognized alpha 2-macroglobulin conformations. *Biochemical Journal, 293*(Pt 2), 443–450.
13. Del Castillo, G., Murillo, M. M., Alvarez-Barrientos, A., Bertran, E., Fernández, M., Sánchez, A., et al. (2006). Autocrine production of TGF-beta confers resistance to apoptosis after an epithelial mesenchymal transition process in hepatocytes: Role of EGF receptor ligands. *Experimental Cell Research, 312*, 2860–2871.
14. Flisiak, R., Maxwell, P., Prokopowicz, D., Timms, P. M., & Panasiuk, A. (2002). Plasma tissue inhibitor of metalloproteinases-1 and transforming growth factor beta 1: Possible non-invasive biomarkers of hepatic fibrosis in patients with chronic B and C hepatitis. *Hepato-Gastroenterology, 49*, 1369–1372.
15. Forbes, S. J., Russo, F. P., Rey, V., Burra, P., Rugge, M., Wright, N. A., et al. (2004). A significant proportion of myofibroblasts are of bone marrow origin in human liver fibrosis. *Gastroenterology, 126*, 955–963.
16. Fujii, H., Hirose, T., Oe, S., Yasuchika, K., Azuma, H., Fujikawa, T., et al. (2002). Contribution of bone marrow cells to liver regeneration after partial hepatectomy in mice. *Journal of Hepatology, 36*, 653–659.
17. Gao, Z., McAlister, V. C., & Williams, G. M. (2001). Repopulation of liver endothelium by bone-marrow-derived cells. *Lancet, 357*, 932–933.
18. George, J., & Tsutsumi, M. (2007). siRNA-mediated knockdown of connective tissue growth factor prevents N-nitroso dimethylamine-induced hepatic fibrosis in rats. *Gene Therapy, 14*, 790–803.

19. Grainger, D. J., Mosedale, E. E., & Metcalfe, J. C. (2000). TGF-beta in blood: A complex problem. *Cytokine & Growth Factor Reviews, 11*, 133–145.

20. Gressner, A. M. (1994). Activation of proteoglycan synthesis in injured liver: A brief review of molecular and cellular aspects. *European Journal of Clinical Chemistry and Clinical Biochemistry, 32*, 225–237.

21. Gressner, A. M., & Weiskirchen, R. (2003). The tightrope of therapeutic suppression of active transforming growth factor-beta: High enough to fall deeply? *Journal of Hepatology, 39*, 856–859.

22. Gressner, A. M., & Weiskirchen, R. (2006). Modern pathogenetic concepts of liver fibrosis suggests stellate cells and TGF-beta as major players and therapeutic targets. *Journal of Cellular and Molecular Medicine, 10*, 76–99.

23. Gressner, A. M., Yagmur, E., Lahme, B., Gressner, O., & Stanzel, S. (2006). Connective tissue growth factor in serum as a new candidate test for assessment of hepatic fibrosis. *Clinical Chemistry, 52*, 1815–1817.

24. Gressner, O. A., Beer, N., Jodlowski, A., & Gressner, A. M. (2009). Impact of quality control accepted inter-laboratory variations on calculated Fibrotest/Actitest scores for the non-invasive biochemical assessment of liver fibrosis. *Clinical Chimica Acta, 409*, 90–95.

25. Gressner, O. A., Fang, M., Li, H., Lu, L. G., Gressner, A. M., & Gao, C. F. (2013). Connective tissue growth factor (CTGF/CCN2) in serum is an indicator of fibrogenic progression and malignant transformation in patients with chronic hepatitis B infection. *Clinical Chimica Acta, 421*, 126–131.

26. Gressner, O. A., Lahme, B., Demirci, I., Gressner, A. M., & Weiskirchen, R. (2007). Differential effects of TGF-beta on connective tissue growth factor (CTGF/CCN2) expression in hepatic stellate cells and hepatocytes. *Journal of Hepatology, 47*, 699–710.

27. Higashiyama, R., Inagaki, Y., Hong, Y. Y., Kushida, M., Nakao, S., Niioka, M., et al. (2007). Bone marrow-derived cells express matrix metalloproteinases and contribute to regression of liver fibrosis in mice. *Hepatology, 45*, 213–222.

28. Hyytiäinen, M., Penttinen, C., & Keski-Oja, J. (2004). Latent TGF-beta binding proteins: Extracellular matrix association and roles in TGFbeta activation. *Critical Reviews in Clinical Laboratory Sciences, 41*, 233–264.

29. Ishii, G., Sangai, T., Sugiyama, K., Ito, T., Hasebe, T., Endoh, Y., et al. (2005). In vivo characterization of bone marrow-derived fibroblasts recruited into fibrotic lesions. *Stem Cells, 23*, 699–706.

30. Kaimori, A., Potter, J., Kaimori, J. Y., Wang, C., Mezey, E., & Koteish, A. (2007). Transforming growth factor-beta1 induces an epithelial-to-mesenchymal transition state in mouse hepatocytes in vitro. *Journal of Biological Chemistry, 282*, 22089–22101.

31. Kalluri, R., & Neilson, E. G. (2003). Epithelial-mesenchymal transition and its implications for fibrosis. *Journal of Clinical Investigation, 112*, 1776–1784.

32. Karasek, M. A. (2007). Does transformation of microvascular endothelial cells into myofibroblasts play a key role in the etiology and pathology of fibrotic disease? *Medical Hypotheses, 68*, 650–655.

33. Kinnman, N., Francoz, C., Barbu, V., Wendum, D., Rey, C., Hultcrantz, R., et al. (2003). The myofibroblastic conversion of peribiliary fibro genic cells distinct from hepatic stellate

cells is stimulated by platelet-derived growth factor during liver fibrogenesis. *Laboratory Investigation, 83*, 163–173.

34. Kinoshita, K., Iimuro, Y., Otogawa, K., Saika, S., Inagaki, Y., Nakajima, Y., et al. (2007). Adenovirus-mediated expression of BMP-7 suppresses the development of liver fibrosis in rats. *Gut, 56*, 706–714.

35. Kisseleva, T., Uchinami, H., Feirt, N., Quintana-Bustamante, O., Segovia, J. C., Schwabe, R. F., et al. (2006). Bone marrow-derived fibrocytes participate in pathogenesis of liver fibrosis. *Journal of Hepatology, 45*, 429–438.

36. Kovalenko, E., Tacke, F., Gressner, O. A., Zimmermann, H. W., Lahme, B., Janetzko, A., et al. (2009). Validation of connective tissue growth factor (CTGF/CCN2) and its gene polymorphisms as noninvasive biomarkers for the assessment of liver fibrosis. *Journal of Viral Hepatitis, 16*, 612–620.

37. Kropf, J., Gressner, A. M., & Tittor, W. (1991). Logistic-regression model for assessing portal hypertension by measuring hyaluronic acid (hyaluronan) and laminin in serum. *Clinical Chemistry, 37*, 30–35.

38. Kubota, A., Okamura, S., Omori, F., Shimoda, K., Otsuka, T., Ishibashi, H., et al. (1995). High serum levels of granulocyte macrophage colony-stimulating factor in patients with liver cirrhosis and granulocytopenia. *Clinical Laboratory Haematology, 17*, 61–63.

39. Kuhn, J., Prante, C., Schön, S., Götting, C., & Kleesiek, K. (2006). Measurement of fibrosis marker xylosyltransferase I activity by HPLC electrospray ionization tandem mass spectrometry. *Clinical Chemistry, 52*, 2243–2249.

40. Leask, A., & Abraham, D. J. (2006). All in the CCN family: Essential matricellular signaling modulators emerge from the bunker. *Journal of Cell Science, 119*, 4803–4810.

41. Lee, J. M., Dedhar, S., Kalluri, R., & Thompson, E. W. (2006). The epithelial-mesenchymal transition: New insights in signaling, development, and disease. *Journal of Cell Biology, 172*, 973–981.

42. Li, G., Xie, Q., Shi, Y., Li, D., Zhang, M., Jiang, S., et al. (2006). Inhibition of connective tissue growth factor by siRNA prevents liver fibrosis in rats. *Journal of Gene Medicine, 8*, 889–900.

43. Liu, D. Y. (2007). Anti-CTGF (CCN2) human antibody therapy: FG-3019 prevents and reverses renal and cardiovascular pathologies in animal models of diabetic complications. *Keystone Symposium on Molecular and Cellular Biology e Abstract Book* (33).

44. Liu, X., Hu, H., & Yin, J. Q. (2006). Therapeutic strategies against TGF-beta signaling pathway in hepatic fibrosis. *Liver International, 26*, 8–22.

45. Lydatakis, H., Hager, I. P., Kostadelou, E., Mpousmpoulas, S., Pappas, S., & Diamantis, I. (2006). Non-invasive markers to predict liver fibrosis in non-alcoholic fatty liver disease. *Liver International, 26*, 864–871.

46. Marra, F. (1999). Hepatic stellate cells and the regulation of liver inflammation. *Journal of Hepatology, 31*, 1120–1130.

47. Marra, F., DeFranco, R., Grappone, C., Milani, S., Pastacaldi, S., Pinzani, M., et al. (1998). Increased expression of monocyte chemotactic protein-1 during active hepatic fibrogenesis: Correlation with monocyte infiltration. *American Journal of Pathology, 152*, 423–430.

48. Marra, F., Valente, A. J., Pinzani, M., & Abboud, H. E. (1993). Cultured human liver fat-storing cells produce monocyte chemotactic protein-1. Regulation by proinflammatory cytokines. *Journal of Clinical Investigation, 92*, 1674–1680.

49. Mehal, W. Z., & Schuppan, D. (2015). Antifibrotic therapies in the liver. *Seminars in Liver Disease, 35*, 184–198.

50. Neilson, E. G. (2005). Setting a trap for tissue fibrosis. *Nature Medicine, 11*, 373–374.

51. Paradis, V., Dargère, D., Vidaud, M., De Gouville, A. C., Huet, S. Martinez, V., et al. (1999). Expression of connective tissue growth factor in experimental rat and human liver fibrosis. *Hepatology, 30*, 968–976.

52. Parkes, J., Guha, I. N., Roderick, P., & Rosenberg, W. (2006). Performance of serum marker panels for liver fibrosis in chronic hepatitis C. *Journal of Hepatology, 44*, 462–474.

53. Patel, K., Bedossa, P., & Castera, L. (2015). Diagnosis of liver fibrosis: Present and future. *Seminars in Liver Disease, 35*, 166–183.

54. Pilling, D., Buckley, C. D., Salmon, M., & Gomer, R. H. (2003). Inhibition of fibrocyte differentiation by serum amyloid P. *Journal of Immunology, 171*, 5537–5546.

55. Pilling, D., Buckley, C. D., Salmon, M., & Gomer, R. H. (2007). *Keystone Symposia on Molecular and Cellular Biology e Abstract Book.*

56. Pinzani, M., Abboud, H. E., Gesualdo, L., & Abboud, S. L. (1992). Regulation of macrophage colony-stimulating factor in liver fat-storing cells by peptide growth factors. *American Journal of Physiology, 262*, C876–C881.

57. Poon, T. C., Hui, A. Y., Chan, H. L., Ang, I. L., Chow, S. M., Wong, N., et al. (2005). Prediction of liver fibrosis and cirrhosis in chronic hepatitis B infection by serum proteomic fingerprinting: A pilot study. *Clinical Chemistry, 51*, 328–335.

58. Poynard, T., Imbert-Bismut, F., Munteanu, M., Messous, D., Myers, R. P., Thabut, D., et al. (2004). Overview of the diagnostic value of biochemical markers of liver fibrosis (FibroTest, HCV FibroSure) and necrosis (ActiTest) in patients with chronic hepatitis C. *Comparative Hepatology, 3*, 8.

59. Poynard, T., Ratziu, V., Naveau, S., Thabut, D., Charlotte, F., Messous, D., et al. (2005). The diagnostic value of biomarkers (SteatoTest) for the prediction of liver steatosis. *Comparative Hepatology, 4*, 10.

60. Quan, T. E., Cowper, S. E., & Bucala, R. (2006). The role of circulating fibrocytes in fibrosis. *Current Rheumatology Reports, 8*, 145–150.

61. Quan, T. E., Cowper, S., Wu, S. P., Bockenstedt, L. K., & Bucala, R. (2004). Circulating fibrocytes: Collagen-secreting cells of the peripheral blood. *International Journal of Biochemistry & Cell Biology, 36*, 598–606.

62. Rachfal, A. W., & Brigstock, D. R. (2003). Connective tissue growth factor (CTGF/CCN2) in hepatic fibrosis. *Hepatology Research, 26*, 1–9.

63. Ramadori, G., & Saile, B. (2004). Portal tract fibrogenesis in the liver. *Laboratory Investigation, 84*, 153–159.

64. Robertson, H., Kirby, J. A., Yip, W. W., Jones, D. E., & Burt, A. D. (2007). Biliary epithelial-mesenchymal transition in post transplantation recurrence of primary biliary cirrhosis. *Hepatology, 45*, 977–981.

65. Romagnani, P., Lasagni, L., & Romagnani, S. (2006). Peripheral blood as a source of stem cells for regenerative medicine. *Expert Opinion on Biological Therapy, 6*, 193–202.

66. Rosenberg, W. M., Voelker, M., Thiel, R., Becka, M., Burt, A., Schuppan, D., et al. (2004). Serum markers detect the presence of liver fibrosis: A cohort study. *Gastroenterology, 127*, 1704–1713.

67. Rosenthal-Allieri, M. A., Peritore, M. L., Tran, A., Halfon, P., Benzaken, S., & Bernard, A. (2005). Analytical variability of the Fibrotest proteins. *Clinical Biochemistry, 38*, 473–478.

68. Ruhnke, M., Nussler, A. K., Ungefroren, H., Hengstler, J. G., Kremer, B., Hoeckh, W., et al. (2005a). Human monocyte-derived neohepatocytes: A promising alternative to primary human hepatocytes for autologous cell therapy. *Transplantation, 79*, 1097–1103.

69. Ruhnke, M., Ungefroren, H., Nussler, A., Martin, F., Brulport, M., Schormann, W., et al. (2005b). Differentiation of in vitro-modified human peripheral blood monocytes into hepatocyte-like and pancreatic islet-like cells. *Gastroenterology, 128*, 1774–1786.

70. Russo, F. P., Alison, M. R., Bigger, B. W., Amofah, E., Florou, A., Amin, F., et al. (2006). The bone marrow functionally contributes to liver fibrosis. *Gastroenterology, 130*, 1807–1821.

71. Rygiel, K. A., Robertson, H., Marshall, H. L., Pekalski, M., Zhao, L., Booth, T. A., et al. (2008). Epithelial-mesenchymal transition contributes to portal tract fibrogenesis during human chronic liver disease. *Laboratory Investigation, 88*, 112–123.

72. Saito, M., Yano, Y., Hirano, H., Momose, K., Yoshida, M., & Azuma, T. (2015). Serum NX-DCP as a new noninvasive model to predict significant liver fibrosis in chronic hepatitis C. *Hepatitis Monthly, 15*, e22978.

73. Saitou, Y., Shiraki, K., Yamanaka, Y., Yamaguchi, Y., Kawakita, T., Yamamoto, N., et al. (2005). Noninvasive estimation of liver fibrosis and response to interferon therapy by a serum fibrogenesis marker, YKL-40, in patients with HCV-associated liver disease. *World Journal of Gastroenterology, 11*, 476–481.

74. Sebastiani, G., Vario, A., Guido, M., Noventa, F., Plebani, M., Pistis, R., et al. (2006). Stepwise combination algorithms of non-invasive markers to diagnose significant fibrosis in chronic hepatitis C. *Journal of Hepatology, 44*, 686–693.

75. Siemens. (2014). ADVIA Centaur Enhanced Liver Fibrosis (ELF) Test Specifications. Siemens Healthcare Diagnostics Inc. Sprenger, H., Kaufmann, A., Garn, H., Lahme, B., Gemsa, D., & Gressner, A. M. (1997). Induction of neutrophil-attracting chemokines in transforming rat hepatic stellate cells. *Gastroenterology, 113*, 277–285.

76. Sugimoto, H., Yang, C., LeBleu, V. S., Soubasakos, M. A., Giraldo, M., Zeisberg, M., et al. (2007). BMP-7 functions as a novel hormone to facilitate liver regeneration. *FASEB Journal, 21*, 256–264.

77. Torok, N. J., Dranoff, J. A., Schuppan, D., & Friedman, S. L. (2015). Strategies and endpoints of antifibrotic drug trials: Summary and recommendations from the AASLD emerging trends conference, Chicago. *Hepatology, 62*, 627–634.

78. Toyoda, H., Kumada, T., Osaki, Y., Tada, T., Kaneoka, Y., & Maeda, A. (2012). Novel method to measure serum levels of des-gamma-carboxy prothrombin for hepatocellular carcinoma in patients taking warfarin: A preliminary report. *Cancer Science, 24*, 52–55.

79. Tran, A., Benzaken, S., Saint-Paul, M. C., Guzman-Granier, E., Hastier, P., Pradier, C., et al. (2000). Chondrex (YKL-40), a potential new serum fibrosis marker in patients with alcoholic liver disease. *European Journal of Gastroenterology & Hepatology, 12*, 989–993.

80. Vega, S., Morales, A. V., Ocaña, O. H., Valdés, F., Fabregat, I., & Nieto, M. A. (2004). Snail blocks the cell cycle and confers resistance to cell death. *Genes & Development, 18*, 1131–1143.

81. Wai, C. T., Greenson, J. K., Fontana, R. J., Kalbfleisch, J. D., Marrero, J. A., Conjeevaram, H. S., et al. (2003). A simple noninvasive index can predict both significant fibrosis and cirrhosis in patients with chronic hepatitis C. *Hepatology, 38*, 518–526.

82. Wang, S., & Hirschberg, R. (2004). Bone morphogenetic protein-7 signals opposing transforming growth factor beta in mesangial cells. *Journal of Biological Chemistry, 279*, 23200–23206.

83. Yang, Y., Pan, X., Lei, W., Wang, J., Shi, J., Li, F., et al. (2006). Regulation of transforming growth factor-beta 1-induced apoptosis and epithelial-to-mesenchymal transition by protein kinase A and signal transducers and activators of transcription 3. *Cancer Research, 66*, 8617–8624.

84. Yannaki, E., Athanasiou, E., Xagorari, A., Constantinou, V., Batsis, I., Kaloyannidis, P., et al. (2005). G-CSF-primed hematopoietic stem cells or G-CSF per se accelerate recovery and improve survival after liver injury, predominantly by promoting endogenous repair programs. *Experimental Hematology, 33*, 108–119.

85. Zeisberg, M. (2006). Bone morphogenic protein-7 and the kidney: Current concepts and open questions. *Nephrology Dialysis Transplantation, 21*, 568–573.

86. Zeisberg, M., & Shah, A. A. (2005). Bone morphogenic protein-7 induces mesenchymal to epithelial transition in adult renal fibroblasts and facilitates regeneration of injured kidney. *Journal of Biological Chemistry, 280*, 8094–8100.

87. Zeisberg, M., Hanai, J., Sugimoto, H., Mammoto, T., Charytan, D., Strutz, F., et al. (2003). BMP-7 counteracts TGF-beta1-induced epithelial-to-mesenchymal transition and reverses chronic renal injury. *Nature Medicine, 9*, 964–968.

Chapter 10

N-ACETYLCYSTEINE AND RESVERATROL AS EFFECTIVE TREATMENTS FOR LIVER DISEASE

Contents

Introduction

Steatosis, steatohepatitis, and in more severe cases, fibrosis and cirrhosis, are among the complex spectrum of stages that comprise liver disease (Massey & Arteel, 2012). Changes in the extracellular matrix's composition and the persistence of parenchyma cell necrosis are hallmarks of the progression of liver fibrosis (ECM). Hepatic stellate cell (HSC) and Kupffer cell activation is a major mechanism that drives this scarring process at the cellular level. Growth factors, cytokines, chemokines, changes in the composition of the extracellular matrix, and molecules linked to oxidative stress also play a pathological role at the molecular level (Friedman, 2000; Friedman et al., 2000). A potent set of enzymes and antioxidant molecules found in the liver aid in preventing the harm caused by various etiological agents. Occasionally, though, these defenses might not be strong enough to restore the redox status to normal during liver damage (Seifried et al., 2007). Because of this, research into and assessment of different exogenous antioxidants is becoming more and more popular. These antioxidants aid in restoring the liver's lost homeostasis following illness and reducing the harm caused by free radical insults. Resveratrol and N-acetylcysteine (NAC) are two of the most effective antioxidants that are used to treat hepatic conditions.

Orientation and Directional Terms

Term	Definition	Illustration
Nonalcoholic fatty liver disease (NAFLD)	Nonalcoholic fatty liver disease (NAFLD) is a condition in which fat builds up in your liver. Nonalcoholic fatty liver (NAFL) and nonalcoholic steatohepatitis (NASH) are types of NAFLD. If you have NASH, you have inflammation and liver damage, along with fat in your liver.	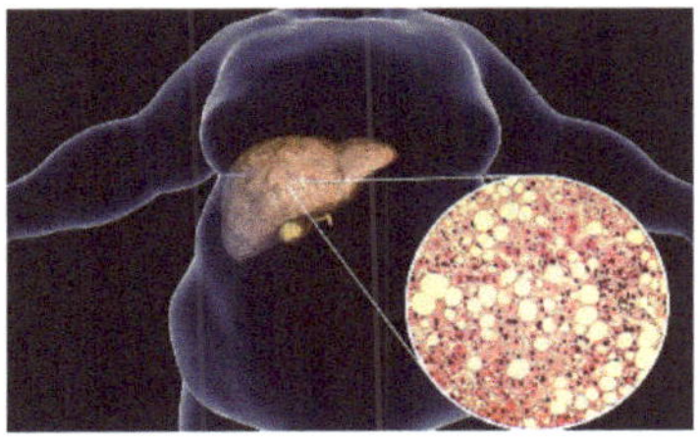
Pentose phosphate pathway (PPP)	Pentose phosphate pathway is a metabolic pathway parallel to glycolysis. It generates NADPH and pentoses (5-carbon sugars) as well as ribose 5-phosphate, a precursor for the synthesis of nucleotides.	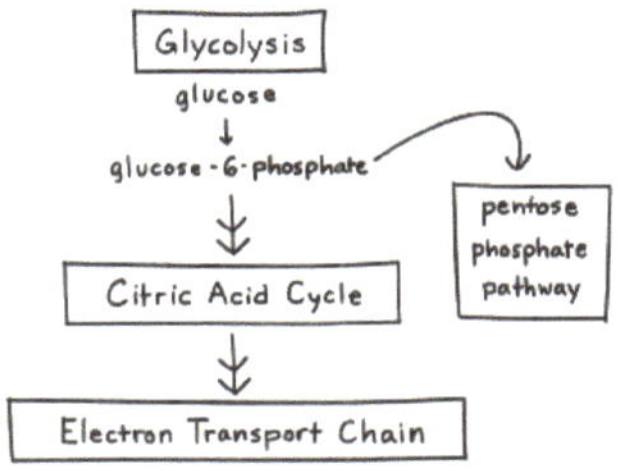
Ursodeoxycholic acid (UDCA)	Ursodeoxycholic acid, also known as ursodiol, is a secondary bile acid, produced in humans and most other species from metabolism by intestinal bacteria. It is synthesized in the liver in some species, and was first identified in bile of bears of genus Ursus, from which its name derived.	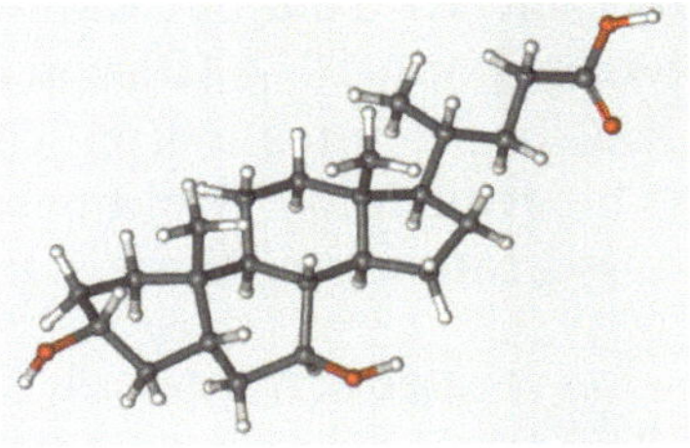
Cystic fibrosis (CF)	Cystic fibrosis affects the cells that produce mucus, sweat and digestive juices. It causes these fluids to become thick and sticky. They then plug up tubes, ducts and passageways.	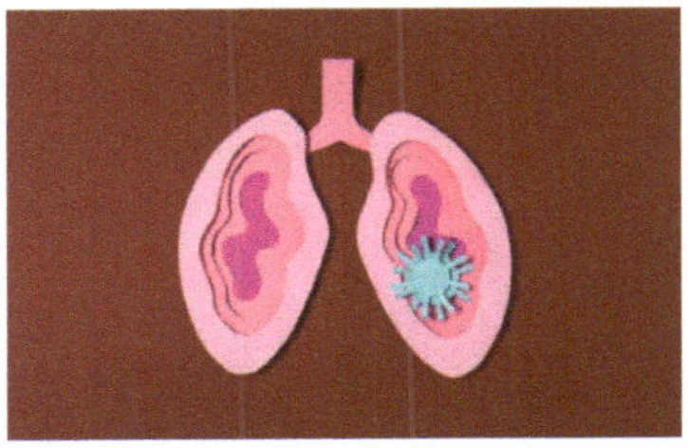
CF-related liver disease (CFLD)	CF-related liver disease (CFLD) is a broad term that has been used to define a spectrum of liver involvement in CF. The recognition of CFLD is increasing due to early diagnosis of CF, improved life expectancy, and greater awareness among clinicians, which leads to screening and monitoring for CFLD.	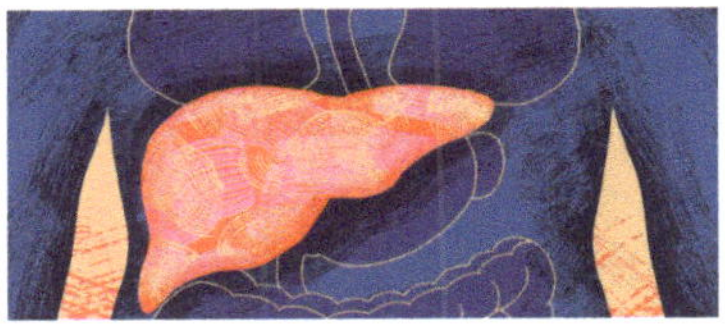

10.1. Overview of NAC and Resveratrol: Chemical Properties and Pharmacokinetic Aspects

NAC, which is the acetylated precursor of L-cysteine and reduced glutathione (GSH), has been used in clinical settings for over three decades. Its main purposes have been as a mucolytic agent for chronic respiratory problems, and as an antidote for acetaminophen overdose-induced hepatotoxicity (Lancaster et al., 2015; Chughlay et al., 2016). Research has demonstrated that NAC is a potent antioxidant and may be used as a therapeutic agent to treat diseases marked by the production of free radicals, such as cancer, heart disease, nephropathy, polycystic ovary, influenza, acute renal failure, and pulmonary fibrosis (Millea, 2009). NAC is a thiol compound with the chemical formula $C_5H_9NO_3S$ and a molecular weight of 163.2 g/mol. These are its chemical and pharmacokinetic characteristics. Oral administration of NAC results in its rapid absorption; first-pass metabolism occurs in the small intestine and liver cells, incorporating NAC into protein peptide chains and forming a variety of metabolites, such as a stable form of L-cysteine, which is the rate-limiting factor for GSH synthesis (Dodd et al., 2008). A very small proportion of intact NAC molecules reach plasma and then tissue. After oral treatment, only 3% of radioactively labeled NAC is eliminated in the feces, suggesting that NAC and its metabolites are almost entirely absorbed. After oral administration, the plasma usually reaches its peak concentration in less than an hour (Holdiness, 1991). Free NAC has a plasma half-life estimated to be about 2.15 h and virtually no NAC is detectable 10–12 h post-administration. The oral bioavailability of intact NAC was estimated to be between 4 and 10 % (Olsson et al., 1988). However, disulfide linking to proteins, and deacetylation of NAC in the intestinal mucosa and lumen are probably the main factors responsible for its low oral bioavailability (Holdiness, 1991). The volume of distribution ranges from 0.33 to 0.47 L/kg and its protein binding is significant, reaching 50% in approximately 4 h after the administration.

Resveratrol (trans-3, 4,′ 5-trihydroxystilbene) is a polyphenol found in grapes, peanuts, and mulberries. As a natural defense mechanism in plants, resveratrol is produced in response to UV irradiation, fungi, rhizobacteria, etc. (Jeandet et al., 2012). Resveratrol has been studied in a wide variety of health areas since the French Paradox was suggested: the French population has a low incidence of cardiovascular diseases although they consume a diet rich in saturated fats (Renaud & De Lorgeril, 1992).

Resveratrol has two isomers: cis- and trans-isomer. However, the trans-isomer appears to be more stable and more prevalent than the cis-isomer (Chen et al., 2007). The low water solubility of resveratrol has an impact on its bioavailability since it absorbs very little when taken orally. After oral administration, resveratrol is absorbed by passive diffusion and passes through a carrier in liver cells, allowing it to accumulate in the liver (Lancon et al., 2004; Bertelli et al., 1998). In studies with humans, resveratrol is primarily metabolized into sulfate- and glucuronide-resveratrol, showing two maximum peaks, with the second peak suggesting enterohepatic recirculation leading to a longer half-life. Absorption is delayed when taken with food. Peak plasma concentrations in healthy volunteers occur 0.8–1.5 hours after dosing in multiple dose regimens. Due to its beneficial effects and instability, there is a growing interest in developing formulations to improve its properties and bioavailability, such as dendrimer nanostructures. Additionally, efforts are being made to create new analogs of resveratrol for optimization. The chemical structures of both drugs can be seen in Figure 10.1.

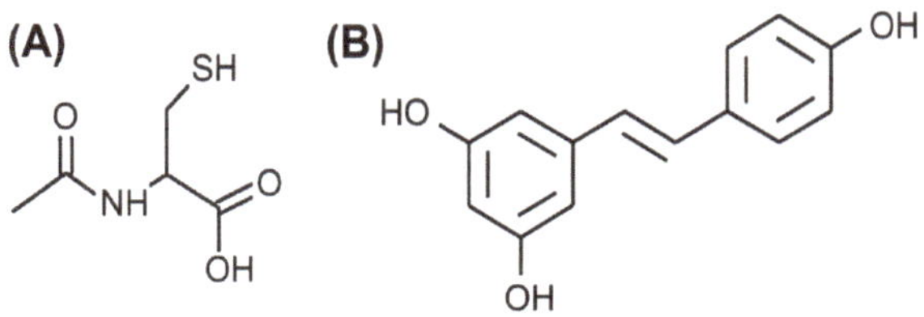

Figure 10.1. *Chemical structures of (A) NAC and (B) Resveratrol.*

Source. E. Cha´vez, et al., 2017, N-Acetylcysteine and Resveratrol Effective Treatments for Liver Disease, http://dx.doi.org/10.1016/B978-0-12-804274-8.00052-7.

10.2. Pharmacodynamic Properties and Clinical Applications

It has been demonstrated that taking NAC supplements raises levels of GSH, the body's main antioxidant (Waring, 2012). The amino acids glutamate, glycine, and cysteine are components of GSH; the latter has the lowest intracellular concentration.

By providing the cysteine required to restore GSH levels, NAC administration can either prevent or reverse GSH depletion, as de novo synthesis is crucial in combating the process of oxidative damage. NAC can lessen the harmful effects of a number of medications. For example, statins, which are the main medications used to lower cholesterol and prevent obstructive cardiovascular events, can cause myopathy and hepatotoxicity, the latter of which is indicated by an increase in plasma transaminases (Kromer and Moosmann, 2009). The exact mechanism underlying this drug's hepatotoxicity is unknown. In a study conducted by Abdoli in 2014, the protective effect of NAC against the cytotoxicity induced by statins in freshly isolated rat hepatocytes was evaluated. NAC treatment reduced reactive oxygen species (ROS) formation, prevented lipid peroxidation assessed by the levels of malondialdehyde (MDA), and improved cell viability and mitochondrial membrane potential; all these changes induced by statins consumption. A possible mechanism by which NAC enhanced mitochondrial integrity is illustrated in Figure 10.2 (Abdoli et al., 2014).

N-acetylcysteine (NAC) is most well-known for its use in treating liver damage caused by acetaminophen (APAP) overdose. When a large amount of acetaminophen is consumed, it can deplete levels of glutathione (GSH). NAC acts as an antidote to APAP intoxication by replenishing intracellular GSH. Additionally, NAC has other important clinical applications such as aiding in recovery from traumatic brain injuries, treating cerebral ischemia, and managing cerebrovascular vasospasm (Bavarsad Shahripour et al., 2014). Moreover, it is an excellent drug to treat idiopathic pulmonary fibrosis, influenza, and polycystic ovary syndrome (Millea, 2009).

Because of the sulfhydryl group in its chemical structure, NAC not only helps to promote the synthesis of GSH but also has an antioxidant effect. As a result, it is an effective scavenger of free radicals and can also lower hydrogen peroxide and hydroxyl radicals (Acharya & Lau-Cam, 2010; Dhouib et al., 2016).

Calorie restriction, also referred to as calorie intake reduction, triggers mechanisms that shield organisms from stress and increase lifespan in various species. Sirtuin 1 (SIRT1) is identified in multiple studies as a key player in the effects of calorie restriction.

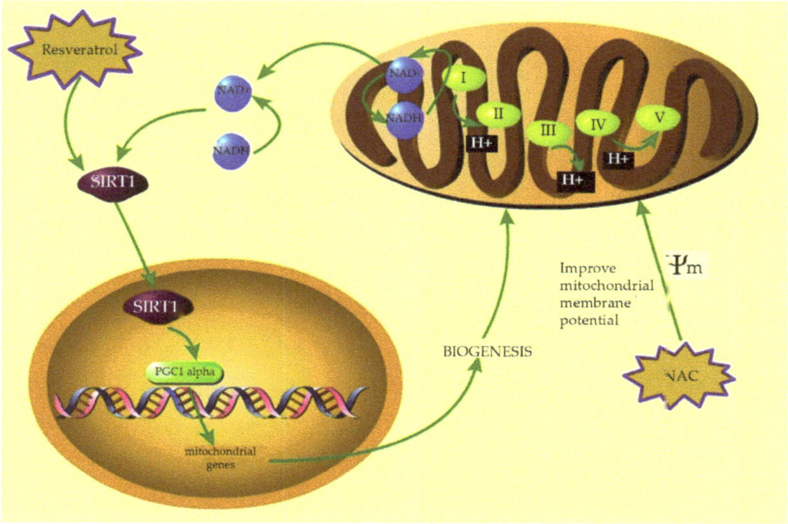

Figure 10.2. *Beneficial effects of NAC and resveratrol in the mitochondrial function and integrity.*

Source: E. Cha´vez, et al., 2017, N-Acetylcysteine and Resveratrol Effective Treatments for Liver Disease, http://dx.doi.org/10.1016/B978-0-12-804274-8.00052-7.

This indicates that resveratrol has been shown to target the same cell receptors as CR to produce positive effects. Additionally, it has been discovered that resveratrol is a strong activator of SIRT1, which can increase the lifespan of certain species (Howitz et al., 2003; Wood et al., 2004; Valenzano et al., 2006).

Additionally, resveratrol inhibits the transcription and activity of cyclooxygenase-2 (COX-2), CYP1A1, and the transcription factor NF-kB. Furthermore, by inhibiting COX and Interleukin-1b (IL-1b), resveratrol has anti-inflammatory effects (Subbaramaiah et al., 1998; Piver et al., 2001; Storz et al., 2004; Chavez et al., 2008).

Pharmacologically several biological actions have been attributed to resveratrol, some of which are the following (Park & Pezzuto, 2015):

- • *Anticarcinogenic:* There are several studies demonstrating its beneficial effect on different kinds of cancer.
- • *Anti-Inflammatory:* Resveratrol treatment in rodents downregulates proinflammatory mediators such as (interleukin) IL-1b, IL-6, tumor necrosis factor-a (TNF-a), interferon-g (IFN-g), NF-kB, COX-2, etc.
- • *Cardioprotective:* Resveratrol has protective effects on restenosis, as antihypertensive, against myocardial ischemia/infarction and atherosclerosis among other vascular effects.
- • *Antidiabetic:* Resveratrol ameliorates diabetic complications with normalized biomarkers in animal models.

The main clinical applications and molecular targets of NAC and resveratrol can be seen in Table 10.1.

Table 10.1. *Molecular Targets and Principal Clinical Applications of NAC and Resveratrol*

Drug	Molecular Target	Clinical Applications
NAC	• inhibits NF-κB activation • decreases the expression of pro inflammatory and pro fibrotic cytokines (IL-2, IL-6, TNF-α, TGF-β) • modulates the expression of iNOS • stimulates Nrf2/HO-1 signal pathway • stimulates GSH synthesis	• antidote for acetaminophen overdose • recovery of traumatic brain injury, cerebral isquemia and cerebrovascular vasospasm • idiopathic pulmonary fibrosis treatment • influenza treatment • polycystic ovary syndrome
Resveratrol	• inhibits COX 2 transcription • inhibits NF-κB activation • decreases the expression of pro fibrotic cytokines (TGF-β). • stimulates Nrf2 signal pathway • inhibits SREBP-1c expression • stimulates PPARγ expression	• Anticarcinogenic • Anti-inflammatory • Cardioprotective • Antidiabetic

Source: E. Cha´vez, et al., 2017, N-Acetylcysteine and Resveratrol Effective Treatments for Liver Disease, http://dx.doi.org/10.1016/B978-0-12-804274-8.00052-7.

10.3. Effects of NAC and Resveratrol in Liver Diseases

Extensive research has been conducted worldwide on the beneficial impact of antioxidant agents in treating various liver diseases. Numerous theories have been proposed regarding how NAC and resveratrol work to combat liver damage, as depicted in Figure 10.3.

The following paragraphs describe the effects and mechanisms used by NAC and resveratrol in several processes of liver damage.

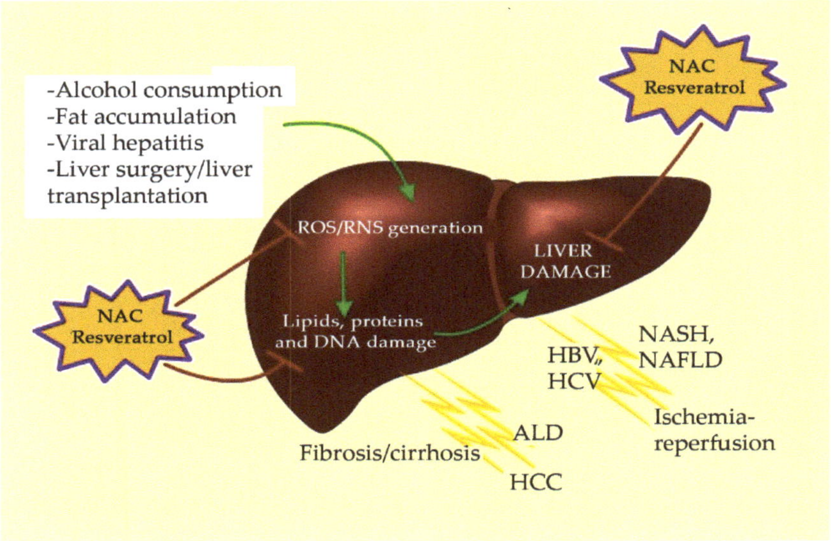

Figure 10.3. *Main action mechanisms of NAC and resveratrol against liver damage.*

Source: E. Cha´vez, et al., 2017, N-Acetylcysteine and Resveratrol Effective Treatments for Liver Disease, http://dx.doi.org/10.1016/B978-0-12-804274-8.00052-7

10.3.1. Effect of NAC and Resveratrol on Liver Fibrosis

Excessive extracellular matrix deposition causes irreversible tissue damage and failure or disruption of normal liver function in liver fibrosis, a nonphysiological scarring process (Richter et al., 2015). Evidence exists to suggest that oxidative stress plays a significant part in this process. A number of growth factors and chemokines are crucial for the development of fibrosis. A major mediator of the fibrotic process, transforming growth factor-b (TGF-b) is essential for liver fibrogenesis. Numerous investigations revealed that distinct signaling pathways connect the development of liver fibrosis to both the generation of ROS and the expression of TGF-b (Galicia-Moreno et al., 2009, 2012); in addition, this cytokine may also deplete the liver GSH content through g-glutamylcysteine synthetase inhibition (Galicia-Moreno et al., 2009, 2012).

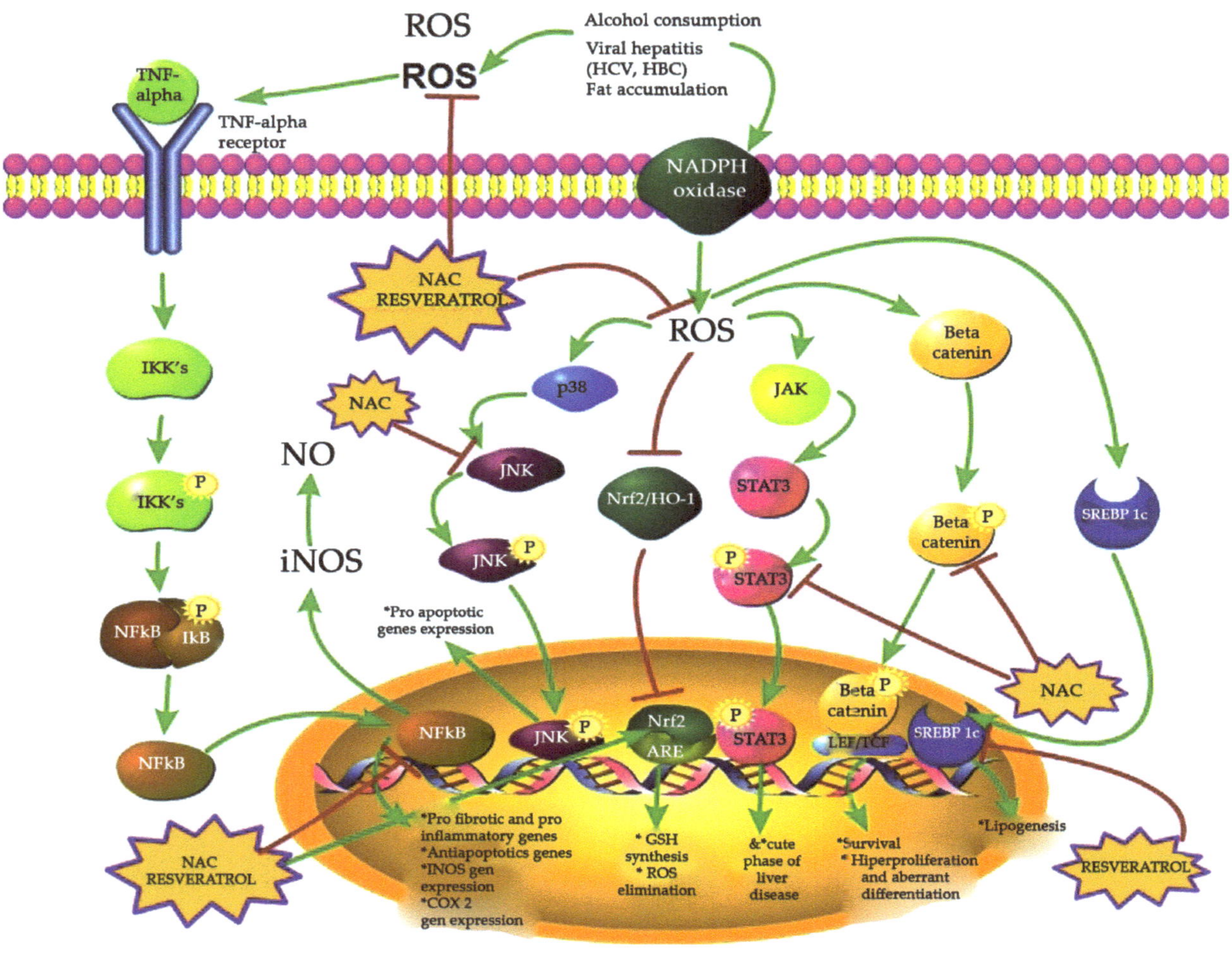

Figure 10.4. *Molecular targets and signal pathways that participate in the antioxidant response exerted by NAC and resveratrol during liver damage.*

Source: E. Cha´vez, et al., 2017, N-Acetylcysteine and Resveratrol Effective Treatments for Liver Disease, http://dx.doi.org/10.1016/B978-0-12-804274-8.00052-7.

Different ROS-induced reactions can be seen during liver fibrosis. For example, liver damage brought on by bile duct ligation (BDL) and carbon tetrachloride (CCl4) causes an increase in hydroxyproline content and a depletion of GSH levels. These responses have also been seen in liver damage brought on by thioacetamide (TAA). It was found that the administration of TAA also inhibits the activity of GSH peroxidase and catalase; the administration of NAC reversed all of these altered parameters brought on by CCl4, BDL, or TAA (Galicia-Moreno et al., 2009, 2012; Nissar et al., 2013).

Lastly, data shows that NAC protected rats from CCl4-induced liver damage by upregulating heme oxygenase-1 and activating the nuclear factor erythroid 2-related factor 2 (Nrf2) pathway; both molecules are associated with the defense against oxidative damage, indicating that NAC is a medication with multiple molecular mechanisms (Cai et al., 2015). Figure 10.4 provides an illustration of these mechanisms.

Resveratrol's antifibrotic qualities have been proven in an experimental model of liver fibrosis brought on by CCl4. Rats given CCl4 show increased TGF-b expression and nuclear localization of NF-kB; remarkably, resveratrol reverses these changes and the buildup of collagen fibers in the liver (Chavez et al., 2008). Resveratrol is known to prevent NF-kB from being activated (Tsai et al., 1999), which as a result reduces the expression of TGF-b.

Since the TGF-b pathway is crucial for the activation of HSC, inhibiting it may help to explain, at least in part, why resveratrol has an antifibrotic effect. When HSC transdifferentiate from a quiescent to a proliferative myofibroblast, these cells produce a lot of extracellular matrix (ECM), which causes liver fibrosis and cirrhosis (Svegliati-Baroni et al., 2008). Additionally, in a cell culture model of transgenic overexpression of the adipogenic factor peroxisome proliferator activated receptor g (PPARg), resveratrol reduces lipid droplet accumulation, a signal of HSC activation; this effect was attributed to the ability of resveratrol to induce SIRT1 (De Souza et al., 2015). Godichaud et al., (2000) have shown that resveratrol can alter the phenotype of liver myofibroblasts by reducing their proliferation, the expression of type I collagen, a-smooth muscle actin, and matrix metalloproteinase-2. Resveratrol inhibits lipopolysaccharide-stimulated Kupffer cells' production of TNF-a and lowers the level of the cell cycle protein cyclin D1 in HSC (Kawada et al., 1998).

Resveratrol not only has immunomodulatory properties but also acts as an antioxidant by scavenging free radicals with its chemical structure, -OH groups, and electron delocalization (Rivera et al., 2008). It can prevent APAP-induced damage by maintaining GSH levels (Sener et al., 2006). Resveratrol also inhibits CYP activation of APAP, activates SIRT1, and downregulates p53 to promote hepatocyte proliferation (Wang et al., 2015). Additionally, it stimulates Nrf2 transportation, inhibiting free radical generation by binding to antioxidant response elements (Bagul et al., 2012; Zini et al., 1999). In a rat model of secondary biliary cirrhosis, resveratrol administration preserves liver function, reduces oxidative damage and inflammation, and inhibits ductular proliferation, showing potential as an anticholestatic agent (Ara et al., 2005).

10.3.2. Effect of NAC and Resveratrol in Alcoholic Liver Disease

Alcohol is the addictive substance that is most socially acceptable worldwide. However, excessive alcohol consumption is associated with major health and financial issues in many societies (Room et al., 2005). According to Gao and Bataller (2011), there are several stages of alcoholic liver disease, such as steatosis, steatohepatitis, and in more extreme situations, fibrosis, cirrhosis, and hepatocellular carcinoma (HCC). When ethanol is consumed, several pathways are triggered which result in an excess of reactive oxygen species. Oxidative stress is the result of such massive production frequently exceeding the ability of the endogenous antioxidant defenses to counteract the generated damage (Arteel, 2003; Galicia-Moreno & Gutierrez-Reyes, 2014).

The emergence of free radical adducts, increased lipid peroxidation, and decreased antioxidant status have all been demonstrated to be correlated with the damage's progression. In liver damage induced by ethanol administration to rats, Ronis et al., (2005) observed that ethanol consumption resulted in steatosis, inflammatory infiltrates, accumulation of MDA, and a decreased antioxidant capacity. When NAC was coadministered with ethanol, the cytosolic antioxidant capacity increased and the ethanol-induced lipid peroxidation was inhibited. Additionally, NAC prevented significant loss of hepatic GSH content and decreased ethanol-induced ALT release and inflammation. NAC treatment decreased the severity of damage due to decreased expression of inflammatory mediators and ceramide accumulation in another study where adult rats were given alcohol to induce steatohepatitis. It also increased the expression of IGF-1 and 2 receptors in the liver, improving hepatic insulin sensibility (Setshedi et al., 2011). Given that the activation of HSC by oxidative stress is a significant factor in the etiopathogenesis of liver cirrhosis, Caro et al., (2014) showed that NAC was useful in suppressing oxidative stress in the liver and promoting mitochondrial biogenesis following a prolonged ethanol diet; this finding indicated that oxidative stress is a trigger for mitochondrial biogenesis. GSH depletion is one of the characteristics of ALD; consequently, several studies have shown that the toxic effects of alcohol consumption can be mitigated or prevented by administering GSH precursor agents, such as NAC, which improve GSH synthesis and shield hepatocytes from oxidative stress damage (Setshedi et al., 2011).

The development of alcoholic hepatitis (AH) is a serious complication among heavy drinkers with liver disease. Clinical studies that examined the effectiveness of NAC in patients with AH took into consideration the fact that heavy alcohol consumption results in oxidative stress and GSH depletion. An investigation conducted by Moreno et al., (2010) found that giving alcoholic patients 100 mg of NAC per kilogram of body weight improved their survival rates, liver dysfunction metrics, and infection rates.

Beneficial characteristics of resveratrol, similar to those seen in experimental models of ethanol administration, have been shown with regard to its effects on patients. Resveratrol primarily prevents alcohol-induced fatty liver by upregulating bile acid synthesis and unsaturated fatty acid elongation genes, which ethanol downregulates (Yao et al., 2014). It's interesting to note that in mice given alcohol, resveratrol increases M2 Kupffer cells polarization and M1 Kupffer cells apoptosis; this effect confers resistance to hepatocyte steatosis and apoptosis, as seen in individuals who drink alcohol but have low hepatic steatosis and high M2 gene expression (Wan et al., 2014). Additionally, resveratrol decreases lipid peroxidation and increases the activity of antioxidant enzymes such as catalase, GSH peroxidase, and superoxide dismutase, which are decreased in rats given ethanol (Kasdallah-Grissa et al., 2007).

10.3.3. Effect of NAC and Resveratrol in Nonalcoholic Fatty Liver Disease and Nonalcoholic Steatohepatitis

One of the most common types of chronic liver disease is nonalcoholic fatty liver disease (NAFLD). Nonalcoholic steatohepatitis (NASH), a subtype of this illness, is defined by persistent, progressive liver damage that can result in cirrhosis, fibrosis, HCC, and even death (Basaranoglu et al., 2013). The buildup of fat in the hepatocytes changes the liver's ability to regenerate itself and makes it more vulnerable to damage. Another stressor is known as the "second hit," and potential candidates for this term are lipid peroxidation, an increase in oxidative stress, and the release of harmful compounds like 4-hydroxynonenal and MDA (Basaranoglu et al., 2013). Research has assessed NAC's capacity to stop lipid peroxidation from spreading and thereby stop NAFLD from developing. Furukawa et al.,(2004) found that giving rats with NASH NAC helped to improve the histology of their livers. Another study found that giving NAC to patients with nonalcoholic fatty liver disease (NAFLD) reduced the size of the spleen, indicating a decrease in fatty infiltration. Additionally, three months of NAC treatment improved liver damage markers like ALT (Khoshbaten et al., 2010; Takaki and Yamamoto, 2015). Numerous studies have demonstrated resveratrol's hepatoprotective properties as well as the value of this anti-inflammatory and antioxidant supplement in the management of liver steatosis. In rat hepatocytes isolated from steatosis, resveratrol decreases the synthesis of triacylglycerols (Gnoni and Paglialonga, 2009); in steatosis induced with palmitate, resveratrol also reduces the expression of the transcription factor important for lipogenesis, sterol regulatory element binding protein 1c (SREBP-1c). These results demonstrate the effectiveness of resveratrol in preventing novo lipogenesis in various in vitro models of hepatic steatosis. , 2009); resveratrol prevents HEPG2 cells from accumulating lipids and triacylglycerol when high glucose concentrations are present (Zang et al., 2006; Shang et al., 2008). The in vivo investigations have produced findings that are consistent with the in vitro research. In several experimental models involving rodents, resveratrol can reduce oxidative stress, lipid droplets, and the buildup of triacylglycerol. An intriguing discovery indicates that resveratrol raises the content of mitochondria, most likely through activating PGC-1a, a transcription factor that is crucial for the oxidation of fatty acids (Baur et al., 2006). It has been shown that resveratrol can increase fatty acid oxidation and decrease certain enzymes that synthesize triacylglycerols (Cho et al., 2012; Ajmo et al., 2008). Yang and Lim demonstrated that resveratrol corrects steatosis caused by a high-fat diet by preventing the NLRP3 inflammasome from activating. This inflammasome is an important modulator of inflammation and metabolism because it can detect insulin resistance and obesity (Yang and Lim, 2014). Kessoku et al., (2016) found that resveratrol inhibits STAT3 signaling, which in turn prevents CD14 expression in Kupffer cells and prevents the cells from going from steatosis to fibrosis.

10.3.4. NAC and Resveratrol in Hepatocellular Carcinoma

It is acknowledged that oxidative stress plays a significant role in the development of chronic liver disease, including hepatocarcinogenesis (Higgs et al., 2014). Numerous antioxidant agents are easily accessible, and research is being done on both their effects in vivo and in vitro.

One pathway that contributes to the development of HCC is the pentose phosphate pathway (PPP). The PPP serves two purposes: (1) it generates NADPH for biosynthetic reactions and (1) it forms ribose 5-phosphate for the synthesis of nucleotides (Perl et al., 2011). This pathway consists of two distinct branches: oxidative and nonoxidative. Transaldolase (TAL) is the limiting enzyme for the nonoxidative branch, while glucose 6-phosphate dehydrogenase (G6PD) is required for the oxidative branch (Qian et al., 2008). Basic research revealed that mice deficient in the TAL enzyme show mitochondrial dysfunction and oxidative stress in their hepatocytes, resulting in liver damage that advances from NAFLD to NASH, cirrhosis, and HCC (Hanczko et al., 2009). NAC treatment avoided the oxidative stress and mitochondrial dysfunction that characterize TAL-deficient livers, which include increased production of lipid peroxidation, 4-HNE, and MDA, as well as the depletion of NADPH and GSH. Conversely, TAL-deficient hepatocyte proliferation is aided by the activation of redox-sensitive transcription factors such as b-catenin, C-Jun N-terminal kinase (JNK), and c-jun. Accordingly, in mice lacking TAL, NAC treatment inhibited the development of NASH, cirrhosis, and HCC by blocking the phosphorylation of b-catenin, JNK, and c-jun activation (Perl et al., 2011).

Only a small number of studies have been conducted in vivo, but an increasing number of studies in vitro systems demonstrate how resveratrol affects various cancer cells. Even though resveratrol has demonstrated positive effects as a chemotherapeutic agent, more research in other models is advised before recommending its use as a therapeutic for humans (Carter et al., 2014).

Resveratrol has been assessed in a few experimental models in relation to HCC. In a study on diethylnitrosamine plus phenobarbital-induced hepatocellular carcinoma (HCC), resveratrol was found to inhibit the formation of hepatocyte nodules by reducing malignant cellular proliferation, promoting apoptosis by decreasing B-cell lymphoma 2 (Bcl2), and upregulating Bax expression. Lowering hepatic cell proliferation is indicated by lower expression of proliferating cell nuclear antigen, which is a sign of resveratrol treatment (Bishayee & Dhir, 2009). Resveratrol administration in the same experimental model increases the hepatic expression of Nrf2, a transcription factor that is important in the expression of genes that are related to antioxidants. In addition, resveratrol has strong anti-inflammatory properties by reducing COX-2 expression and nuclear translocation of NF-kB to the nucleus, and it is an excellent free radical scavenger (Bishayee et al., 2010).

Remarkably, a clinical study showed that resveratrol could cause cancerous cells to undergo apoptosis in patients who had liver metastases and colorectal cancer (Howells et al., 2011). Resveratrol has been shown in certain in vitro experiments to be able to inhibit human hepatoblastoma cells' (HepG2) ability to proliferate in a dose-dependent manner. Resveratrol also stops the cells from going through mitosis and arrests them in the S and G2/M phases (Delmas et al., 2000). Additionally, resveratrol inhibits the expression of vascular endothelial growth factor (VEGF) in HepG2 cells, downregulates NF-kB signaling pathways, and overexpresses Caveolin-1. These actions increase the amount of apoptosis that resveratrol induces in a manner that is dependent on the expression of caspase-3 and the p38 mitogen-activated protein kinase pathway (Zhang et al., 2005; Yu et al., 2008; Yang et al., 2009).

10.3.5. NAC and Resveratrol in Viral Hepatitis

Alcohol, NASH, and the hepatitis C virus (HCV) are the main causes of cirrhosis in the developed world, while viral hepatitis caused by the hepatitis B virus (HBV) is thought to be the main cause in developing nations (Zakhari, 2013). Hepatitis A virus (HAV) is thought to be the cause of acute liver failure (ALF) in 26% of cases, according to reports from hepatic transplant centers. However, the exact mortality rate of HAV infection is unknown and is not regarded as a public health concern (Lim and Kim, 2008; Blachier et al., 2013). The application of NAC in the treatment of viral hepatitis is supported by a number of different mechanisms, including: (1) aiding in the synthesis of GSH that has been depleted during ALF; (2) acting as a particular substrate for hepatic microsomal GSH transferase; and (3) having antioxidant and immunomodulatory properties (Harrison et al., 1991; Alipour et al., 2007; Kortsalioudaki et al., 2008; Lee et al., 2009).

Acute chronic hepatitis brought on by HCV infection carries a high risk of developing end-stage cirrhosis and HCC. Oxidative stress brought on by HCV replication exacerbates insulin and INF resistance. NS5A in particular has attracted a lot of attention as a potential cellular target. A serine phosphoprotein called NS5A is found in the cytoplasm of the endoplasmic reticulum membrane's perinuclear reticular network. Because of its potential involvement in IFN resistance, NS5A gained notoriety (Gong et al., 2001). It has been documented that the disruption of intracellular calcium is caused by NS5A. Ca^{2+} signaling then causes an increase in ROS in mitochondria, which in turn causes NF-kB and STAT-3 to translocate into the nucleus. In the case of NF-kB, this results in the expression of antiapoptotic genes like IAP protein or genes that promote proliferation like myc and Bcl-2 (Mercurio and Manning, 1999). In the case of STAT-3, this causes the acute phase of liver disease, which may be related to the acute hepatitis brought on by HCV infection. The activation of STAT-3 and NF-kB was inhibited in the presence of NAC (Gong et al., 2001). Ultimately, HCV also damages mitochondria and triggers the production of ROS and NO, which break down double-stranded DNA; these reactions are all neutralized by ROS and NO inhibitors (Zakhari, 2013).

Another research that demonstrates the beneficial effects of NAC is a meta-analysis carried out by Long et al., (2015), wherein they came to the conclusion that, in order to improve liver function, the combination of hepatoprotective agents and antiviral drugs is preferable than antiviral drugs alone. In patients with chronic hepatitis B, NAC administration lowers serum levels of aminotransferases and total bilirubin while increasing prothrombin activity (Long et al., 2015). Lastly, nitric oxide (NO) plays a role in the pathophysiology of autoimmune and viral hepatitis. Interestingly, NAC influences the expression of iNOS in human hepatocytes that have been stimulated by proinflammatory cytokines (Majano et al., 2004; Moreno-Otero and Trapero-Marugan, 2010).

Mice's liver damage caused by Concanavalin-A (Con-A) is similar to human hepatitis caused by viruses and autoimmune diseases. Con-treated mice produce more TNF-a, IL-2, and IL-6 as well as higher levels of ALT and AST; however, resveratrol dramatically suppresses these increases in transaminases and inflammatory cytokines. Resveratrol has been shown through immunohistochemistry to decrease CD4, which suggests that it can lessen inflammation and cell aggregation (Zhou et al., 2015). Remarkably, Jiang et al., (2012) have demonstrated how resveratrol can replenish the PPAR-a and SIRT1 expression that was lost as a result of a chronic HCV infection in mice, thereby halting the progression of hepatic steatosis.

10.3.6. Effect of NAC and Resveratrol in Hepatic Ischemia-Reperfusion Injury

Both liver resectional surgery and liver transplantation result in hepatic ischemia followed by reperfusion (HIR) (Jegatheeswaran and Siriwardena, 2010). The activation of Kupffer cells, the release of cytokines and chemokines, the change in mitochondrial permeability, the recruitment of neutrophils, and the generation of reactive oxygen species (ROS) are all elements of the liver damage process known as HIR, which ultimately leads to hepatocyte death (Wang et al., 2014).

A comprehensive review of the literature encompassing 19 studies evaluating the effects of NAC administration in experimental HIR revealed that 15 of the studies demonstrated improved outcomes, primarily a decrease in transaminase, when NAC (150 mg/kg) was administered prior to the induction of IR. Additionally, two out of four transplantation models demonstrated an improvement in hepatic function (Jegatheeswaran and Siriwardena, 2010). Conversely, Wang and colleagues (2014) discovered that the administration of NAC not only improved the serum markers of liver damage in a mouse model of segmental hepatic warm ischemia, but also improved the autophagy and apoptosis that occurred during HIR. The results of the study demonstrated that the protective effects of NAC are associated with ROS scavenging and JNK pathway targeting through the JNK/Bcl-2 pathway, which phosphorylates Bcl-2 and promotes autophagic cell death.

Resveratrol has been shown to be able to reduce the quantity of VEGF and HIF-1a that are seen in HIR in rats that have had their portal pedicle clamped and then reperfused. These proteins were therefore proposed as crucial molecular targets to stop the spread of tumors and their metastases (Zhang et al., 2014). However, in rats with HIR, resveratrol protects against hepatocyte apoptosis by upregulating Bcl-2 expression and downregulating Bax and caspase-3 expression (Shen et al., 2013). These effects are significant because they indicate that resveratrol has the capacity to discriminate between normal and tumor cells.

Through the inhibition of thioredoxin (Trx), a protein known as thioredoxin-interacting protein (Txnip) may mediate oxidative stress. Antoine Nivet et al., (2010) discovered that an HIR model overexpresses Txnip. Remarkably, resveratrol increases liver Trx redox activity by suppressing Txnip expression; this finding suggests a different antioxidant mechanism.

10.4. Side-Effects and Toxicology of NAC and Resveratrol

Even at high dosages, NAC is a medication that is widely acknowledged to be safe and well tolerated. NAC is safe to take in small doses of 1200 mg twice a day or less. Side effects are uncommon at these doses, but they can include nausea, vomiting, diarrhea, flushing, pain in the epigastrium, and constipation (Atkuri in al. 2007). Rarely, parenteral administration has resulted in allergic reactions, typically in the form of a brief skin rash or angioedema (Tenenbein, 1984). While NAC overdoses have been linked to fatalities, no such overdoses at normal dosages have been documented (Mant et al., 1984). Appelboam et al. (2002) detail the 40-year-old woman who visited the emergency room after purposefully overdosing on paracetamol, which resulted in the first fatal response to the therapeutic use of NAC. Her severe asthma was a past health issue. Following the administration of a 150 mg/kg NAC infusion, the patient experienced a severe bronchospasm-only anaphylactoid reaction. It is well known that NAC induces bronchospasm, most likely through inhibition of allergen tachyphylaxis or localized histamine release (Dorsch et al., 1987). Patients brittle asthma contributed to the severity of reaction; the author also suggests that it is important to take into account the dose and rate of NAC infusion to prevent lethal responses by NAC administration (Appelboam et al., 2002).

It is well known that resveratrol is safe; in fact, several clinical studies have shown that patients tolerate resveratrol well. Doses less than 1 g typically have no negative effects. Carneiro Tome et al., (2012) found that giving resveratrol in the form of grape extract for a year does not cause any negative side effects. Furthermore, in healthy individuals, a single 500 mg oral dose (tablet) was well tolerated and no negative side effects were noted (Sergides et al., 2016). Another study (Timmers et al.,2011) that administered 150 mg of resveratrol for a month in an attempt to mimic the effects of calorie restriction did not find any adverse effects.

Digestive disorders have been reported when resveratrol is administered at doses above 1 g; however, these results are not conclusive since the same effects were exhibited by patients that received placebo (Howells et al., 2011; Brown et al., 2010). Further studies are needed to find out if resveratrol possesses side-effects.

10.5. NAC and Resveratrol Formulations

The enteral pharmaceutical formulations of NAC include pills and capsules, as well as a range of effervescent formulations that can be mixed with juice, water, or other beverages to produce a drink that tastes good, is easily tolerated, and absorbs quickly (Atkuri et al., 2007). NAC must be oxidized to produce di-NAC, which is pharmacologically active at very low concentrations and is needed for the production of NAC. It is crucial to remember that the processes used in the production of these NAC preparations might not have included safeguards against NAC oxidizing to its dimeric form while the product is being manufactured or stored. To reduce the possible toxicity of acetaminophen, it has been proposed that NAC and acetaminophen be coadministered and possibly coformulated (Andrus et al., 2001). Equimolar doses of NAC and acetaminophen may be administered to achieve this aim, according to basic research (Atkuri et al., 2007).

Conversely, the FDA has approved the intravenous treatment of paracetamol poisoning within 8–10 hours of ingestion of sterile, pyrogen-free NAC. A sterile solution containing 200 mg/mL (20% w/v) in a 30 mL vial is also offered for this formulation. NAC 6 g is contained in each vial (Culley and Krenzelok, 2005).

As mentioned above, resveratrol is characterized by its low aqueous solubility and poor bioavailability. In order to improve its pharmacokinetics, different pharmaceutical approaches have been developed. According to this, the ability of nanocarrier systems to increase the resveratrol bioavailability has been demonstrated. Resveratrol formulated as nanosuspension was showed to increase the solubility and dissolution rate (Kobierski et al., 2009). Moreover, solid nanoparticles enhanced cellular uptake and allowed the sustained release of resveratrol (Teskac & Kristl, 2010).

Another approach to improve stability and the beneficial effects of resveratrol is the microparticle system; additionally, this system led to controlled release of the drug (Cho et al., 2014). As a manner of protection from metabolism, resveratrol has been formulated as liposomes: interestingly, efficacy is improved in this way (Mignet et al., 2013).

To investigate the stability and bioavailability of resveratrol, more studies on dosage and formulation design are required. This suggests that a system of solid-lipid-based nanoparticles enhanced stability and bioavailability; additionally, in an experimental model of paracetamol-induced liver cirrhosis, this system decreased serum markers of liver disease (Singh et al., 2016).

We suggest that NAC and resveratrol be used to treat acute or chronic liver diseases because of their strong antioxidant qualities, which are supported by a large body of research, and because oxidative stress is a major factor in the development of liver damage. In addition to its antioxidant qualities, a number of fundamental and clinical investigations have demonstrated the intricate mechanisms of action of resveratrol and NAC on the pathophysiological process implicated in the majority of liver diseases. Among these activities are the blocking or opening of significant signaling pathways associated with liver damage. It is recommended that these medications be assessed in upcoming clinical trials for hepatitis C or HCC. It is obvious that more research in the pharmaceutical field will be helpful in determining the best formulation to increase the drugs' stability and bioavailability while avoiding any potential toxicity.

10.6. Ursodeoxycholic Acid for the Treatment of Liver Diseases

10.6.1. History of Ursodeoxycholic Acid

Several chronic cholestatic liver diseases are commonly treated with ursodeoxycholic acid (UDCA). It has been used for centuries to treat liver diseases in traditional Chinese medicine. In fact, hepatobiliary disorders were treated with the Chinese medication yutan, a powder preparation made from the dried bile of adult bears (Bachrach and Hofmann, 1982). Ursocholeinic acid, as it was initially named by Hammarsten, was an unidentified bile acid found in polar bear bile that was first discovered in 1902. Shoda was the first to identify the chemical form of UDCA from Chinese black bear bile in 1927.

Because Shoda initially discovered this bile acid in the bile of the bear (called ursus in Latin), he named it ursodeoxycholic acid, based on his belief that it was a chemical isomer of deoxycholic acid. Iwasaki's 1936 definition of the chemical structure of UDCA made it possible for its adequate synthesis to be used in clinical research (Lazaridis et al., 2001). In 1975, Makino reported the first prospective study of patients with gallbladder stones treated with UDCA demonstrating gallstone dissolution (Makino et al., 1975). In 1985, Leuschner first observed improved liver tests of patients with chronic active hepatitis treated with UDCA for gallstone dissolution (Leuschner et al., 1985). In 1987, Poupon suggested that long-term use of UDCA is safe and effective in patients suffering from primary biliary cirrhosis (PBC) (Poupon et al., 1987). Since then, a variety of studies have shown the beneficial effect of UDCA in liver disorders. In clinical practice today, UDCA possesses a defined role in treating patients with cholestatic liver diseases. At present, it is the only drug approved by the United States Food and Drug Administration for the treatment of PBC.

10.6.2. Physicochemical Properties and Pharmacokinetics of UDCA

Hepatocytes use cholesterol as a raw material to make bile acids, which are acidic steroids. Protonated, or unionized, natural bile acids are highly soluble in water. It is more hydrophilic than the predominant bile acids in bile, such as chenodeoxycholic and deoxycholic, and goes by the name 3a, 7b-dihydroxy-5b-cholan-24-oic acid. The hydrophilic groups in UDCA are responsible for this feature. Because it is not produced in the liver, bacterial 7b epimerization of the primary bile acid, chenodeoxycholic, is most likely the source of UDCA, which makes up to 4% of the bile acid pool in humans (Bachrach and Hofmann, 1982). After UDCA is formed, the colonic mucosa passively absorbs it, allowing it to enter the portal circulation and eventually the bile acid pool.

When taken orally, UDCA is quickly absorbed by passive transport in the upper ileum and jejunum and by active transport in the terminal ileum. Usually, 60–80% of the dose that is given is absorbed. When UDCA is administered with a meal, absorption may be increased; however, in patients who have decreased biliary secretion of endogenous bile acids (e.g., in those suffering from cholestasis). Following intestinal absorption, UDCA travels via the portal circulation before being absorbed by the hepatocytes at their sinusoidal domain through particular bile acid transporters, such as the organic anion transporting polypeptide (OATP) and the Na^+-dependent taurocholate (NTCP) (Kullak-Ublick et al., (2000). UDCA is conjugated to taurine or glycine (primarily) within the hepatocyte (Hofmann, 1994). It is then carried into the bile ducts using another bile acid carrier molecule called the bile salt export pump (BSEP; Kullak-Ublick et al., (2000). The liver can clear up to 60% of the drug in its first pass. In the intestine, certain bacteria break down to produce lithocholic acid and 7-ketolithocholic acid. Hepatotoxic, lithocholic acid damages the liver parenchyma in a variety of animal species. Only a very small amount is absorbed by humans, and this is detoxified by the liver through sulfation before being eliminated with the bile and eventually in the feces. UDCA has a biological half-life of 30.5–50.8 days.

10.6.3. Pharmacological Activities of UDCA

When UDCA is taken orally, the intestinal absorption of cholesterol is inhibited, and the amount of cholesterol secreted into the bile is decreased, resulting in a reduction in cholesterol saturation. Indeed, UDCA reduces the biliary cholesterol by40 ± 60%. In terms of bile acid metabolism, research has demonstrated that in patients with hyperlipidemia, cholestatic liver diseases, and healthy individuals, UDCA increases the metabolic conversion of cholesterol to bile acids (Hofmann, 1994). One mechanism for UDCA's protective effect in the treatment of cholestatic liver disease is its ability to both prevent and reduce the downregulation of BSEP caused by deoxycholic acid (Paolini et al., 2002). The putative jejunal facilitated and the ileal active bile acid uptake can both be decreased by UDCA, according to studies utilizing intestinal brush border membrane vesicles (Aldini et al., 1996).

Based on current understanding, the mechanism of action of UDCA in hepatic and cholestatic diseases likely involves the hydrophilic, cytoprotective, nontoxic UDCA replacing the lipophilic, detergent-like, toxic bile acids, improving hepatocyte secretory function, and influencing immunoregulatory processes.

10.6.4. Mechanisms of UDCA Action

UDCA, a water-soluble bile acid that is non-toxic, becomes the main bile acid present in the bloodstream and bile by blocking the absorption of harmful natural bile salts in the intestines (Stiehl et al., 1990; Crosignani et al., 1991; Beuers et al., 1992b; Rudolph et al., 1993). This alteration of balance between toxic hydrophobic bile salts and nontoxic hydrophilic bile salts in the bile acid pool is probably the most important mode of action of UDCA (Stiehl et al., 1999).

Although potential mechanisms of action, such as increased hydrophilic bile acid pool, hepatobiliary secretion stimulation, immune modulation, membrane stabilizing, antioxidative, and cytoprotective mechanisms, have been studied, the precise mechanism of action of UDCA in cholestatic diseases remains unclear.

- ***Stimulation of Hepatobiliary Secretion***: The quantity and activity of carrier proteins in the canalicular membrane, which are controlled at the transcriptional and posttranscriptional levels in the hepatocyte, determine the secretory capacity of the cells. UDCA causes transcriptional and posttranscriptional alterations that improve the expression and functionality of basolateral and canalicular transporters. UDCA administration increases the expression of genes for the canalicular transporters MRP2 (divalent bile acids and anionic conjugate transporter) and BSEP (monovalent bile acids transporter) in mice (Paolini et al., 2002). The expression of genes for basolateral bile acid efflux pumps, MRP3 and MRP4, is also enhanced by UDCA in mice (Zollner et al., 2003). In rodents, UDCA induces posttranscriptional processes via calcium-dependent (protein kinase C-a) PKC-a and MAP-kinases, which in turn cause vesicular exocytosis and transporter targeting to the canalicular membrane (Paumgartner and Beuers, 2002, 2004). UDCA enhances excretory function in PBC patients (Poupon et al., 1991) and it has been demonstrated that UDCA therapy increases MRP2 expression (Poupon et al., 1993). The hepatobiliary bicarbonate secretion in PBC patients may be enhanced by UDCA treatment by upregulating the chloride-bicarbonate anion exchanger AE2, which is found in the apical membrane of both hepatocytes and cholangiocytes (Medina et al., 1997; Prieto et al., 1993, 1999).

Short-term secretion regulation may be determined by UDCA's effects on transporter activity and insertion into the canalicular membrane, even though long-term regulation may be influenced by the effects on transporter mRNA and protein levels. The synthesis, apical insertion, and activation of the AE2, MRP2, and BSEP are all increased by UDCA, which may improve both bile salt-dependent and -independent bile flow (Paumgartner and Beuers, 2004).

- ***Expansion of Hydrophilic Bile Acid Pool:*** At concentrations found in bile, hydrophobic bile acids cause extracellular cytotoxicity and harm cell membranes. The UDCA treatment lessens the toxic potential of bile that could exacerbate any primary disease-specific duct lesion by changing the hydrophobic and hydrophilic nature of bile acid composition.

UDCA is a natural bile acid devoid of any cytotoxicity up to concentrations of 500 mmol/L, according to several models in vitro. The amidated forms of UDCA inhibit the intestinal absorption of endogenous bile acids (Lanzini et al., 2003) as well as the fraction absorbed in the small bile ducts. This effect in concert with stimulation of hepatocellular bile acid secretion (with no change in bile acid synthesis) (Beuers et al., 1992b; Jazrawi et al., 1994) leads to permanent interruption of the enterohepatic circulation and a fall in concentrations of endogenous hydrophobic bile acids in the blood, liver, and extrahepatic tissues. As a consequence, UDCA becomes the major circulating bile acid and the hydrophobicity of the circulating bile acid pool is thereby reduced.

The precise role that UDCA plays in preventing liver damage through the displacement of endogenous bile acids is still unknown. Interestingly, several studies have demonstrated that in patients with cholestatic liver diseases, there was no difference in the pool size of bile acids or the serum concentration of the primary endogenous hydrophobic bile acids before or after UDCA therapy (Beuers et al., 1992b; Rudolph and others. 1993).

These findings suggest that UDCA is unlikely to enhance cholestatic patients' liver function by merely moving endogenous bile acids to a different location in the bile acid pool or by increasing the amount of hydrophilic bile acids already present.

- ***Cytoprotective Effects:*** At the cellular and molecular levels, UDCA can directly protect cells by stabilizing hepatocyte membranes, bolstering defenses against oxidative stress, and preventing apoptosis brought on by a variety of agents.

a. *Membrane Stabilizing Effect:* UDCA conjugates have been demonstrated to counteract the membrane-damaging effects of lipophilic bile acids (Heuman and Bajaj, 1994). While UDCA conjugates integrate into the membranes' interface, lower their polarity, and shield them from the lipophilic bile acids' detergent action, UDCA binds to the polar domain of the membranes (Guldutuna et al., 1993). Toxic bile salts also change the permeability of mitochondrial membranes, which results in hepatocyte necrosis. The bile salt-induced modification of mitochondrial membrane permeability is inhibited by UDCA (Rodrigues et al., 1998). Because of its ability to stabilize membranes, UDCA thereby protects mitochondrial, basolateral, and canalicular membranes from damage caused by toxic bile acid.

b. *Antioxidative Effect:* Reactive oxygen species are secreted by Kupffer's cells, which can be activated by toxic bile salts. Hepatocytes are susceptible to damage from reactive oxygen species due to lipid peroxidation. As an antioxidant, UDCA prevents toxic bile salts from activating Kupffer's cells, as reported by Sokol et al., 1993).

The markedly increased production of mitochondrial peroxide and hydroxynonenal protein adducts observed during chronic cholestasis is prevented by UDCA-induced enhancement of liver glutathione levels and the upregulation of g-glutamylcysteine synthetase and methionine S-adenosyl transferase (Bernstein et al., 2002; Lapenna et al., 2002; Ljubuncic et al., 2000; Mitsuyoshi et al., 1999; Rodriguez-Ortigosa et al., 2002). UDCA also stimulates (Nf-E2 related factor 2) NRF2- mediated hepatocellular transport, detoxification, and antioxidative-stress systems in mice, and enhances hepatic NRF2 and thioredoxin in PBC (Kawata et al., 2010).

c. *Inhibition of Apoptosis*: One significant method of cell death in liver diseases is apoptosis. According to research conducted in vitro, UDCA can prevent both hepatic and nonhepatic cells from going through apoptosis when they are exposed to a range of stimuli, including ethanol, hydrophobic bile acids, transforming growth factor beta 1 (TGF-b1), Fas ligand, and okadaic acid. UDCA has antiapoptotic effects on cholangiocytes in PBC patients (Koga et al., 1997) and so may inhibit the availability of mitochondrial antigens in dendritic cells and macrophages, the trigger of the autoimmune process (Allina et al., 2006). In virtue of its antiapoptotic properties, UDCA has also been proposed as an additional treatment for viral hepatitis (Kountouras et al., 2003). This concept might be supported by an improved response rate to alpha-interferon in nonresponder patients with hepatitis C virus (HCV) related chronic hepatitis (Fabbri et al., 2000). Although intriguing, the significance of antiapoptotic mechanisms in the beneficial effects of UDCA in liver disease remains unclear at present.

Targeting mitochondrial function and integrity, lowering endoplasmic reticulum stress, and interacting with survival signals in the cAMP, Akt, nuclear factor kappa-B (NF-kB), mitogen-activated protein kinases (MAPK), and phosphatidylinositol 3-kinase signaling pathways are some of the mechanisms underlying UDCA's antiapoptotic qualities (Poupon, 2012). Another way UDCA prevents cell death is through activating the epidermal growth factor receptor (EGFR), which stops bile acid-induced apoptosis in rat liver cells. EGFR triggers MAPK to send a survival signal and prevent apoptosis (Qiao et al., 2002). While UDCA interferes with E2F-1 transcriptional activation of apoptosis, thereby modulating p53 stabilization, NF-kB activation, and the expression of Bcl-2 family members through a mechanism involving nuclear glucocorticoid and mineralocorticoid receptors, TGF-b1-induced hepatocyte apoptosis is linked to activation of E2F transcription factors and p53 stabilization through its inhibitor Mdm2. 2004).

- ***Immunomodulatory Properties:*** In patients with PBC and extra hepatic cholestasis, the expression of (human leukocyte antigen) HLA class I and II antigens increases on both hepatocytes and bile ducts. UDCA treatment has been shown to significantly reduce HLA class I and II expression in PBC patients (Hirano et al., 1996; Terasaki et al., 1991) and inhibited interferon-g-inducible activation of (major histocompatibility complex) MHC class II in vitro via a glucocorticoid-receptor-dependent pathway (Tanaka et al., 1996), thereby suggesting that UDCA may be interfering with the basic mechanisms of autoimmunity.

In several experimental models, UDCA exerted immunosuppressive properties by modifying Toll-like receptor (TLR) 4 and TLR9-signaling pathways, leading to immune cell activation and inflammation (Unitt & Hornigold, 2011). These effects could be related to the glucocorticoid receptor agonist activity of UDCA. In addition, UDCA corrects natural killer T cell activity by inhibiting prostaglandin E2 production in PBC (Nishigaki et al., 1996), and UDCA administration in PBC blunts the accumulation of endotoxin in bile and suppresses the immune reaction against lipid A (Ballot et al., 2004).

10.6.5. Clinical Use and Efficacy of UDCA

Cholestatic and other liver diseases have been treated with UDCA. Here, we go over the key research done on these hepatic disorders and talk about how UDCA is used in clinical settings.

1. ***UDCA as Therapeutic Agents for Cholestatic Liver Diseases***

- *Primary Biliary Cirrhosis*: PBC is a chronic liver disease that is typified by the small-to-medium-sized bile ducts being gradually destroyed by the immune system. This leads to chronic cholestasis, inflammation of the portal tract, and fibrosis, which can eventually cause cirrhosis and liver failure (Selmi et al., 2011). The only approved therapy for PBC by the US FDA is UDCA at a dose of 13–15 mg/kg/day. This treatment is also recommended by the practice guidelines of both the European and American Associations for the Study of Liver Diseases for PBC patients with abnormal biochemical values (European Association for the Study of the Liver, 2009; Lindor et al., 2009a) as well as "Guidelines

> for the management of PBC issued by the Intractable Hepatobiliary Disease Study Group supported by the Ministry of Health, Labor and Welfare of Japan" (Working Subgroup for Clinical Practice Guidelines for Primary Biliary Cirrhosis, 2014). Although a wide variety of agents other than UDCA, including methotrexate, malotilate, silymarin, cyclosporine A, colchicine, thalidomide, and chlorambucil, have been studied in clinical trials for the treatment of PBC, the results have not been encouraging (Pares, 2014).

The first account of the effectiveness of UDCA was published in 1987 by Poupon et al., found that when PBC patients received the medication for two years, there was a significant improvement in the biochemical parameters gamma-glutamyl transpeptidase (GGT), alkaline phosphatase (ALP), alanine aminotransferase (ALT), and bilirubin. Since then, several randomized controlled trials have been carried out to assess the effectiveness of UDCA in PBC. Studies have consistently shown a decrease in antimitochondrial antibody titers and immunoglobulin M (IgM) levels, along with a significant improvement in serum markers of cholestasis and biliary injury (Heathcote et al., 1994; Lindor et al., 1994; Poupon et al., 1991; Combes et al., 1995; Eriksson et al., 1997; Angulo et al., 1999; Pares et al., 2000; Papatheodoridis et al., 2002). In general, UDCA has been associated with a reduced risk of developing varices and slower histological progression (Lindor et al., 2009a). Additionally, research has shown that patients with stage 1 or 2 disease who received long-term UDCA had a similar survival rate to that of a healthy control population (Corpechot et al., 2005). Some studies have raised doubts about the survival benefits of UDCA in PBC (Goulis et al., 1999; Gong et al., 2007; Rudic et al., 2012). However, many of these studies only lasted 2 years, which may not have been long enough to assess the effectiveness of any medical treatment on survival (Floreani et al., 2015). Conversely, a separate meta-analysis that excluded short-term studies (<24 months) and those using a low dosage of UDCA (<10 mg/kg/day) found that long-term UDCA significantly improved transplant-free survival and delayed histological progression in early-stage patients (Shi et al., 2006). The prognosis of primary biliary cholangitis (PBC) is influenced by the therapeutic impact of UDCA. Extensive work has been done in the past decade to establish criteria for assessing the response to UDCA, particularly in terms of prognostic biomarkers and validating the predictive value of UDCA on transplant-free survival in PBC. Multiple studies have demonstrated that the biochemical response to UDCA at 1 year and 6 months can effectively predict long-term outcomes (Pares et al., 2006; Corpechot et al., 2008; Kuiper et al., 2009; Kumagi et al., 2010). The efficiency of several combinations of serum bilirubin, ALP, and aspartate aminotransferase (AST) threshold values to predict outcomes was assessed after 1 year of treatment in 292 patients with PBC. Patients showing ALP < 3 upper limit of normal (ULN), AST < 2 ULN, and bilirubin 1 mg/dL after 1 year of UDCA had a significantly higher 10-year transplant-free survival rate than those who did not (90% vs. 51%) (Corpechot et al., 2008). Zhang et al., (2013) compared the Paris, Barcelona, Toronto, and Ehime criteria for predicting the outcome of UDCA treatment in a 14-year cohort of PBC patients, and the results demonstrated that biochemical responses at the sixth month can be used in place of those evaluated after 1 year of UDCA therapy.

Patients who respond positively to UDCA treatment typically experience improved biochemistry after 6–9 months. However, those who do not reach these milestones are more likely to deteriorate over time. Response to treatment is also influenced by factors such as sex and age at initial presentation, with women under the age of 50 showing the lowest response rates and more severe symptoms (Carbone et al., 2013). Such patients should the focus on novel therapy to improve outcomes. Men with PBC have a lower likelihood of responding to therapy but with a lower symptom burden and the age at presentation is not important (Carbone et al., 2013). Kumagi's study showed that ductopenia on baseline biopsy as a predictive factor for histological progression and treatment failure (Kumagi et al., 2010). As UDCA slows down the disease's progression and, consequently, lowers the chance of developing cirrhosis—the primary risk factor for primary liver cancer—it may also help patients with PBC avoid developing hepatocellular carcinoma (Jackson et al., 2007; Cavazza et al., 2009).

- *Primary Sclerosing Cholangitis:* With 70–80% of patients also having concurrent inflammatory bowel disease (IBD), primarily ulcerative colitis, primary sclerosing cholangitis (PSC) is a chronic immune-mediated disease of the liver with an unclear etiology. PSC is characterized by chronic inflammation and bile duct fibrosis (Singh and Talwalkar, 2013). Moreover, PSC should be regarded as a premalignant condition since it significantly raises the risk of colorectal cancer and cholangiocarcinoma (CCA) in comparison to the general population, with cancer being the primary cause of death for PSC patients (Bergquist et al., in 2002). Since the first (randomized controlled trial) RCT (UDCA 13–15 mg/kg/day) reported in 1992, which demonstrated significant improvement in multiple biochemical endpoints as well as liver histology (Beuers et al., 1992a), UDCA has been evaluated repeatedly for management of patients with PSC. Low-dose (10–15 mg/ kg/ day) and intermediate-dose (17–23 mg/kg/day) were associated with significant biochemical improvement, but no difference in death, liver transplantation, or CCA. However, high-dose (28–30 mg/kg/day) was associated with a twofold increase in serious adverse events (Lindor et al., 2009b). A 2010 guideline issued by AASLD recommends against UDCA use in the treatment of PSC (Chapman et al., 2010). EASL guidelines suggested that UDCA be only offered to patients with PSC who have advanced colitis (European Association for the Study of the Liver, 2009). The Cochrane systematic review evaluated UDCA in eight RCTs (592 patients with PSC were treated for 3 months to 6 years) (Poropat et al., 2011). The results showed UDCA treatment did not significantly reduce the risk of death. The authors concluded that they did not find enough evidence to support or refuse the use of UDCA in the treatment of PSC, however, UDCA seems to lead to a significant improvement in liver biochemistry (Poropat et al., 2011). Therefore, more RCTs are needed before UDCA can be recommended for this indication.

On the other hand, a study prospectively assessed the impact of a three-month UDCA withdrawal on quality of life and serum biochemical tests (Wunsch et al., 2014). The results unequivocally demonstrated that stopping long-term UDCA treatment causes a substantial and quick decline in biochemical cholestasis, which is accompanied by a higher Mayo risk score (MRS) (Wunsch et al., 2014). Tabibian et al. (2014) suggested that patients with well-compensated PSC may still benefit from the prudent use of UDCA. They recommended that PSC patients may use UDCA 17–23 mg/kg/day if they exhibit symptoms associated with PSC and/or ALP > 1.5 × ULN. Treatment could be continued for six months if the patient tolerates it well in order to track ALP normalization, a reduction of more than 40% from baseline, and/or improvement in symptoms. They might terminate UDCA if they don't (Tabibian and Lindor, 2014). The American College of Gastroenterology's 2015 guidelines state that UDCA should not be used in doses greater than 28 mg/kg/day, but they do not offer any recommendations regarding its use (Lindor et al., 2015). There is some evidence to suggest that UDCA may alter the risk of colorectal neoplasia; at standard doses, the risk may be reduced, but at high doses, it may be increased (Eaton et al., 2011; Pardi et al., 2003). Based on a meta-analysis of six studies reporting 41 cases of advanced colorectal neoplasia in 546 patients with (primary sclerosing cholangitis - inflammatory bowel disease) PSC-IBD, it has been shown that standard dose UDCA was associated with a 63% risk reduction (Lindstrom et al., 2012). Therefore, standard dose UDCA has been recommended as a chemopreventive agent for reduction in colorectal cancer in PSC in high-risk groups such as those with a strong family history of colorectal cancer, previous colorectal neoplasia, or long-standing extensive colitis by EASL (European Association for the Study of the Liver, 2009) and the American Gastroenterological Association (Farraye et al., 2010).

- *Intrahepatic Cholestasis of Pregnancy*: The most common liver disease during pregnancy is called intrahepatic cholestasis of pregnancy (ICP), which is characterized by elevated bile acids and/or transaminases and otherwise unexplained pruritus in the late second and third trimesters of pregnancy. ICP is linked to a higher chance of the mother developing hepatobiliary disease later in life and of the fetus experiencing unfavorable perinatal outcomes (Marschall, 2015). In ICP, stimulation of impaired hepatocellular secretion could be crucial for rapid relief of pruritus and improvement of serum liver tests, as it is in some forms of drug-induced cholestasis (Beuers, 2006). UDCA was found to increase the expression of placental bile acid transporters and their regulating nuclear factors, which may enhance maternal-fetal bile acid transfer and to reduce bile acid levels in cord blood, amniotic fluid, and colostrum (Beuers, 2006; Geenes et al., 2011). UDCA was also found to correct the reversed feto-maternal bile acid gradient in ICP (Geenes et al., 2014).

The first report of UDCA efficacy in ICP was published in 1991 showing an improvement in serum bile salts and pruritus with the treatment (Mazzella et al., 1991). This preliminary observation was later confirmed by other groups (Brites et al., 1998; Palma et al., 1992) and until 2015, a total of 11 randomized controlled trials have been published in English that compared UDCA to other drugs, placebo, or no treatment (Marschall, 2015). The Cochrane systematic review published in 2013 suggested that UDCA significantly improves pruritus. Fewer instances of fetal distress/ asphyxial events were seen in the UDCA groups when compared with placebo but the difference was not statistically significant (Gurung et al., 2013). The latest placebo-controlled trial of UDCA (450 mg/day) in 20 Finnish women with ICP confirmed improvement of pruritus scores and liver transaminases (Joutsiniemi et al., 2014). A meta-analysis included 11 RCTs (n = 625) and six nonrandomized studies (n = 211) for articles published from 1966 to June 2012 (Grand'Maison et al., 2014). Overall, women treated with UDCA had decreased pruritus in 73% of RCTs and in 100% of nonrandomized studies with available data. Liver function tests were improved in 82% of RCTs and in 100% of (numerical rating scale) NRSs with available data. UDCA use did not affect the cesarean section rate, but was associated with less prematurity, less use of neonatal intensive care units, and trends toward increased birth weight and decreased meconium staining (Grand'Maison et al., 2014). Therefore, both at low and standard doses, UDCA is effective in attenuating ICP pruritus and improving maternal transaminases and serum bile salts.

Furthermore, there have been no published studies to date that have documented any negative effects of UDCA on puerpera or fetuses, indicating that it is safe to use during the third trimester. Moreover, the finding that UDCA lowers the levels of primary bile acids in colostrum and that the amount of this acid in breast milk is less than 0.01% of the amount given to the mother lends credence to the safety of its application (Brites and Rodrigues, 1998). To sum up, UDCA is regarded as the initial course of treatment for ICP. The ideal daily dosage for prescription medication until delivery is 15 mg/kg.

- *Liver Disease in Cystic Fibrosis:* The most prevalent genetic illness affecting Caucasians, with an autosomal recessive inheritance pattern, is cystic fibrosis (CF). Even though lung disease is the primary cause of morbidity and death, advances in medical treatment and patient care have changed the trajectory of cystic fibrosis (CF) and significantly increased life expectancy. Other organ manifestations therefore gain greater clinical significance. For nearly 30% of patients with CF, liver disease is a contributing factor. Neonatal cholestasis, hepatic steatosis, and focal or multilobular cirrhosis are among the conditions in the spectrum. After lung illness and complications from organ transplantation, CF-associated liver disease (CFLD) is currently thought to be the third most common cause of death for patients with CF (Moyer and Balistreri, 2009). For the long-term prognosis of CFLD, there is no known treatment that is beneficial. There is debate regarding UDCA's function in CFLD. Moderate doses of UDCA may improve biochemical parameters in patients with CFLD, according to limited clinical evidence. Around 1990, UDCA was introduced for the therapy of CFLD (Colombo et al., 1990; Cotting et al., 1990). Its use in CFLD is justified by the desire to replace toxic bile acids that build up in the hepatocytes and to lessen the viscosity of bile (Colombo et al., 1992). Research indicates that the optimal dosage of UDCA is 20–30 mg/kg/

day, which is greater than the dosages prescribed for other liver conditions. Additionally, it has been demonstrated that long-term UDCA treatment can halt the development of cirrhotic alterations and even reverse those that already exist in cases of focal biliary cirrhosis (Lamireau et al., 2004; Siano et al., 2010). A retrospective analysis of 278 adult CF patients revealed 27 (9.7%) to have liver disease; of these, 22 had taken UDCA, which was linked to significant reductions in serum ALT, GGT, and ALP activities as well as improvement in hepatobiliary symptoms in half of the patients (Desmond et al., 2007). A retrospective long-term follow-up case-control study showed that UDCA treatment normalized serum liver enzyme levels and reduced the incidence of overt liver disease in CF patients. Furthermore, over an extended observation period, UDCA-treated CF patients demonstrated stable lung function comparable to that of non-UDCA-treated CF patients (Kappler et al., 2012). There isn't any solid proof, though, that it enhances other results. According to a Cochrane review, there is not enough data to say whether UDCA is beneficial for treating or preventing CFLD (Cheng et al., 2014).

As a result, the function of UDCA in the treatment of subclinical or other early forms of CFLD remains unclear, as does its role in the disease overall. Moderate doses of UDCA may improve biochemical parameters in patients with CFLD, according to limited clinical evidence. However, there's no solid proof that it enhances other outcomes, and more research is desperately needed before definitive recommendations supporting or opposing the use of UDCA can be made.

- *Progressive Familial Intrahepatic Cholestasis:* A collection of uncommon conditions known as progressive familial intrahepatic cholestasis (PFIC) are brought on by abnormalities in bile secretion and typically manifest as intrahepatic cholestasis in early childhood and infancy. Their inheritance pattern is autosomal recessive. PFIC is classified into three distinct types based on subtle variations in their clinical, biochemical, and histological characteristics. These types are linked to mutations in ATP8B1 (PFICI), ABCB11 (PFICII), and ABCB4 (PFICIII) (Jacquemin et al., 2001; van Mil et al., 2005; Davit-Spraul et al., 2010). The optimal course of action for treating PFIC remains to be fully determined and is likely to depend on the specific type of PFIC, the severity of the disease at diagnosis, and primarily the penetrance of gene defects. With a 5-year survival rate of roughly 92%, liver transplantation is regarded as a conclusive therapeutic approach (Wanty et al., 2004). When combined with standard nutritional support, UDCA is the most important medical treatment. In 39 children treated with 20–30 mg/kg/day of UDCA for 2–4 years, the most significant and persuasive study showed a significant decrease in ALT and GGT levels and an improved nutritional state, with a corresponding improvement in hepatosplenomegaly and pruritus (Jacquemin et al., 1997). Moreover it has been shown that UDCA efficacy is related to early initiation of the therapy, low penetrance of the genetic defect and less severe preexisting liver damage (Wanty et al., 2004). The therapeutic effect appears to be dependent on the type of mutation, with premature stop codons leading to a truncated protein being associated with nearly no response to therapy (Jacquemin et al., 2001).

Chronic UDCA treatment normalizes liver function tests and improves clinical parameters in as many as 50% of patients with ABCB4 deficiency (PFIC III) (Jacquemin et al., 2001, 1997). Therefore, when it comes to the initial therapeutic management of patients with ABCB4 deficiency, especially in cases where a missense mutation in the corresponding gene is discovered, UDCA should be the first option. Nevertheless, the effects of UDCA treatment in patients with ATP8B1 or ABCB11 deficiency are inconsistent, ranging from a noticeable improvement to none at all (Davit-Spraul et al., 2010; Lykavieris et al., 2003; van Ooteghem et al., 2002; Whitington et al., 1994).

- *Other Pediatric Cholestatic Disorders:* Alagille's syndrome, biliary atresia, and other syndromes involving the disappearance of bile ducts are among these syndromes. Before a liver transplant, patients with improved or stabilized cholestasis should be considered candidates for UDCA therapy (Ullrich et al., 1987). For the majority of pediatric cholestatic syndromes, UDCA is currently the only available medical treatment; in certain cases, it serves as a bridge therapy before liver transplantation (Festi et al., 2007).
- *Chronic Graft-Versus-Host Disease Involving the Liver*: After receiving an allogeneic bone marrow transplant, graft-versus-host disease (GVHD) can affect the liver, resulting in cholestatic symptoms and veno-occlusive disease. Short-term UDCA treatment has been shown in pilot studies to improve cholestasis in hepatic GVHD patients (Fried et al., 1992; Wulffraat et al., 1997). In patients receiving a bone marrow transplant and following a preparative regimen of busulfan plus cyclophosphamide, prophylactic administration of UDCA reduced the incidence of cholestasis and hepatic complications, according to a randomized, placebo-controlled trial (Essell et al., 1998).
- *Drug-Induced Cholestasis:* The beneficial effect of UDCA in drug-induced cholestasis has been demonstrated in small case series (Lazaridis et al., 2001). Anecdotal evidence of the effectiveness of UDCA, albeit in certain circumstances, in drug-induced cholestasis, specifically disappearing bile duct syndrome, has been reported (Smith et al., 2005). In order to confirm the possible beneficial impact of UDCA in drug-induced cholestasis, controlled investigations are necessary. However, because these cases are isolated and involve a variety of drugs, conducting such trials can be challenging.
- *Total Parenteral Nutrition-Associated Liver Disease:* Individuals receiving long-term total parenteral nutrition may experience hepatic disease, which typically presents as cholestatic abnormalities with elevated serum

ALP and bilirubin levels. Liver disease can be temporary or chronic (Calmus et al., 1990). A number of small studies have demonstrated the potential benefits of oral UDCA administration at doses of 10–30 mg/kg body weight per day in neonates with parenteral nutrition-associated cholestasis (Spagnuolo et al., 1996; Levine et al., 1999; Chen et al., 2004; De Marco et al., 2006). A controlled trial of erythromycin and UDCA in premature infants during parenteral nutrition observed that UDCA was effective in preventing cholestasis in very low birth weight infants (Gokmen et al., 2012). A retrospective study conducted on newborns recently showed that UDCA therapy was linked to increased weight gain and a quicker decline in conjugated bilirubin, but it was not linked to how long parenteral nutrition-associated liver disease would last (Thibault et al., 2014). UDCA is recommended as a treatment for elevated liver enzymes in children with parenteral nutrition-associated liver disease in the 2014 Clinical Guidelines of the American Society for Parenteral and Enteral Nutrition (Wales et al., 2014). Nevertheless, the evidence is of extremely poor quality and complicated by the use of enteral feeding in addition to UDCA treatment (Wales et al., 2014). Adult patients have more conflicting data regarding the benefits of UDCA. One study found that treatment with an average of 11± mg oral UDCA/kg body weight per day is linked to a decrease in GGT and ALT levels but not in AST, bilirubin, or ALP levels (Beau et al., 1994).

2. ***UDCA as Therapeutic Agents for Noncholestatic Liver Diseases***

- *Chronic Viral Hepatitis*: Bile acids significantly increase serum transaminase activities in hepatitis B and C, but they have no effect on the virus's ability to clear. This is according to the 2007 Cochrane systematic review (Chen et al., 2007). Effects on long-term outcomes such as hepatocellular carcinoma, hepatic decompensation, and liver-related mortality are not sufficiently supported or refuted by available data. There were 29 randomized trials using bile acids to treat hepatitis B or C in specific Cochrane systematic reviews. None, nevertheless, had excellent methodological quality (Chen et al., 2007). A prospective cohort study demonstrated that UDCA might prevent HCC development in HCV-related liver cirrhosis (Tarao et al., 2005). The cumulative 5-year incidence of HCC in the patients treated with UDCA was 17.9% (10 of 56) and was significantly lower than that in patients not treated with UDCA (39.1%, 18 of 46; $p = .025$) (Tarao et al., 2005).
- *Nonalcoholic Steatohepatitis:* Larger studies were unable to corroborate the early reports of beneficial effects of low (12–15 mg/kg/day) and high (28–35 mg/kg/day) UDCA on liver biochemistries, steatosis, and histology in nonalcoholic fatty liver disease (NAFLD) (Dufour et al., 2006; Laurin et al., 1996; Pietu et al., 2012; Ratziu et al., 2011). Two large randomized studies in patients with biopsy-confirmed nonalcoholic steatohepatitis (NASH) showed no significant effects for UDCA on NASH histology with low (13–15 mg/kg/day for 2 years, $n = 166$) or high-dose (23–28 mg/kg/day for 1.5 years, $n = 185$) UDCA (Lindor et al., 2004; Leuschner et al., 2010). These findings were confirmed

in our meta-analysis (Wu et al., 2012) and a Cochrane Review by Orlando et al. (2007), which concluded that there was no clear evidence to support or refute the effect of UDCA in adult patients with NASH. A single randomized controlled trial in children confirmed the lack of efficacy found in adults (Vajro et al., 2000).

- *Liver Transplantation:* A common issue that arises after liver transplantation is biliary lesions. Toxic bile acids can result in severe bile tract injury in addition to ischemic and immunologic factors (Cursio and Gugenheim, 2012). Early hepatobiliary injury following orthotopic liver transplantation (OLT) may be attributed to a high bile acid/phospholipid ratio and intrahepatic bile retention, according to research (Yska et al., 2008). Hydrophobic bile acids can cause hepatobiliary injury, but UDCA can prevent it by altering the composition of bile acids early after OLT, according to a recent randomized, placebo-controlled trial. Following OLT, more than 100 patients were given either UDCA or a placebo for four weeks. According to the authors, UDCA treatment had no effect on the overall outcome as assessed by graft and patient survival after five years. However, after UDCA was administered, not only were liver enzymes significantly reduced, but also the incidence of biliary sludge and casts (Wang et al., 2012).

UDCA was recommended as a treatment for acute cellular rejection due to its immunomodulatory qualities, which have been supported by encouraging results from uncontrolled studies. Following liver transplantation, UDCA was evaluated in four randomized, placebo-controlled trials to see if it could be used as a preventative measure to lower the incidence of acute cellular rejection (Pageaux et al., 1995; Barnes et al., 1997; Keiding et al., 1997; Fleckenstein et al., 1998). When compared to the control group in three of these studies, UDCA was unable to stop acute cellular rejection in the treatment group (Pageaux et al., 1995; Keiding et al., 1997; Fleckenstein et al., 1998). However, in one study, the addition of UDCA to the immunosuppression regimen led to improved 90-day and 1-year survival, a reduction in acute cellular rejection episodes, and a shorter hospital stay (Barnes et al., 1997).

- *Alcoholic Liver Disease:* In a human hepatocyte cell line and in rat liver mitochondria, UDCA prevented the damage caused by ethanol (Lazaridis et al., 2001). UDCA (15 mg/kg per day) for 4 weeks improved liver tests in the treatment group compared to the control subjects in a placebo-controlled cross-over study of patients with alcoholic cirrhosis (Plevris et al., 1991). However, in order to assess this preliminary report, randomized controlled trials are required.

A Closer Look

Non-Alcoholic Fatty Liver Disease (NAFLD)

Non-alcoholic fatty Liver Disease (NAFLD) is a condition characterized by excessive fat accumulation in the liver not caused by alcohol consumption. It encompasses a spectrum of liver conditions ranging from simple steatosis, where fat builds up in liver cells without causing significant inflammation or damage, to non-alcoholic steatohepatitis (NASH), which involves inflammation and liver cell damage. Over time, NASH can progress to fibrosis (scarring), cirrhosis, and liver cancer. NAFLD is increasingly recognized as the most common liver disorder in Western countries, with its prevalence closely linked to the rising rates of obesity, type 2 diabetes, and metabolic syndrome. The condition is often asymptomatic in its early stages, making it challenging to diagnose without medical screening. Symptoms, if they do appear, may include fatigue, weakness, and right upper abdominal pain.

Risk factors for NAFLD include obesity, insulin resistance, high blood sugar (as seen in type 2 diabetes), and elevated levels of fats in the blood (such as triglycerides). Genetics and lifestyle factors, such as diet and physical inactivity, also play significant roles. The pathogenesis of NAFLD involves a complex interplay of metabolic, genetic, and environmental factors. The "two-hit" hypothesis is a widely accepted explanation, where the "first hit" involves insulin resistance leading to fat accumulation in the liver, and the "second hit" includes oxidative stress, inflammation, and mitochondrial dysfunction, which contribute to liver injury and NASH development.

Diagnosis of NAFLD typically starts with blood tests that reveal elevated liver enzymes, although normal enzyme levels do not exclude the disease. Imaging studies, such as ultrasound, CT scans, or MRI, can detect liver fat, but liver biopsy remains the gold standard for diagnosing NASH and assessing liver fibrosis. Given the invasive nature of biopsy, non-invasive methods like transient elastography (FibroScan) and blood markers are increasingly used for assessing liver stiffness and fibrosis.

Treatment for NAFLD focuses primarily on lifestyle modifications, as there are no specific medications approved for the condition. Weight loss through diet and exercise is the cornerstone of management and can significantly reduce liver fat, inflammation, and fibrosis. A weight reduction of 7–10% is often recommended for meaningful improvement. Dietary changes, particularly the adoption of a Mediterranean diet rich in fruits, vegetables, whole grains, and healthy fats, are beneficial. Regular physical activity, aiming for at least 150 minutes of moderate-intensity exercise per week, is also crucial. In some cases, medications that improve insulin sensitivity, such as metformin or pioglitazone, and those targeting dyslipidemia, like statins, may be used, although their efficacy specifically for NAFLD remains under investigation.

Ongoing research is exploring novel therapeutic targets, including agents that reduce liver fat, alleviate inflammation, and prevent fibrosis. Given the potential for NAFLD to progress to severe liver disease, early detection and intervention are vital. Public health strategies to combat obesity and metabolic syndrome, along with individual patient management, are essential components in addressing the growing burden of NAFLD. As understanding of the disease improves, a multifaceted approach integrating lifestyle changes, medical management, and possibly new pharmacological treatments holds promise for better outcomes in patients with NAFLD.

Summary

- Liver disease covers a complex spectrum of stages that includes steatosis, steatohepatitis, and in severe cases fibrosis and cirrhosis. Liver fibrosis progression is characterized by the perpetuation of necrosis of the parenchyma cells and alterations in the composition of the extracellular matrix (ECM).
- NAC, the acetylated precursor of both the amino acid L-cysteine and reduced glutathione (GSH) has been in clinical use for more than 30 years, mainly as a mucolytic agent in chronic respiratory illnesses, as well as an antidote for hepatotoxicity caused by acetaminophen overdose.
- Liver fibrosis is a nonphysiological scarring process where an excessive ECM deposition leads to irreversible tissue damage and failure or disturbance of proper liver function.
- Nonalcoholic fatty liver disease (NAFLD) is one of the most prevalent forms of chronic liver disease. Within this disease, nonalcoholic steatohepatitis (NASH), is a condition characterized by chronic and progressive liver damage that may lead to fibrosis, cirrhosis, HCC, and death.
- NAC is a drug generally recognized as safe and well tolerated even at high doses. At oral dosages of 1200 mg twice daily or lower, NAC is well-tolerated and permitted. At these doses, side effects are unusual but may include vomiting, nausea, diarrhea, flushing, epigastric pain, and constipation.
- Ursodeoxycholic acid (UDCA) is widely used for the treatment of a variety of chronic cholestatic liver diseases. It has been used for centuries in traditional Chinese medicine as a remedy for liver diseases.
- Bile acids are acidic steroids that are synthesized from cholesterol within the hepatocytes. Natural bile acids in their protonated (or unionized) form are quite insoluble in water.
- UDCA, a hydrophilic nontoxic bile acid, becomes the predominant bile acid in serum and bile by competitively inhibiting the ileal absorption of natural, toxic endogenous bile salts
- Hydrophobic bile acids damage cell membranes and exert extracellular cytotoxicity at concentrations that are present in bile.
- PBC is a chronic liver disease characterized by progressive immune-mediated destruction of the small-to-mediumsized bile ducts, resulting in chronic cholestasis, portal inflammation, and fibrosis that can lead to cirrhosis and, ultimately, liver failure

References

1. Abdoli, N., Azarmi, Y., & Eghbal, M. A. (2014). Protective effects of N-acetylcysteine against the statin's cytotoxicity in freshly isolated rat hepatocytes. *Advances in Pharmacological Sciences, 4*, 249–254.
2. Acharya, M., & Lau-Cam, C. A. (2010). Comparison of the protective actions of N-acetylcysteine, hypotaurine, and taurine against acetaminophen-induced hepatotoxicity in the rat. *Journal of Biomedical Science, 17*(Suppl. 1), S35.
3. Ajmo, J. M., Liang, X., Rogers, C. Q., Pennock, B., & You, M. (2008). Resveratrol alleviates alcoholic fatty liver in mice. *American Journal of Physiology–Gastrointestinal and Liver Physiology, 295*, G833–G842.

4. Alipour, M., Omri, A., Smith, M. G., & Suntres, Z. E. (2007). Prophylactic effect of liposomal N-acetylcysteine against LPS-induced liver injuries. *Journal of Endotoxin Research, 13*, 297–304.

5. Allina, J., Hu, B., Sullivan, D. M., Fiel, M. I., Thung, S. N., Bronk, S. F., et al. (2006). T cell targeting and phagocytosis of apoptotic biliary epithelial cells in primary biliary cirrhosis. *Journal of Autoimmunity, 27*, 232–241.

6. Almeida, L., Vaz-Da-Silva, M., Falcao, A., Soares, E., Costa, R., Loureiro, A. I., Fernandes-Lopes, C., Rocha, J. F., Nunes, T., Wright, L., & Soares-Da-Silva, P. (2009). Pharmacokinetic and safety profile of trans-resveratrol in a rising multiple-dose study in healthy volunteers. *Molecular Nutrition & Food Research, 53*(Suppl. 1), S7–S15.

7. Andrus, J. P., Herzenberg, L. A., & Derosa, S. C. (2001). Effects of legislation restricting pack sizes of paracetamol on self-poisoning. Paracetamol should be packaged with its antidote. *BMJ, 323*, 634.

8. Angulo, P., Batts, K. P., Therneau, T. M., Jorgensen, R. A., Dickson, E. R., & Lindor, K. D. (1999). Long-term ursodeoxycholic acid delays histological progression in primary biliary cirrhosis. *Hepatology, 29*, 644–647.

9. Appelboam, A. V., Dargan, P. I., & Knighton, J. (2002). Fatal anaphylactoid reaction to N-acetylcysteine: Caution in patients with asthma. *Emergency Medicine Journal, 19*, 594–595.

10. Ara, C., Kirimlioglu, H., Karabulut, A. B., Coban, S., Ay, S., Harputluoglu, M., Kirimlioglu, V., & Yilmaz, S. (2005). Protective effect of resveratrol against oxidative stress in cholestasis. *Journal of Surgical Research, 127*, 112–117.

11. Arteel, G. E. (2003). Oxidants and antioxidants in alcohol-induced liver disease. *Gastroenterology, 124*, 778–790.

12. Atkuri, K. R., Mantovani, J. J., & Herzenberg, L. A. (2007). N-Acetylcysteine: A safe antidote for cysteine/glutathione deficiency. *Current Opinion in Pharmacology, 7*, 355–359.

13. Bachrach, W. H., & Hofmann, A. F. (1982). Ursodeoxycholic acid in the treatment of cholesterol cholelithiasis. Part I. *Digestive Diseases and Sciences, 27*, 737–761.

14. Bagul, P. K., Middela, H., Matapally, S., Padiya, R., Bastia, T., Madhusudana, K., Reddy, B. R., Chakravarty, S., & Banerjee, S. K. (2012). Attenuation of insulin resistance, metabolic syndrome, and hepatic oxidative stress by resveratrol in fructose-fed rats. *Pharmacological Research, 66*, 260–268.

15. Ballot, E., Bandin, O., Chazouilleres, O., Johanet, C., & Poupon, R. (2004). Immune response to lipopolysaccharide in primary biliary cirrhosis and autoimmune diseases. *Journal of Autoimmunity, 22*, 153–158.

16. Barnes, D., Talenti, D., Cammell, G., Goormastic, M., Farquhar, L., Henderson, M., et al. (1997). A randomized clinical trial of ursodeoxycholic acid as adjuvant treatment to prevent liver transplant rejection. *Hepatology, 26*, 853–857.

17. Basaranoglu, M., Basaranoglu, G., & Senturk, H. (2013). From fatty liver to fibrosis: A tale of "second hit". *World Journal of Gastroenterology, 19*, 1158–1165.

18. Baur, J. A., Pearson, K. J., Price, N. L., Jamieson, H. A., Lerin, C., Kalra, A., Prabhu, V. V., Allard, J. S., Lopez-Lluch, G., Lewis, K., Pistell, P. J., Poosala, S., Becker, K. G., Boss, O., Gwinn, D., Wang, M., Ramaswamy, S., Fishbein, K. W., Spencer, R. G., Lakatta, E. G., Le Couteur, D., Shaw,

R. J., Navas, P., Puigserver, P., Ingram, D. K., De Cabo, R., & Sinclair, D. A. (2006). Resveratrol improves health and survival of mice on a high-calorie diet. *Nature, 444*, 337–342.

19. Bavarsad Shahripour, R., Harrigan, M. R., & Alexandrov, A. V. (2014). N-acetylcysteine (NAC) in neurological disorders: Mechanisms of action and therapeutic opportunities. *Brain and Behavior, 4*, 108–122.

20. Beau, P., Labat-Labourdette, J., Ingrand, P., & Beauchant, M. (1994). Is ursodeoxycholic acid an effective therapy for total parenteral nutrition-related liver disease? *Journal of Hepatology, 20*, 240–244.

21. Bergquist, A., Ekbom, A., Olsson, R., Kornfeldt, D., Loof, L., Danielsson, A., et al. (2002). Hepatic and extrahepatic malignancies in primary sclerosing cholangitis. *Journal of Hepatology, 36*, 321–327.

22. Bernstein, C., Payne, C. M., Bernstein, H., & Garewal, H. (2002). Activation of the metallothionein IIA promoter and other key stress response elements by ursodeoxycholate in HepG2 cells: Relevance to the cytoprotective function of ursodeoxycholate. *Pharmacology, 65*, 2–9.

23. Bertelli, A., Bertelli, A. A., Gozzini, A., & Giovannini, L. (1998). Plasma and tissue resveratrol concentrations and pharmacological activity. *Drugs Experimental and Clinical Research, 24*, 133–138.

24. Beuers, U. (2006). Drug insight: Mechanisms and sites of action of ursodeoxycholic acid in cholestasis. *Nature Clinical Practice Gastroenterology & Hepatology, 3*, 318–328.

25. Beuers, U., Spengler, U., Kruis, W., Aydemir, U., Wiebecke, B., Heldwein, W., et al. (1992a). Ursodeoxycholic acid for treatment of primary sclerosing cholangitis: A placebo-controlled trial. *Hepatology, 16*, 707–714.

26. Beuers, U., Spengler, U., Zwiebel, F. M., Pauletzki, J., Fischer, S., & Paumgartner, G. (1992b). Effect of ursodeoxycholic acid on the kinetics of the major hydrophobic bile acids in health and in chronic cholestatic liver disease. *Hepatology, 15*, 603–608.

27. Bishayee, A., & Dhir, N. (2009). Resveratrol-mediated chemoprevention of diethyl nitrosamine-initiated hepatocarcinogenesis: Inhibition of cell proliferation and induction of apoptosis. *Chemical Biology & Interactions, 179*, 131–144.

28. Bishayee, A., Waghray, A., Barnes, K. F., Mbimba, T., Bhatia, D., Chatterjee, M., & Darvesh, A. S. (2010). Suppression of the inflammatory cascade is implicated in resveratrol chemoprevention of experimental hepatocarcinogenesis. *Pharmaceutical Research, 27*, 1080–1091.

29. Blachier, M., Leleu, H., Peck-Radosavljevic, M., Valla, D. C., & Roudot-Thoraval, F. (2013). The burden of liver disease in Europe: A review of available epidemiological data. *Journal of Hepatology, 58*, 593–608.

30. Brites, D., & Rodrigues, C. M. (1998). Elevated levels of bile acids in colostrum of patients with cholestasis of pregnancy are decreased following ursodeoxycholic acid therapy. *Journal of Hepatology, 29*, 743–751.

31. Brites, D., Rodrigues, C. M., Oliveira, N., Cardoso, M., & Graca, L. M. (1998). Correction of maternal serum bile acid profile during ursodeoxycholic acid therapy in cholestasis of pregnancy. *Journal of Hepatology, 28*, 91–98.

32. Brown, V. A., Patel, K. R., Viskaduraki, M., Crowell, J. A., Perloff, M., Booth, T. D., Vasilinin, G., Sen, A., Schinas, A. M., Piccirilli, G., Brown, K., Steward, W. P., Gescher, A. J., & Brenner, D.

E. (2010). Repeat dose study of the cancer chemo preventive agent resveratrol in healthy volunteers: Safety, pharmacokinetics, and effect on the insulin-like growth factor axis. *Cancer Research, 70*, 9003–9011.

33. Cai, Z., Lou, Q., Wang, F., Li, E., Sun, J., Fang, H., Xi, J., & Ju, L. (2015). N-acetylcysteine protects against liver injury induced by carbon tetrachloride via activation of the Nrf2/HO-1 pathway. *International Journal of Clinical and Experimental Pathology, 8*, 8655–8662.

34. Calmus, Y., Gane, P., Rouger, P., & Poupon, R. (1990). Hepatic expression of class I and class II major histocompatibility complex molecules in primary biliary cirrhosis: Effect of ursodeoxycholic acid. *Hepatology, 11*, 12–15.

35. Carbone, M., Mells, G. F., Pells, G., Dawwas, M. F., Newton, J. L., Heneghan, M. A., et al. (2013). Sex and age are determinants of the clinical phenotype of primary biliary cirrhosis and response to ursodeoxycholic acid. *Gastroenterology, 144*, 560–569, e567; quiz e513–564.

36. Caro, A. A., Bell, M., Ejiofor, S., Zurcher, G., Petersen, D. R., & Ronis, M. J. (2014). N-acetylcysteine inhibits the up-regulation of mitochondrial biogenesis genes in livers from rats fed ethanol chronically. *Alcoholism: Clinical and Experimental Research, 38*, 2896–2906.

37. Carter, L. G., D'Orazio, J. A., & Pearson, K. J. (2014). Resveratrol and cancer: Focus on in vivo evidence. *Endocrine-Related Cancer, 21*, R209–R225.

38. Cavazza, A., Caballeria, L., Floreani, A., Farinati, F., Bruguera, M., Caroli, D., et al. (2009). Incidence, risk factors, and survival of hepatocellular carcinoma in primary biliary cirrhosis: Comparative analysis from two centers. *Hepatology, 50*, 1162–1168.

39. Chapman, R., Fevery, J., Kalloo, A., Nagorney, D. M., Boberg, K. M., Shneider, B., et al. (2010). Diagnosis and management of primary sclerosing cholangitis. *Hepatology, 51*, 660–678.

40. Chapter 10

41. Chauhan, A. S. (2015). Dendrimer nanotechnology for enhanced formulation and controlled delivery of resveratrol. *Annals of the New York Academy of Sciences, 1348*, 134–140.

42. Chavez, E., Reyes-Gordillo, K., Segovia, J., Shibayama, M., Tsutsumi, V., Vergara, P., Moreno, M. G., & Muriel, P. (2008). Resveratrol prevents fibrosis, NF-kB activation and TGF-b increases induced by chronic CCl4 treatment in rats. *Journal of Applied Toxicology, 28*, 35–43.

43. Chen, C. Y., Tsao, P. N., Chen, H. L., Chou, H. C., Hsieh, W. S., & Chang, M. H. (2004). Ursodeoxycholic acid (UDCA) therapy in very low-birth-weight infants with parenteral nutrition-associated cholestasis. *Journal of Pediatrics, 145*, 317–321.

44. Chen, W., Liu, J., & Gluud, C. (2007). Bile acids for viral hepatitis. *Cochrane Database of Systematic Reviews*, CD003181.

45. Chen, X., He, H., Wang, G., Yang, B., Ren, W., Ma, L., & Yu, Q. (2007). Stereospecific determination of cis- and trans-resveratrol in rat plasma by HPLC: Application to pharmacokinetic studies. *Biomedical Chromatography, 21*, 257–265.

46. Cheng, K., Ashby, D., & Smyth, R. L. (2014). Ursodeoxycholic acid for cystic fibrosis-related liver disease. *Cochrane Database of Systematic Reviews*, 12, CD000222.

47. Cho, A. R., Chun, Y. G., Kim, B. K., & Park, D. J. (2014). Preparation of chitosan-TPP microspheres as resveratrol carriers. *Journal of Food Science, 79*, E568–E576.

48. Cho, S. J., Jung, U. J., & Choi, M. S. (2012). Differential effects of low-dose resveratrol on adiposity and hepatic steatosis in diet-induced obese mice. *British Journal of Nutrition, 108*, 2166–2175.

49. Chughlay, M. F., Kramer, N., Spearman, C. W., Werfalli, M., & Cohen, K. (2016). N-acetylcysteine for non-paracetamol drug-induced liver injury: A systematic review. *British Journal of Clinical Pharmacology*. https://doi.org/10.1111/bcp.12880.

50. Colombo, C., Apostolo, M. G., Assaisso, M., Roman, B., & Bottani, P. (1992). Liver disease in cystic fibrosis. *Netherlands Journal of Medicine, 41*, 119–122.

51. Colombo, C., Setchell, K. D., Podda, M., Crosignani, A., Roda, A., Curcio, L., et al. (1990). Effects of ursodeoxycholic acid therapy for liver disease associated with cystic fibrosis. *Journal of Pediatrics, 117*, 482–489.

52. Combes, B., Carithers Jr., R. L., Maddrey, W. C., Lin, D., McDonald, M. F., Wheeler, D. E., et al. (1995). A randomized, double-blind, placebo-controlled trial of ursodeoxycholic acid in primary biliary cirrhosis. *Hepatology, 22*, 759–766.

53. Corpechot, C., Abenavoli, L., Rabahi, N., Chretien, Y., Andreani, T., Johanet, C., et al. (2008). Biochemical response to ursodeoxycholic acid and long-term prognosis in primary biliary cirrhosis. *Hepatology, 48*, 871–877.

54. Corpechot, C., Carrat, F., Bahr, A., Chretien, Y., Poupon, R. E., & Poupon, R. (2005). The effect of ursodeoxycholic acid therapy on the natural course of primary biliary cirrhosis. *Gastroenterology, 128*, 297–303.

55. Cotting, J., Lentze, M. J., & Reichen, J. (1990). Effects of ursodeoxycholic acid treatment on nutrition and liver function in patients with cystic fibrosis and longstanding cholestasis. *Gut, 31*, 918–921.

56. Crosignani, A., Podda, M., Battezzati, P. M., Bertolini, E., Zuin, M., Watson, D., et al. (1991). Changes in bile acid composition in patients with primary biliary cirrhosis induced by ursodeoxycholic acid administration. *Hepatology, 14*, 1000–1007.

57. Culley, C. M., & Krenzelok, E. P. (2005). A clinical and pharmacoeconomic justification for intravenous acetylcysteine: A US perspective. *Toxicology Reviews, 24*, 131–143.

58. Cursio, R., & Gugenheim, J. (2012). Ischemia-reperfusion injury and ischemic-type biliary lesions following liver transplantation. *Journal of Transplantation, 2012*, 164329.

59. Davit-Spraul, A., Fabre, M., Branchereau, S., Baussan, C., Gonzales, E., Stieger, B., et al. (2010). ATP8B1 and ABCB11 analysis in 62 children with normal gamma-glutamyl transferase progressive familial intrahepatic cholestasis (PFIC): Phenotypic differences between PFIC1 and PFIC2 and natural history. *Hepatology, 51*, 1645–1655.

60. De Marco, G., Sordino, D., Bruzzese, E., Di Caro, S., Mambretti, D., Tramontano, A., et al. (2006). Early treatment with ursodeoxycholic acid for cholestasis in children on parenteral nutrition because of primary intestinal failure. *Alimentary Pharmacology & Therapeutics, 24*, 387–394.

61. De Souza, I. C., Martins, L. A., De Vasconcelos, M., De Oliveira, C. M., Barbe-Tuana, F., Andrade, C. B., Pettenuzzo, L. F., Borojevic, R., Margis, R., Guaragna, R., & Guma, F. C. (2015). Resveratrol regulates the quiescence-like induction of activated stellate cells by modulating the PPARγ/SIRT1 ratio. *Journal of Cellular Biochemistry, 116*, 2304–2312.

62. Delmas, D., Jannin, B., Cherkaoui Malki, M., & Latruffe, N. (2000). Inhibitory effect of resveratrol on the proliferation of human and rat hepatic derived cell lines. *Oncology Reports, 7*, 847–852.

63. Desmond, C. P., Wilson, J., Bailey, M., Clark, D., & Roberts, S. K. (2007). The benign course of liver disease in adults with cystic fibrosis and the effect of ursodeoxycholic acid. *Liver International, 27*, 1402–1408.

64. Dhouib, I. E., Annabi, A., Jallouli, M., Elfazaa, S., & Lasram, M. M. (2016). A minireview on N-acetylcysteine: An old drug with new approaches. *Life Sciences, 2*, 30152–30157.

65. Dodd, S., Dean, O., Copolov, D. L., Malhi, G. S., & Berk, M. (2008). N-acetylcysteine for antioxidant therapy: Pharmacology and clinical utility. *Expert Opinion on Biological Therapy, 8*, 1955–1962.

66. Dorsch, W., Auch, E., & Powerlowicz, P. (1987). Adverse effects of acetylcysteine on human and guinea pig bronchial asthma in vivo and on human fibroblasts and leukocytes in vitro. *International Archives of Allergy and Applied Immunology, 82*, 33–39.

67. Dufour, J. F., Oneta, C. M., Gonvers, J. J., Bihl, F., Cerny, A., Cereda, J. M., et al. (2006). Randomized placebo-controlled trial of ursodeoxycholic acid with vitamin E in nonalcoholic steatohepatitis. *Clinical Gastroenterology and Hepatology, 4*, 1537–1543.

68. Eaton, J. E., Silveira, M. G., Pardi, D. S., Sinakos, E., Kowdley, K. V., Luketic, V. A., et al. (2011). High-dose ursodeoxycholic acid is associated with the development of colorectal neoplasia in patients with ulcerative colitis and primary sclerosing cholangitis. *American Journal of Gastroenterology, 106*, 1638–1645.

69. Eriksson, L. S., Olsson, R., Glauman, H., Prytz, H., Befrits, R., Ryden, B. O., et al. (1997). Ursodeoxycholic acid treatment in patients with primary biliary cirrhosis: A Swedish multicenter, double-blind, randomized controlled study. *Scandinavian Journal of Gastroenterology, 32*, 179–186.

70. Essell, J. H., Schroeder, M. T., Harman, G. S., Halvorson, R., Lew, V., Callander, N., et al. (1998). Ursodiol prophylaxis against hepatic complications of allogeneic bone marrow transplantation: A randomized, double-blind, placebo-controlled trial. *Annals of Internal Medicine, 128*, 975–981.

71. European Association for the Study of the Liver. (2009). EASL Clinical Practice Guidelines: Management of cholestatic liver diseases. *Journal of Hepatology, 51*, 237–267.

72. Fabbri, C., Marchetto, S., Pezzoli, A., Accogli, E., Fusaroli, P., Azzaroli, F., et al. (2000). Efficacy of ursodeoxycholic acid in association with alpha-interferon for chronic hepatitis C in alpha-interferon non-responder patients. *European Journal of Gastroenterology & Hepatology, 12*, 511–515.

73. Farraye, F. A., Odze, R. D., Eaden, J., Itzkowitz, S. H., McCabe, R. P., Dassopoulos, T., et al. (2010). AGA medical position statement on the diagnosis and management of colorectal neoplasia in inflammatory bowel disease. *Gastroenterology, 138*, 738–745.

74. Festi, D., Montagnani, M., Azzaroli, F., Lodato, F., Mazzella, G., Roda, A., et al. (2007). Clinical efficacy and effectiveness of ursodeoxycholic acid in cholestatic liver diseases. *Current Clinical Pharmacology, 2*, 155–177.

75. Fleckenstein, J. F., Paredes, M., & Thuluvath, P. J. (1998). A prospective, randomized, double-blind trial evaluating the efficacy of ursodeoxycholic acid in prevention of liver transplant rejection. *Liver Transplantation and Surgery, 4*, 276–279.

76. Floreani, A., Franceschet, I., Perini, L., Cazzagon, N., Gershwin, M. E., & Bowlus, C. L. (2015). New therapies for primary biliary cirrhosis. *Clinical Reviews in Allergy & Immunology, 48*, 263–272.

77. Fried, R. H., Murakami, C. S., Fisher, L. D., Willson, R. A., Sullivan, K. M., & McDonald, G. B. (1992). Ursodeoxycholic acid treatment of refractory chronic graft-versus-host disease of the liver. *Annals of Internal Medicine, 116*, 624–629.

78. Friedman, S. L. (2000). Molecular regulation of hepatic fibrosis, an integrated cellular response to tissue injury. *Journal of Biological Chemistry, 275*, 2247–2250.

79. Friedman, S. L., Maher, J. J., & Bissell, D. M. (2000). Mechanisms and therapy of hepatic fibrosis: Report of the AASLD Single Topic Basic Research Conference. *Hepatology, 32*, 1403–1408.

80. Furukawa, S., Fujita, T., Shimabukuro, M., Iwaki, M., Yamada, Y., Nakajima, Y., Nakayama, O., Makishima, M., Matsuda, M., & Shimomura, I. (2004). Increased oxidative stress in obesity and its impact on metabolic syndrome. *Journal of Clinical Investigation, 114*, 1752–1761.

81. Galicia-Moreno, M., & Gutierrez-Reyes, G. (2014). The role of oxidative stress in the development of alcoholic liver disease. *Revista de Gastroenterología de México, 79*, 135–144.

82. Galicia-Moreno, M., Favari, L., & Muriel, P. (2012). Antifibrotic and antioxidant effects of N-acetylcysteine in an experimental cholestatic model. *European Journal of Gastroenterology & Hepatology, 24*, 179–185.

83. Galicia-Moreno, M., Rodriguez-Rivera, A., Reyes-Gordillo, K., Segovia, J., Shibayama, M., Tsutsumi, V., Vergara, P., Moreno, M. G., & Muriel, P. (Eds.). (2009). N-Acetylcysteine prevents carbon tetrachloride-induced liver cirrhosis: Role of liver transforming growth factor-beta and oxidative stress. *Journal of Hepatology, 51*(Supplement), 135–144.

84. Gao, B., & Bataller, R. (2011). Alcoholic liver disease: Pathogenesis and new therapeutic targets. *Gastroenterology, 141*, 1572–1585.

85. Geenes, V. L., Dixon, P. H., Chambers, J., Raguz, S., Marin, J. J., Bhakoo, K. K., et al. (2011). Characterisation of the nuclear receptors FXR, PXR and CAR in normal and cholestatic placenta. *Placenta, 32*, 535–537.

86. Geenes, V., Lovgren-Sandblom, A., Benthin, L., Lawrance, D., Chambers, J., Gurung, V., et al. (2014). The reversed feto-maternal bile acid gradient in intrahepatic cholestasis of pregnancy is corrected by ursodeoxycholic acid. *PLoS One, 9*, e83828.

87. Gnoni, G. V., & Paglialonga, G. (2009). Resveratrol inhibits fatty acid and triacylglycerol synthesis in rat hepatocytes. *European Journal of Clinical Investigation, 39*, 211–218.

88. Godichaud, S., Krisa, S., Couronne, B., Dubuisson, L., Merillon, J. M., Desmouliere, A., & Rosenbaum, J. (2000). Deactivation of cultured human liver myofibroblasts by trans-resveratrol, a grapevine-derived polyphenol. *Hepatology, 31*, 922–931.

89. Gokmen, T., Oguz, S. S., Bozdag, S., Erdeve, O., Uras, N., & Dilmen, U. (2012). A controlled trial of erythromycin and UDCA in premature infants during parenteral nutrition in minimizing feeding intolerance and liver function abnormalities. *Journal of Perinatology, 32*, 123–128.

90. Gong, G., Waris, G., Tanveer, R., & Siddiqui, A. (2001). Human hepatitis C virus NS5A protein alters intracellular calcium levels, induces oxidative stress, and activates STAT-3 and NF-kB. *Proceedings of the National Academy of Sciences U.S.A., 98*, 9599–9604.

91. Gong, Y., Huang, Z., Christensen, E., & Gluud, C. (2007). Ursodeoxycholic acid for patients with primary biliary cirrhosis: An updated systematic review and meta-analysis of randomized clinical trials using Bayesian approach as sensitivity analyses. *American Journal of Gastroenterology, 102*, 1799–1807.
92. Goulis, J., Leandro, G., & Burroughs, A. K. (1999). Randomized controlled trials of ursodeoxycholic-acid therapy for primary biliary cirrhosis: A meta-analysis. *Lancet, 354*, 1053–1060.
93. Grand'Maison, S., Durand, M., & Mahone, M. (2014). The effects of ursodeoxycholic acid treatment for intrahepatic cholestasis of pregnancy on maternal and fetal outcomes: A meta-analysis including non-randomized studies. *Journal of Obstetrics and Gynaecology Canada, 36*, 632–641.
94. Guldutuna, S., Zimmer, G., Imhof, M., Bhatti, S., You, T., & Leuschner, U. (1993). Molecular aspects of membrane stabilization by ursodeoxycholate. *Gastroenterology, 104*, 1736–1744.
95. Gurung, V., Middleton, P., Milan, S. J., Hague, W., & Thornton, J. G. (2013). Interventions for treating cholestasis in pregnancy. *Cochrane Database of Systematic Reviews, 6*, CD000493.
96. Hanczko, R., Fernandez, D. R., Doherty, E., Qian, Y., Vas, G., Niland, B., Telarico, T., Garba, A., Banerjee, S., Middleton, F. A., Barrett, D., Barcza, M., Banki, K., Landas, S. K., & Perl, A. (2009). Prevention of hepatocarcinogenesis and increased susceptibility to acetaminophen-induced liver failure in transaldolase-deficient mice by N-acetylcysteine. *Journal of Clinical Investigation, 119*, 1546–1557.
97. Harrison, P. M., Wendon, J. A., Gimson, A. E., Alexander, G. J., & Williams, R. (1991). Improvement by acetylcysteine of hemodynamics and oxygen transport in fulminant hepatic failure. *New England Journal of Medicine, 324*, 1852–1857.
98. Heathcote, E. J., Cauch-Dudek, K., Walker, V., Bailey, R. J., Elendis, L. M., Ghent, C. N., et al. (1994). The Canadian multicenter double-blind randomized controlled trial of ursodeoxycholic acid in primary biliary cirrhosis. *Hepatology, 19*, 1149–1156.
99. Heuman, D. M., & Bajaj, R. (1994). Ursodeoxycholate conjugates protect against disruption of cholesterol-rich membranes by bile salts. *Gastroenterology, 106*, 1333–1341.
100. Higgs, M. R., Chouteau, P., & Lerat, H. (2014). "Liver let die": Oxidative DNA damage and hepatotropic viruses. *Journal of General Virology, 95*, 991–1004.
101. Hirano, F., Tanaka, H., Makino, Y., Okamoto, K., & Makino, I (1996). Effects of ursodeoxycholic acid and chenodeoxycholic acid on major histocompatibility complex class I gene expression. *Journal of Gastroenterology, 31*, 55–60.
102. Hofmann, A. F. (1994). Pharmacology of ursodeoxycholic acid, an enterohepatic drug. *Scandinavian Journal of Gastroenterology. Supplement, 204*, 1–15.
103. Holdiness, M. R. (1991). Clinical pharmacokinetics of N-acetylcysteine. *Clinical Pharmacokinetics, 20*, 123–134.
104. Howells, L. M., Berry, D. P., Elliott, P. J., Jacobson, E. W., Hoffmann, E., Hegarty, B., Brown, K., Steward, W. P., & Gescher, A. J. (2011). Phase I randomized, double-blind pilot study of micronized resveratrol (SRT501) in patients with hepatic metastases: Safety, pharmacokinetics, and pharmacodynamics. *Cancer Prevention Research (Phila), 4*, 1419–1425.

105. Howitz, K. T., Bitterman, K. J., Cohen, H. Y., Lamming, D. W., Lavu, S., Wood, J. G., Zipkin, R. E., Chung, P., Kisielewski, A., Zhang, L. L., Scherer, B., & Sinclair, D. A. (2003). Small molecule activators of sirtuins extend *Saccharomyces cerevisiae* lifespan. *Nature, 425*, 191–196.

106. Jackson, H., Solaymani-Dodaran, M., Card, T. R., Aithal, G. P., Logan, R., & West, J. (2007). Influence of ursodeoxycholic acid on the mortality and malignancy associated with primary biliary cirrhosis: A population-based cohort study. *Hepatology, 46*, 1131–1137.

107. Jacquemin, E., De Vree, J. M., Cresteil, D., Sokal, E. M., Sturm, E., Dumont, M., et al. (2001). The wide spectrum of multidrug resistance 3 deficiency: From neonatal cholestasis to cirrhosis of adulthood. *Gastroenterology, 120*, 1448–1458.

108. Jacquemin, E., Hermans, D., Myara, A., Habes, D., Debray, D., Hadchouel, M., et al. (1997). Ursodeoxycholic acid therapy in pediatric patients with progressive familial intrahepatic cholestasis. *Hepatology, 25*, 519–523.

109. Jazrawi, R. P., de Caestecker, J. S., Goggin, P. M., Britten, A. J., Joseph, A. E., Maxwell, J. D., et al. (1994). Kinetics of hepatic bile acid handling in cholestatic liver disease: Effect of ursodeoxycholic acid. *Gastroenterology, 106*, 134–142.

110. Jeandet, P., Delaunois, B., Aziz, A., Donnez, D., Vasserot, Y., Cordelier, S., & Courot, E. (2012). Metabolic engineering of yeast and plants for the production of the biologically active hydroxystilbene, resveratrol. *Journal of Biomedical Biotechnology, 2012*, 579089.

111. Jegatheeswaran, S., & Siriwardena, A. K. (2010). Experimental and clinical evidence for modification of hepatic ischemia-reperfusion injury by N-acetylcysteine during major liver surgery. *HPB (Oxford), 13*, 71–78.

112. Jiang, L., Gu, Y., Ye, J., Liu, F., Zhao, Y., Wang, C., Xu, Y., Cao, X., Zhang, L., Dong, W., Li, F., Wang, J., Wang, H., & Li, Q. (2012). Resveratrol prevents hepatic steatosis induced by hepatitis C virus core protein. *Biotechnology Letters, 34*, 2205–2212.

113. Joutsiniemi, T., Timonen, S., Leino, R., Palo, P., & Ekblad, U. (2014). Ursodeoxycholic acid in the treatment of intrahepatic cholestasis of pregnancy: A randomized controlled trial. *Archives of Gynecology and Obstetrics, 289*, 541–547.

114. Kappler, M., Espach, C., Schweiger-Kabesch, A., Lang, T., Hartl, D., Hector, A., et al. (2012). Ursodeoxycholic acid therapy in cystic fibrosis liver disease: A retrospective long-term follow-up case-control study. *Alimentary Pharmacology & Therapeutics, 36*, 266–273.

115. Kasdallah-Grissa, A., Mornagui, B., Aouani, E., Hammami, M., El May, M., Gharbi, N., Kamoun, A., & El-Fazaa, S. (2007). Resveratrol, a red wine polyphenol, attenuates ethanol-induced oxidative stress in rat liver. *Life Sciences, 80*, 1033–1039.

116. Kawada, N., Seki, S., Inoue, M., & Kuroki, T. (1998). Effect of antioxidants, resveratrol, quercetin, and N-acetylcysteine, on the functions of cultured rat hepatic stellate cells and Kupffer cells. *Hepatology, 27*, 1265–1274.

117. Kawata, K., Kobayashi, Y., Souda, K., Kawamura, K., Sumiyoshi, S., Takahashi, Y., et al. (2010). Enhanced hepatic Nrf2 activation after ursodeoxycholic acid treatment in patients with primary biliary cirrhosis. *Antioxidants & Redox Signaling, 13*, 259–268.

118. Keiding, S., Hockerstedt, K., Bjoro, K., Bondesen, S., Hjortrup, A., Isoniemi, H., et al. (1997). The Nordic multicenter double-blind randomized controlled trial of prophylactic ursodeoxycholic acid in liver transplant patients. *Transplantation, 63*, 1591–1594.

119. Kessoku, T., Imajo, K., Honda, Y., Kato, T., Ogawa, Y., Tomeno, W., Kato, S., Mawatari, H., Fujita, K., Yoneda, M., Nagashima, Y., Saito, S., Wada, K., & Nakajima, A. (2016). Resveratrol ameliorates fibrosis and inflammation in a mouse model of nonalcoholic steatohepatitis. *Scientific Reports, 6*, 22251.

120. Khoshbaten, M., Aliasgarzadeh, A., Masnadi, K., Tarzamani, M. K., Farhang, S., Babaei, H., Kiani, J., Zaare, M., & Najafipoor, F. (2010). N-acetylcysteine improves liver function in patients with nonalcoholic fatty liver disease. *Hepatitis Monthly, 10*, 12–16.

121. Kobierski, S., Ofori-Kwakye, K., Muller, R. H., & Keck, C. M. (2009). Resveratrol nanosuspensions for dermal application: Production, characterization, and physical stability. *Pharmazie, 64*, 741–747.

122. Koga, H., Sakisaka, S., Ohishi, M., Sata, M., & Tanikawa, K. (1997). Nuclear DNA fragmentation and expression of Bcl-2 in primary biliary cirrhosis. *Hepatology, 25*, 1077–1084.

123. Kortsalioudaki, C., Taylor, R. M., Cheeseman, P., Bansal, S., Mieli-Vergani, G., & Dhawan, A. (2008). Safety and efficacy of N-acetylcysteine in children with non-acetaminophen-induced acute liver failure. *Liver Transplantation, 14*, 25–30.

124. Kountouras, J., Zavos, C., & Chatzopoulos, D. (2003). Apoptosis in hepatitis C. *Journal of Viral Hepatitis, 10*, 335–342.

125. Kromer, A., & Moosmann, B. (2009). Statin-induced liver injury involves cross-talk between cholesterol and selenoprotein biosynthetic pathways. *Molecular Pharmacology, 75*, 1421–1429.

126. Kuiper, E. M., Hansen, B. E., de Vries, R. A., den Ouden-Muller, J. W., van Ditzhuijsen, T. J., Haagsma, E. B., et al. (2009). Improved prognosis of patients with primary biliary cirrhosis that have a biochemical response to ursodeoxycholic acid. *Gastroenterology, 136*, 1281–1287.

127. Kullak-Ublick, G. A., Stieger, B., Hagenbuch, B., & Meier, P. J. (2000). Hepatic transport of bile salts. *Seminars in Liver Disease, 20*, 273–292.

128. Kumagi, T., Guindi, M., Fischer, S. E., Arenovich, T., Abdalian, R., Coltescu, C., et al. (2010). Baseline ductopenia and treatment response predict long-term histological progression in primary biliary cirrhosis. *American Journal of Gastroenterology, 105*, 2186–2194.

129. Lamireau, T., Monnereau, S., Martin, S., Marcotte, J. E., Winnock, M., & Alvarez, F. (2004). Epidemiology of liver disease in cystic fibrosis: A longitudinal study. *Journal of Hepatology, 41*, 920–925.

130. Lancaster, E. M., Hiatt, J. R., & Zarrinpar, A. (2015). Acetaminophen hepatotoxicity: An updated review. *Archives of Toxicology, 89*, 193–199.

131. Lancon, A., Delmas, D., Osman, H., Thenot, J. P., Jannin, B., & Latruffe, N. (2004). Human hepatic cell uptake of resveratrol: Involvement of both passive diffusion and carrier-mediated process. *Biochemistry and Biophysics Research Communications, 316*, 1132–1137.

132. Lanzini, A., De Tavonatti, M. G., Panarotto, B., Scalia, S., Mora, A., Benini, F., et al. (2003). Intestinal absorption of the bile acid analogue 75Se-homocholic acid-taurine is increased in primary biliary cirrhosis, and reverts to normal during ursodeoxycholic acid administration. *Gut, 52*, 1371–1375.

133. Lapenna, D., Ciofani, G., Festi, D., Neri, M., Pierdomenico, S. D., Giamberardino, M. A., et al. (2002). Antioxidant properties of ursodeoxycholic acid. *Biochemical Pharmacology, 64*, 1661–1667.

134. Laurin, J., Lindor, K. D., Crippin, J. S., Gossard, A., Gores, G. J., Ludwig, J., et al. (1996). Ursodeoxycholic acid or clofibrate in the treatment of non-alcohol-induced steatohepatitis: A pilot study. *Hepatology, 23*, 1464–1467.

135. Lazaridis, K. N., Gores, G. J., & Lindor, K. D. (2001). Ursodeoxycholic acid: Mechanisms of action and clinical use in hepatobiliary disorders. *Journal of Hepatology, 35*, 134–146.

136. Lee, W. M., Hynan, L. S., Rossaro, L., Fontana, R. J., Stravitz, R. T., Larson, A. M., Davern II, T. J., Murray, N. G., McCashland, T., Reisch, J. S., & Robuck, P. R. (2009). Intravenous N-acetylcysteine improves transplant-free survival in early-stage non-acetaminophen acute liver failure. *Gastroenterology, 137*, 856–864.

137. Leuschner, U. F., Lindenthal, B., Herrmann, G., Arnold, J. C., Rossle, M., Cordes, H. J., et al. (2010). High-dose ursodeoxycholic acid therapy for nonalcoholic steatohepatitis: A double-blind, randomized, placebo-controlled trial. *Hepatology, 52*, 472–479.

138. Leuschner, U., Leuschner, M., Sieratzki, J., Kurtz, W., & Hubner, K. (1985). Gallstone dissolution with ursodeoxycholic acid in patients with chronic active hepatitis and two years follow-up. A pilot study. *Digestive Diseases and Sciences, 30*, 642–649.

139. Levine, A., Maayan, A., Shamir, R., Dinari, G., Sulkes, J., & Sirotta, L. (1999). Parenteral nutrition-associated cholestasis in preterm neonates: Evaluation of ursodeoxycholic acid treatment. *Journal of Pediatric Endocrinology & Metabolism, 12*, 549–553.

140. Lim, Y. S., & Kim, W. R. (2008). The global impact of hepatic fibrosis and end-stage liver disease. *Clinical Liver Disease, 12*, 733–746.

141. Lindor, K. D., Dickson, E. R., Baldus, W. P., Jorgensen, R. A., Ludwig, J., Murtaugh, P. A., et al. (1994). Ursodeoxycholic acid in the treatment of primary biliary cirrhosis. *Gastroenterology, 106*, 1284–1290.

142. Lindor, K. D., Gershwin, M. E., Poupon, R., Kaplan, M., Bergasa, N. V., Heathcote, E. J., et al. (2009a). Primary biliary cirrhosis. *Hepatology, 50*, 291–308.

143. Lindor, K. D., Kowdley, K. V., & Harrison, M. E., American College of Gastroenterology. (2015). ACG clinical guideline: Primary sclerosing cholangitis. *American Journal of Gastroenterology, 110*, 646–659, quiz 660.

144. Lindor, K. D., Kowdley, K. V., Heathcote, E. J., Harrison, M. E., Jorgensen, R., Angulo, P., et al. (2004). Ursodeoxycholic acid for treatment of nonalcoholic steatohepatitis: Results of a randomized trial. *Hepatology, 39*, 770–778.

145. Lindor, K. D., Kowdley, K. V., Luketic, V. A., Harrison, M. E., McCashland, T., Befeler, A. S., et al. (2009b). High-dose ursodeoxycholic acid for the treatment of primary sclerosing cholangitis. *Hepatology, 50*, 808–814.

146. Lindstrom, L., Boberg, K. M., Wikman, O., Friis-Liby, I., Hultcrantz, R., Prytz, H., et al. (2012). High dose ursodeoxycholic acid in primary sclerosing cholangitis does not prevent colorectal neoplasia. *Alimentary Pharmacology & Therapeutics, 35*, 451–457.

147. Ljubuncic, P., Tanne, Z., & Bomzon, A. (2000). Ursodeoxycholic acid suppresses extent of lipid peroxidation in diseased liver in experimental cholestatic liver disease. *Digestive Diseases and Sciences, 45*, 1921–1928.

148. Long, L. H., Xue, C. Q., Shi, J. F., Dong, J. N., & Wang, L. (2015). Efficacy of hepatoprotective agents with or without antiviral drugs on liver function and fibrosis in patients with hepatitis B: A meta-analysis. *Hepatitis Monthly, 15*, 29052.

149. Lykavieris, P., van Mil, S., Cresteil, D., Fabre, M., Hadchouel, M., Klomp, L., et al. (2003). Progressive familial intrahepatic cholestasis type 1 and extrahepatic features: No catch-up of stature growth, exacerbation of diarrhea, and appearance of liver steatosis after liver transplantation. *Journal of Hepatology, 39*, 447–452.

150. Majano, P. L., Medina, J., Zubia, I., Sunyer, L., Lara-Pezzi, E., Maldonado-Rodriguez, A., Lopez-Cabrera, M., & Moreno-Otero, R. (2004). N-Acetyl-cysteine modulates inducible nitric oxide synthase gene expression in human hepatocytes. *Journal of Hepatology, 40*, 632–637.

151. Makino, I., Shinozaki, K., Yoshino, K., & Nakagawa, S. (1975). Dissolution of cholesterol gallstones by long-term administration of ursodeoxycholic acid. *Nihon Shokakibyo Gakkai Zasshi, 72*, 690–702.

152. Mant, T. G., Tempowski, J. H., Volans, G. N., & Talbot, J. C. (1984). Adverse reactions to acetylcysteine and effects of overdose. *British Medical Journal (Clinical Research Ed.), 289*, 217–219.

153. Marschall, H. U. (2015). Management of intrahepatic cholestasis of pregnancy. *Expert Review of Gastroenterology & Hepatology, 9*, 1273–1279.

154. Massey, V. L., & Arteel, G. E. (2012). Acute alcohol-induced liver injury. *Frontiers in Physiology, 3*, 193.

155. Mazzella, G., Rizzo, N., Salzetta, A., Iampieri, R., Bovicelli, L., & Roda, E. (1991). Management of intrahepatic cholestasis in pregnancy. *Lancet, 338*, 1594–1595.

156. Medina, J. F., Martinez, A., Vazquez, J. J., & Prieto, J. (1997). Decreased anion exchanger 2 immunoreactivity in the liver of patients with primary biliary cirrhosis. *Hepatology, 25*, 12–17.

157. Mercurio, F., & Manning, A. M. (1999). NF-kB as a primary regulator of the stress response. *Oncogene, 18*, 6163–6171.

158. Mignet, N., Seguin, J., & Chabot, G. G. (2013). Bioavailability of polyphenol liposomes: A challenge ahead. *Pharmaceutics, 5*, 457–471.

159. Millea, P. J. (2009). N-acetylcysteine: Multiple clinical applications. *American Family Physician, 80*, 265–269.

160. Mitsuyoshi, H., Nakashima, T., Sumida, Y., Yoh, T., Nakajima, Y., Ishikawa, H., et al. (1999). Ursodeoxycholic acid protects hepatocytes against oxidative injury via induction of antioxidants. *Biochemical and Biophysical Research Communications, 263*, 537–542.

161. Moreno-Otero, R., & Trapero-Marugan, M. (2010). Hepatoprotective effects of antioxidants in chronic hepatitis C. *World Journal of Gastroenterology, 16*, 1937–1938.

162. Moreno, C., Langlet, P., Hittelet, A., Lasser, L., Degre, D., Evrard, S., Colle, I., Lemmers, A., Deviere, J., & Le Moine, O. (2010). Enteral nutrition with or without N-acetylcysteine in the treatment of severe acute alcoholic hepatitis: A randomized multicenter controlled trial. *Journal of Hepatology, 53*, 1117–1122.

163. Moyer, K., & Balistreri, W. (2009). Hepatobiliary disease in patients with cystic fibrosis. *Current Opinion in Gastroenterology, 25*, 272–278.

164. Nishigaki, Y., Ohnishi, H., Moriwaki, H., & Muto, Y. (1996). Ursodeoxycholic acid corrects defective natural killer activity by inhibiting prostaglandin E2 production in primary biliary cirrhosis. *Digestive Diseases and Sciences, 41*, 1487–1493.

165. Nissar, A. U., Farrukh, M. R., Kaiser, P. J., Rafiq, R. A., Afnan, Q., & Bhushan, S. (2013). Effect of N-acetyl cysteine (NAC), an organosulfur compound from Allium plants, on experimentally induced hepatic prefibrogenic events in Wistar rats. *Phytomedicine, 20*, 828–833.

166. Nivet-Antoine, V., Cottart, C. H., Lemarechal, H., Vamy, M., Margaill, I., Beaudeux, J. L., Bonnefont-Rousselot, D., & Borderie, D. (2010). Transresveratrol downregulates Txnip overexpression occurring during liver ischemia-reperfusion. *Biochimie, 92*, 1766–1771.

167. Olsson, B., Johansson, M., Gabrielsson, J., & Bolme, P. (1988). Pharmacokinetics and bioavailability of reduced and oxidized N-acetylcysteine. *European Journal of Clinical Pharmacology, 34*, 77–82.

168. Orlando, R., Azzalini, L., Orando, S., & Lirussi, F. (2007). Bile acids for nonalcoholic fatty liver disease and/or steatohepatitis. *Cochrane Database of Systematic Reviews, CD005160*.

169. Pageaux, G. P., Blanc, P., Perrigault, P. F., Navarro, F., Fabre, J. M., Souche, B., et al. (1995). Failure of ursodeoxycholic acid to prevent acute cellular rejection after liver transplantation. *Journal of Hepatology, 23*, 119–122.

170. Palma, J., Reyes, H., Ribalta, J., Iglesias, J., Gonzalez, M. C., Hernandez, I., et al. (1992). Effects of ursodeoxycholic acid in patients with intrahepatic cholestasis of pregnancy. *Hepatology, 15*, 1043–1047.

171. Paolini, M., Pozzetti, L., Montagnani, M., Potenza, G., Sabatini, L., Antelli, A., et al. (2002). Ursodeoxycholic acid (UDCA) prevents DCA effects on male mouse liver via up-regulation of CYP and preservation of BSEP activities. *Hepatology, 36*, 305–314.

172. Papatheodoridis, G. V., Hadziyannis, E. S., Deutsch, M., & Hadziyannis, S. J. (2002). Ursodeoxycholic acid for primary biliary cirrhosis: Final results of a 12-year, prospective, randomized, controlled trial. *American Journal of Gastroenterology, 97*, 2063–2070.

173. Pardi, D. S., Loftus Jr., E. V., Kremers, W. K., Keach, J., & Lindor, K. D. (2003). Ursodeoxycholic acid as a chemopreventive agent in patients with ulcerative colitis and primary sclerosing cholangitis. *Gastroenterology, 124*, 889–893.

174. Pares, A. (2014). Old and novel therapies for primary biliary cirrhosis. *Seminars in Liver Disease, 34*, 341–351.

175. Pares, A., Caballeria, L., & Rodes, J. (2006). Excellent long-term survival in patients with primary biliary cirrhosis and biochemical response to ursodeoxycholic acid. *Gastroenterology, 130*, 715–720.

176. Pares, A., Caballeria, L., Rodes, J., Bruguera, M., Rodrigo, L., Garcia-Plaza, A., et al. (2000). Long-term effects of ursodeoxycholic acid in primary biliary cirrhosis: Results of a double-blind controlled multicentric trial. UDCA-Cooperative Group from the Spanish Association for the Study of the Liver. *Journal of Hepatology, 32*, 561–566.

177. Park, E. J., & Pezzuto, J. M. (2015). The pharmacology of resveratrol in animals and humans. *Biochimica et Biophysica Acta, 1852*, 1071–1113.

178. Paumgartner, G., & Beuers, U. (2002). Ursodeoxycholic acid in cholestatic liver disease: Mechanisms of action and therapeutic use revisited. *Hepatology, 36*, 525–531.

179. Paumgartner, G., & Beuers, U. (2004). Mechanisms of action and therapeutic efficacy of ursodeoxycholic acid in cholestatic liver disease. *Clinical Liver Disease, 8*, 67–81 vi.

180. Perl, A., Hanczko, R., Telarico, T., Oaks, Z., & Landas, S. (2011). Oxidative stress, inflammation, and carcinogenesis are controlled through the pentose phosphate pathway by transaldolase. *Trends in Molecular Medicine, 17*, 395–403.

181. Pietu, F., Guillaud, O., Walter, T., Vallin, M., Hervieu, V., Scoazec, J. Y., et al. (2012). Ursodeoxycholic acid with vitamin E in patients with nonalcoholic steatohepatitis: Long-term results. *Clinical Research in Hepatology & Gastroenterology, 36*, 146–155.

182. Piver, B., Berthou, F., Dreano, Y., & Lucas, D. (2001). Inhibition of CYP3A, CYP1A, and CYP2E1 activities by resveratrol and other non-volatile red wine components. *Toxicology Letters, 125*, 83–91.

183. Plevris, J. N., Hayes, P. C., & Bouchier, I. A. (1991). Ursodeoxycholic acid in the treatment of alcoholic liver disease. *European Journal of Gastroenterology & Hepatology, 3*, 653–656.

184. Poropat, G., Giljaca, V., Stimac, D., & Gluud, C. (2011). Bile acids for primary sclerosing cholangitis. *Cochrane Database of Systematic Reviews, CD003626*.

185. Poupon, R. (2012). Ursodeoxycholic acid and bile-acid mimetics as therapeutic agents for cholestatic liver diseases: An overview of their mechanisms of action. *Clinical Research in Hepatology & Gastroenterology, 36*(Suppl. 1), S3–S12.

186. Poupon, R. E., Balkau, B., Eschwege, E., & Poupon, R. (1991). A multicenter, controlled trial of ursodiol for the treatment of primary biliary cirrhosis. UDCA-PBC Study Group. *New England Journal of Medicine, 324*, 1548–1554.

187. Poupon, R. E., Chretien, Y., Poupon, R., & Paumgartner, G. (1993). Serum bile acids in primary biliary cirrhosis: Effect of ursodeoxycholic acid therapy. *Hepatology, 17*, 599–604.

188. Poupon, R., Chretien, Y., Poupon, R. E., Ballet, F., Calmus, Y., & Darnis, F. (1987). Is ursodeoxycholic acid an effective treatment for primary biliary cirrhosis? *Lancet, 1*, 834–836.

189. Prieto, J., Garcia, N., Marti-Climent, J. M., Penuelas, I., Richter, J. A., & Medina, J. F. (1999). Assessment of biliary bicarbonate secretion in humans by positron emission tomography. *Gastroenterology, 117*, 167–172.

190. Prieto, J., Qian, C., Garcia, N., Diez, J., & Medina, J. F. (1993). Abnormal expression of anion exchanger genes in primary biliary cirrhosis. *Gastroenterology, 105*, 572–578.

191. Qian, Y., Banerjee, S., Grossman, C. E., Amidon, W., Nagy, G., Barcza, M., Niland, B., Karp, D. R., Middleton, F. A., Banki, K., & Perl, A. (2008). Transaldolase deficiency influences the pentose phosphate pathway, mitochondrial homeostasis, and apoptosis signal processing. *Biochemical Journal, 415*, 123–134.

192. Qiao, L., Yacoub, A., Studer, E., Gupta, S., Pei, X. Y., Grant, S., et al. (2002). Inhibition of the MAPK and PI3K pathways enhances UDCA-induced apoptosis in primary rodent hepatocytes. *Hepatology, 35*, 779–789.

193. Ratziu, V., de Ledinghen, V., Oberti, F., Mathurin, P., Wartelle-Bladou, C., Renou, C., et al. (2011). A randomized controlled trial of high-dose ursodesoxycholic acid for nonalcoholic steatohepatitis. *Journal of Hepatology, 54*, 1011–1019.

194. References

195. Renaud, S., & De Lorgeril, M. (1992). Wine, alcohol, platelets, and the French paradox for coronary heart disease. *Lancet, 339*, 1523–1526.

196. Richter, K., Konzack, A., Pihlajaniemi, T., Heljasvaara, R., & Kietzmann, T. (2015). Redox-fibrosis: Impact of TGFβ1 on ROS generators, mediators, and functional consequences. *Redox Biology, 6*, 344–352.

197. Rivera, H., Morales-Rios, M. S., Bautista, W., Shibayama, M., Tsutsumi, V., Muriel, P., & Perez-Alvarez, V. (2011). A novel fluorinated stilbene exerts hepatoprotective properties in CCl4-induced acute liver damage. *Canadian Journal of Physiology and Pharmacology, 89*, 759–766.

198. Rivera, H., Shibayama, M., Tsutsumi, V., Perez-Alvarez, V., & Muriel, P. (2008). Resveratrol and trimethylated resveratrol protect from acute liver damage induced by CCl4 in the rat. *Journal of Applied Toxicology, 28*, 147–155.

199. Rodrigues, C. M., Fan, G., Ma, X., Kren, B. T., & Steer, C. J. (1998). A novel role for ursodeoxycholic acid in inhibiting apoptosis by modulating mitochondrial membrane perturbation. *Journal of Clinical Investigation, 101*, 2790–2799.

200. Rodriguez-Ortigosa, C. M., Cincu, R. N., Sanz, S., Ruiz, F., Quiroga, J., & Prieto, J. (2002). Effect of ursodeoxycholic acid on methionine adenosyl transferase activity and hepatic glutathione metabolism in rats. *Gut, 50*, 701–706.

201. Ronis, M. J., Butura, A., Sampey, B. P., Shankar, K., Prior, R. L., Korourian, S., Albano, E., Ingelman-Sundberg, M., Petersen, D. R., & Badger, T. M. (2005). Effects of N-acetylcysteine on ethanol-induced hepatotoxicity in rats fed via total enteral nutrition. *Free Radical Biology and Medicine, 39*, 619–630.

202. Room, R., Babor, T., & Rehm, J. (2005). Alcohol and public health. *Lancet, 365*, 519–530.

203. Rotches-Ribalta, M., Andres-Lacueva, C., Estruch, R., Escribano, E., & Urpi-Sarda, M. (2012). Pharmacokinetics of resveratrol metabolic profile in healthy humans after moderate consumption of red wine and grape extract tablets. *Pharmacological Research, 66*, 375–382.

204. Rudic, J. S., Poropat, G., Krstic, M. N., Bjelakovic, G., & Gluud, C. (2012). Ursodeoxycholic acid for primary biliary cirrhosis. *Cochrane Database of Systematic Reviews, 12*, CD000551.

205. Rudolph, G., Endele, R., Senn, M., & Stiehl, A. (1993). Effect of ursodeoxycholic acid on the kinetics of cholic acid and chenodeoxycholic acid in patients with primary sclerosing cholangitis. *Hepatology, 17*, 1028–1032.

206. Seifried, H. E., Anderson, D. E., Fisher, E. I., & Milner, J. A. (2007). A review of the interaction among dietary antioxidants and reactive oxygen species. *Journal of Nutritional Biochemistry, 18*, 567–579.

207. Selmi, C., Bowlus, C. L., Gershwin, M. E., & Coppel, R. L. (2011). Primary biliary cirrhosis. *Lancet, 377*, 1600–1609.

208. Sener, G., Toklu, H. Z., Sehirli, A. O., Velioglu-Ogunc, A., Cetinel, S., & Gedik, N. (2006). Protective effects of resveratrol against acetaminophen-induced toxicity in mice. *Hepatology Research, 35*, 62–68.

209. Sergides, C., Chirila, M., Silvestro, L., Pitta, D., & Pittas, A. (2016). Bioavailability and safety study of resveratrol 500 mg tablets in healthy male and female volunteers. *Experimental and Therapeutic Medicine, 11*, 164–170.

210. Setshedi, M., Longato, L., Petersen, D. R., Ronis, M., Chen, W. C., Wands, J. R., & De La Monte, S. M. (2011). Limited therapeutic effect of N-acetylcysteine on hepatic insulin resistance in an experimental model of alcohol-induced steatohepatitis. *Alcoholism: Clinical and Experimental Research, 35*, 2139–2151.

211. Shang, J., Chen, L. L., Xiao, F. X., Sun, H., Ding, H. C., & Xiao, H. (2008). Resveratrol improves non-alcoholic fatty liver disease by activating AMP-activated protein kinase. *Acta Pharmacologica Sinica, 29*, 698–706.

212. Shen, X., Zhao, G., Wang, R., Liu, T., & Liu, L. (2013). Protective effect of propofol and resveratrol pretreatment against hepatocyte apoptosis in rats with hepatic ischemia-reperfusion injury. *Nan Fang Yi Ke Da Xue Xue Bao, 33*, 80–85.

213. Shi, J., Wu, C., Lin, Y., Chen, Y. X., Zhu, L., & Xie, W. F. (2006). Long-term effects of mid-dose ursodeoxycholic acid in primary biliary cirrhosis: A meta-analysis of randomized controlled trials. *American Journal of Gastroenterology, 101*, 1529–1538.

214. Siano, M., De Gregorio, F., Boggia, B., Sepe, A., Ferri, P., Buonpensiero, P., et al. (2010). Ursodeoxycholic acid treatment in patients with cystic fibrosis at risk for liver disease. *Digestive and Liver Disease, 42*, 428–431.

215. Singh, A., Ahmad, I., Ahmad, S., Iqbal, Z., & Ahmad, F. J. (2016). A novel monolithic controlled-delivery system of resveratrol for enhanced hepatoprotection: Nano formulation development, pharmacokinetics, and pharmacodynamics. *Drug Development and Industrial Pharmacy*, 1–51.

216. Singh, S., & Talwalkar, J. A. (2013). Primary sclerosing cholangitis: Diagnosis, prognosis, and management. *Clinical Gastroenterology and Hepatology, 11*, 898–907.

217. Smith, L. A., Ignacio, J. R., Winesett, M. P., Kaiser, G. C., Lacson, A. G., Gilbert-Barness, E., et al. (2005). Vanishing bile duct syndrome: Amoxicillin-clavulanic acid associated intra-hepatic cholestasis responsive to ursodeoxycholic acid. *Journal of Pediatric Gastroenterology and Nutrition, 41*, 469–473.

218. Sokol, R. J., Devereaux, M., Khandwala, R., & O'Brien, K. (1993). Evidence for involvement of oxygen free radicals in bile acid toxicity to isolated rat hepatocytes. *Hepatology, 17*, 869–881.

219. Sola, S., Castro, R. E., Kren, B. T., Steer, C. J., & Rodrigues, C. M. (2004). Modulation of nuclear steroid receptors by ursodeoxycholic acid inhibits TGF-beta1-induced E2F-1/p53-mediated apoptosis of rat hepatocytes. *Biochemistry, 43*, 8429–8438.

220. Spagnuolo, M. I., Iorio, R., Vegnente, A., & Guarino, A. (1996). Ursodeoxycholic acid for treatment of cholestasis in children on long-term total parenteral nutrition: A pilot study. *Gastroenterology, 111*, 716–719.

221. Stiehl, A., Benz, C., & Sauer, P. (1999). Mechanism of hepatoprotective action of bile salts in liver disease. *Gastroenterology Clinics of North America, 28*, 195–209.

222. Stiehl, A., Rudolph, G., Raedsch, R., Moller, B., Hopf, U., Lotterer, E., et al. (1990). Ursodeoxycholic acid-induced changes of plasma and urinary bile acids in patients with primary biliary cirrhosis. *Hepatology, 12*, 492–497.

223. Storz, P., Doppler, H., & Toker, A. (2004). Activation loop phosphorylation controls protein kinase D-dependent activation of nuclear factor kappaB. *Molecular Pharmacology, 66*, 870–879.

224. Subbaramaiah, K., Chung, W. J., Michaluart, P., Telang, N., Tanabe, T., Inoue, H., Jang, M., Pezzuto, J. M., & Dannenberg, A. J. (1998). Resveratrol inhibits cyclooxygenase-2 transcription

and activity in phorbol ester-treated human mammary epithelial cells. *Journal of Biological Chemistry, 273*, 21875–21882.

225. Svegliati-Baroni, G., De Minicis, S., & Marzioni, M. (2008). Hepatic fibrogenesis in response to chronic liver injury: Novel insights on the role of cell-to-cell interaction and transition. *Liver International, 28*, 1052–1064.
226. Tabibian, J. H., & Lindor, K. D. (2014). Ursodeoxycholic acid in primary sclerosing cholangitis: If withdrawal is bad, then administration is good (right?). *Hepatology, 60*, 785–788.
227. Takaki, A., & Yamamoto, K. (2015). Control of oxidative stress in hepatocellular carcinoma: Helpful or harmful? *World Journal of Hepatology, 7*, 968–979.
228. Tanaka, H., Makino, Y., Miura, T., Hirano, F., Okamoto, K., Komura, K., et al. (1996). Ligand-independent activation of the glucocorticoid receptor by ursodeoxycholic acid. Repression of IFN-gamma-induced MHC class II gene expression via a glucocorticoid receptor-dependent pathway. *Journal of Immunology, 156*, 1601–1608.
229. Tarao, K., Fujiyama, S., Ohkawa, S., Miyakawa, K., Tamai, S., Hirokawa, S., et al. (2005). Ursodiol use is possibly associated with lower incidence of hepatocellular carcinoma in hepatitis C virus-associated liver cirrhosis. *Cancer Epidemiology, Biomarkers & Prevention, 14*, 164–169.
230. Tenenbein, M. (1984). Hypersensitivity-like reactions to N-acetylcysteine. *Veterinary and Human Toxicology, 26*(Suppl. 2), 3–5.
231. Terasaki, S., Nakanuma, Y., Ogino, H., Unoura, M., & Kobayashi, K. (1991). Hepatocellular and biliary expression of HLA antigens in primary biliary cirrhosis before and after ursodeoxycholic acid therapy. *American Journal of Gastroenterology, 86*, 1194–1199.
232. Teskac, K., & Kristl, J. (2010). The evidence for solid lipid nanoparticles mediated cell uptake of resveratrol. *International Journal of Pharmaceutics, 390*, 61–69.
233. Thibault, M., McMahon, J., Faubert, G., Charbonneau, J., Malo, J., Ferreira, E., et al. (2014). Parenteral nutrition-associated liver disease: A retrospective study of ursodeoxycholic acid use in neonates. *Journal of Pediatric Pharmacology and Therapeutics, 19*, 42–48.
234. Timmers, S., Konings, E., Bilet, L., Houtkooper, R. H., Van De Weijer, T., Goossens, G. H., Hoeks, J., Van Der Krieken, S., Ryu, D., Kersten, S., Moonen-Kornips, E., Hesselink, M. K., Kunz, I., Schrauwen-Hinderling, V. B., Blaak, E. E., Auwerx, J., & Schrauwen, P. (2011). Calorie restriction-like effects of 30 days of resveratrol supplementation on energy metabolism and metabolic profile in obese humans. *Cell Metabolism, 14*, 612–622.
235. Tome-Carneiro, J., Gonzalvez, M., Larrosa, M., Yanez-Gascon, M. J., Garcia-Almagro, F. J., Ruiz-Ros, J. A., Garcia-Conesa, M. T., Tomas-Barberan, F. A., & Espin, J. C. (2012). One-year consumption of a grape nutraceutical containing resveratrol improves the inflammatory and fibrinolytic status of patients in primary prevention of cardiovascular disease. *American Journal of Cardiology, 110*, 356–363.
236. Tsai, S. H., Lin-Shiau, S. Y., & Lin, J. K. (1999). Suppression of nitric oxide synthase and the down-regulation of the activation of NFkB in macrophages by resveratrol. *British Journal of Pharmacology, 126*, 673–680.
237. Ullrich, D., Rating, D., Schroter, W., Hanefeld, F., & Bircher, J. (1987). Treatment with ursodeoxycholic acid renders children with biliary atresia suitable for liver transplantation. *Lancet, 2*, 1324.

238. Unitt, J., & Hornigold, D. (2011). Plant lectins are novel Toll-like receptor agonists. *Biochemical Pharmacology, 81*, 1324–1328.

239. Vajro, P., Franzese, A., Valerio, G., Iannucci, M. P., & Aragione, N. (2000). Lack of efficacy of ursodeoxycholic acid for the treatment of liver abnormalities in obese children. *Journal of Pediatrics, 136*, 739–743.

240. Valenzano, D. R., Terzibasi, E., Genade, T., Cattaneo, A., Domenici, L., & Cellerino, A. (2006). Resveratrol prolongs lifespan and retards the onset of age-related markers in a short-lived vertebrate. *Current Biology, 16*, 296–300.

241. van Mil, S. W., Houwen, R. H., & Klomp, L. W. (2005). Genetics of familial intrahepatic cholestasis syndromes. *Journal of Medical Genetics, 42*, 449–463.

242. van Ooteghem, N. A., Klomp, L. W., van Berge-Henegouwen, G. P., & Houwen, R. H. (2002). Benign recurrent intrahepatic cholestasis progressing to progressive familial intrahepatic cholestasis: Low GGT cholestasis is a clinical continuum. *Journal of Hepatology, 36*, 439–443.

243. Vaz-Da-Silva, M., Loureiro, A. I., Falcao, A., Nunes, T., Rocha, J. F., Fernandes-Lopes, C., Soares, E., Wright, L., Almeida, L., & Soares-DaSilva, P. (2008). Effect of food on the pharmacokinetic profile of transresveratrol. *International Journal of Clinical Pharmacology and Therapeutics, 46*, 564–570.

244. Wales, P. W., Allen, N., Worthington, P., George, D., Compher, C., & American Society for Parenteral and Enteral Nutrition, et al. (2014). A.S.P.E.N. clinical guidelines: Support of pediatric patients with intestinal failure at risk of parenteral nutrition-associated liver disease. *JPEN Journal of Parenteral and Enteral Nutrition, 38*, 538–557.

245. Wan, J., Benkdane, M., Teixeira-Clerc, F., Bonnafous, S., Louvet, A. Lafdil, F., Pecker, F., Tran, A., Gual, P., Mallat, A., Lotersztajn, S., & Pavoine, C. (2014). M2 Kupffer cells promote M1 Kupffer cell apoptosis: A protective mechanism against alcoholic and nonalcoholic fatty liver disease. *Hepatology, 59*, 130–142.

246. Wang, C., Chen, K., Xia, Y., Dai, W., Wang, F., Shen, M., Cheng, P., Wang, J., Lu, J., Zhang, Y., Yang, J., Zhu, R., Zhang, H., Li, J., Zheng, Y., Zhou, Y., & Guo, C. (2014). N-acetylcysteine attenuates ischemia-reperfusion-induced apoptosis and autophagy in mouse liver via regulation of the ROS/JNK/Bcl-2 pathway. *PLoS One, 9*, e108855.

247. Wang, G. L., Fu, Y. C., Xu, W. C., Feng, Y. Q., Fang, S. R., & Zhou, X. H. (2009). Resveratrol inhibits the expression of SREBP1 in a cell model of steatosis via the Sirt1-FOXO1 signaling pathway. *Biochemical and Biophysical Research Communications, 380*, 644–649.

248. Wang, S. Y., Tang, H. M., Chen, G. Q., Xu, J. M., Zhong, L., Wang, Z. W., et al. (2012). Effect of ursodeoxycholic acid administration after liver transplantation on serum liver tests and biliary complications: A randomized clinical trial. *Digestion, 86*, 208–217.

249. Wang, Y., Jiang, Y., Fan, X., Tan, H., Zeng, H., Chen, P., Huang, M., & Bi, H. (2015). Hepatoprotective effect of resveratrol against acetaminophen-induced liver injury is associated with inhibition of CYP-mediated bioactivation and regulation of SIRT1-p53 signaling pathways. *Toxicology Letters, 236*, 82–89.

250. Wanty, C., Joomye, R., Van Hoorebeek, N., Paul, K., Otte, J. B., Reding, R., et al. (2004). Fifteen years single center experience in the management of progressive familial intrahepatic cholestasis of infancy. *Acta Gastroenterologica Belgica, 67*, 313–319.

251. Waring, W. S. (2012). Novel acetylcysteine regimens for treatment of paracetamol overdose. *Therapeutic Advances in Drug Safety, 3*, 305–315.

252. Whitington, P. F., Freese, D. K., Alonso, E. M., Schwarzenberg, S. J., & Sharp, H. L. (1994). Clinical and biochemical findings in progressive familial intrahepatic cholestasis. *Journal of Pediatric Gastroenterology and Nutrition, 18*, 134–141.

253. Wood, J. G., Rogina, B., Lavu, S., Howitz, K., Helfand, S. L., Tatar, M., & Sinclair, D. (2004). Sirtuin activators mimic caloric restriction and delay ageing in metazoans. *Nature, 430*, 686–689.

254. Working Subgroup for Clinical Practice Guidelines for Primary Biliary Cirrhosis. (2014). Guidelines for the management of primary biliary cirrhosis: The intractable hepatobiliary disease study group supported by the ministry of health, labor and welfare of Japan. *Hepatology Research, 44*(Suppl. S1), 71–90.

255. Wu, S. D., Li, L., & Wang, J. Y. (2012). Ursodeoxycholic acid for nonalcoholic steatohepatitis. *European Journal of Gastroenterology & Hepatology, 24*, 1247–1253.

256. Wulffraat, N. M., Haddad, E., Benkerrou, M., Spliet, W. G., Patey, N., Fischer, A., et al. (1997). Hepatic GVHD after HLA-haploidentical bone marrow transplantation in children with severe combined immunodeficiency: The effect of ursodeoxycholic acid. *British Journal of Haematology, 96*, 776–780.

257. Wunsch, E., Trottier, J., Milkiewicz, M., Raszeja-Wyszomirska, J., Hirschfield, G. M., Barbier, O., et al. (2014). Prospective evaluation of ursodeoxycholic acid withdrawal in patients with primary sclerosing cholangitis. *Hepatology, 60*, 931–940.

258. Yang, H. L., Chen, W. Q., Cao, X., Worschech, A., Du, L. F., Fang, W. Y., Xu, Y. Y., Stroncek, D. F., Li, X., Wang, E., & Marincola, F. M. (2009). Caveolin-1 enhances resveratrol-mediated cytotoxicity and transport in a hepatocellular carcinoma model. *Journal of Translational Medicine, 7*, 22.

259. Yang, S. J., & Lim, Y. (2014). Resveratrol ameliorates hepatic metaflammation and inhibits NLRP3 inflammasome activation. *Metabolism, 63*, 693–701.

260. Yao, R., Yasuoka, A., Kamei, A., Ushiama, S., Kitagawa, Y., Rogi, T., Shibata, H., Abe, K., & Misaka, T. (2014). Nuclear receptor-mediated alleviation of alcoholic fatty liver by polyphenols contained in alcoholic beverages. *PLoS One, 9*, e87142.

261. Yska, M. J., Buis, C. I., Monbaliu, D., Schuurs, T. A., Gouw, A. S., Kahmann, O. N., et al. (2008). The role of bile salt toxicity in the pathogenesis of bile duct injury after non-heart-beating porcine liver transplantation. *Transplantation, 85*, 1625–1631.

262. Yu, H., Pan, C., Zhao, S., Wang, Z., Zhang, H., & Wu, W. (2008). Resveratrol inhibits tumor necrosis factor-alpha-mediated matrix metalloproteinase-9 expression and invasion of human hepatocellular carcinoma cells. *Biomedicine & Pharmacotherapy, 62*, 366–372.

263. Zakhari, S. (2013). Bermuda triangle for the liver: Alcohol, obesity, and viral hepatitis. *Journal of Gastroenterology and Hepatology, 28*(Suppl. 1), 18–25.

264. Zang, M., Xu, S., Maitland-Toolan, K. A., Zuccollo, A., Hou, X., Jiang, B., Wierzbicki, M., Verbeuren, T. J., & Cohen, R. A. (2006). Polyphenols stimulate AMP-activated protein kinase, lower lipids, and inhibit accelerated atherosclerosis in diabetic LDL receptor-deficient mice. *Diabetes, 55*, 2180–2191.

265. Zhang, L. N., Shi, T. Y., Shi, X. H., Wang, L., Yang, Y. J., Liu, B., et al. (2013). Early biochemical response to ursodeoxycholic acid and long-term prognosis of primary biliary cirrhosis: Results of a 14-year cohort study. *Hepatology, 58*, 264–272.

266. Zhang, M., Li, W., Yu, L., & Wu, S. (2014). The suppressive effect of resveratrol on HIF-1α and VEGF expression after warm ischemia and reperfusion in rat liver. *PLoS One, 9*, e109589.

267. Zhang, Q., Tang, X., Lu, Q. Y., Zhang, Z. F., Brown, J., & Le, A. D. (2005). Resveratrol inhibits hypoxia-induced accumulation of hypoxia inducible factor-1alpha and VEGF expression in human tongue squamous cell carcinoma and hepatoma cells. *Molecular Cancer Therapeutics, 4*, 1465–1474.

268. Zhou, Y., Chen, K., He, L., Xia, Y., Dai, W., Wang, F., Li, J., Li, S., Liu, T., Zheng, Y., Wang, J., Lu, W., Yin, Q., Lu, J., Teng, H., & Guo, C. (2015). The protective effect of resveratrol on Concanavalin A-induced acute hepatic injury in mice. *Gastroenterology Research and Practice, 2015*, 506390.

269. Zini, R., Morin, C., Bertelli, A., Bertelli, A. A., & Tillement, J. P. (1999). Effects of resveratrol on the rat brain respiratory chain. *Drugs of Experimental and Clinical Research, 25*, 87–97.

270. Zollner, G., Fickert, P., Fuchsbichler, A., Silbert, D., Wagner, M., Arbeiter, S., et al. (2003). Role of nuclear bile acid receptor, FXR, in adaptive ABC transporter regulation by cholic and ursodeoxycholic acid in mouse liver, kidney and intestine. *Journal of Hepatology, 39*, 480–488.

INDEX

E

F

G

H

I

K

L

M

N

O

P

FSC
www.fsc.org
MIX
Papier | Fördert gute Waldnutzung
FSC® C083411

Kolibri 360 GmbH
Ferdinand-Jühlke-Straße 7
99095 Erfurt, Deutschland
produktsicherheit@kolibri360.de